# Clinical Anesthesiology
## Board Review

# Clinical Anesthesiology Board Review

## Second Edition

## A Test Simulation and Self-Assessment Tool


**Larry Chu, MD, MS**

Assistant Professor of Anesthesia
Department of Anesthesiology and Critical Care Medicine
Stanford University School of Medicine
Stanford, California

**Bassam Kadry, MD**

Associate Editor
Stanford University Medical Centre
Stanford, California


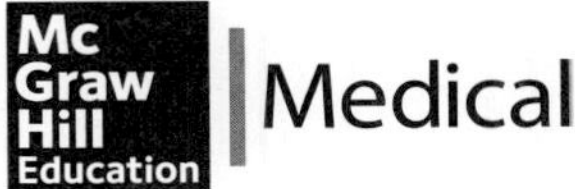


New York / Chicago / San Francisco / Athens / London / Madrid / Mexico City
Milan / New Delhi / Singapore / Sydney / Toronto

This book was set in Times Roman by Cenveo® Publisher Services.
The editors were Brian Belval and Regina Y. Brown.
The production supervisor was Catherine Saggese.
Project management was provided by Vastavikta Sharma, Cenveo Publisher Services.
RR Donnelley was printer and binder.

This book is printed on acid-free paper.


**Cataloguing in Publication data is on file at the Library of Congress.**

# Contents

# Contributing Authors


**Aileen Adriano**
Stanford University School of Medicine
Stanford, California

**Gail Boltz**
Stanford University School of Medicine
Stanford, California

**Ian Carroll**
Stanford University School of Medicine
Stanford, California

**Jerry Chao**
Stanford University School of Medicine
Stanford, California

**Marianne Chen**
Stanford University School of Medicine
Stanford, California

**Larry Chu**
Stanford University School of Medicine
Stanford, California

**Dave Clark**
Stanford University School of Medicine
Stanford, California

**Alimorad Djalali**
Stanford University School of Medicine
Stanford, California

**Genevieve D'souza**
Stanford University School of Medicine
Stanford, California

**Reuben Eng**
Stanford University School of Medicine
Stanford, California

**Roy Esaki**
Stanford University School of Medicine
Stanford, California

**Andrea Fuller**
University of Colorado
Denver, Colorado

**Maria Cristina Gutierrez**
Stanford University School of Medicine
Stanford, California

**Leland Hanowell**
Stanford University School of Medicine
Stanford, California

**Kyle Harrison**
Stanford University School of Medicine
Stanford, California

**James Janik**
Stanford University School of Medicine
Stanford, California

**Shanthala Keshavacharya**
Stanford University School of Medicine
Stanford, California

**Calvin Kuan**
Stanford University School of Medicine
Stanford, California

**Jody Leng**
Stanford University School of Medicine
Stanford, California

**Yun-Sheen Liu**
Stanford University School of Medicine
Stanford, California

**Jeannie Lo**
Stanford University School of Medicine
Stanford, California

**Kevin Malott**
Stanford University School of Medicine
Stanford, California

**Ed Mariano**
Stanford University School of Medicine
Stanford, California

**Vanessa Moll**
Stanford University School of Medicine
Stanford, California

**Caro Monico**
Stanford University School of Medicine
Stanford, California

**Christie Brown Munoz**
Stanford University School of Medicine
Stanford, California

**Megan Olejniczak**
Stanford University School of Medicine
Stanford, California

**Bridget Philip**
Stanford University School of Medicine
Stanford, California

**Rohith Piyaratna**
Stanford University School of Medicine
Stanford, California

**Andy Powell**
Stanford University School of Medicine
Stanford, California

**Zoel Quinonez**
Stanford University School of Medicine
Stanford, California

**Chandra Ramamoorthy**
Stanford University School of Medicine
Stanford, California

**Suma Ramzan**
Stanford University School of Medicine
Stanford, California

**Loren Riskin**
Stanford University School of Medicine
Stanford, California

**Jeannie Seybold**
Stanford University School of Medicine
Stanford, California

**Steve Shafer**
Stanford University School of Medicine
Stanford, California

**Chris Stasny**
Stanford University School of Medicine
Stanford, California

**Elizabeth Steele**
University of New Mexico
Albuquerque, New Mexico

**Naiyi Sun**
Stanford University School of Medicine
Stanford, California

**Pedro Tanaka**
Stanford University School of Medicine
Stanford, California

**Christopher Tirce**
Stanford University School of Medicine
Stanford, California

**Katherine Vuong**
Stanford Quiversity School of Medicine
Stanford, California

**Tammy Nai-yen Wang**
Stanford University School of Medicine
Stanford, California

**Heidi Witherell**
Stanford University School of Medicine
Stanford, California

**Cristina Wood**
Stanford University School of Medicine
Stanford, California

# How to Use This Book

This text is designed as a test simulation and self-assessment tool. It is not intended to replace a comprehensive topical review of anesthesia that is the foundation of high-quality anesthesia education and clinical practice. Readers who have already completed a rigorous topical review may wish to use this text as a simulation of an actual American Board of Anesthesiology (ABA) examination. The actual ABA test booklets are reprinted in this text and should be completed sequentially by the reader. Time restrictions should be followed strictly to assist the reader in assessing the pacing of an actual examination.

## OPTIONAL QUESTIONS

The ABA occasionally tests knowledge of controversial topics in anesthesia. In addition, some aspects of clinical knowledge and the practice of anesthesiology have changed significantly since this examination was first administered. Accordingly, some questions that were written in 1993 cannot be answered in 2013. In addition, certain drugs (e.g., pipecuronium and enflurane) are no longer used commonly by anesthesiologists in the United States. We have prepared detailed answers and explanations for all these questions and encourage the reader to review them. We have indicated these questions as "optional" on the examination answer sheets for readers who wish to omit them from their test simulation or self-assessment exercises. Our answers provide useful information that can be reviewed after these exercises have been completed.

*The 1993 ABA/ASA In-Training Examination is reprinted with permission of The American Board of Anesthesiology, Inc, 4208 Six Forks Road, Suite 1500, Raleigh, NC 27609-5765. The ABA does not attest to the current veracity of the items presented.*

# AMERICAN BOARD OF ANESTHESIOLOGY

# AMERICAN SOCIETY OF ANESTHESIOLOGISTS

## IN-TRAINING EXAMINATION

### Book A
### $3^1/_2$ hours

*Do not break the seal until you are told to do so.*

*Read the directions on the back cover.*

**PREPARED IN COOPERATION WITH NATIONAL BOARD OF MEDICAL EXAMINERS®**



ABA/ASA 93SA
pp 40, qtn 175

Printed in
U.S.A.

1. During mechanical ventilation, factors that influence the correlation between set tidal volume and exhaled tidal volume include

   (1) inspiratory time
   (2) fresh gas flow
   (3) compliance of the breathing circuit
   (4) addition of positive end-expiratory pressure to the circuit


2. In a 45-year-old man with adult respiratory distress syndrome, which of the following will result from institution of mechanical ventilation with positive end-expiratory pressure?

   (1) Decreased intrapulmonary shunt
   (2) Increased pulmonary compliance
   (3) Increased ventilation-perfusion ratio in the dependent portion of the lung
   (4) Decreased dead space to tidal volume ratio


3. A 58-year-old man with suspected carcinoma of the lung requires postoperative ventilation following general anesthesia for mediastinoscopy. Preoperatively, his shoulder muscles are weak bilaterally, but strength improves with exercise. This patient will show

   (1) inadequate reversal of neuromuscular block with an anticholinesterase drug
   (2) increased sensitivity to both depolarizing and nondepolarizing muscle relaxants
   (3) increased muscle strength following plasmapheresis
   (4) resolution of symptoms following administration of hydrocortisone

FOR EACH ITEM FILL IN ONLY ONE CIRCLE ON YOUR ANSWER SHEET

DIRECTIONS SUMMARIZED

| A | B | C | D | E |
|---|---|---|---|---|
| 1, 2, 3 | 1, 3 | 2, 4 | 4 | All are |
| only | only | only | only | correct |

4. Which of the following statements concerning postoperative shivering is true?

    (1) It increases carbon dioxide production
    (2) It is suppressed by intravenous meperidine
    (3) It accentuates halothane-related tremors
    (4) It increases heat loss

5. In which of the following conditions is the elimination half-life of an amide local anesthetic prolonged?

    (1) Liver disease
    (2) Term pregnancy
    (3) Heart failure
    (4) Kidney disease

6. A 10-year-old child with asthma is undergoing anesthesia with nitrous oxide, oxygen, and halothane. Effects of the accidental injection of atropine 2 mg in this patient would include

    (1) postoperative delirium
    (2) ventricular dysrhythmias
    (3) increased body temperature
    (4) bronchospasm

7. True statements concerning the oculocardiac reflex include the following:

    (1) It is more likely to occur in a patient with hypercarbia than in a patient with normocarbia
    (2) It is not seen during operative procedures on an empty orbit
    (3) Its afferent limb is the trigeminal nerve
    (4) It does not occur in the awake patient

8. Phase II succinylcholine block is characterized by

    (1) a train-of-four ratio less than 0.7
    (2) nonsustained response to tetanic stimulation
    (3) post-tetanic facilitation
    (4) improvement by edrophonium

9. Advantages of closed-circuit anesthesia over a semiclosed anesthesia system include the ability to

    (1) more quickly alter the inspired anesthetic concentration
    (2) decrease the total amount of inhalational anesthetic used
    (3) more easily increase $Paco_2$ during emergence
    (4) decrease heat loss to a greater extent

| DIRECTIONS SUMMARIZED | | | | |
|---|---|---|---|---|
| A | B | C | D | E |
| 1, 2, 3 | 1, 3 | 2, 4 | 4 | All are |
| only | only | only | only | correct |

10. Chronic hyperglycemia from excessive glucose administration during parenteral hyperalimentation causes

    (1) retinal degeneration
    (2) depression of granulocyte function
    (3) inhibition of platelet aggregation
    (4) hypercarbia

11. Which of the following produces effective transtracheal jet ventilation through a 14-gauge intravenous catheter?

    (1) Oxygen through a 50-psi pressure regulator
    (2) An Ambu bag with oxygen flow at 15 L/min
    (3) Oxygen flush from the fresh gas outlet from the anesthesia machine
    (4) The reservoir bag from the anesthesia circle system

12. During intraoperative mapping of a seizure focus under general anesthesia, electroencephalogram (EEG) activation may be enhanced or seizures induced by the use of

    (1) ketamine
    (2) methohexital
    (3) enflurane
    (4) thiopental

13. Transthoracic resistance to DC defibrillation is decreased by

    (1) use of conductive gel
    (2) multiple attempts at defibrillation
    (3) defibrillation during expiration
    (4) larger electrodes

14. Compared with a healthy 20-year-old, respiratory function in a healthy 1-year-old is characterized by

    (1) greater chest wall compliance
    (2) lesser lung compliance
    (3) greater small airway resistance
    (4) similar functional residual capacity/total lung volume (FRC/TLC) ratio

15. True statements concerning insertion of a total hip prosthesis with methylmethacrylate cement include the following:

    (1) Hypotension is more likely with placement in the acetabulum than with insertion in the femoral shaft
    (2) Absorbed volatile monomer causes vasodilation
    (3) A deliberate hypotensive technique is contraindicated
    (4) Arterial hemoglobin desaturation may result from fat embolization

FOR EACH ITEM FILL IN ONLY ONE CIRCLE ON YOUR ANSWER SHEET

| | DIRECTIONS SUMMARIZED | | | |
| :---: | :---: | :---: | :---: | :---: |
| A | B | C | D | E |
| 1, 2, 3 | 1, 3 | 2, 4 | 4 | All are |
| only | only | only | only | correct |

16. True statements concerning *direct* ventricular defibrillation during cardiopulmonary bypass include the following:

    (1) Shocks greater than 30 J are associated with myocardial damage
    (2) Hypokalemia increases the chance of defibrillation
    (3) Myocardial impedance decreases after a single shock
    (4) Thin-walled ventricles defibrillate more easily than hypertrophied ventricles

17. The indications for administration of fresh frozen plasma include

    (1) acute volume expansion in a hypovolemic patient
    (2) bleeding in a patient with a normal activated clotting time after cardiopulmonary bypass
    (3) transfusion of 6 units of red blood cells in a 70-kg patient
    (4) bleeding in a patient with a prolonged bleeding time and abnormal factor VIII

18. Immediately after sustaining a traumatic cord transection with a T4 level, a patient requires emergency laparotomy. Disease-related factors affecting anesthetic management include

    (1) venous pooling
    (2) hypothermia
    (3) decreased peripheral vascular resistance
    (4) decreased alveolar ventilation

19. Trigeminal neuralgia is characterized by

    (1) unilateral, intense, paroxysmal pain of sudden onset
    (2) diminished sensation in the distribution of the maxillary division of the trigeminal nerve
    (3) normal function of the glossopharyngeal nerve
    (4) resolution of symptoms by injection of local anesthetic at trigger points

20. During general anesthesia in a healthy patient, hypothermia to 33°C results in

    (1) prolongation of vecuronium action
    (2) protection against cerebral ischemia
    (3) potentiation of isoflurane
    (4) increased risk for ventricular dysrhythmias

21. Factors that decrease the incidence of deep vein thrombosis following total hip replacement include

    (1) external compression of the lower extremities
    (2) epidural anesthesia intraoperatively
    (3) prophylactic aspirin
    (4) deliberate hypotension intraoperatively

FOR EACH ITEM FILL IN ONLY ONE CIRCLE ON YOUR ANSWER SHEET

**DIRECTIONS SUMMARIZED**

| A | B | C | D | E |
|---|---|---|---|---|
| 1, 2, 3 | 1, 3 | 2, 4 | 4 | All are |
| only | only | only | only | correct |

22. Ketamine administered in anesthetic doses

    (1)  increases intracranial pressure
    (2)  does not cause respiratory depression
    (3)  is eliminated by hepatic metabolism
    (4)  increases bronchomotor tone

23. During laser excision of a sublaryngeal tumor, the risk of airway ignition would be decreased by using

    (1)  water-based lubricants
    (2)  jet ventilation without an endotracheal tube
    (3)  saline solution in the endotracheal tube cuff
    (4)  nitrous oxide

24. A 24-year-old patient with hypertension and hypercalcemia is scheduled for a parathyroidectomy. Serum calcium concentration may be decreased by the administration of

    (1)  calcium channel blocker
    (2)  magnesium sulfate
    (3)  sodium bicarbonate
    (4)  vigorous volume expansion

25. Effects of open cholecystectomy under general anesthesia with mechanical ventilation include

    (1)  increased intrapulmonary shunting
    (2)  decreased lung volumes up to 48 hours postoperatively
    (3)  decreased FRC
    (4)  decreased dead space

26. Features of the neonate's prompt adjustment to extrauterine life include

    (1)  lung expansion resulting in increased pulmonary vascular resistance
    (2)  nonshivering thermogenesis as a response to cold stress
    (3)  anatomic closure of the ductus arteriosus
    (4)  initial expansion of airless collapsed lungs by creation of negative pressures of 40 to 80 $cmH_2O$

27. Landmarks used in performing a superior laryngeal nerve block include the

    (1)  transverse process of C6
    (2)  cricoid cartilage
    (3)  angle of the mandible
    (4)  greater cornu of the hyoid cartilage

FOR EACH ITEM FILL IN ONLY ONE CIRCLE ON YOUR ANSWER SHEET

| | DIRECTIONS SUMMARIZED | | | |
|:---:|:---:|:---:|:---:|:---:|
| A | B | C | D | E |
| 1, 2, 3 | 1, 3 | 2, 4 | 4 | All are |
| only | only | only | only | correct |

28. Blood products that transmit viruses include

    (1) factor IX concentrate
    (2) plasma protein fraction
    (3) cryoprecipitate
    (4) albumin

29. Compared with healed cascade-type humidifiers, heated nebulizers used for humidification are associated with a greater risk for

    (1) bacterial transmission
    (2) increased airway resistance
    (3) water intoxication
    (4) inspissated secretions in large airways

30. Landmarks for caudal block include the

    (1) sciatic notch
    (2) posterior-superior iliac spines
    (3) iliac crests
    (4) sacral cornu

31. Changes in pulmonary function associated with advanced age include

    (1) decreased lung compliance
    (2) increased alveolar dead space
    (3) decreased FRC
    (4) decreased maximum voluntary ventilation

32. The minimum alveolar concentration (MAC) of isoflurane is decreased by

    (1) ethanol-induced enzyme induction
    (2) hyperventilation to a $Pa_{CO_2}$ of 25 mm Hg
    (3) chronic anemia to a hematocrit of 20%
    (4) decreased body temperature to 34°C

33. Compared with fentanyl, characteristics of alfentanil include

    (1) greater protein binding
    (2) more rapid clearance
    (3) shorter elimination half-life
    (4) greater volume of distribution

| DIRECTIONS SUMMARIZED | | | | |
|---|---|---|---|---|
| A | B | C | D | E |
| 1, 2, 3 | 1, 3 | 2, 4 | 4 | All are |
| only | only | only | only | correct |

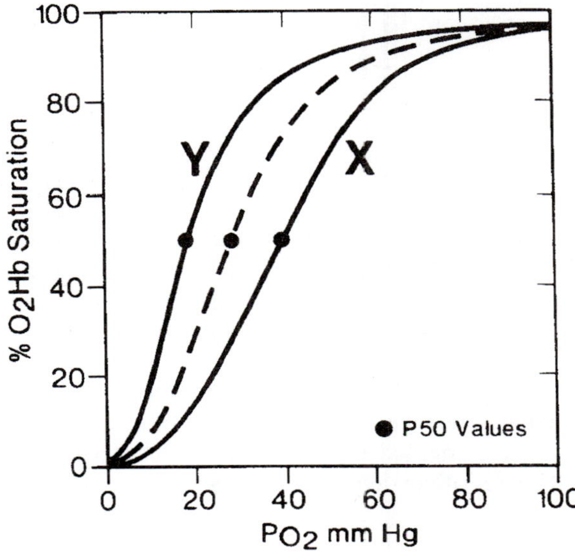


34. The oxygen-dissociation curve in the center of the graph represents normal adult hemoglobin. True statements concerning curves X and Y include the following:

    (1) Curve Y represents hemoglobin characteristic of a normal neonate
    (2) Curve X represents hemoglobin characteristic of 3-week-old banked blood
    (3) Curve Y represents hemoglobin characteristic of an alkalotic patient
    (4) Curve X represents hemoglobin characteristic of a hypothermic patient

35. A 45-year-old man who is scheduled for coronary artery bypass grafting is receiving heparin and nitroglycerin infusions for preinfarction angina. True statements concerning use of heparin during coronary revascularization in this patient include the following:

    (1) The anticoagulant effect is enhanced by the nitroglycerin
    (2) Platelet count should be determined before the operation
    (3) Activated coagulation time is unreliable after prolonged administration of heparin
    (4) The dose of heparin necessary to provide adequate systemic anticoagulation is likely to be increased

36. True statements concerning negative-pressure pulmonary edema include the following:

    (1) It is associated with airway obstruction
    (2) It responds to diuretic therapy
    (3) Resolution occurs within 24 hours
    (4) Debilitated adults are predisposed to it

| DIRECTIONS SUMMARIZED | | | | |
|---|---|---|---|---|
| A | B | C | D | E |
| 1, 2, 3 | 1, 3 | 2, 4 | 4 | All are |
| only | only | only | only | correct |

37. Landmarks for the sciatic nerve via a posterior approach include the

    (1) posterior superior iliac spine
    (2) coccyx
    (3) greater trochanter of the femur
    (4) iliac crest

38. Epidural anesthesia for cesarean delivery is planned for a 30-year-old woman in labor. She has preeclampsia and takes propranolol for mitral valve prolapse. A test dose of 3 mL of 2% lidocaine containing 15 µg of epinephrine is administered, and no change in heart rate is noted by palpation of the pulse. Before injection of more local anesthetic, blood is freely aspirated from the catheter. Explanations for failure of the intravenous test dose include the following:

    (1) The pain of labor masked the change usually seen with the test dose
    (2) Preexisting β-adrenergic blockade blunted the tachycardia from the intravenous epinephrine
    (3) Changes in pulse rate were too brief to be noted by palpation of the pulse
    (4) Preeclampsia decreased the sensitivity to exogenously administered catecholamines

39. A 76-year-old man with a history of angina, dyspnea on exertion, and syncope attributable to aortic stenosis is brought to the operating room for open reduction of an ankle fracture. An electrocardiogram (ECG) shows sinus rhythm. Anesthetic considerations include the following:

    (1) Nitroglycerin is contraindicated
    (2) Atrial fibrillation should be treated with synchronized cardioversion
    (3) The risk for cardiac complications is the same as that of patients with coronary artery stenosis
    (4) Spinal anesthesia is relatively contraindicated

40. Use of hyperventilation to decrease brain swelling also decreases

    (1) $P_{50}$ of hemoglobin
    (2) serum-ionized calcium concentration
    (3) serum potassium concentration
    (4) cerebral metabolic rate

41. A neonate born at 32 weeks' gestation has cyanosis, tachypnea, a scaphoid abdomen, and a cardiac impulse on the right. Immediate management of this child should include

    (1) insertion of a chest tube
    (2) limiting inspired oxygen concentration to 50%
    (3) administration of rapid positive-pressure ventilation by mask
    (4) insertion of a nasogastric tube

FOR EACH ITEM FILL IN ONLY ONE CIRCLE ON YOUR ANSWER SHEET

| DIRECTIONS SUMMARIZED | | | | |
|:---:|:---:|:---:|:---:|:---:|
| A | B | C | D | E |
| 1, 2, 3 | 1, 3 | 2, 4 | 4 | All are |
| only | only | only | only | correct |

42. The principle underlying diffusion hypoxia also explains

    (1) apneic oxygenation
    (2) the concentration effect
    (3) the solubility effect
    (4) the second gas effect

43. True statements concerning carbon dioxide absorption in breathing-system canisters include the following:

    (1) The major reactant of baralyme is barium hydroxide
    (2) Baralyme contains silica to minimize dust
    (3) The major component of soda lime is sodium hydroxide
    (4) Both baralyme and soda lime contain calcium hydroxide

44. Factors that decrease local anesthetic concentration in the fetus include

    (1) maternal hypotension
    (2) maternal acidemia
    (3) maternal serum alpha acid glycoprotein concentration
    (4) fetal acidosis

45. An oxygen analyzer sensor placed in the inspiratory limb of a circle system

    (1) is useful as a disconnect alarm if placed near the patient
    (2) will increase dead space
    (3) will be more pressure sensitive than one placed in the expiratory limb
    (4) should not be placed distal to an in-circuit humidifier

46. Agents that produce an acute withdrawal response in patients addicted to heroin include

    (1) pentazocine
    (2) nalbuphine
    (3) buprenorphine
    (4) naloxone

47. A 68-year-old man has had severe, constant burning and aching in the right forehead and anterior scalp for 6 weeks after an episode of herpes zoster. True statements concerning this patient's condition include the following:

    (1) It is more common in elderly patients
    (2) The neuralgia involves the supraorbital branches of the ophthalmic division of the facial nerve
    (3) Tricyclic antidepressants often provide effective pain relief
    (4) Opioid analgesics are the first-line treatment

<table>
<tr><td colspan="5" align="center"><u>DIRECTIONS SUMMARIZED</u></td></tr>
<tr><td align="center">A</td><td align="center">B</td><td align="center">C</td><td align="center">D</td><td align="center">E</td></tr>
<tr><td align="center">1, 2, 3</td><td align="center">1, 3</td><td align="center">2, 4</td><td align="center">4</td><td align="center">All are</td></tr>
<tr><td align="center">only</td><td align="center">only</td><td align="center">only</td><td align="center">only</td><td align="center">correct</td></tr>
</table>

48. Three weeks after exposure to toxic levels of an organophosphate insecticide, a farm worker is scheduled for inguinal herniorrhaphy. Which of the following should be avoided?

    (1) Spinal anesthesia with tetracaine
    (2) Epidural anesthesia with 2-chloroprocaine
    (3) Atracurium neuromuscular block
    (4) Succinylcholine infusion

49. The addition of halothane 0.5% to nitrous oxide and oxygen 50% each for cesarean delivery

    (1) increases the incidence of low Apgar scores
    (2) increases operative blood loss
    (3) increases the incidence of maternal hypotension
    (4) decreases the incidence of maternal awareness

50. Stellate ganglion block is associated with ipsilateral

    (1) mydriasis
    (2) diaphoresis
    (3) exophthalmos
    (4) scleral hyperemia

51. A 22-year-old man is unconscious after free-basing "crack." Likely findings include

    (1) depressed ST segments
    (2) hyperthermia
    (3) premature ventricular contractions
    (4) pinpoint pupils

52. Administration of halothane to a healthy patient causes

    (1) decreased myocardial contractility
    (2) depressed baroreceptor response
    (3) increased venous capacitance
    (4) decreased systemic vascular resistance

53. Indications for administration of calcium chloride during cardiopulmonary resuscitation include

    (1) acute hyperkalemia
    (2) electromechanical dissociation
    (3) verapamil toxicity
    (4) digoxin toxicity

<table>
<tr><td colspan="5" align="center">DIRECTIONS SUMMARIZED</td></tr>
<tr><td align="center">A<br>1, 2, 3<br>only</td><td align="center">B<br>1, 3<br>only</td><td align="center">C<br>2, 4<br>only</td><td align="center">D<br>4<br>only</td><td align="center">E<br>All are<br>correct</td></tr>
</table>

54. A 27-year-old man is undergoing emergency bronchoscopy with propofol-vecuronium anesthesia after aspirating a peanut. Intervals of apneic oxygenation are used to facilitate the procedure. Initial blood gas values while breathing pure oxygen are $Pa_{O_2}$ 400 mm Hg and $Pa_{CO_2}$ 30 mm Hg. Effects of 10 minutes of apneic oxygenation at a flow rate of 10 L/min include

    (1) decreased heart rate
    (2) decreased $Pa_{O_2}$ to 50 mm Hg
    (3) cutaneous vasoconstriction
    (4) increased $Pa_{CO_2}$ to 60 mm Hg

55. In a patient with normal hemodynamics, systemic blood pressure is measured using a radial artery catheter and a noninvasive oscillometric blood pressure (NIBP) monitor on the same arm. Compared with the readings from the NIBP monitor, the indwelling catheter would show

    (1) the same or higher systolic blood pressure
    (2) lower diastolic pressure if the transducer is damped
    (3) the same mean blood pressure
    (4) lower blood pressure values if the catheter is replaced by one with a larger diameter

56. A 20-kg, 4-year-old boy receives atropine 0.3 mg intramuscularly 1 hour before inguinal herniorrhaphy under general anesthesia. Forty minutes later while still in the preoperative preparation room, his temperature is 38.6°C. Likely causes of the temperature elevation include

    (1) malignant hyperthermia
    (2) alteration of central temperature regulation
    (3) release of catecholamines
    (4) suppression of sweating

57. If ketorolac 30 mg were substituted for meperidine 100 mg after an outpatient inguinal herniorrhaphy, the patient would experience less

    (1) respiratory depression
    (2) analgesia
    (3) nausea
    (4) bleeding

58. An asymptomatic 22-year-old man with asthma undergoes herniorrhaphy under 1.5% lidocaine epidural anesthesia to a sensory level of T2-3. Which of the following will occur with this level of anesthesia?

    (1) The ability to cough will be normal
    (2) Vital capacity will be unchanged
    (3) Intraoperative bronchospasm will be prevented
    (4) Tidal volume will be unchanged

FOR EACH ITEM FILL IN ONLY ONE CIRCLE ON YOUR ANSWER SHEET

| | DIRECTIONS SUMMARIZED | | | |
|---|---|---|---|---|
| A | B | C | D | E |
| 1, 2, 3 | 1, 3 | 2, 4 | 4 | All are |
| only | only | only | only | correct |

59. True statements concerning epidurally administered morphine include the following:

    (1) The long duration of analgesia results from high lipid solubility
    (2) Pruritus is completely reversed by naloxone
    (3) Plasma morphine levels are lower than those seen after intramuscular administration
    (4) Analgesia is inadequate for the pain of labor

60. A 36-year-old woman is scheduled for cholecystectomy. She is 65 in tall and weighs 180 kg. Compared with a patient of the same height who weighs 60 kg, this patient is at increased risk for

    (1) hypoxemia in the supine position
    (2) fasting hypoglycemia
    (3) acid aspiration syndrome
    (4) difficult reversal of neuromuscular block

61. Radiologic findings in advanced emphysema include

    (1) ground-glass appearance of lung fields
    (2) increased cardiothoracic ratio
    (3) increased bronchial markings
    (4) flattening of the hemidiaphragms

62. Anesthetic agents that are safe for use in a patient with acute intermittent porphyria include

    (1) ketamine
    (2) isoflurane
    (3) pancuronium
    (4) etomidate

63. Recurrent laryngeal nerve paralysis is a recognized complication of which of the following procedures?

    (1) Ligation of a patent ductus arteriosus
    (2) Stellate ganglion block
    (3) Mediastinoscopy
    (4) Use of a topical ice slush during heart surgery

64. Clinical situations associated with an increase in parasympathetic activity include

    (1) manipulation of the carotid sinus
    (2) intestinal insufflation during colonoscopy
    (3) traction on the superior oblique muscle during strabismus surgery
    (4) caudal anesthesia for excision of a pilonidal cyst

FOR EACH ITEM FILL IN ONLY ONE CIRCLE ON YOUR ANSWER SHEET

| | DIRECTIONS SUMMARIZED | | | |
|---|---|---|---|---|
| A | B | C | D | E |
| 1, 2, 3 | 1, 3 | 2, 4 | 4 | All are |
| only | only | only | only | correct |

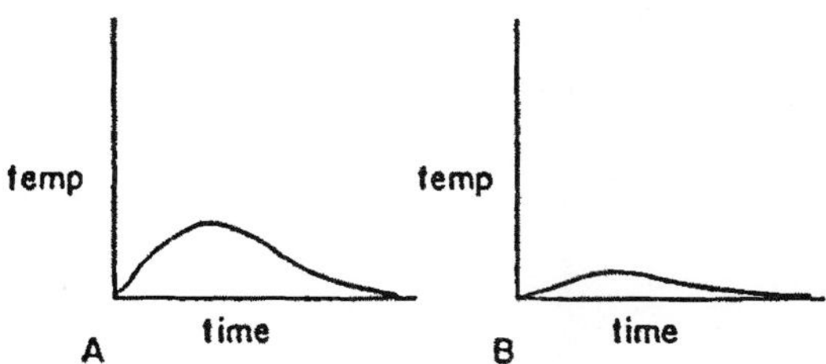


65. Curve A shown here is an accurate thermodilution curve from a patient with a cardiac output of 4 L/min. Curve B was obtained at the same time from the same patient. Curve B is consistent with

    (1) an opening at the syringe-catheter junction that allows some injectate to leak out of the system
    (2) use of room-temperature injectate when the computer is programmed for iced injectate
    (3) injection of cold indicator solution through a long extension tube rather than directly into the correct catheter lumen
    (4) use of 10 mL of cold indicator solution when the cardiac output computer is programmed for 5 mL of injectate

---

66. While oliguria is evaluated after operative repair of an aortic aneurysm, large "V" waves are noted in a pulmonary artery occlusion pressure trace. With which of the following disorders is this finding consistent?

    (1) Tricuspid regurgitation
    (2) Mitral regurgitation
    (3) Aortic regurgitation
    (4) Coronary artery disease

67. Under which of the following conditions is the output of an agent-specific vaporizer higher than the dial setting?

    (1) The vaporizer is filled with an agent of higher vapor pressure
    (2) Ambient temperature increases from 20°C to 24°C
    (3) The vaporizer is used at an elevation of 5000 ft
    (4) The inspiratory valve is incompetent

68. The advantages of colloid over crystalloid for massive volume replacement include

    (1) lower incidence of pulmonary edema
    (2) greater urine output
    (3) less disruption of hemostasis
    (4) greater potency in restoring circulatory homeostasis

FOR EACH ITEM FILL IN ONLY ONE CIRCLE ON YOUR ANSWER SHEET

| DIRECTIONS SUMMARIZED | | | | |
|:---:|:---:|:---:|:---:|:---:|
| A | B | C | D | E |
| 1, 2, 3 | 1, 3 | 2, 4 | 4 | All are |
| only | only | only | only | correct |

69. A 24-year-old man has constant burning pain 3 months after sustaining a crush injury to the arm. The injured muscles and joints are healed. Findings consistent with a diagnosis of causalgia include

    (1) beads of perspiration on the skin
    (2) skin discoloration
    (3) hypersensitivity to touch
    (4) warm extremity

70. A 45-year-old patient who takes tranylcypromine (Parnate), a monoamine oxidase (MAO) inhibitor, is scheduled for elective surgery under general anesthesia. True statements include the following:

    (1) Meperidine can produce hyperthermia
    (2) Surgery must be delayed for 2 weeks after discontinuation of MAO inhibitor therapy
    (3) An exaggerated response to ephedrine should be expected
    (4) A decrease in pressor response to phenylephrine should be expected

71. A 52-year-old man with a chronic cough associated with a long history of smoking is scheduled for elective cholecystectomy. Cessation of smoking for 48 hours will result in

    (1) decreased bronchial secretions
    (2) shift of the oxyhemoglobin dissociation curve to the right
    (3) decreased airway irritability
    (4) decreased carboxyhemoglobin level

72. A 55-year-old woman has a urine output of 15 mL during the first 2 hours following a radical hysterectomy. Findings consistent with a prerenal cause include

    (1) urine osmolality 590 mOsm/L
    (2) plasma creatinine concentration 1.1 mg/dL
    (3) urine specific gravity 1.025
    (4) urine sodium concentration 40 mEq/L

DIRECTIONS: Each of the numbered items or incomplete statements in this section is followed by answers or by completions of the statement. Select the ONE lettered answer or completion that is BEST in each case and fill in the circle containing the corresponding letter or the answer sheet.

73. An 8-kg, 1-year-old child has a measured blood loss of 50 mL during the first 2 hours of a rectal pull-through operation. Preoperative hematocrit was 31%. Balanced saline solution 150 mL has been administered for replacement. Urine output has been 2 mL for the last hour, heart rate is 160 bpm (beats per minute), and blood pressure is 40/15 mm Hg. The most appropriate fluid therapy is

   (A) 25% albumin
   (B) balanced salt solution
   (C) balanced salt solution and mannitol
   (D) 5% dextrose in 0.45% saline solution
   (E) packed red blood cells

74. An increased initial dose and a decreased maintenance dose of pancuronium are required in patients with

   (A) advanced age
   (B) burns
   (C) cirrhosis
   (D) chronic renal failure
   (E) fever

75. Which of the following statements concerning banked blood is true?

   (A) Red blood cells preserved with CPDA-1 (citrate phosphate dextrose adenine 1) have a shelf life of approximately 21 days
   (B) Packed red blood cells deliver oxygen normally immediately after administration
   (C) Packed red blood cells contain most of the leukocytes present in the donated unit
   (D) Citrate is used as a source of energy for whole blood
   (E) Stored whole blood contains all coagulation factors except II and VIII

76. A 73-year-old woman with a preoperative serum creatinine concentration of 2.1 mg/dL develops oliguria during enflurane anesthesia. Urine sodium concentration is 10 mEq/L and urine osmolality is 450 mOsm/L. The most likely cause of these findings is

   (A) acute renal failure
   (B) chronic renal insufficiency
   (C) decreased renal perfusion
   (D) fluoride nephrotoxicity
   (E) intraoperative administration of furosemide

77. During active labor, 10 mL of bupivacaine 0.5% with epinephrine 1:200,000 is administered epidurally. Fifteen minutes later, maternal blood pressure is 70/50 mm Hg and heart rate is 70 bpm; fetal heart rate is 90 bpm for 45 seconds, with loss of beat-to-beat variability. The most likely explanation for the fetal vital signs is

   (A) fetal bupivacaine cardiotoxicity
   (B) maternal bupivacaine cardiotoxicity
   (C) maternal hypotension
   (D) uterine artery vasoconstriction
   (E) umbilical cord compression

78. Compared with diazepam, midazolam

    (A) is more lipid soluble
    (B) has a longer elimination half-life
    (C) has a larger volume of distribution
    (D) has a greater clearance
    (E) undergoes slower hepatic metabolism

79. A 30-year-old woman has difficulty talking 15 minutes after initiation of interscalene block for closed reduction of a dislocated shoulder. The most likely cause is

    (A) cervical sympathetic block
    (B) delayed systemic toxic reaction
    (C) phrenic nerve paralysis
    (D) pneumothorax
    (E) recurrent laryngeal nerve block

80. An acutely ill 65-year-old man with sepsis has severe hypophosphatemia. Which of the following is most likely to result from this electrolyte disorder?

    (A) Bronchospasm
    (B) Diarrhea
    (C) Muscle weakness
    (D) Seizures
    (E) Ventricular ectopy

81. During a right lower lobe resection, $Sp_{O_2}$ decreases from 99% to 70% after institution of one-lung ventilation. $F_{IO_2}$ is 1.0. The most appropriate management is to

    (A) administer an inhaled bronchodilator
    (B) apply continuous positive airway pressure to the right lung
    (C) apply positive end-expiratory pressure to the left lung
    (D) increase tidal volume
    (E) reinflate the right lung

82. Carbon dioxide retention first occurs when the ratio of forced expiratory volume in 1 second to vital capacity ($FEV_1/VC$) decreases below

    (A) 15%
    (B) 35%
    (C) 50%
    (D) 65%
    (E) 75%

83. During recovery from halothane anesthesia, an alveolar concentration of 0.1% will have the greatest effect on

    (A) myocardial contractility
    (B) ventilatory response to hypercarbia
    (C) atrioventricular conduction
    (D) ventilatory response to hypoxia
    (E) neuromuscular transmission

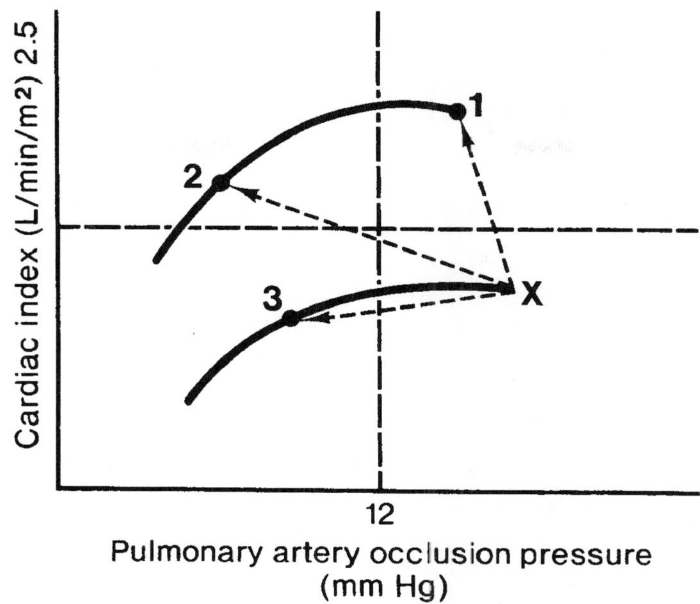


84. In this diagram, point "X" represents a patient with severe left ventricular dysfunction. The points labeled 1, 2, and 3 each represent the results of a different therapeutic intervention. Which of the following represents the most likely intervention at each point?

|       | **Point 1**   | **Point 2**   | **Point 3**   |
|-------|---------------|---------------|---------------|
| (A)   | Dopamine      | Furosemide    | Nitroprusside |
| (B)   | Dopamine      | Nitroprusside | Furosemide    |
| (C)   | Furosemide    | Dopamine      | Nitroprusside |
| (D)   | Nitroprusside | Dopamine      | Furosemide    |
| (E)   | Nitroprusside | Furosemide    | Dopamine      |

---

85. With long-term administration, which of the following drugs produces the most prolonged sedative effect of diazepam?

(A) Cimetidine
(B) Famotidine
(C) Metoclopramide
(D) Ranitidine
(E) Warfarin

86. During uncomplicated mask induction with halothane and 50% nitrous oxide in oxygen in a 6-month-old infant with a large ventricular septal defect and valvular pulmonic stenosis, $SpO_2$ decreases from 85% (room air) to 60%; heart rate is 100 bpm and blood pressure is 62/40 mm Hg. The most appropriate management is to

(A) administer atropine
(B) administer phenylephrine
(C) administer propranolol
(D) increase anesthetic depth
(E) intubate the trachea

87. Which of the following statements concerning variable decelerations of fetal heart rate is true?

     (A)  It indicates compression of the umbilical cord
     (B)  It indicates compression of the fetal head
     (C)  It indicates prematurity
     (D)  It is obliterated by atropine
     (E)  It occurs normally following epidural anesthesia

88. During enflurane anesthesia for colectomy in a 75-year-old man with sepsis, urine output decreases to 10 mL/h. Heart rate is 120 bpm, blood pressure is 100/50 mm Hg, central venous pressure is 10 mm Hg, and pulmonary artery occlusion pressure is 15 mm Hg. The most appropriate management at this time is to

     (A)  measure cardiac output
     (B)  increase fluid administration
     (C)  infuse dopamine
     (D)  administer propranolol
     (E)  switch from enflurane to isoflurane

89. The effect of neomycin at the neuromuscular junction is

     (A)  decreased by depolarizing relaxants
     (B)  partially reversed by calcium
     (C)  potentiated by anticholinesterases
     (D)  prevented by pretreatment with magnesium
     (E)  primarily prejunctional

90. A patient is bleeding excessively after routine transurethral resection of the prostate. Reexploration discloses diffuse oozing. The most appropriate management is administration of

     (A)  platelets
     (B)  fresh frozen plasma
     (C)  desmopressin
     (D)  epsilon-aminocaproic acid
     (E)  cryoprecipitate

91. Which of the following statements concerning FRC is true?

     (A)  It decreases linearly during a 3-hour anesthetic
     (B)  It decreases in pregnancy primarily because of a decrease in the expiratory reserve volume
     (C)  It increases in patients with a history of heavy smoking
     (D)  It increases with pulmonary contusions
     (E)  It is smaller (mL/kg) in children than in adults

92. After 2 hours of anesthesia with halothane 1.2% and oxygen, nitrous oxide 75% is added to the inspired gas mixture. This addition would

     (A)  increase the alveolar halothane and oxygen concentrations above inspired
     (B)  increase the alveolar halothane concentration only
     (C)  cause no change in alveolar gas concentrations compared with inspired
     (D)  decrease alveolar oxygen concentration compared with inspired
     (E)  decrease alveolar oxygen and halothane concentrations below inspired

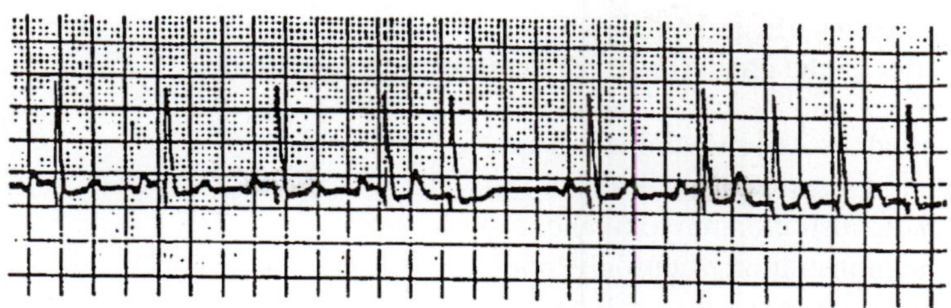

93. The ECG tracing shown here shows

    (A) aberrant intraventricular conduction
    (B) acceleration of phase 4 depolarization of the sinus node
    (C) a compensatory pause
    (D) initiation of reentrant supraventricular tachycardia
    (E) paroxysmal atrial fibrillation

---

94. One hour after an open cholecystectomy, a 42-year-old patient is hemodynamically stable and breathing spontaneously (rate 10/min and regular) at an $F_{IO_2}$ of 0.4. Fentanyl, isoflurane, nitrous oxide, and pancuronium were used during the procedure. Analysis of arterial blood gases is most likely to show the following:

| | pH | $P_{CO_2}$ (mm Hg) | $P_{O_2}$ (mm Hg) |
|---|---|---|---|
| (A) | 7.18 | 40 | 100 |
| (B) | 7.18 | 60 | 140 |
| (C) | 7.28 | 50 | 85 |
| (D) | 7.40 | 26 | 220 |
| (E) | 7.40 | 40 | 40 |

95. A 6-year-old child with asthma begins wheezing during anesthesia with halothane and nitrous oxide in oxygen. A loading dose of aminophylline is administered followed by continuous infusion. Premature ventricular contractions appear on the ECG. The most appropriate management is to

    (A) administer fentanyl
    (B) discontinue aminophylline
    (C) increase exhalation time
    (D) increase the inspired concentration of halothane
    (E) switch the inhalational agent to isoflurane

96. Oxygen 100 mL/min is bubbled through a vaporizer containing an anesthetic with a vapor pressure of 150 mm Hg, and this mixture is added to a fresh gas flow of 5 L/min. The delivered anesthetic concentration is

    (A) 0.25%
    (B) 0.5%
    (C) 1%
    (D) 2.5%
    (E) 5%

97. A 50-year-old man who takes aspirin and nifedipine is scheduled for thoracotomy with one-lung ventilation. Which of the following is associated with the greatest risk for intraoperative hypoxemia?

(A) Preoperative withdrawal of nifedipine therapy
(B) Intraoperative mild respiratory acidosis
(C) Intraoperative administration of isoflurane
(D) Intraoperative administration of nitroglycerin
(E) Intraoperative thoracic epidural morphine

98. A 35-year-old woman with severe myasthenia gravis is scheduled for thymectomy. Which of the following preoperative pulmonary function tests is most likely to be normal?

(A) Forced expiratory volume in 1 second ($FEV_1$)
(B) Forced vital capacity (FVC)
(C) $FEV_1$/FVC
(D) Maximum voluntary ventilation
(E) Peak inspiratory force

99. A 66-year-old man with aortic regurgitation is brought to the operating room for aortic valve replacement after having received morphine, scopolamine premedication. $Po_2$ is 40 mm Hg in a sample of pulmonary artery blood drawn 10 minutes after the patient started breathing pure oxygen. This finding is compatible with

(A) wedging of the catheter tip
(B) left-to-right intracardiac shunting
(C) increased intrapulmonary shunting
(D) excessively depressed ventilation
(E) normal cardiac output

100. Which of the following statements concerning metoclopramide is true?

(A) It is antagonized by concomitant administration of atropine
(B) It decreases gastrointestinal motility
(C) It decreases gastric secretion
(D) It lacks antiemetic properties
(E) It stimulates dopamine receptors

101. During halothane anesthesia with spontaneous ventilation, the most reliable sign of malignant hyperthermia is

(A) hypertension
(B) increased temperature
(C) increased minute ventilation
(D) muscle rigidity
(E) tachycardia

102. Which of the following is the most appropriate action after an anesthetic vaporizer is tipped?

(A) Return to the manufacturer for recalibration
(B) Flush the vaporizer with oxygen at 5 L/min for 24 hours
(C) Store the vaporizer for 24 hours at room temperature
(D) Set the vaporizer at low concentration and flush with oxygen at 10 L/min for 30 minutes
(E) Verify the vaporizer output with mass spectrography

103. Following pneumonectomy, a paralyzed patient being mechanically ventilated has the following arterial blood gas values: $Pao_2$ 71 mm Hg, $Paco_2$ 55 mm Hg, pH 7.29. $Svo_2$ is 45%. The most likely explanation for this $Svo_2$ is

    (A) decreased red cell mass
    (B) high cardiac output
    (C) hypothermia
    (D) peripheral left-to-right arteriovenous shunt
    (E) ventilation/perfusion mismatch

104. Which of the following is a sign of cyclosporine toxicity?

    (A) Abnormal hepatic enzyme activity
    (B) Decreased hemoglobin concentration
    (C) Increased serum creatinine concentration
    (D) Nodular density on radiograph of the chest
    (E) ST–T-wave changes on ECG

105. Myofascial pain is an example of

    (A) a central pain state
    (B) neuropathic pain
    (C) psychogenic pain
    (D) somatic pain
    (E) visceral pain

106. In children with preoperative upper respiratory tract infection, which of the following is associated with the greatest risk for postoperative airway obstruction?

    (A) Age less than 1 year
    (B) Endotracheal intubation
    (C) Head and neck surgery
    (D) Inadequate airway humidification
    (E) Surgery for more than 2 hours

107. In an anesthetized patient being mechanically ventilated, end-expired carbon dioxide is 58 mm Hg and peak inspiratory airway pressure is 15 $cmH_2O$. Ventilator settings indicate a delivered tidal volume of 800 mL, but the expiratory flow meter shows a tidal volume of 360 mL. Which of the following is the most likely cause of this discrepancy?

    (A) Fresh gas flow of 0.5 L/min
    (B) Incompetence of the pressure-relief valve
    (C) Low ventilatory rate
    (D) Presence of a hole in the ventilator bellows
    (E) Prolongation of the inspiratory phase

108. Which of the following statements concerning pipecuronium is true?

    (A) It has a faster onset than pancuronium
    (B) It increases systemic vascular resistance
    (C) It induces tachycardia
    (D) It is eliminated by the kidney
    (E) It induces histamine release

109. Left ventricular end-diastolic volume is most likely to be underestimated by pulmonary artery occlusion pressure in patients with

   (A) acute myocardial ischemia
   (B) aortic insufficiency
   (C) mitral stenosis
   (D) primary pulmonary hypertension
   (E) tricuspid stenosis


110. Which of the following statements concerning the cardiovascular effects of intravenous bupivacaine is true?

   (A) Bretylium is effective in treating bupivacaine-induced ventricular arrhythmias
   (B) Cardiovascular toxicity is decreased during pregnancy
   (C) Cardiovascular toxicity occurs at lower blood levels than central nervous system toxicity
   (D) Systemic vascular resistance is unchanged
   (E) The rate of impulse conduction through the heart is increased


111. Which of the following is indicated by an alarm condition in the line-isolation monitor?

   (A) An electric shock to the patient
   (B) A power surge in the main hospital power supply
   (C) Disconnection of the patient from an electrocautery grounding pad
   (D) Overload of the operating room circuits
   (E) The presence of a current leak between an operating room electric device and ground


112. Which of the following statements concerning ketorolac is true?

   (A) It binds to opioid receptors
   (B) It causes dose-related thrombocytopenia
   (C) It decreases heart rate during isoflurane anesthesia
   (D) It is eliminated unchanged in urine
   (E) It reversibly inhibits cyclooxygenase


113. Postoperatively, a patient is being mechanically ventilated by a constant-flow, pressure-cycled ventilator with the following initial settings: inspiratory/expiratory (I/E) ratio of 1:2, peak inspiratory pressure (PIP) of 25 $cmH_2O$, and rate of 10/min. One hour later, the I/E ratio is 1:4. Which of the following would ensure that the minute ventilation is the same as that initially set?

   (A) Inflate the endotracheal tube cuff to prevent leakage
   (B) Double the respiratory rate
   (C) Decrease the expiratory pause until the I/E ratio is 1.0
   (D) Increase the PIP until the I/E ratio is 1:2
   (E) Increase the PIP to 50 $cmH_2O$


114. Left ventricular subendocardial perfusion pressure is best estimated by the difference between

   (A) mean arterial and central venous pressures
   (B) diastolic arterial and pulmonary artery occlusion pressures
   (C) mean arterial and pulmonary artery occlusion pressures
   (D) systolic arterial and pulmonary artery occlusion pressures
   (E) diastolic arterial and central venous pressures

115. A 29-year-old man who has been nasotrachealy intubated for 2 weeks following a motor vehicle accident has a fever (39°C) and a constant headache. Leukocyte count is 18,000/mm³. The most likely cause is

    (A) fractured nasal septum
    (B) retropharyngeal abscess
    (C) maxillary sinusitis
    (D) meningitis
    (E) rhinovirus infection

116. Surgery is cancelled 10 minutes after initiation of intravenous regional anesthesia with 50 mL of lidocaine 0.5%. To terminate anesthesia safely, what is the most appropriate timing for deflating the tourniquet?

    (A) Immediately if benzodiazepines have been administered
    (B) Immediately after intravenous administration of ephedrine 10 mg
    (C) Immediately, followed by repeated reinflation and deflation
    (D) In no less than 20 minutes after initial injection
    (E) In no less than 45 minutes after initial injection

117. A 2500-g, 12-hour-old infant is tracheally intubated and mechanically ventilated at a rate of 20/min with an $F_{IO_2}$ of 0.4 and PIP of 25 cmH$_2$O. At birth, amniotic fluid was meconium stained and Apgar scores were 2 and 7. The most recent arterial blood gas levels are $Pa_{O_2}$ 50 mm Hg, $Pa_{CO_2}$ 55 mm Hg, and pH 7.20. The most appropriate management is to

    (A) administer sodium bicarbonate
    (B) begin intravenous infusion of prostaglandin $E_1$
    (C) increase $F_{IO_2}$
    (D) increase ventilation
    (E) perform bronchial lavage

118. A 60-year-old woman who is taking propranolol for hypertension and is allergic to penicillin is anesthetized with thiopental and halothane for resection of an abdominal aortic aneurysm. Shortly after intubation she is given vancomycin 500 mg intravenously, after which her blood pressure decreases from 140/80 to 70/50 mm Hg while her heart rate remains steady at 64 bpm. The most likely explanation for the decrease in blood pressure is

    (A) cross-sensitivity of penicillin and vancomycin
    (B) interaction of vancomycin and propranolol
    (C) vancomycin-induced anaphylactoid reaction
    (D) interaction of halothane and propranolol
    (E) interaction of halothane and vancomycin

119. During a reoperative total hip arthroplasty requiring transfusion of 8 units of packed red blood cells, blood begins to ooze from the operative field and intravenous catheter sites. Urine is pink. The most likely cause is

    (A) citrate intoxication
    (B) factor V and VIII deficiencies
    (C) rhabdomyolysis
    (D) thrombocytopenia
    (E) transfusion reaction

120. Eight hours after abdominal surgery, a 51-year-old patient becomes increasingly somnolent. Epidural morphine 5 mg was administered immediately following the procedure. Postoperatively, respiratory rate has not decreased below 12/min and $SpO_2$ has remained greater than 92%. Arterial blood gas analysis shows $PaO_2$ 80 mm Hg, $PaCO_2$ 82 mm Hg, and pH 7.1. Which of the following is the most appropriate conclusion?

    (A) Analysis of the blood sample was delayed
    (B) The blood sample was venous rather than arterial
    (C) The patient is receiving supplemental oxygen
    (D) The pulse oximeter readings are falsely high
    (E) No treatment is required at this time

121. A 76-year-old patient is restless and hallucinating in the preoperative holding area. He received morphine 5 mg and scopolamine 0.4 mg intramuscularly as premedication and is now breathing oxygen 2 L/min through nasal prongs. $SpO_2$ is 98%. Which of the following is the most appropriate next step?

    (A) Administration of naloxone
    (B) Administration of physostigmine
    (C) Induction of general anesthesia
    (D) Determination of serum electrolyte concentrations
    (E) Computed tomographic (CT) scan of the head

122. For any given $FIO_2$ and $PaCO_2$, the $PaO_2$ is lower in a healthy paralyzed patient anesthetized with isoflurane than in the same patient unanesthetized and breathing spontaneously. The primary cause of this difference is

    (A) controlled ventilation
    (B) increased airway resistance
    (C) inhibition of hypoxic pulmonary vasoconstriction
    (D) intraoperative hypothermia
    (E) preferential ventilation of nondependent lung

123. Normal pseudocholinesterase

    (A) is highly concentrated at the motor end-plate
    (B) hydrolyzes succinylcholine by Hofmann elimination
    (C) is produced primarily at nerve terminals
    (D) is antagonized by acetylcholinesterase inhibitors
    (E) resists dibucaine inhibition more than its atypical variant

124. Thirty-six hours after primary repair of meningomyelocele, a term newborn has frequent periods of apnea lasting 25 seconds and associated with oxygen desaturation to 80%. The most likely explanation is

    (A) hyperglycemia
    (B) loss of cerebrospinal fluid
    (C) obstructive hydrocephalus
    (D) residual anesthetic effect
    (E) normal postoperative events

125. Inhalation induction of anesthesia is more rapid in a 6-month-old infant than in an adult because infants have

      (A) greater ratio of alveolar ventilation to FRC
      (B) greater ratio of blood volume to body weight
      (C) greater solubility of anesthetic in blood
      (D) lower anesthetic requirement
      (E) lower distribution of cardiac output to vessel-rich organs

126. Which of the following findings is most hazardous in premature infants?

      (A) Hematocrit of 55%
      (B) Rectal temperature of 35°C
      (C) Umbilical arterial blood $P_{O_2}$ of 50 mm Hg
      (D) Umbilical arterial blood $P_{CO_2}$ of 45 mm Hg
      (E) Umbilical arterial systolic pressure of 60 mm Hg

127. A 40-year-old patient has pain following injection of 8 mL of thiopental 2.5% through a right radial artery catheter. His hand remains pink. Which of the following is the most appropriate next step?

      (A) Injection of lidocaine through the catheter
      (B) Injection of nitroglycerin through the catheter
      (C) Injection of papaverine through the catheter
      (D) Right stellate ganglion block
      (E) No intervention

128. During nitrous oxide anesthesia, which of the following expands most rapidly?

      (A) Air bubble in the blood
      (B) Air in the intestine
      (C) Endotracheal tube cuff
      (D) Pneumothorax
      (E) Sulfahexafluoride bubble in the vitreal cavity

129. While an anesthesia machine is checked, opening the oxygen flow–control valve yields no oxygen flow, although the wall-mounted oxygen pipeline supply gauge reads 50 psi (pounds per square inch gauge). Opening the backup oxygen cylinder results in normal oxygen flow. The most likely cause is

      (A) failure of the oxygen pipeline supply
      (B) failure of the second-stage oxygen pressure regulator
      (C) a malfunctioning check valve in the oxygen pipeline supply inlet
      (D) a malfunctioning fail-safe valve
      (E) a malfunctioning oxygen flow–control valve

130. Which of the following statements concerning pulmonary function in patients with pulmonary fibrosis is true?

      (A) Diffusion capacity is decreased
      (B) Pulmonary artery diastolic-to-occlusion pressure gradients are normal
      (C) Ventilation-perfusion relationships are normal
      (D) Static pulmonary compliance is unchanged
      (E) Mechanical ventilation with slow rate and large tidal volume is optimal

131. In which of the following situations is mismatching of ventilation to perfusion in the lung greatest?

    (A) Awake patient, spontaneous ventilation, lateral decubitus position
    (B) Anesthetized patient, controlled ventilation, supine position
    (C) Anesthetized patient, controlled ventilation, lateral decubitus position
    (D) Anesthetized patient, controlled ventilation, sitting position
    (E) Anesthetized patient, spontaneous ventilation, prone position

132. The following hemodynamic profile is from a 62-year-old man in the intensive care unit (ICU) after coronary artery bypass grafting.

| | Entering ICU | + 30 Minutes |
|---|---|---|
| Heart rate (bpm) | 90 | 120 |
| Blood pressure (mm Hg) | 125/75 | 80/30 |
| PADP (mm Hg) | 12 | 25 |
| PAOP (mm Hg) | 10 | 25 |
| CVP (mm Hg) | 6 | 8 |

Which of the following is the most likely cause of the changes occurring after 30 minutes?

    (A) Anaphylactic reaction
    (B) Left ventricular ischemia
    (C) Pericardial tamponade
    (D) Pulmonary embolism
    (E) Septic shock

133. The odor of isoflurane is noted during isoflurane anesthesia with an endotracheal tube and mechanical ventilation. Mean airway pressure is unchanged. A scavenging system with an open interface and an active disposal system is being used. The most likely cause of the isoflurane odor is

    (A) a leak in the inspiratory limb of the anesthesia circuit
    (B) application of excessive negative pressure to the scavenging interface
    (C) malfunction of the pop-off valve of the anesthesia machine
    (D) obstruction of the gas disposal tubing leading from the scavenging interface
    (E) obstruction of the transfer tubing to the scavenging interface

134. Which of the following statements concerning the volume of distribution of a drug is true?

    (A) It is equal to the sum of the volumes of the tissue spaces into which it diffuses
    (B) It is equal to the volume to which it is distributed outside the plasma volume
    (C) It is unaltered by the amount bound to red blood cells and plasma proteins
    (D) It depends on elimination from plasma
    (E) It relates the total amount of the drug in the body to the plasma concentration

135. Which of the following statements concerning propofol is true?

    (A) Active metabolites can produce residual postoperative sedation
    (B) It causes less cardiovascular depression than an equivalent induction dose of thiopental
    (C) It causes less respiratory depression than an equivalent induction dose of thiopental
    (D) It has analgesic properties
    (E) The vehicle emulsion is associated with hypersensitivity reactions

136. The ECG strip shown here is recorded as a patient with a permanent transvenous DDD pacemaker enters the operating room. These changes indicate that the pacemaker is

(A) sensing the T waves
(B) sensing the retrograde P waves
(C) triggering off the intrinsic atrial activity
(D) malfunctioning in the atrial pacing mechanism
(E) prematurely stimulating the ventricle

---

137. Acute epiglottitis usually

(A) requires a lateral radiograph of the neck for diagnosis
(B) occurs in children 2 to 4 years of age
(C) is treated effectively with racemic epinephrine
(D) has a viral etiology
(E) requires immediate awake intubation by direct laryngoscopy in the emergency department

138. Characteristics of postdural puncture headache include

(A) incidence unrelated to the timing of ambulation
(B) increased severity with addition of vasoconstrictors to the anesthetic
(C) less frequent occurrence if the needle bevel is perpendicular to the direction of dural fibers
(D) more frequent occurrence in men
(E) prevention by prophylactic epidural blood patch

139. Which of the following statements concerning the superior laryngeal nerve is true?

(A) It provides sensory innervation to the subglottic surface of the vocal cord
(B) It provides sensory innervation to the inferior surface of the epiglottis
(C) It is a branch of the glossopharyngeal nerve
(D) It is blocked by injection of anesthetic near the lateral portion of the cricothyroid membrane
(E) It is the most commonly injured nerve during thyroid surgery

140. Which of the following is a complication of glycine used for irrigation during transurethral resection of the prostate?

(A) Epileptiform activity on EEG
(B) Peripheral neuropathy
(C) Tachycardia
(D) Transient blindness
(E) Transient deafness

141. In the event of a leak in the air flowmeter, which flowmeter arrangement produces the lowest risk for delivering hypoxic gas mixtures?

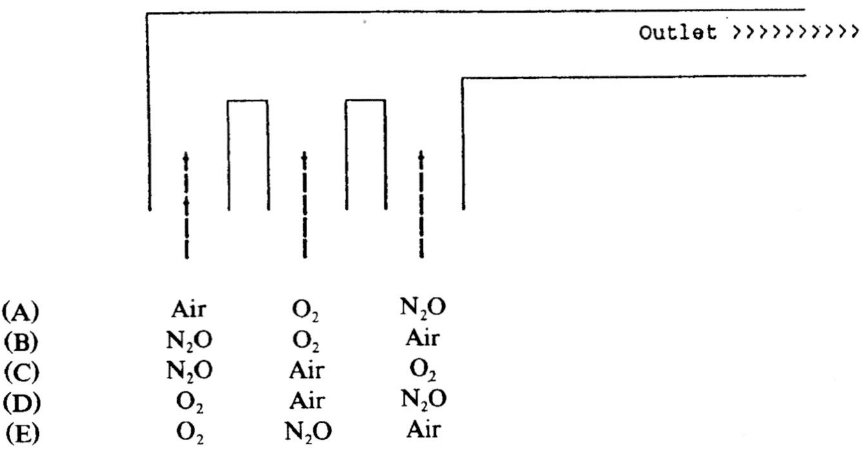


|  |  |  |  |
|-----|------|------|------|
| (A) | Air  | $O_2$ | $N_2O$ |
| (B) | $N_2O$ | $O_2$ | Air |
| (C) | $N_2O$ | Air | $O_2$ |
| (D) | $O_2$ | Air | $N_2O$ |
| (E) | $O_2$ | $N_2O$ | Air |

---

142. A 100-kg, 42-year-old woman received enflurane and oxygen for clipping of an intracranial aneurysm lasting 8 hours. In the first 2 postoperative hours, urine output is 2 L. Serum sodium concentration is 152 mEq/L. Urine osmolality and central venous pressure are low. Which of the following is best used to establish the diagnosis?

(A) Pulmonary artery occlusion pressure
(B) Serum fluoride concentration
(C) Serum osmolality
(D) Response to antidiuretic hormone
(E) Response to fluid restriction

143. The drug that causes dose-dependent EEG evidence of both central nervous system excitation and depression is

(A) lidocaine
(B) halothane
(C) thiopental
(D) nitrous oxide
(E) midazolam

144. Which of the following findings differentiates the pickwickian syndrome from morbid obesity?

(A) Carbon dioxide retention
(B) Upper airway obstruction
(C) Decreased forced expiratory volume
(D) Increased shunt fraction
(E) Increased FRC

145. Which of the following is the most likely sequela of interscalene brachial plexus block?

    (A) Cervical epidural block
    (B) Hemidiaphragmatic paralysis
    (C) Pneumothorax
    (D) Seizure
    (E) Vocal cord paralysis

146. Which of the following is the most reliable indicator of adequate reversal of neuromuscular block?

    (A) Inspiratory force equal to $-30$ cmH$_2$O
    (B) Sustained head lift for 5 seconds
    (C) Train-of-four ratio of 0.7
    (D) Twitch height at 100% of control
    (E) Vital capacity of 15 mL/kg

147. A 25-year-old man requires exploratory laparotomy following a motor vehicle accident. He is acutely intoxicated with alcohol. Which of the following is the most likely result of the alcohol ingestion?

    (A) Hyperdynamic circulation
    (B) Hyperglycemia
    (C) Hyperthermia
    (D) Increased respiratory depression from opioids
    (E) Increased sensitivity to neuromuscular blocking drugs

148. The decreased duration of action of an intravenous dose of fentanyl compared with an intravenous dose of morphine is best explained by

    (A) greater lipid solubility
    (B) increased hepatic metabolism
    (C) less protein binding
    (D) shorter elimination half-life
    (E) smaller volume of distribution

149. Which of the following complications of caudal anesthesia with 0.25% bupivacaine is more likely in children than in adults?

    (A) Intravascular injection
    (B) Neurotoxicity
    (C) Profound motor block
    (D) Systemic toxicity
    (E) Total spinal block

150. After an axillary brachial plexus block, the patient feels pain when the surgeon clips the skin over the thenar eminence. The most likely cause is inadequate anesthesia in the distribution of the

    (A) intercostobrachial nerve
    (B) median nerve
    (C) musculocutaneous nerve
    (D) radial nerve
    (E) ulnar nerve

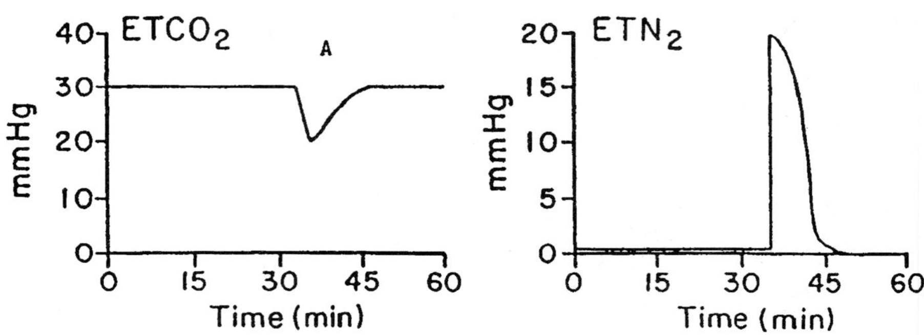



151. This trend plot shows end-tidal gases measured during a radical neck dissection. The event occurring at A is most likely

    (A)  acute hypotension
    (B)  endobronchial intubation
    (C)  kinking of the endotracheal tube
    (D)  rupture of the endotracheal tube cuff
    (E)  venous air embolism

---

152. A 36-year-old woman develops acute airway obstruction 24 hours after total thyroidectomy. The most likely cause is

    (A)  bilateral recurrent laryngeal nerve injury
    (B)  unilateral recurrent laryngeal nerve injury
    (C)  hypocalcemia
    (D)  subglottic edema
    (E)  tracheomalacia

153. Arterial pressure in the radial artery is 155/70 mm Hg measured by a correctly calibrated catheter-transducer system. At the same time, aortic pressure is 140/75 mm Hg using a high-fidelity catheter tip transducer. The most likely cause of this discrepancy is

    (A)  a large amount of air in the dome of the radial artery transducer
    (B)  coarctation of the aorta
    (C)  peripheral vascular constriction produced by sympathetic stimulation
    (D)  physiologic amplification of the waveform from the aorta to the radial artery
    (E)  too high a frequency response in the catheter-transducer system

154. During insertion of a Harrington rod with deliberate hypotension for correction of spinal scoliosis, accurate interpretation of somatosensory evoked potentials requires

    (A)  core temperature greater than 35°C
    (B)  hematocrit of at least 25%
    (C)  mean arterial pressure greater than 70 mm Hg
    (D)  $P_{O_2}$ of at least 80 mm Hg
    (E)  reversal of neuromuscular block

155. During insufflation of the peritoneal cavity with carbon dioxide at the start of laparoscopy, heart rate increases to 140 bpm, blood pressure decreases to 70/40 mm Hg, and a loud murmur is heard through the esophageal stethoscope. The most appropriate immediate step is to

    (A) administer a vasoconstrictor
    (B) infuse crystalloid solution rapidly
    (C) discontinue the inhaled anesthetic
    (D) insert a central venous catheter
    (E) deflate the abdomen

156. A 35-year-old man has acute onset of low back pain, lower extremity weakness, and bladder dysfunction. He had a lumbar laminectomy 2 years ago. A myelogram shows disk herniation at L4-5. The most appropriate management is

    (A) bed rest
    (B) administration of a nonsteroidal anti-inflammatory agent
    (C) epidural administration of a corticosteroid
    (D) epidural administration of a local anesthetic
    (E) surgical decompression

157. A patient with chronic obstructive pulmonary disease is undergoing spinal anesthesia to a T6 sensory level. The most pronounced effect on pulmonary function will be a decrease in

    (A) minute ventilation
    (B) peak expiratory flow
    (C) physiologic dead space
    (D) tidal volume
    (E) vital capacity

158. A 70-year-old patient is shivering and has chest pain in the PACU following a cholecystectomy. Heart rate is 120 bpm, and blood pressure is 220/120 mm Hg. $Sp_{O_2}$ is 97% at an $F_{IO_2}$ of 0.4. An ECG shows ST–T-wave changes, which are not affected by intravenous administration of nitroglycerin. Which of the following is the most appropriate next step?

    (A) Administration of esmolol
    (B) Administration of hydralazine
    (C) Administration of nitroprusside
    (D) Application of a warming blanket
    (E) Increasing $F_{IO_2}$

159. A 24-year-old man who sustained multiple rib fractures in a motor vehicle accident has air leaks through bilateral chest tubes. Which of the following is most likely following initiation of high-frequency jet ventilation?

    (A) Airway pressure will be measured most reliably at the proximal (external) end of the endotracheal tube
    (B) Atelectatic areas of the lungs will reexpand
    (C) Changes in end-tidal carbon dioxide tension measured at the tip of the endotracheal tube will match changes in $Pa_{CO_2}$
    (D) Hypercarbia will develop
    (E) The air leaks will be proportional to peak airway pressure

160. Which of the following statements concerning the risk of acquiring hepatitis from a blood transfusion is true?

    (A) Most patients with posttransfusion hepatitis become clinically jaundiced
    (B) Most cases of posttransfusion hepatitis are caused by the hepatitis B virus
    (C) The risk for hepatitis is less than that for AIDS
    (D) The risk for posttransfusion hepatitis is less than 1% per unit transfused
    (E) The incidence of posttransfusion hepatitis has remained unchanged over the past decade


161. Which of the following is more likely to occur with use of trimethaphan to induce hypotension than with use of nitroprusside?

    (A) A predictable decrease in mean arterial pressure
    (B) Increased mixed venous $Po_2$
    (C) Increased serum lactate concentration
    (D) Mydriasis
    (E) Reflex tachycardia


162. Local anesthetics block nerve conduction by

    (A) closing calcium channels
    (B) decreasing intracellular calcium concentration
    (C) decreasing potassium conductance
    (D) causing extrusion of intracellular potassium
    (E) inhibiting cellular influx of sodium


163. Which of the following drugs decreases lower esophageal sphincter tone?

    (A) Edrophonium
    (B) Glycopyrrolate
    (C) Metoclopramide
    (D) Prochlorperazine
    (E) Succinylcholine


164. In patients homozygous for atypical pseudocholinesterase, which of the following best explains the prolonged action of succinylcholine?

    (A) An increased proportion of the dose reaches the neuromuscular junction
    (B) Diffusion away from the neuromuscular junction is slowed
    (C) Hepatic clearance of succinylcholine is decreased
    (D) Prejunctional activity is unopposed
    (E) Succinylmonocholine induces neuromuscular block


165. Recognized side effects of magnesium sulfate used for the treatment of preeclampsia that would be of anesthetic concern include each of the following *except*

    (A) maternal pulmonary edema
    (B) neonatal hypotonia
    (C) increased maternal sensitivity to succinylcholine
    (D) increased maternal sensitivity to vecuronium
    (E) maternal hypokalemia

166. A comatose 40-year-old man is to undergo evacuation of an acute subdural hematoma. His left pupil is dilated and blood is present behind the left tympanic membrane. Each of the following is an acceptable intervention *except*

    (A) application of 5 cmH$_2$O positive end-expiratory pressure
    (B) blind nasotracheal intubation
    (C) use of isoflurane
    (D) use of nitrous oxide
    (E) use of succinylcholine

167. A jaundiced patient requires general anesthesia for portocaval shunt. He has a long history of alcohol abuse and is cirrhotic with ascites. Special considerations relevant to induction of anesthesia for this patient include each of the following *except* that

    (A) Denitrogenation by mask may be more rapid than expected
    (B) The risk of aspiration is increased
    (C) The dose of thiopental necessary for induction will be predictably reduced
    (D) The duration of succinylcholine action may be prolonged
    (E) Alfentanil would be an appropriate supplement

168. A patient being mechanically ventilated in the ICU requires wound debridement twice daily. Each of the following agents would be appropriate for induction of brief general anesthesia *except*

    (A) nitrous oxide
    (B) etomidate
    (C) ketamine
    (D) methohexital
    (E) midazolam

169. A computer program for hemodynamic calculations has the following input values: body surface area, arterial blood pressure, heart rate, pulmonary artery occlusion pressure, pulmonary artery pressure, and cardiac output. Each of the following values can be derived with this program *except*

    (A) cardiac index
    (B) stroke volume index
    (C) systemic vascular resistance
    (D) pulmonary vascular resistance
    (E) left ventricular stroke work index

170. A successful ankle block for transmetatarsal amputation of the first and second toes should include each of the following nerves *except* the

    (A) saphenous
    (B) deep peroneal
    (C) superficial peroneal
    (D) sural
    (E) tibial

171. Each of the following contributes to hypotension following induction of anesthesia with propofol *except*

    (A) central vagal stimulation
    (B) decreased central sympathetic tone
    (C) direct myocardial depression
    (D) resetting of arterial baroreceptors
    (E) systemic vasodilation

172. Inhibition of labor by terbutaline causes each of the following maternal side effects *except*

    (A) hyperkalemia
    (B) hypotension
    (C) ventricular dysrhythmias
    (D) hyperglycemia
    (E) pulmonary edema

173. A 66-year-old man with chronic obstructive pulmonary disease who underwent colectomy 12 hours ago has been receiving an epidural infusion of fentanyl at a rate of 100 μg/h. Which of the following is *least* likely to develop?

    (A) Hypotension
    (B) Nausea
    (C) Pruritus
    (D) Respiratory depression
    (E) Urinary retention

174. A 65-year-old man is disoriented and has a headache and nausea in the recovery room 30 minutes after transurethral resection of the prostate with glycine irrigation performed under spinal anesthesia. Heart rate is 50 bpm and blood pressure is 180/110 mm Hg. Which of the following is *least* likely?

    (A) Decreased serum osmolality
    (B) Serum sodium concentration 132 mEq/L
    (C) Increased serum ammonia concentration
    (D) Bibasilar rales
    (E) Jugular venous distention

175. A 70-year-old man sustains injuries to both carotid bodies during bilateral carotid endarterectomies performed 4 days apart. Two hours after the second procedure, the patient is breathing room air in the PACU. Which of the following sets of arterial blood gas values is *least* likely?

| | pH | $P_{CO_2}$ (mm Hg) | $P_{O_2}$ (mm Hg) |
|---|---|---|---|
| (A) | 7.3 | 50 | 58 |
| (B) | 7.3 | 50 | 86 |
| (C) | 7.4 | 40 | 86 |
| (D) | 7.4 | 42 | 58 |
| (E) | 7.5 | 32 | 58 |

# GENERAL INSTRUCTIONS

1. Please write your name and identification number in the space provided on the front of this test book. If you are taking the examination for Board Certification, your identification number is printed on your notification card. If you are an In-Training Resident, use your U.S. Social Security Number. If you do not have a U.S. Social Security Number, use your Canadian Social Insurance Number.

2. Your name and identification number and all of your answers must be recorded on the separate answer sheet enclosed in this booklet.

   The sample on the right shows how to record your identification number on the answer sheet. Be sure to enter your number in the boxes provided and also to mark it in the appropriate spaces as illustrated.

3. Credit will be given only for answers marked on the answer sheet. You may make any preliminary notes or calculations in the test books, but be sure that all of your answers are marked on the answer sheet. Only one choice should be marked for each question. Multiple answers for the same question are treated as wrong answers. In marking your answer sheet use only a soft (#2) lead pencil. Do NOT use a pen or pencil with hard lead. Make each mark heavy and black enough to obliterate completely the letter within the circle. Marks should fill the circle; if marks are light or outside the circle, you may not receive credit for your answers. Make no stray marks on the answer sheet, as these could lower your score. If you wish to change an answer, be sure to erase your first mark completely.

4. This test book contains two different types of questions, each of which is preceded by special directions. You are advised to study the directions carefully. Even though you may be in doubt about the correct answer, select the choice that you consider to be the best. Your score is the number of questions you answered correctly.

5. You will have 3½ hours to work on this section of the test which contains 175 questions.

---

# RULES OF CONDUCT FOR EXAMINEES DURING ABA/ASA IN-TRAINING EXAMINATION

1. Do not falsify information required for admission to the examination or impersonate another ABA/ASA examinee.

2. Do not bring calculators, watches with memory capability, books, papers, or memoranda of any kind into the examination room.

3. Do not break the seal on your test books until you are instructed to do so by the proctor.

4. Do not tear any pages or portions of pages from the test books or tear your answer sheet.

5. Do not disturb the examination process by talking, smoking, or interfering with others who are taking the examination.

6. Do not attempt to observe the test books or answer sheets of other examinees. Do not copy the answers of another examinee, permit answers to be copied, or in any way provide or receive unauthorized information about the content of the examination while it is in progress.

7. Terminate the examination immediately upon instruction by the proctor to do so.

8. Do not take the test books, answer sheets, or any documents, examination material, or memoranda from the room.

Failure to abide by these rules of conduct during this examination may result in disciplinary actions by the ABA/ASA In-Training Council or by the American Board of Anesthesiology. Statistical analyses may be used to verify observations and/or reports of suspected irregularities in conduct.

# AMERICAN BOARD OF ANESTHESIOLOGY

# AMERICAN SOCIETY OF ANESTHESIOLOGISTS

## IN-TRAINING EXAMINATION

### Book B
### 3½ hours

*Do not break the seal until you are told to do so.*

*Read the directions on the back cover.*

**PREPARED IN COOPERATION WITH NATIONAL BOARD OF MEDICAL EXAMINERS®**



ABA/ASA 93TB
pp 40, qtn 174

Printed in
U.S.A.

DIRECTIONS: Each of the numbered items or incomplete statements in this section is followed by answers or by completions of the statement. Select the ONE lettered answer or completion that is BEST in each case and fill in the circle containing the corresponding letter on the answer sheet.


1. The need for increased doses of nondepolarizing muscle relaxants in patients with extensive burns is best explained by

    (A) increased protein binding
    (B) hypermetabolism
    (C) increased glomerular filtration rate
    (D) proliferation of receptors on burned muscle
    (E) decreased volume of distribution


2. Which of the following parts of the infant's airway determines the appropriate diameter of a nasotracheal tube?

    (A) Nares
    (B) Glottis
    (C) Vocal cords
    (D) Cricoid cartilage
    (E) Third tracheal ring


3. Administration of 200 mEq of sodium bicarbonate during cardiopulmonary resuscitation is associated with

    (A) Cerebrospinal fluid (CSF) alkalosis
    (B) hypercalcemia
    (C) hypercarbia
    (D) hyperkalemia
    (E) shift of the oxyhemoglobin dissociation curve to the right


4. When compared with diazepam, midazolam

    (A) metabolites contribute more significantly to the sedative effect
    (B) elimination is less dependent on hepatic metabolism
    (C) has more predictable action after intramuscular administration
    (D) produces less respiratory depression
    (E) produces less hypotension during induction of anesthesia with opioids


5. Which of the following statements concerning a patient who has been receiving nitroprusside for several days is true?

    (A) Biotransformation of cyanide requires a sulfur donor
    (B) Formation of methemoglobin increases cyanide toxicity
    (C) Increased serum thiocyanate concentrations are innocuous
    (D) Mixed venous $P_{O_2}$ decreases as cyanide toxicity develops
    (E) Serum thiocyanate concentrations reflect the degree of cyanide toxicity

6. Which of the following increases the cephalad spread of hyperbaric intrathecal local anesthetics?

    (A)  Cephalad-directed needle bevel
    (B)  Coughing
    (C)  Lithotomy position
    (D)  Obesity
    (E)  Rapid injection


7. Compared with a patient without liver disease, a patient with cirrhosis will have

    (A)  greater accumulation of vecuronium with infusion
    (B)  increased unbound plasma vecuronium concentration
    (C)  more frequent occurrence of phase II block after succinylcholine administration
    (D)  prolonged elimination half-life of atracurium
    (E)  unchanged volume of distribution for pancuronium


8. Intrathecally administered opioids exert their analgesic effects primarily in the

    (A)  brain stem
    (B)  fourth ventricle
    (C)  spinal nerve roots
    (D)  spinothalamic tracts
    (E)  substantia gelatinosa


9. During laser excision of vocal cord polyps in a 5-year-old boy, dark smoke suddenly appears in the surgical field. The trachea is intubated and anesthesia is being maintained with halothane, nitrous oxide, and oxygen. The most appropriate initial step is to

    (A)  change from oxygen and nitrous oxide to air
    (B)  fill the oropharynx with water
    (C)  instill water into the endotracheal tube
    (D)  remove the endotracheal tube
    (E)  ventilate with carbon dioxide


10. During craniotomy in the sitting position, end-tidal carbon dioxide tension suddenly decreases. Ventilatory excursion of the chest is normal. Further evaluation is most likely to show a decrease in

    (A)  alveolar-to-arterial oxygen tension difference
    (B)  alveolar-to-arterial carbon dioxide tension difference
    (C)  dead space ventilation
    (D)  pulmonary artery pressure
    (E)  pulmonary artery occlusion pressure (PAOP)


11. Which of the following is a cardiorespiratory effect of epidural block to a T4 sensory level?

    (A)  Decreased expiratory reserve volume
    (B)  Decreased tidal volume
    (C)  Increased circulating catecholamine concentrations
    (D)  Increased heart rate
    (E)  Unchanged vital capacity

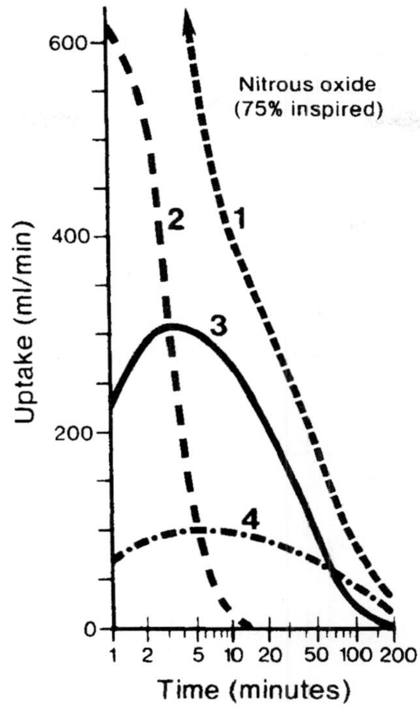



12. This figure describes the uptake of nitrous oxide 75% by individual tissue groups (vessel-rich group [VRG], muscle group [MG], fat group [FG]) and their sum (total uptake, [TU]). Which set of labels accurately describes the curves?

|     | **1** | **2** | **3** | **4** |
|-----|-----|-----|-----|-----|
| (A) | MG  | FG  | VRG | TU  |
| (B) | VRG | MG  | FG  | TU  |
| (C) | FG  | MG  | TU  | VRG |
| (D) | TU  | FG  | MG  | VRG |
| (E) | TU  | VRG | MG  | FG  |

---

13. A 67-year-old man undergoes spinal anesthesia with hyperbaric tetracaine 10 mg for transurethral resection of the prostate. At the end of the 50-minute procedure, the level of anesthesia is T6 and blood pressure is 120/70 mm Hg. Within 2 minutes after transfer to a stretcher, the patient has nausea and blood pressure decreases to 76/42 mm Hg. Which of the following is the most likely cause of the acute hypotension?

(A) Acute congestive heart failure
(B) Decreased venous return
(C) Dilutional hyponatremia
(D) Progression of sympathetic block
(E) Unrecognized bladder perforation

14. A 26-year-old woman has persistent uterine bleeding following a normal spontaneous delivery without anesthesia. The uterus is firm on manual examination. Which of the following anesthetics is most appropriate for manual extraction of the placenta?

    (A) Halothane
    (B) Pudendal block with lidocaine
    (C) Subarachnoid tetracaine
    (D) Thiopental
    (E) Vecuronium

15. Compared with intermittent positive-pressure ventilation (IPPV), intermittent mandatory ventilation (IMV)

    (A) better maintains cardiac output
    (B) provides less than full mechanical ventilatory support
    (C) requires a greater level of sedation
    (D) requires a higher $F_{IO_2}$
    (E) requires a lower inspiratory flow rate

16. Which of the following findings would be considered normal in the electroencephalogram (EEG) of an adult?

    (A) Decreased frequency during induction with halogenated anesthetics
    (B) Decreased frequency in frontal areas with administration of nitrous oxide 50%
    (C) Dominance of beta rhythm at 20 to 30 Hz during the awake relaxed state
    (D) Electrical silence with administration of isoflurane 2.5 minimum alveolar concentration (MAC)
    (E) The presence of burst suppression during natural sleep

17. Proper zeroing of an arterial pressure transducer attached to a supine anesthetized patient is best accomplished by

    (A) continuous flow of fluid through the intravascular catheter
    (B) opening the system to air at heart level
    (C) placement of the transducer diaphragm at heart level
    (D) proper damping of the transducer system
    (E) zeroing the transducer during the expiration phase of mechanical ventilation

18. A 1-month-old infant becomes hypoxemic faster during apnea than an adult. Which of the following is the primary cause of this difference?

    (A) Functional residual capacity in an infant is half that of an adult
    (B) Metabolic rate in an infant is twice that of an adult
    (C) Resting $Pa_{O_2}$ in an infant is lower than that in an adult
    (D) The number of alveoli in an infant is 12% the number in an adult
    (E) The hemoglobin dissociation curve in an infant is shifted to the right

19. During extracorporeal shock wave lithotripsy, the shock wave should be synchronized with

    (A) the P wave of the (electrocardiogram) ECG
    (B) the R wave of the ECG
    (C) the T wave of the ECG
    (D) peak inspiration
    (E) end expiration

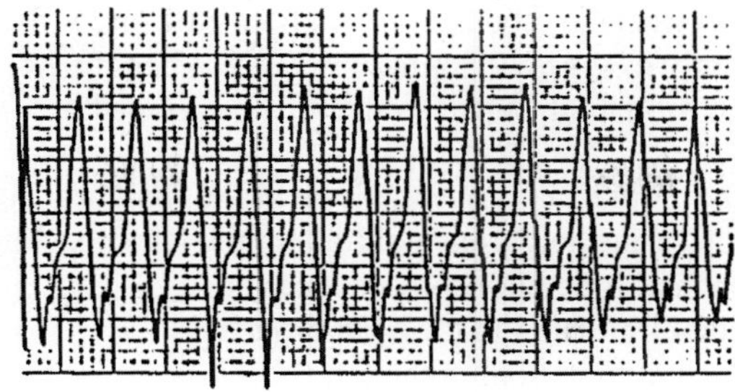

20. The cardiac rhythm illustrated shown here appeared suddenly in an anesthetized patient. The most appropriate management is

   (A) administration of adenosine
   (B) administration of digoxin
   (C) administration of epinephrine
   (D) overdrive pacing
   (E) synchronous cardioversion

---

21. Which of the following statements concerning hyperkalemia after succinylcholine administration to a patient with a spinal cord injury is true?

   (A) It is unlikely to occur if the lesion is located below T6
   (B) It is unlikely to occur within 24 hours of the injury
   (C) It is unlikely to occur more than 60 days after the initial injury
   (D) It is prevented by pretreatment with small doses of a nondepolarizing agent
   (E) It is decreased in magnitude by pretreatment with calcium chloride

22. The severity of chronic bronchitis is best assessed by measuring

   (A) tidal volume
   (B) carbon dioxide diffusion capacity
   (C) sputum production over 24 hours
   (D) forced vital capacity
   (E) arterial blood gases

23. An 8-kg, 1-year-old boy is scheduled for a bilateral inguinal hernia repair. If regional anesthesia is to be used for postoperative analgesia, which of the following statements is true?

   (A) Caudal administration of 0.25% bupivacaine will provide analgesia without evidence of motor block
   (B) Caudal administration of 0.125% bupivacaine is as effective as caudal administration of 0.25% bupivacaine
   (C) Caudal analgesia is more difficult to achieve in young children than in adults
   (D) The recommended volume of local anesthetic used for caudal analgesia in children is 3 mL per year of age
   (E) The volume of 0.25% bupivacaine required for bilateral ilioinguinal and iliohypogastric nerve blocks would be too large

24. After a left-sided double-lumen endotracheal tube is inserted, both cuffs are inflated. When the right (tracheal) lumen is clamped, breath sounds are heard only in the lower right lung field. When the left (bronchial) lumen is clamped, breath sounds are heard over the entire left lung field. Where is the tube positioned?

(A) Tracheal orifice above the carina and bronchial limb in the right bronchus
(B) Tracheal orifice above the carina and bronchial limb in the left bronchus
(C) Tracheal orifice and bronchial limb both above the carina
(D) Tracheal cuff and bronchial limb both in the right bronchus
(E) Tracheal orifice and bronchial limb both in the left bronchus

25. A 27-year-old man with type I von Willebrand disease requires internal fixation of an open fracture of the femur. Prothrombin time, partial thromboplastin time, and platelet count are normal. During surgery, there is significant oozing from the wound and the surgeon notes poor clot quality. The most appropriate therapy at this time is administration of

(A) cryoprecipitate
(B) desmopressin
(C) fresh frozen plasma
(D) lyophilized factor VII concentrate
(E) platelets

26. A 30-year-old man is brought to the emergency department after being rescued from a house fire. With the trachea intubated and $F_{IO_2}$ at 1.0, arterial blood gas values are $P_{aO_2}$ 495 mm Hg, $P_{aCO_2}$ 28 mm Hg, and pH 7.28. Hemoglobin saturation measured by co-oximeter is 50%. The most appropriate next step is to

(A) add positive end-expiratory pressure
(B) add *n*-acetylcysteine to the inhaled gases
(C) administer sodium bicarbonate intravenously
(D) transfuse 2 units of packed red blood cells
(E) transfer to a hyperbaric chamber

27. A 60-kg, 45-year-old woman who takes digoxin for atrial fibrillation receives furosemide 40 mg and mannitol 60 g during resection of a supratentorial meningioma. After initiation of hyperventilation to decrease $P_{aCO_2}$ from 35 to 20 mm Hg, multifocal premature ventricular contractions are noted on the ECG. The most likely cause is

(A) acute hypokalemia
(B) cerebral ischemia
(C) impending herniation of the brain stem
(D) paradoxical air embolism
(E) surgical manipulation of the meningioma

28. A 50-year-old woman with subarachnoid hemorrhage and left hemiparesis undergoes clipping of a right cerebral aneurysm. On the second postoperative day, mental status deteriorates. Blood pressure is 110/70 mm Hg. A cerebral angiogram shows vasospasm. The most appropriate management is to

(A) administer dexamethasone
(B) administer mannitol
(C) administer phentolamine
(D) expand intravascular volume
(E) intubate and hyperventilate to a $P_{aCO_2}$ of 28 mm Hg

29. Which of the following statements concerning cerebral blood flow (CBF) during anesthesia is true?

(A) CBF changes minimally when $Pa_{CO_2}$ increases from 30 to 40 mm Hg
(B) CBF changes minimally when $P_{O_2}$ decreases from 160 to 100 mm Hg
(C) CBF is autoregulated when mean arterial pressure is 40 mm Hg
(D) CBF is coupled to cerebral metabolism during isoflurane anesthesia
(E) CBF is unaffected by 1.2% isoflurane at a $Pa_{CO_2}$ of 40 mm Hg

30. Which of the following drugs is contraindicated in patients with Parkinson disease?

(A) Atropine
(B) Dopamine
(C) Droperidol
(D) Fentanyl
(E) Isoflurane

31. A 70-kg patient with no acute bleeding has a preoperative platelet count of 40,000/mm³. Following preoperative transfusion of platelets 10 units, the predicted platelet count would be

(A) 50,000/mm³
(B) 80,000/mm³
(C) 90,000/mm³
(D) 140,000/mm³
(E) 190,000/mm³

32. Two hours after coronary artery bypass grafting, a 60-year-old man has a heart rate of 140 bpm and blood pressure of 80/60 mm Hg. Cardiac index is 1.5 L/min/m². Central venous pressure is 23 mm Hg with large *a* waves in the right atrial pressure tracing. A pulsus paradoxus of 6 mm Hg is noted. Which of the following is the most likely diagnosis?

(A) Atrial flutter
(B) Cardiac tamponade
(C) Hypovolemia
(D) Junctional tachycardia
(E) Tension pneumothorax

33. Which of the following is the strongest indication for one-lung ventilation?

(A) Descending thoracic aortic aneurysm
(B) Esophageal resection
(C) Lobectomy for lung abscess
(D) Lobectomy for tumor
(E) Pneumonectomy for tumor

34. In a 65-year-old man, which of the following findings on preoperative pulmonary function testing is associated with the highest risk for respiratory insufficiency following pneumonectomy?

(A) Maximum voluntary ventilation at 65% of predicted
(B) Mean pulmonary artery pressure of 28 mm Hg
(C) Predicted postoperative forced expiratory volume in 1 second ($FEV_1$) of 800 mL
(D) Residual volume to total lung capacity (RV/TLC) ratio of 0.35
(E) Vital capacity of 3 L

35. During transurethral resection of the prostate, intravascular absorption of glycine irrigant most commonly produces

    (A) alkalosis
    (B) hemolysis
    (C) hypertension
    (D) tachycardia
    (E) wheezing

36. A 2.2-kg, 6-hour-old neonate is to undergo gastrostomy followed by repair of a tracheoesophageal fistula. During induction with halothane, air, and oxygen, the abdomen becomes distended. Appropriate management is to

    (A) intubate and assist spontaneous ventilation
    (B) intubate and control ventilation
    (C) insert an orogastric tube
    (D) allow the patient to breathe spontaneously by mask until gastrostomy
    (E) control ventilation by mask until gastrostomy

37. Which of the following is an advantage of a circle system over a Mapleson D system?

    (A) Better anesthetic conservation
    (B) Lower dead space
    (C) Lower circuit resistance
    (D) More efficient scavenging
    (E) More rapid changes in inspired gas concentration

38. A 27-year-old man with a 1-month history of quadriplegia at a C6 level is given general anesthesia for cystoscopy. During the cystoscopy, blood pressure suddenly increases to 220/120 mm Hg. Further evaluation is most likely to show

    (A) atrial fibrillation (ventricular rate 100 bpm)
    (B) paroxysmal atrial tachycardia (150 bpm)
    (C) sinus bradycardia
    (D) piloerection above the level of C6
    (E) sweating above the level of C6

39. Which of the following is the primary factor regulating normal coronary blood flow?

    (A) Aortic diastolic pressure
    (B) Coronary perfusion pressure
    (C) Heart rate
    (D) Myocardial oxygen consumption
    (E) Systolic wall tension

40. Which of the following statements concerning pressure support ventilation is true?

    (A) Continuous positive airway pressure is provided during inspiration and expiration
    (B) Delivered tidal volume remains the same with decreasing lung compliance
    (C) Inspiratory effort less than $-2$ cmH$_2$O is not assisted
    (D) The overall work of breathing decreases when weaning from mechanical ventilation
    (E) The patient will need more sedation than during IMV

41. If administered epidurally in equipotent doses, which of the following opioids will produce analgesia over the greatest number of dermatomes?

    (A)  Fentanyl
    (B)  Hydromorphone
    (C)  Meperidine
    (D)  Morphine
    (E)  Sufentanil

42. Which of the following is decreased by alkalinization of a 1.5% lidocaine solution?

    (A)  Concentration of free base
    (B)  Dose required for anesthesia
    (C)  Duration of anesthesia
    (D)  Intracellular concentration of ionized lidocaine
    (E)  Time to onset of anesthesia

43. Cyanide toxicity from nitroprusside is unlikely in patients with renal dysfunction because

    (A)  renal excretion of thiosulfate is decreased
    (B)  metabolic acidosis inactivates cyanide
    (C)  anemia inhibits breakdown of nitroprusside by oxyhemoglobin
    (D)  thiocyanate is formed in the liver
    (E)  the dose of nitroprusside necessary to lower blood pressure is greatly decreased

44. Twelve hours after an uneventful hysterectomy with lidocaine epidural anesthesia, a 70-year-old woman has partial paralysis of the lower extremities. She is receiving morphine 0.5 mg/h through an epidural catheter and is pain free. On examination, definite motor loss is noted in the lower extremities, but no other deficits are apparent. The most appropriate action at this time is to

    (A)  administer naloxone
    (B)  substitute fentanyl for morphine infusion
    (C)  remove the epidural catheter
    (D)  obtain an MRI of the lumbar spine
    (E)  reassure the patient

45. Equipment that is attached to a patient should have leakage current no greater than

    (A)  10 microamps
    (B)  100 microamps
    (C)  1 milliamp
    (D)  10 milliamps
    (E)  100 milliamps

46. When the inspired gas is changed from air to 20% oxygen and 80% nitrous oxide, $Pao_2$ increases because

    (A)  increased pulmonary artery pressure perfuses alveoli that previously enhanced dead space
    (B)  nitrous oxide stimulates the respiratory center
    (C)  rapid absorption of nitrous oxide increases alveolar oxygen concentration
    (D)  replacement of nitrogen by nitrous oxide expands atelectatic alveoli
    (E)  respiratory depression from nitrous oxide shifts the oxyhemoglobin dissociation curve

47. Which of the following characteristics of local anesthetics is associated with long duration of action?

    (A) High degree of lipid solubility
    (B) High degree of protein binding
    (C) High molecular weight
    (D) High $pK_a$
    (E) Presence of ester linkage

48. Which of the following drugs used to produce or reverse muscle relaxation has the greatest prolongation of action in a patient with end-stage renal disease?

    (A) Atracurium
    (B) Neostigmine
    (C) Pancuronium
    (D) Succinylcholine
    (E) Vecuronium

49. In a patient with chronic congestive heart failure, the safest pharmacologic approach to brain swelling during a craniotomy is

    (A) dexamethasone
    (B) furosemide
    (C) mannitol
    (D) thiopental
    (E) urea

50. In clinical anesthesia practice, the term "informed consent" is best described as a legal concept in which patients

    (A) agree to anesthesia care based on full disclosure of facts needed to make the decision intelligently
    (B) are told of all possible risks of anesthesia and anesthetic procedures
    (C) delegate all decisions regarding anesthesia care to the anesthesiologist
    (D) release the physicians from liability
    (E) sign global consent forms for surgical procedures that cover the administration of anesthesia care

51. The low fetal/maternal plasma ratio of bupivacaine compared with lidocaine is due to

    (A) fetal tissue binding
    (B) fetal plasma protein binding
    (C) maternal plasma protein binding
    (D) ionization in maternal blood
    (E) ionization in fetal blood

52. A previously healthy 28-year-old man is admitted to the emergency department with a probable opioid overdose. Arterial blood gas values are $Pa_{O_2}$ 49 mm Hg, $Pa_{CO_2}$ 76 mm Hg, and pH 7.12 while breathing room air. Which of the following statements is true?

    (A) Aspiration of gastric contents must have occurred
    (B) Hypoventilation alone can explain the acidosis and hypoxemia
    (C) The hypoxemia is probably due to noncardiogenic pulmonary edema
    (D) Naloxone should be administered only if the patient is normothermic
    (E) Pure oxygen is contraindicated

53. In which of the following clinical circumstances does downregulation of β-adrenergic receptors occur?

    (A) Chronic congestive heart failure
    (B) Hypothyroidism
    (C) Long-term clonidine administration
    (D) Long-term metoprolol administration
    (E) Stable angina

54. Which of the following is the most likely cause of apnea occurring after a retrobulbar block?

    (A) Epidural injection
    (B) Increased intracranial pressure
    (C) Oculopontine reflex
    (D) Ophthalmic artery injection
    (E) Subarachnoid injection

55. A 40-year-old man is undergoing open reduction and internal fixation of a fractured femur. During anesthesia with fentanyl, enflurane, and oxygen, heart rate decreases to 20 bpm and 6 premature ventricular contractions per minute are noted. No pulse is detected. The most appropriate next step is to

    (A) administer atropine
    (B) administer epinephrine
    (C) administer lidocaine
    (D) apply a transthoracic pacemaker
    (E) start cardiopulmonary resuscitation

56. A 35-year-old woman with systemic lupus erythematosus is admitted to the critical care unit following sudden onset of severe chest pain. Examination shows tachycardia, hypotension, pulmonary edema, and a blowing systolic murmur in the left parasternal region. The most appropriate management is

    (A) aerosol administration of terbutaline
    (B) intravenous infusion of phenylephrine and nitroglycerin
    (C) intravenous infusion of esmolol
    (D) intravenous infusion of epinephrine and nitroprusside
    (E) volume loading with lactated Ringer solution

57. The following table shows the pharmacokinetic effects of a new neuromuscular blocker.

|                        | **Normal**   | **Renal Failure** |
| ---------------------- | ------------ | ----------------- |
| Volume of distribution | 15 L         | 21 L              |
| Clearance              | 200 mL/min   | 100 mL/min        |

In a patient with renal failure, which of the following will result in a response to this drug most similar to that of a normal individual?

    (A) Increased loading dose
    (B) The same maintenance dose
    (C) Decreased maintenance dose interval
    (D) Avoidance of continuous infusion
    (E) Increased dose of anticholinesterase for reversal

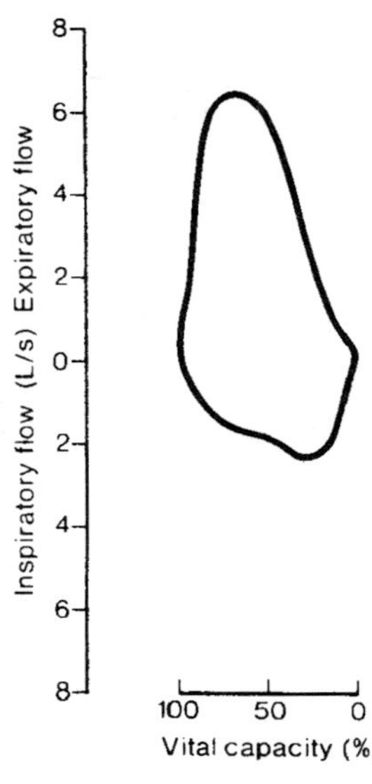


58. The flow-volume loop shown here is most likely from a patient with which of the following?

    (A) Bilateral vocal cord paralysis
    (B) Chronic bronchitis
    (C) Tracheal stenosis six months after a previous tracheostomy
    (D) Tumor of the lower trachea
    (E) Normal respiratory status

---

59. A 66-year-old patient with aortic stenosis is scheduled for aortic valve replacement. Examination shows blood pressure of 110/60 mm Hg and sinus rhythm at a rate of 75 bpm. PAOP is 20 mm Hg with a prominent *a* wave on the tracing. Which of the following is the most appropriate management?

    (A) Increasing myocardial contractility
    (B) Maintaining PAOP below 20 mm Hg
    (C) Maintaining sinus rhythm
    (D) Promoting mild tachycardia
    (E) Decreasing peripheral resistance

60. During rapid-sequence induction prior to an emergency surgical procedure, a 20-year-old patient vomits gastric contents containing particulate matter. An endotracheal tube is easily inserted and ventilation with pure oxygen is initiated. Despite the presence of bilateral breath sounds, $SpO_2$ is 90%. Which of the following is the most appropriate next step?

    (A) Administration of broad-spectrum antibiotics
    (B) Intravenous administration of high-dose methylprednisolone
    (C) Bronchial lavage with normal saline solution
    (D) Bronchoscopy to remove particulate matter
    (E) Cancellation of the surgical procedure

61. A radial artery catheter is to be used for blood pressure measurement during a sitting craniotomy. When zeroing the transducer, which of the following describes the best levels for placement of the transducer and opening of the system to air?

|       | Transducer | Opening to Air |
|-------|-----------|----------------|
| (A)   | Head      | Wrist          |
| (B)   | Head      | Head           |
| (C)   | Head      | Heart          |
| (D)   | Heart     | Heart          |
| (E)   | Heart     | Wrist          |

62. The gauge pressure on a cylinder of nitrous oxide

   (A) varies with the size of the cylinder
   (B) is the same for full and half-full cylinders
   (C) is the same as that of a full cylinder of oxygen if both are full
   (D) is independent of the temperature of the cylinder
   (E) reliably indicates the amount of nitrous oxide in the cylinder

63. Immediately after sustaining severe head injury, a 20-year-old man has a blood pressure of 150/90 mm Hg and an intracranial pressure of 35 mm Hg. After 1 hour of thiopental infusion, blood pressure is 105/60 mm Hg, intracranial pressure is 20 mm Hg, central venous pressure is 5 mm Hg, and temperature is 36°C. The EEG shows slow-wave activity. The most appropriate next step is administration of

   (A) additional thiopental
   (B) a corticosteroid
   (C) furosemide
   (D) nimodipine
   (E) phenylephrine

64. Following induction of anesthesia with sufentanil and pancuronium, a patient with left main coronary artery disease has a decrease in blood pressure from 110/70 to 60/40 mm Hg. There is no change in heart rate or ECG. The most appropriate management of the hypotension is administration of

   (A) calcium chloride
   (B) ephedrine
   (C) epinephrine
   (D) isoproterenol
   (E) phenylephrine

65. In a 35-year-old patient, which of the following is associated with an increased duration of clinical narcosis following infusion of a total dose of 10 mg/kg thiopental over 3 hours?

   (A) Alcoholism in remission
   (B) Asthma
   (C) Fever
   (D) Obesity
   (E) Use of appetite suppressants

66. A previously healthy, 60-kg, 17-year-old boy is undergoing emergency surgery for a gunshot wound involving the iliac vein. Ventilation is controlled with a tidal volume of 700 mL/breath, rate of 10/min, and peak inspiratory pressure of 30 cmH₂O. Body temperature is normal. The most likely cause of an end-tidal carbon dioxide partial pressure of 16 mm Hg is

    (A) endobronchial intubation
    (B) excessive expiratory time
    (C) excessive tidal volume
    (D) low cardiac output
    (E) pulmonary aspiration

67. Which of the following statements concerning anesthetic management for MRIs is true?

    (A) ECG wires are associated with patient burns
    (B) Mechanical ventilation of the lungs is not feasible
    (C) Monitors with ferromagnetic components may be used
    (D) Oxygen analysis of inspired gas is inaccurate
    (E) Pulse oximetry is not reliable near the MR scanner

68. Intraocular pressure is

    (A) decreased by glycopyrrolate
    (B) increased by hyperventilation
    (C) decreased by halothane
    (D) increased by nondepolarizing muscle relaxants
    (E) increased by phenylephrine eye drops

69. Compared with adult hemoglobin, which of the following is a characteristic of fetal hemoglobin?

    (A) It has a greater oxygen-carrying capacity
    (B) It has a lower $P_{50}$
    (C) It is more likely to cause an artifactual increase in $SpO_2$
    (D) It is more likely to sickle
    (E) It unloads oxygen more readily at the tissues

70. Which of the following is most effective in decontaminating an anesthesia machine that was splattered with HIV-contaminated blood?

    (A) Bleach
    (B) De-ionized water
    (C) Ethylene oxide
    (D) Hydrogen peroxide
    (E) Isopropyl alcohol

71. Which of the following is greater in an obese patient than in a nonobese patient of equal height?

    (A) Milliliters of local anesthetic required for epidural block
    (B) Milligrams of succinylcholine required for intubation
    (C) Clearance of diazepam
    (D) Clearance of fentanyl
    (E) Oxygen consumption per body surface area

72. The best premedication regimen for a known active narcotic addict would include

    (A) secobarbital
    (B) diazepam
    (C) nalbuphine
    (D) morphine
    (E) droperidol

73. During cardiopulmonary bypass at a nasopharyngeal temperature of 28°C and a hematocrit of 20%, temperature-corrected $Pa_{CO_2}$ is 50 mm Hg and uncorrected $Pa_{CO_2}$ is 60 mm Hg. The most appropriate management is to

    (A) administer additional opioid
    (B) administer packed red blood cells to increase hematocrit to 25%
    (C) further decrease the patient's temperature
    (D) increase fresh gas flow to the oxygenator
    (E) institute mechanical ventilation

74. Two days after coronary artery bypass grafting, a 62-year-old man remains sedated, tracheally intubated, and mechanically ventilated with full neuromuscular block. Over the next 3 hours, $Pa_{O_2}$ decreases from 90 to 70 mm Hg at an $FI_{O_2}$ of 0.7, peak inspiratory pressure measured proximally in the ventilatory circuit increases from 40 to 66 $cmH_2O$, and plateau pressure remains unchanged at 30 $cmH_2O$. Which of the following is the most likely cause of these changes?

    (A) Adult respiratory distress syndrome
    (B) Bronchial mucus plugging
    (C) Left ventricular failure
    (D) Lobar pneumonia
    (E) Tension pneumothorax

75. A combined epidural and general anesthetic is used for aortofemoral bypass surgery. Just before extubation, the patient received morphine 5 mg through the epidural catheter. Eleven hours later, he is unresponsive while breathing 40% oxygen from a face mask. Respiratory rate is 6/min and $Sp_{O_2}$ is 92%. Arterial blood gas analysis shows $Pa_{O_2}$ 80 mm Hg, $Pa_{CO_2}$ 84 mm Hg, and pH 7.16. Which of the following statements concerning this patient is true?

    (A) Hypercarbia is contributing to the decreased level of consciousness
    (B) Naloxone is ineffective for reversing the respiratory depression
    (C) The oxygen saturation is higher than expected because of the pH
    (D) The risk for respiratory depression would have been lower with subarachnoid administration of 0.5 mg morphine
    (E) Residual local anesthetic is contributing to the respiratory depression

76. A rapid shallow ventilatory pattern is most energy efficient for a patient who

    (A) has a low ratio of forced expiratory volume in 1 second to vital capacity ($FEV_1/VC$)
    (B) has a high ratio of tidal volume to vital capacity and diminished vital capacity
    (C) has increased pulmonary compliance
    (D) is using the accessory muscles of respiration
    (E) has increased airway resistance

77. A 70-year-old patient has absence of the left radial pulse 1 month after repair of an aortic aneurysm. Arterial pressure was monitored perioperatively with a 20-gauge left radial artery catheter. Which of the following statements concerning this complication is true?

    (A)  A preoperative Allen test would have predicted this complication
    (B)  Stellate ganglion block should be performed
    (C)  This complication would have been less likely with an 18-gauge catheter
    (D)  This patient has poor collateral circulation in the hand
    (E)  The pulse will likely return

78. Five minutes after intrathecal administration of tetracaine 12 mg in hyperbaric solution, a 60-year-old man has a weak hand grasp. Respirations are normal, heart rate has decreased from 80 to 45 bpm, and blood pressure has decreased from 150/80 to 90/50 mm Hg. The most appropriate management at this time is

    (A)  administration of atropine
    (B)  administration of ephedrine
    (C)  administration of phenylephrine
    (D)  placement of the patient in the head-down position
    (E)  observation

79. A burn is found at the site of the electrocautery pad. Which of the following is most likely?

    (A)  The electrosurgical unit was in the bipolar mode
    (B)  The electrocautery pad became partially detached
    (C)  The electrosurgical unit ground wire was severed
    (D)  The line-isolation monitor alarmed
    (E)  The patient became grounded

80. Which property of oxygen is detected by the fail-safe device on the anesthesia machine?

    (A)  Concentration
    (B)  Flow
    (C)  Pressure
    (D)  Partial pressure
    (E)  Reserve volume

81. Which of the following nerves should be blocked for an operation at the medial aspect of the lower leg?

    (A)  Femoral
    (B)  Sciatic
    (C)  Obturator
    (D)  Common peroneal
    (E)  Tibial

82. Which of the following is most effective in preventing intraoperative hypothermia in adults?

    (A)  Heating and humidifying inspired gases
    (B)  Maintaining a warm operating room
    (C)  Using a circulating warm-water mattress
    (D)  Using reflective coverings
    (E)  Warming intravenous fluids

83. Which of the following shaded areas most accurately represents the dead space of a properly functioning circle system?

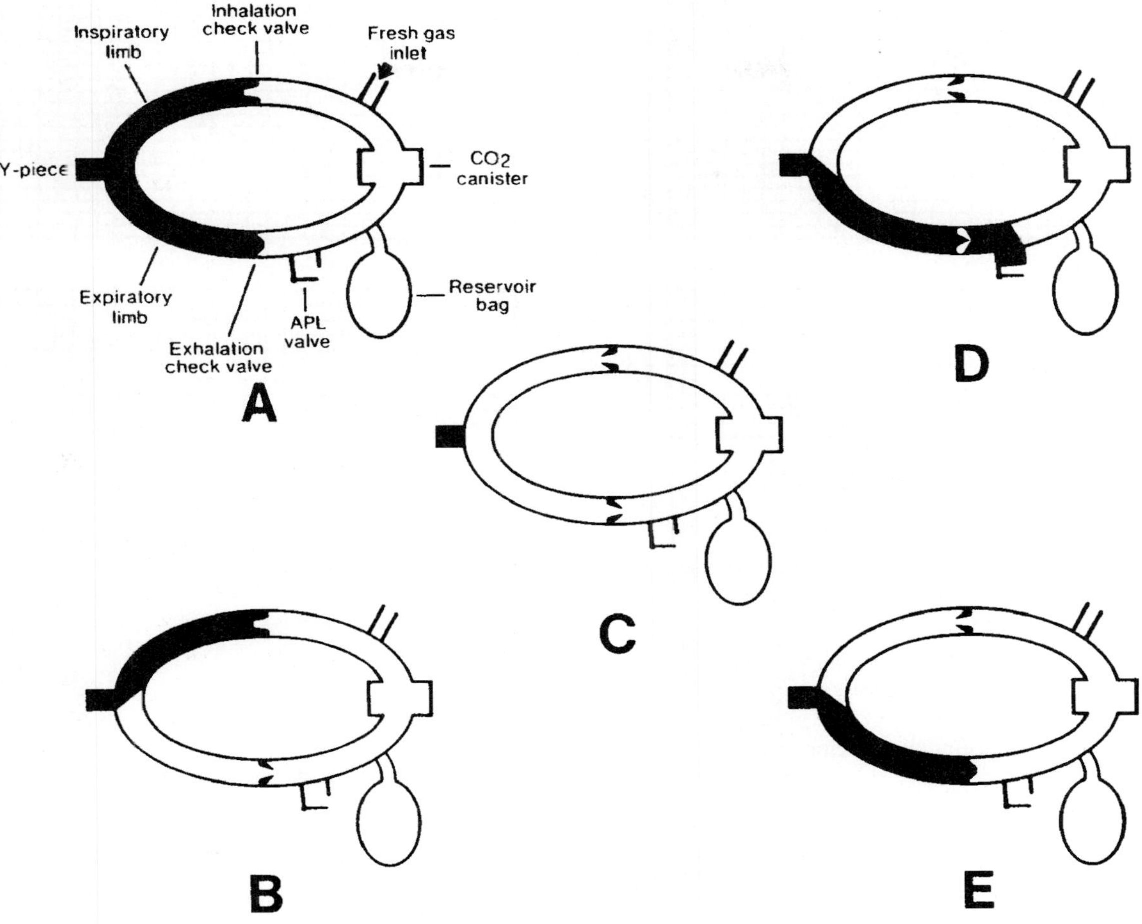


---

84. The effect of succinylcholine is terminated at postsynaptic effector cells by

(A) binding and uptake by effector cells
(B) diffusion into capillaries
(C) hydrolysis by junctional cholinesterase
(D) hydrolysis by pseudocholinesterase
(E) spontaneous degradation to succinylmonocholine

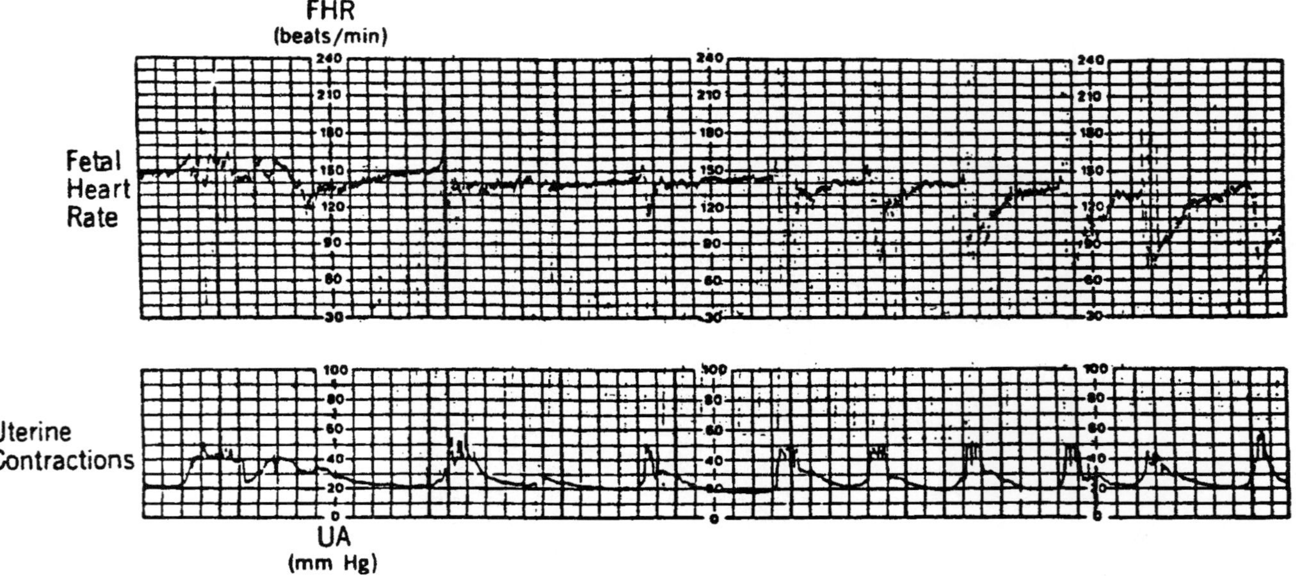



85. The fetal heart rate and uterine contraction tracings shown here are most consistent with

    (A) fetal acidosis
    (B) fetal cerebral hemorrhage
    (C) fetal head compression
    (D) fetal hypoxia
    (E) uteroplacental insufficiency

---

86. The cardiovascular effects of an inhalational anesthetic are evaluated in 10 normal volunteers in the awake resting state and after 15 minutes of constant inspired concentration. Results were analyzed by $t$ test for paired data and are presented below as mean ± standard deviation.

| | Mean Arterial Pressure (mm Hg) | Heart Rate (bpm) | Cardiac Output (L/min) |
| --- | --- | --- | --- |
| Awake | 94 ± 5 | 82 ± 2 | 4.2 ± 0.5 |
| Anesthetized | 83 ± 9 | 90 ± 2[a] | 3.9 ± 0.7 |

[a] $p < .05$

Based on these data, which of the following conclusions is most valid?

    (A) A decrease in cardiac output would have been evident if more subjects were included in the study
    (B) The anesthetic decreases mean arterial pressure
    (C) The anesthetic does not cause cardiac depression
    (D) The anesthetic is unsafe for patients with coronary artery disease
    (E) There is a 95% to 100% chance that the anesthetic increases heart rate

87. A patient with alcoholic cirrhosis, ascites, and gastrointestinal bleeding receives 4 units of red blood cells prior to anesthesia with isoflurane in oxygen for emergency exploratory laparotomy. After the peritoneum is opened and the fluid is drained, blood pressure decreases to 60/40 mm Hg and $Spo_2$ decreases to 90%. The most likely cause of the hypoxemia is

    (A) acute myocardial ischemia
    (B) decreased 2,3-diphosphoglycerate in transfused blood
    (C) increased intrapulmonary shunting
    (D) relative hypovolemia
    (E) venous air embolism

88. Which of the following statements concerning barbiturate protection from cerebral ischemia is true?

    (A) It may be achieved with dosages low enough to avoid cardiovascular effects
    (B) It is linearly dose-related
    (C) It improves neurologic outcome following cardiac arrest
    (D) It is most useful in patients with focal ischemia
    (E) It is unrelated to EEG activity

89. A 77-year-old woman is still intubated and breathing spontaneously following a total hip replacement. The muscle relaxant has been reversed. Tidal volume is 400 mL, end-tidal carbon dioxide tension is 45 mm Hg, and $Spo_2$ is 98% at an $Fio_2$ of 1.0. On transfer from the operating table to the gurney, heart rate increases from 65 to 100 bpm and blood pressure decreases from 130/80 to 80/50 mm Hg. End-tidal carbon dioxide tension is 30 mm Hg and $Spo_2$ is 94%. The most likely diagnosis is

    (A) anaphylactic reaction
    (B) bronchospasm
    (C) myocardial infarction
    (D) pulmonary embolism
    (E) unreplaced blood loss

90. A 40-year-old woman has continuous nondermatomal burning pain of the distal foot 4 weeks after sustaining a metatarsal fracture. On examination, the foot is mildly swollen, tender, and cool. Which of the following statements concerning this condition is true?

    (A) A radiograph of the distal bones of the painful foot will show severe osteoporosis
    (B) A technetium scan of the distal joints of the painful foot will show decreased uptake
    (C) Early use of opioid analgesia will prevent progression of the symptoms
    (D) Intravenous phentolamine will relieve the pain
    (E) The chance of spontaneous recovery within 8 weeks is greater than 80%

91. Evaluation of a postoperative neurologic deficit discloses inability to oppose the thumb and little finger, weakness of abduction of the thumb, and loss of flexion of the distal phalanx of the index finger. This problem is most likely related to

    (A) paresthesia occurring during an interscalene brachial plexus block
    (B) attempted radial artery cannulation at the wrist
    (C) inadequate padding under the elbow
    (D) attempted venipuncture in the antecubital fossa
    (E) abduction of the upper humerus against an "ether screen"

92. Arterial oxyhemoglobin desaturation develops more rapidly following apnea in a pregnant patient at term than in a nonpregnant patient with a large intra-abdominal tumor. Which of the following findings in pregnancy is the most likely cause?

    (A)  Higher cardiac output
    (B)  Higher oxygen consumption
    (C)  Larger anatomic dead space
    (D)  Smaller blood volume
    (E)  Smaller functional residual capacity

93. Which of the following best describes the relationship between cerebral perfusion pressure and CBF in a patient with untreated chronic hypertension?

    (A)  It is constant at mean blood pressures between 50 and 150 mm Hg
    (B)  It is linear for all blood pressures
    (C)  Flow versus pressure curve is hyperbolic
    (D)  Flow versus pressure curve is shifted to the right
    (E)  Flow versus pressure curve is shifted to the left

94. The accuracy of oxyhemoglobin saturation determined by digital pulse oximetry is affected significantly by each of the following *except*

    (A)  movement of the patient
    (B)  isovolemic hemodilution to a hematocrit of 23%
    (C)  position of the operating room light
    (D)  intravenous administration of methylene blue
    (E)  infusion of phenylephrine

95. The use of droperidol as a preanesthetic medication has been associated with each of the following *except*

    (A)  acute anxiety
    (B)  anterograde amnesia
    (C)  hypotension
    (D)  extrapyramidal signs
    (E)  catalepsy

96. Each of the following changes is expected with deliberate hypothermia *except*

    (A)  decreased unloading of oxygen from hemoglobin
    (B)  a 5% decrease in MAC for each 1°C decrease in temperature
    (C)  increased arterial oxygen and carbon dioxide contents
    (D)  a 50% decrease in cerebral metabolic rate at 28°C
    (E)  spike and dome EEG activity at temperatures below 30°C

97. Each of the following drugs is a cause of central anticholinergic syndrome *except*

    (A)  amitriptyline
    (B)  atropine
    (C)  diphenhydramine
    (D)  promethazine
    (E)  ranitidine

98. A 24-year-old woman requires anesthesia for emergency repair of open fractures of the tibia and fibula. She used cocaine 2 hours ago. Blood pressure is 170/110 mm Hg. Each of the following is useful in managing the hypertension *except*

> (A) hydralazine
> (B) labetalol
> (C) nitroprusside
> (D) phentolamine
> (E) propranolol

99. Carbon monoxide poisoning with a carboxyhemoglobin concentration of 20% is characterized by each of the following *except*

> (A) decreased oxygen-carrying capacity of hemoglobin
> (B) decreased $Pao_2$
> (C) shift of the oxyhemoglobin dissociation curve to the left
> (D) normal minute volume of ventilation
> (E) headache and nausea

100. A 40-year-old woman receives alfentanil 75 µg/kg followed by an infusion of 1.5 µg/kg/min for a 1-hour cholecystectomy and cholangiogram. This regimen could be associated with each of the following *except*

> (A) muscle rigidity
> (B) increased biliary tract pressure
> (C) inadequate anesthesia
> (D) postoperative respiratory depression
> (E) 2 to 4 hours of postoperative analgesia

101. Monitoring sensory evoked potentials may be useful in detecting functional derangement of each of the following *except*

> (A) cranial nerve pathways during posterior fossa operations
> (B) motor pathways during anterior cervical diskectomy
> (C) dorsal column pathways during operations for spinal tumors
> (D) visual pathways during operations on the sphenoid wing
> (E) cortical pathways during carotid artery operations

102. Which of the following drugs is *least* likely to cross the placenta?

> (A) Lidocaine
> (B) Meperidine
> (C) Midazolam
> (D) Thiopental
> (E) Vecuronium

DIRECTIONS: For each of the questions or incomplete statements below, ONE or MORE of the answers or completions given is correct. On the answer sheet fill in the circle containing

A if only *1, 2, and 3* are correct,
B if only *1 and 3* are correct,
C if only *2 and 4* are correct,
D if only *4* is correct,
E if all are correct.

FOR EACH ITEM FILL IN ONLY ONE CIRCLE ON YOUR ANSWER SHEET

| DIRECTIONS SUMMARIZED | | | | |
|---|---|---|---|---|
| A | B | C | D | E |
| 1, 2, 3 | 1, 3 | 2, 4 | 4 | All are |
| only | only | only | only | correct |

103. Characteristics of a depolarizing neuromuscular block include

(1) tetanic fade at 50 Hz for 5 seconds
(2) decreased train-of-four ratio
(3) post-tetanic facilitation
(4) decreased twitch height

104. Before awake nasal intubation in a patient who has been NPO, areas to be anesthetized are supplied by which of the following nerves?

(1) Glossopharyngeal
(2) Superior laryngeal
(3) Recurrent laryngeal
(4) Hypoglossal

105. A 40-year-old patient is referred to a pain clinic for evaluation of right upper quadrant pain 6 months after cholecystectomy performed through a subcostal incision. Which of the following procedures would provide diagnostic information?

(1) Intercostal nerve blocks
(2) Celiac plexus block
(3) Differential spinal block
(4) Lumbar sympathetic block

106. Compared with intermittent injections of intramuscular opioids for postoperative pain relief, patient-controlled analgesia is associated with

(1) lower incidence of nausea and vomiting
(2) increased risk for ventilatory depression
(3) greater variability in opioid pharmacokinetics
(4) lower total opioid requirement

FOR EACH ITEM FILL IN ONLY ONE CIRCLE ON YOUR ANSWER SHEET

<table>
<tr><td colspan="5" align="center">DIRECTIONS SUMMARIZED</td></tr>
<tr><td align="center">A</td><td align="center">B</td><td align="center">C</td><td align="center">D</td><td align="center">E</td></tr>
<tr><td align="center">1, 2, 3</td><td align="center">1, 3</td><td align="center">2, 4</td><td align="center">4</td><td align="center">All are</td></tr>
<tr><td align="center">only</td><td align="center">only</td><td align="center">only</td><td align="center">only</td><td align="center">correct</td></tr>
</table>

107. Adverse reactions to protamine include

    (1) markedly increased pulmonary vascular resistance
    (2) anaphylaxis
    (3) decreased systemic vascular resistance
    (4) noncardiogenic pulmonary edema

108. Causes of the hypoxemia that occurs in patients with advanced cirrhosis include

    (1) decreased total lung capacity
    (2) decreased cardiac output
    (3) right-to-left pulmonary shunting
    (4) decreased 2,3-diphosphoglycerate concentration in erythrocytes

109. In a patient who is spontaneously breathing room air at the conclusion of a nitrous oxide (70%)-opioid anesthetic, causes of hypoxemia include

    (1) decreased functional residual capacity
    (2) dilution of alveolar oxygen by outpouring of nitrous oxide
    (3) opioid-induced respiratory depression
    (4) increased physiologic dead space

110. Compared with an induction dose of midazolam, an induction dose of thiopental causes a greater decrease in

    (1) blood pressure
    (2) cerebral blood flow (CBF)
    (3) cerebral metabolic rate
    (4) cortical EEG activity

111. The $F_{IO_2}$ achieved by nasal prongs with oxygen flowing at 8 L/min depends on

    (1) tidal volume
    (2) respiratory frequency
    (3) inspiratory flow rate
    (4) volume of the nasopharynx

112. The administration of mannitol 1 g/kg over 15 minutes produces an acute increase in

    (1) serum potassium concentration
    (2) central venous pressure
    (3) systemic vascular resistance
    (4) serum osmolality

FOR EACH ITEM FILL IN ONLY ONE CIRCLE ON YOUR ANSWER SHEET

| DIRECTIONS SUMMARIZED | | | | |
|---|---|---|---|---|
| A | B | C | D | E |
| 1, 2, 3 | 1, 3 | 2, 4 | 4 | All are |
| only | only | only | only | correct |

113. Compared with a term infant, an infant born at 32 weeks' gestation who receives anesthesia at 2 months of age is at increased risk for

    (1) pulmonary oxygen toxicity
    (2) postoperative apnea
    (3) renal failure
    (4) retrolental fibroplasia

114. Advantages of performing spinal anesthesia via the lateral approach include

    (1) larger opening for needle insertion than for the midline approach
    (2) avoidance of the calcified interspinous ligament in the elderly
    (3) less flexion of the spine required than for the midline approach
    (4) less likelihood of peridural vein puncture than for the midline approach

115. In meralgia paresthetica

    (1) there is pain in the anterolateral aspect of the thigh
    (2) the obturator nerve is involved
    (3) obesity is an associated factor
    (4) neurolytic alcohol block is the treatment of choice

116. In patients undergoing transsphenoidal hypophysectomy for acromegaly, anesthesia is complicated by

    (1) decreased subglottic diameter
    (2) temporomandibular joint dysfunction
    (3) glucose intolerance
    (4) diabetes insipidus

117. In which of the following ways does the infant airway differ from that of the adult?

    (1) The larynx is more cephalad
    (2) The vocal cords are perpendicular to the plane of the trachea
    (3) The cricoid cartilage is the narrowest part of the airway
    (4) The larynx is more anterior

118. The duration of an epidural block can be increased clinically by

    (1) use of a local anesthetic with low protein binding
    (2) use of a local anesthetic with low $pK_a$
    (3) addition of sodium bicarbonate to the local anesthetic
    (4) increasing the total dose of the local anesthetic

<table>
<tr><td colspan="5" align="center"><u>DIRECTIONS SUMMARIZED</u></td></tr>
<tr><td align="center">A</td><td align="center">B</td><td align="center">C</td><td align="center">D</td><td align="center">E</td></tr>
<tr><td align="center">1, 2, 3</td><td align="center">1, 3</td><td align="center">2, 4</td><td align="center">4</td><td align="center">All are</td></tr>
<tr><td align="center">only</td><td align="center">only</td><td align="center">only</td><td align="center">only</td><td align="center">correct</td></tr>
</table>

119. Prior to vaginal delivery at term, a primiparous woman receives epidural anesthesia administered through a catheter inserted at L2-3. The following day she has left footdrop and sensory loss over the left outer calf. Causes of these complications include

    (1) compression of the obturator nerve by excessive thigh flexion
    (2) compression of the lumbosacral trunk by the fetal head
    (3) nerve root injury by the epidural needle
    (4) compression of the common peroneal nerve by the stirrup

120. A 2-year-old boy with tetralogy of Fallot is scheduled for repair of bilateral inguinal hernias. True statements concerning this child include the following:

    (1) Oxygen saturation will improve with crying
    (2) Cyanosis will increase with use of halothane
    (3) Resistance to pulmonary outflow will be fixed
    (4) An increased red cell mass will compensate for right-to-left shunt

121. A previously healthy 28-year-old woman who had a subarachnoid hemorrhage 2 days ago is scheduled for a craniotomy and clipping of an anterior communicating artery aneurysm. She is awake, oriented, and neurologically intact. True statements concerning anesthetic management include the following:

    (1) The arterial pressure should be maintained above the preoperative values during induction
    (2) Hyperventilation to a $Paco_2$ of 25 to 30 mm Hg should be initiated prior to endotracheal intubation
    (3) Mannitol should be given immediately following induction
    (4) The mean arterial pressure should be decreased to 50 mm Hg if necessary for surgical exposure

122. A 45-year-old man is scheduled for elective antrectomy and vagotomy. He has drunk a six-pack beer daily for 20 years. Laboratory evaluation shows the following findings:

| | **Patient** | **Normal** |
|---|---|---|
| AST (SGOT) (U/L) | 75 | 0-45 |
| ALT (SGPT) (U/L) | 56 | 0-45 |
| LDH (U/L) | 300 | 50-250 |
| Alkaline phosphatase (U/L) | 120 | 25-115 |
| Bilirubin (mg/dL) | 1.2 | 0.1-1.2 |

Based on these laboratory findings, anticipated problems in anesthetic management include

    (1) increased risk for halothane hepatotoxicity
    (2) coagulation disorders
    (3) large peripheral arteriovenous shunts
    (4) increased anesthetic requirements

| DIRECTIONS SUMMARIZED | | | | |
|---|---|---|---|---|
| A | B | C | D | E |
| 1, 2, 3 | 1, 3 | 2, 4 | 4 | All are |
| only | only | only | only | correct |

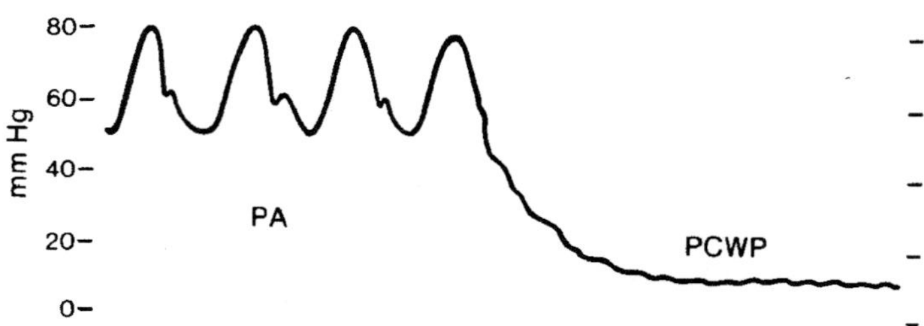



123. Causes of the pulmonary artery pressure and pulmonary artery occlusion pressure waveforms shown here include

    (1) catheter overwedging
    (2) protamine reaction
    (3) acute mitral regurgitation
    (4) primary pulmonary hypertension

---

124. Electrolyte profiles consistent with pyloric stenosis in a 6-week-old infant include the following:

| | $Na^+$ (mEq/L) | $K^+$ (mEq/L) | $Cl^-$ (mEq/L) | $HCO_3^-$ (mEq/L) |
|---|---|---|---|---|
| (1) | 145 | 3.5 | 108 | 24 |
| (2) | 145 | 2.5 | 85 | 15 |
| (3) | 160 | 5.5 | 120 | 36 |
| (4) | 128 | 2.5 | 85 | 32 |

| DIRECTIONS SUMMARIZED | | | | |
|---|---|---|---|---|
| A | B | C | D | E |
| 1, 2, 3 | 1, 3 | 2, 4 | 4 | All are |
| only | only | only | only | correct |

125. True statements concerning regional anesthesia with peripheral nerve blocks for an operation on the knee using a tourniquet include the following:

    (1) The inguinal perivascular block includes the obturator nerve
    (2) Paresthesias are required during sciatic block
    (3) The lateral femoral cutaneous nerve must be blocked
    (4) Block of the lumbar plexus in the psoas compartment provides adequate anesthesia

126. Proximal spread of a local anesthetic solution placed in the axillary perivascular space is promoted by

    (1) increased volume of the local anesthetic agent
    (2) digital pressure distal to the injection site
    (3) cephalad direction of the needle
    (4) adduction of the shoulder after the injection

| DIRECTIONS SUMMARIZED | | | | |
|:---:|:---:|:---:|:---:|:---:|
| A | B | C | D | E |
| 1, 2, 3 | 1, 3 | 2, 4 | 4 | All are |
| only | only | only | only | correct |

127. Indications for neurolytic celiac plexus ablation include pain due to carcinoma of the

  (1) sigmoid colon
  (2) kidney
  (3) ovary
  (4) pancreas

128. Compared with a 20-year-old patient, an 80-year-old patient will

  (1) have similar EEG sensitivity to the same blood concentrations of thiopental
  (2) require lower induction doses (mg/kg) of thiopental
  (3) have increased sensitivity to volatile anesthetics
  (4) require lower doses (mg/kg) of succinylcholine

129. Induction of anesthesia with usual drug dosages and concentrations may lead to cardiovascular signs of overdose in patients with hypothyroidism because of expected decreases in

  (1) respiratory quotient
  (2) minute volume of breathing
  (3) circulating blood volume
  (4) cardiac output

130. The duration of the anticoagulant effect of heparin is

  (1) independent of body temperature
  (2) determined primarily by renal excretion
  (3) prolonged two to three times with hypoalbuminemia
  (4) dose dependent

131. During general endotracheal anesthesia, early signs of an acute asthma attack include

  (1) alteration of the expiratory plateau on capnography
  (2) increased $Paco_2$
  (3) increased peak airway pressure
  (4) hypoxemia

132. At the placental interface, the efficiency of oxygen transport to the fetus is enhanced by

  (1) movement of the maternal oxyhemoglobin dissociation curve to the right
  (2) diffusion of carbon dioxide from fetal blood
  (3) movement of the fetal oxyhemoglobin dissociation curve to the left
  (4) maternal hyperventilation

| DIRECTIONS SUMMARIZED | | | | |
|---|---|---|---|---|
| A | B | C | D | E |
| 1, 2, 3 | 1, 3 | 2, 4 | 4 | All are |
| only | only | only | only | correct |

133. During a carbon dioxide challenge test in a healthy patient, the $Pa_{CO_2}$ increases to 60 mm Hg. Expected effects include

    (1) decreased pulmonary vascular resistance
    (2) increased cardiac output
    (3) renovascular dilation
    (4) sympathetic stimulation

134. Which of the following peripheral nerves must be blocked for removal of a glass splinter from the plantar surface of the heel?

    (1) Tibial
    (2) Saphenous
    (3) Sural
    (4) Superficial peroneal

135. A 26-year-old woman is to undergo emergency laparotomy for a ruptured appendix. She has been taking propylthiour-acil and an oral β-adrenergic blocker for 2 days for acute hyperthyroidism. Appropriate perioperative therapy includes administration of

    (1) potassium iodide
    (2) hydrocortisone
    (3) propranolol
    (4) propylthiouracil

136. A previously healthy 55-year-old patient is spontaneously breathing oxygen, nitrous oxide, and halothane during a minor surgical procedure. The end-tidal halothane concentration measured by mass spectrometry is 0.7%, end-tidal nitrous oxide concentration is 50%, and end-tidal carbon dioxide concentration is 9%. Findings consistent with these concentrations include

    (1) tachycardia
    (2) decreased requirement for halothane
    (3) premature ventricular contractions
    (4) serum bicarbonate concentration of 35 mEq/L

137. A 48-year-old man who is undergoing a right upper lobectomy for cancer has a $Pa_{O_2}$ of 67 mm Hg while his left lung is being ventilated at 10 mL/kg at a rate of 10 breaths/min. Measures to increase $Pa_{O_2}$ include

    (1) hyperventilation to a $Pa_{CO_2}$ of 30 mm Hg
    (2) insufflation of the right lung with continuous positive airway pressure
    (3) application of positive end-expiratory pressure 15 $cmH_2O$ to the left lung
    (4) partial occlusion of right pulmonary blood flow

| DIRECTIONS SUMMARIZED | | | | |
|:---:|:---:|:---:|:---:|:---:|
| A | B | C | D | E |
| 1, 2, 3 | 1, 3 | 2, 4 | 4 | All are |
| only | only | only | only | correct |

138. Uterine contractility is decreased by

    (1) epidural lidocaine
    (2) terbutaline
    (3) ketamine anesthesia
    (4) halothane

139. During induction of anesthesia for removal of a large intracranial tumor, effects of adding 1 MAC of isoflurane at normocarbia include

    (1) decreased cerebral metabolic rate
    (2) attenuated cerebrovascular response to $Paco_2$
    (3) increased intracranial pressure
    (4) abolished cerebral autoregulation

140. Intraoperative events that may cause an increased arterial to end-tidal carbon dioxide tension difference include

    (1) pulmonary embolus
    (2) induced hypotension
    (3) application of positive end-expiratory pressure
    (4) atelectasis

141. Factors that decrease beat-to-beat variability of the fetal heart rate include

    (1) epidural administration of lidocaine
    (2) maternal hypotension
    (3) intravenous administration of ephedrine
    (4) intravenous administration of glycopyrrolate

142. Neural fibers that transmit pain include

    (1) B fibers
    (2) C fibers
    (3) A-alpha fibers
    (4) A-delta fibers

143. Gas flow through an endotracheal tube is

    (1) directly related to the change in pressure along the length of the tube
    (2) inversely related to the viscosity of the gas
    (3) inversely related to the length of the tube
    (4) directly related to the square of the radius of the tube

FOR EACH ITEM FILL IN ONLY ONE CIRCLE ON YOUR ANSWER SHEET

| DIRECTIONS SUMMARIZED | | | | |
|:---:|:---:|:---:|:---:|:---:|
| A | B | C | D | E |
| 1, 2, 3 | 1, 3 | 2, 4 | 4 | All are |
| only | only | only | only | correct |

144. Hetastarch

   (1) produces a hypercoagulable state
   (2) complicates blood crossmatching
   (3) is contraindicated in patients with diabetes mellitus
   (4) is metabolized by amylase

145. During pelvic laparoscopy under epidural anesthesia, the patient is placed in the Trendelenburg position and the abdomen is distended by insufflation of carbon dioxide. Anticipated responses include

   (1) hyperpnea to maintain normal minute ventilation
   (2) pain despite sensory block to T4
   (3) decreased venous return and cardiac output
   (4) metabolic acidosis from absorption of carbon dioxide

146. When triggered by the R wave, the intra-aortic balloon pump is likely to be ineffective with

   (1) prolonged use of electrocautery
   (2) development of rapid atrial fibrillation
   (3) sudden onset of aortic regurgitation
   (4) sudden onset of mitral regurgitation

147. An asymptomatic 40-year-old woman with a systolic click and a late systolic murmur is scheduled for total abdominal hysterectomy. Anesthetic considerations include the following:

   (1) Prophylactic antibiotics are recommended
   (2) Intraoperative fluid restriction is indicated
   (3) The patient is predisposed to tachyarrhythmias
   (4) Myocardial depressant inhalational agents are contraindicated

148. A 24-year-old woman who is receiving magnesium sulfate for severe preeclampsia requires emergency cesarean delivery. True statements concerning succinylcholine-induced muscle relaxation in this patient include the following:

   (1) It will be potentiated by the magnesium sulfate
   (2) Fasciculations will be absent following succinylcholine administration
   (3) It will be prolonged
   (4) It can be antagonized by calcium chloride

<table>
<tr><td colspan="5" align="center"><u>DIRECTIONS SUMMARIZED</u></td></tr>
<tr><td align="center">A</td><td align="center">B</td><td align="center">C</td><td align="center">D</td><td align="center">E</td></tr>
<tr><td align="center">1, 2, 3</td><td align="center">1, 3</td><td align="center">2, 4</td><td align="center">4</td><td align="center">All are</td></tr>
<tr><td align="center">only</td><td align="center">only</td><td align="center">only</td><td align="center">only</td><td align="center">correct</td></tr>
</table>

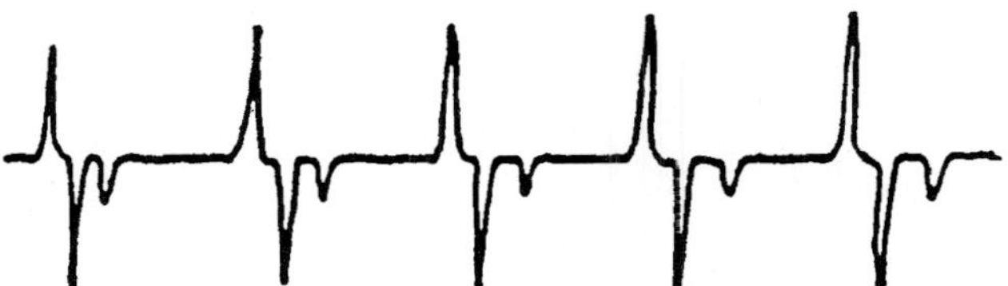

149. During posterior fossa surgery in the sitting position

(1) a single-lumen central venous catheter should display the ECG shown above
(2) PAOPs greater than 10 mm Hg prevent paradoxical air embolism
(3) if venous air embolism occurs, pulmonary artery pressure increases before precordial Doppler sounds change
(4) if venous air embolism occurs, aspiration of air from the distal lumen of a pulmonary artery catheter is less effective than aspiration from a multiorificed central venous catheter

---

150. A patient undergoing strabismus repair develops acute bradycardia during traction on an eye muscle. This response is

(1) mediated by a facial nerve afferent
(2) also manifested by ventricular ectopy
(3) prevented by preanesthetic intramuscular administration of atropine
(4) treated by stopping the surgical stimulus

151. In a patient treated with propranolol and phenoxybenzamine prior to resection of a solitary pheochromocytoma, factors contributing to postoperative hypotension include

(1) residual $\alpha$-adrenergic block
(2) heart failure
(3) residual $\beta$-adrenergic block
(4) adrenal insufficiency

152. Anesthesia is induced with isoflurane and nitrous oxide in a patient with low cardiac output. Compared with a patient with normal cardiac function, which of the following will occur?

(1) Alveolar isoflurane concentration will approach the inspired concentration more rapidly
(2) Total uptake of isoflurane will be higher during the first 11 minutes
(3) The rate of rise in the alveolar concentration of isoflurane will be affected more than that of nitrous oxide
(4) Induction will be slower

<table>
<tr><td colspan="5" align="center"><u>DIRECTIONS SUMMARIZED</u></td></tr>
<tr><td align="center">A</td><td align="center">B</td><td align="center">C</td><td align="center">D</td><td align="center">E</td></tr>
<tr><td align="center">1, 2, 3</td><td align="center">1, 3</td><td align="center">2, 4</td><td align="center">4</td><td align="center">All are</td></tr>
<tr><td align="center">only</td><td align="center">only</td><td align="center">only</td><td align="center">only</td><td align="center">correct</td></tr>
</table>

153. Factors associated with postintubation croup in children include

    (1) age less than 3 months
    (2) history of recent upper respiratory infection
    (3) use of a nasotracheal tube
    (4) surgery of the head and neck

154. True statements concerning the effects of amrinone include the following:

    (1) Systemic vascular resistance is decreased
    (2) Intracellular levels of cyclic adenosine monophosphate (cAMP) are increased
    (3) It acts independently of $\beta_1$-adrenergic receptors
    (4) Simultaneous administration of norepinephrine enhances ventricular dysrhythmias

155. Deflation of a leg tourniquet after 2 hours of inflation decreases

    (1) mixed venous oxygen saturation
    (2) core temperature
    (3) systemic vascular resistance
    (4) end-tidal carbon dioxide tension

156. Compared with those of isoflurane, the respiratory effects of enflurane include

    (1) similar decrease in airway resistance
    (2) greater attenuation of hypoxic pulmonary vasoconstriction
    (3) greater increase in $Paco_2$ during spontaneous ventilation at 1 MAC
    (4) less inhibition of hypoxic ventilatory drive at "MAC awake" concentrations

157. Intravenous drugs that produce central nervous system effects by modulating $\gamma$-aminobutyric acid receptor activity include

    (1) midazolam
    (2) thiopental
    (3) flumazenil
    (4) ketamine

158. Findings consistent with heparin-induced thrombocytopenia include

    (1) platelet count of $25,000/mm^3$
    (2) subcutaneous route of heparin administration
    (3) thrombosis
    (4) onset within 4 hours of initiating heparin therapy

FOR EACH ITEM FILL IN ONLY ONE CIRCLE ON YOUR ANSWER SHEET

DIRECTIONS SUMMARIZED

| A | B | C | D | E |
|---|---|---|---|---|
| 1, 2, 3 | 1, 3 | 2, 4 | 4 | All are |
| only | only | only | only | correct |

159. An anephric 12-year-old patient with a large pericardial effusion is to have pericardiocentesis under general anesthesia. Appropriate anesthetic management includes

    (1) maintenance of a high venous pressure
    (2) prevention of tachycardia
    (3) avoidance of positive end-expiratory pressure
    (4) reduction of systemic vascular resistance

160. Reliable indicators of left ventricular function in a patient with severe chronic obstructive pulmonary disease include

    (1) left ventricular end-diastolic volume
    (2) pulmonary artery diastolic pressure
    (3) left atrial pressure
    (4) cardiac index

161. A 38-year-old woman who takes verapamil for idiopathic hypertrophic subaortic stenosis is anesthetized with enflurane, nitrous oxide, oxygen, and fentanyl for laparoscopic cholecystectomy. After inflation of the abdomen with carbon dioxide, heart rate increases to 140 bpm, blood pressure decreases to 85/60 mm Hg, and ST-segment depression occurs. End-tidal carbon dioxide concentration is unchanged. Appropriate pharmacologic management includes intravenous administration of

    (1) phenylephrine
    (2) nitroglycerin
    (3) esmolol
    (4) calcium chloride

162. Compared with intermittent bolus administration, effects of continuous infusion of a short-acting anesthetic include

    (1) increased therapeutic index
    (2) decreased serum concentration required
    (3) prolonged recovery time
    (4) decreased total amount of anesthetic required

163. During abdominal closure for gastroschisis in a 1-day-old infant, airway pressure increases and oxygen saturation decreases. Breath sounds are bilateral, and endotracheal suctioning does not improve ventilation. After increasing $F_{IO_2}$, appropriate management includes

    (1) deepening volatile anesthesia
    (2) administering additional muscle relaxant
    (3) adding positive end-expiratory pressure
    (4) foregoing primary abdominal closure

FOR EACH ITEM FILL IN ONLY ONE CIRCLE ON YOUR ANSWER SHEET

<table>
<tr><td colspan="5" align="center"><u>DIRECTIONS SUMMARIZED</u></td></tr>
<tr><td align="center">A</td><td align="center">B</td><td align="center">C</td><td align="center">D</td><td align="center">E</td></tr>
<tr><td align="center">1, 2, 3</td><td align="center">1, 3</td><td align="center">2, 4</td><td align="center">4</td><td align="center">All are</td></tr>
<tr><td align="center">only</td><td align="center">only</td><td align="center">only</td><td align="center">only</td><td align="center">correct</td></tr>
</table>

164. True statements concerning airway management in a patient with suspected injury to the cervical spine following head and chest trauma include the following:

    (1) Cricothyroidotomy is the preferred method of securing the airway
    (2) Injuries at C1 or C2 place the patient at greatest risk for neurologic injury during laryngoscopy
    (3) Cricoid pressure is contraindicated
    (4) A normal lateral, anteroposterior (AP), and open-mouth view of the cervical spine rules out spinal cord injury

165. A 30-year-old man with gunshot wounds receives an emergency transfusion of 4 units of uncrossmatched O, Rh-negative blood. His blood type is AB, Rh-positive. For further intraoperative transfusion he should receive

    (1) O, Rh-negative red cells
    (2) AB, Rh-positive red cells
    (3) AB, Rh-positive plasma
    (4) O, Rh-negative plasma

166. A 46-year-old man who takes clonidine for essential hypertension undergoes a 12-hour limb reimplantation under general anesthesia. Which of the following should be anticipated during the perioperative course?

    (1) Decreased anesthetic requirements
    (2) Postoperative hypertension
    (3) Blunting of tachycardia with tracheal intubation
    (4) Excessive postoperative drowsiness

167. Defective expiratory unidirectional valves in a circle system result in

    (1) increased dead space
    (2) decreased $F_{IO_2}$
    (3) prolonged anesthetic induction
    (4) transformation to a nonrebreathing system

168. In the absence of a change in the ventilator settings, the measured exhaled tidal volume on the machine spirometer decreases when

    (1) the endotracheal tube migrates into the right main stem bronchus
    (2) fresh gas flow is decreased
    (3) a heated humidifier is added
    (4) the endotracheal tube cuff begins to leak

| DIRECTIONS SUMMARIZED | | | | |
|---|---|---|---|---|
| A | B | C | D | E |
| 1, 2, 3 | 1, 3 | 2, 4 | 4 | All are |
| only | only | only | only | correct |

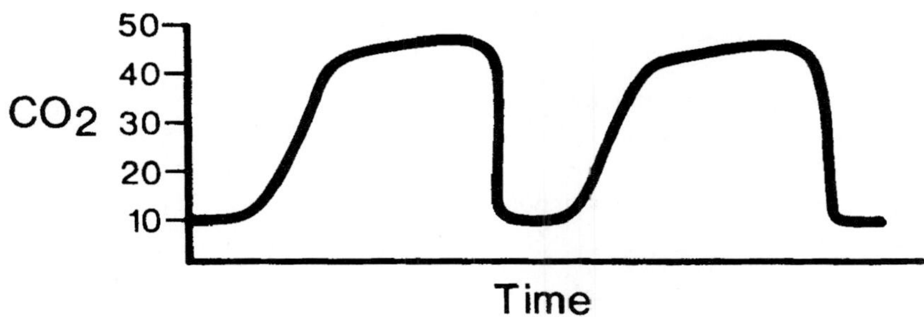


169. The capnographic waveform shown above was obtained during anesthesia using a semiclosed circle system and mechanical ventilation. This waveform is consistent with

    (1) increased body temperature to 40°C
    (2) kinking of the endotracheal tube
    (3) inadequate minute ventilation
    (4) an incompetent expiratory valve

170. A 45-year-old woman is scheduled for a cholecystectomy following an episode of acute cholecystitis. Thirty minutes after premedication with morphine and midazolam, she has nausea and acute right upper quadrant pain. Drugs that alleviate these symptoms include

    (1) glucagon
    (2) nitroglycerin
    (3) naloxone
    (4) flumazenil

171. During a blood transfusion, a patient develops sudden hypotension and oozing from the puncture sites. Laboratory studies useful in establishing the diagnosis include

    (1) serum-free hemoglobin concentration
    (2) direct antiglobulin (Coombs') test
    (3) urine hemoglobin concentration
    (4) serum haptoglobin concentration

172. A continuous infusion of atracurium for 60 hours has been associated with

    (1) seizure activity
    (2) histamine release
    (3) increased anesthetic requirements
    (4) adrenal suppression

| DIRECTIONS SUMMARIZED | | | | |
|---|---|---|---|---|
| A | B | C | D | E |
| 1, 2, 3 | 1, 3 | 2, 4 | 4 | All are |
| only | only | only | only | correct |

173. The anesthetic recovery of a newborn infant is complicated by the slow return of neuromuscular function. Factors that would cause this complication include

    (1) an inadequate dose of anticholinesterase
    (2) active maternal myasthenia gravis
    (3) a core temperature of 35°C
    (4) intraoperative administration of cefamandole

174. Complications of stellate ganglion block include

    (1) elevation of the ipsilateral hemidiaphragm
    (2) total spinal anesthesia
    (3) seizures
    (4) hoarseness

# GENERAL INSTRUCTIONS

1. Please write your name and identification number in the space provided on the front of this test book. If you are taking the examination for Board Certification, your identification number is printed on your notification card. If you are an In-Training Resident, use your U.S. Social Security Number. If you do not have a U.S. Social Security Number, use your Canadian Social Insurance Number.

2. Your name and identification number and all of your answers must be recorded on the separate answer sheet enclosed in this booklet.

   The sample on the right shows how to record your identification number on the answer sheet. Be sure to enter your number in the boxes provided and also to mark it in the appropriate spaces as illustrated.

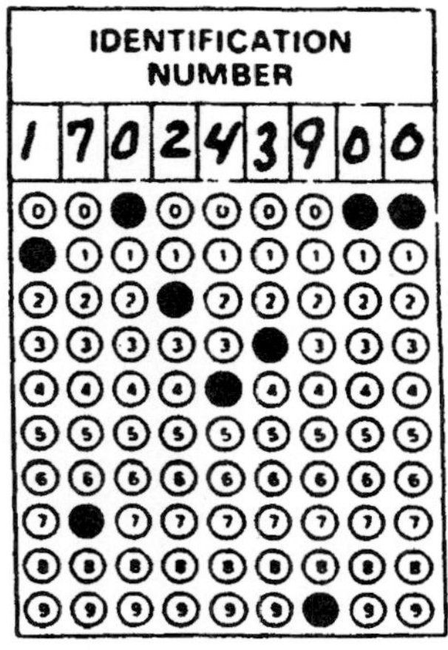

3. Credit will be given only for answers marked on the answer sheet. You may make any preliminary notes or calculations in the test books, but be sure that all of your answers are marked on the answer sheet. Only one choice should be marked for each question. Multiple answers for the same question are treated as wrong answers. In marking your answer sheet use only a soft (#2) lead pencil. Do NOT use a pen or pencil with hard lead. Make each mark heavy and black enough to obliterate completely the letter within the circle. Marks should fill the circle; if marks are light or outside the circle, you may not receive credit for your answers. Make no stray marks on the answer sheet, as these could lower your score. If you wish to change an answer, be sure to erase your first mark completely.

4. This test book contains two different types of questions, each of which is preceded by special directions. You are advised to study the directions carefully. Even though you may be in doubt about the correct answer, select the choice that you consider to be the best. Your score is the number of questions you answered correctly.

5. You will have 3½ hours to work on this section of the test which contains 174 questions.

---

# RULES OF CONDUCT FOR EXAMINEES DURING ABA/ASA IN-TRAINING EXAMINATION

1. Do not falsify information required for admission to the examination or impersonate another ABA/ASA examinee.

2. Do not bring calculators, watches with computer capability, books, papers, or memoranda of any kind into the examination room.

3. Do not break the seal on your test books until you are instructed to do so by the proctor.

4. Do not tear any pages or portions of pages from the test books or tear your answer sheet.

5. Do not disturb the examination process by talking, smoking, or interfering with others who are taking the examination.

6. Do not attempt to observe the test books or answer sheets of other examinees. Do not copy the answers of another examinee, permit answers to be copied, or in any way provide or receive unauthorized information about the content of the examination while it is in progress.

7. Terminate the examination immediately upon instruction by the proctor to do so.

8. Do not take the test books, answer sheets, or any documents, examination material, or memoranda from the room.

Failure to abide by these rules of conduct during this examination may result in disciplinary actions by the ABA/ASA In-Training Council or by the American Board of Anesthesiology. Statistical analyses may be used to verify observations and /or reports of suspected irregularities in conduct.

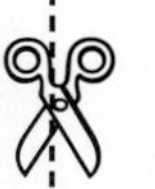

# Book A Answer Sheet

| | | | | | | | | | | | | | | | | |
|---|---|---|---|---|---|---|---|---|---|---|---|---|---|---|---|---|
| 1) | 1 | 2 | 3 | 4 | | 45) | 1 | 2 | 3 | 4 | | 89) | A | B | C | D | E |
| 2) | 1 | 2 | 3 | 4 | | 46) | 1 | 2 | 3 | 4 | | 90) | A | B | C | D | E |
| 3) | 1 | 2 | 3 | 4 | | 47) | 1 | 2 | 3 | 4 | | 91) | A | B | C | D | E |
| 4) | 1 | 2 | 3 | 4 | | 48) | 1 | 2 | 3 | 4 | | 92) | A | B | C | D | E |
| 5) | 1 | 2 | 3 | 4 | | 49) | 1 | 2 | 3 | 4 | | 93) | A | B | C | D | E |
| 6) | 1 | 2 | 3 | 4 | | 50) | 1 | 2 | 3 | 4 | | 94) | A | B | C | D | E |
| 7) | 1 | 2 | 3 | 4 | | 51) | 1 | 2 | 3 | 4 | | 95) | A | B | C | D | E |
| 8) | 1 | 2 | 3 | 4 | | 52) | 1 | 2 | 3 | 4 | | 96) | A | B | C | D | E |
| 9) | 1 | 2 | 3 | 4 | | 53) | 1 | 2 | 3 | 4 | | 97) | A | B | C | D | E |
| 10) | 1 | 2 | 3 | 4 | | 54) | 1 | 2 | 3 | 4 | | 98) | A | B | C | D | E |
| 11) | 1 | 2 | 3 | 4 | | 55) | 1 | 2 | 3 | 4 | | 99) | A | B | C | D | E |
| 12) | 1 | 2 | 3 | 4 | | 56) | 1 | 2 | 3 | 4 | | 100) | A | B | C | D | E |
| 13) | 1 | 2 | 3 | 4 | | 57) | 1 | 2 | 3 | 4 | | 101) | A | B | C | D | E |
| 14) | 1 | 2 | 3 | 4 | | 58) | 1 | 2 | 3 | 4 | | 102) | A | B | C | D | E |
| 15) | 1 | 2 | 3 | 4 | | 59) | 1 | 2 | 3 | 4 | | 103) | A | B | C | D | E |
| 16) | 1 | 2 | 3 | 4 | | 60) | 1 | 2 | 3 | 4 | | 104) | A | B | C | D | E |
| 17) | 1 | 2 | 3 | 4 | | 61) | 1 | 2 | 3 | 4 | | 105) | A | B | C | D | E |
| 18) | 1 | 2 | 3 | 4 | | 62) | 1 | 2 | 3 | 4 | | 106) | A | B | C | D | E |
| 19) | 1 | 2 | 3 | 4 | | 63) | 1 | 2 | 3 | 4 | | 107) | A | B | C | D | E |
| 20) | 1 | 2 | 3 | 4 | | 64) | 1 | 2 | 3 | 4 | | 108) | A | B | C | D | E |
| 21) | 1 | 2 | 3 | 4 | | 65) | 1 | 2 | 3 | 4 | | 109) | A | B | C | D | E |
| 22) | 1 | 2 | 3 | 4 | | 66) | 1 | 2 | 3 | 4 | | 110) | A | B | C | D | E |
| 23) | 1 | 2 | 3 | 4 | | 67) | 1 | 2 | 3 | 4 | | 111) | A | B | C | D | E |
| 24) | 1 | 2 | 3 | 4 | | 68) | 1 | 2 | 3 | 4 | | 112) | A | B | C | D | E |
| 25) | 1 | 2 | 3 | 4 | | 69) | 1 | 2 | 3 | 4 | | 113) | A | B | C | D | E |
| 26) | 1 | 2 | 3 | 4 | | 70) | 1 | 2 | 3 | 4 | | 114) | A | B | C | D | E |
| 27) | 1 | 2 | 3 | 4 | | 71) | 1 | 2 | 3 | 4 | | 115) | A | B | C | D | E |
| 28) | 1 | 2 | 3 | 4 | | 72) | 1 | 2 | 3 | 4 | | 116) | A | B | C | D | E |
| 29) | 1 | 2 | 3 | 4 | | 73) | A | B | C | D | E | 117) | A | B | C | D | E |
| 30) | 1 | 2 | 3 | 4 | | 74) | A | B | C | D | E | 118) | A | B | C | D | E |
| 31) | 1 | 2 | 3 | 4 | | 75) | A | B | C | D | E | 119) | A | B | C | D | E |
| 32) | 1 | 2 | 3 | 4 | | 76) | A | B | C | D | E | 120) | A | B | C | D | E |
| 33) | 1 | 2 | 3 | 4 | | 77) | A | B | C | D | E | 121) | A | B | C | D | E |
| 34) | 1 | 2 | 3 | 4 | | 78) | A | B | C | D | E | 122) | A | B | C | D | E |
| 35) | 1 | 2 | 3 | 4 | | 79) | A | B | C | D | E | 123) | A | B | C | D | E |
| 36) | 1 | 2 | 3 | 4 | | 80) | A | B | C | D | E | 124) | A | B | C | D | E |
| 37) | 1 | 2 | 3 | 4 | | 81) | A | B | C | D | E | 125) | A | B | C | D | E |
| 38) | 1 | 2 | 3 | 4 | | 82) | A | B | C | D | E | 126) | A | B | C | D | E |
| 39) | 1 | 2 | 3 | 4 | | 83) | A | B | C | D | E | 127) | A | B | C | D | E |
| 40) | 1 | 2 | 3 | 4 | | 84) | A | B | C | D | E | 128) | A | B | C | D | E |
| 41) | 1 | 2 | 3 | 4 | | 85) | A | B | C | D | E | 129) | A | B | C | D | E |
| 42) | 1 | 2 | 3 | 4 | | 86) | A | B | C | D | E | 130) | A | B | C | D | E |
| 43) | 1 | 2 | 3 | 4 | | 87) | A | B | C | D | E | 131) | A | B | C | D | E |
| 44) | 1 | 2 | 3 | 4 | | 88) | A | B | C | D | E | 132) | A | B | C | D | E |

| 133) | A | B | C | D | E |
| 134) | A | B | C | D | E |
| 135) | A | B | C | D | E |
| 136) | A | B | C | D | E |
| 137) | A | B | C | D | E |
| 138) | A | B | C | D | E |
| 139) | A | B | C | D | E |
| 140) | A | B | C | D | E |
| 141) | A | B | C | D | E |
| 142) | A | B | C | D | E |
| 143) | A | B | C | D | E |
| 144) | A | B | C | D | E |
| 145) | A | B | C | D | E |
| 146) | A | B | C | D | E |
| 147) | A | B | C | D | E |
| 148) | A | B | C | D | E |
| 149) | A | B | C | D | E |
| 150) | A | B | C | D | E |
| 151) | A | B | C | D | E |
| 152) | A | B | C | D | E |
| 153) | A | B | C | D | E |
| 154) | A | B | C | D | E |
| 155) | A | B | C | D | E |
| 156) | A | B | C | D | E |
| 157) | A | B | C | D | E |
| 158) | A | B | C | D | E |
| 159) | A | B | C | D | E |
| 160) | A | B | C | D | E |
| 161) | A | B | C | D | E |
| 162) | A | B | C | D | E |
| 163) | A | B | C | D | E |
| 164) | A | B | C | D | E |
| 165) | A | B | C | D | E |
| 166) | A | B | C | D | E |
| 167) | A | B | C | D | E |
| 168) | A | B | C | D | E |
| 169) | A | B | C | D | E |
| 170) | A | B | C | D | E |
| 171) | A | B | C | D | E |
| 172) | A | B | C | D | E |
| 173) | A | B | C | D | E |
| 174) | A | B | C | D | E |
| 175) | A | B | C | D | E |

# 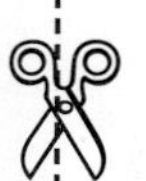 Book B Answer Sheet

| | | | | | | | | | | | | | | | | | | |
|---|---|---|---|---|---|---|---|---|---|---|---|---|---|---|---|---|---|---|
| 1) | A | B | C | D | E | 45) | A | B | C | D | E | 89) | A | B | C | D | E |
| 2) | A | B | C | D | E | 46) | A | B | C | D | E | 90) | A | B | C | D | E |
| 3) | A | B | C | D | E | 47) | A | B | C | D | E | 91) | A | B | C | D | E |
| 4) | A | B | C | D | E | 48) | A | B | C | D | E | 92) | A | B | C | D | E |
| 5) | A | B | C | D | E | 49) | A | B | C | D | E | 93) | A | B | C | D | E |
| 6) | A | B | C | D | E | 50) | A | B | C | D | E | 94) | A | B | C | D | E |
| 7) | A | B | C | D | E | 51) | A | B | C | D | E | 95) | A | B | C | D | E |
| 8) | A | B | C | D | E | 52) | A | B | C | D | E | 96) | A | B | C | D | E |
| 9) | A | B | C | D | E | 53) | A | B | C | D | E | 97) | A | B | C | D | E |
| 10) | A | B | C | D | E | 54) | A | B | C | D | E | 98) | A | B | C | D | E |
| 11) | A | B | C | D | E | 55) | A | B | C | D | E | 99) | A | B | C | D | E |
| 12) | A | B | C | D | E | 56) | A | B | C | D | E | 100) | A | B | C | D | E |
| 13) | A | B | C | D | E | 57) | A | B | C | D | E | 101) | A | B | C | D | E |
| 14) | A | B | C | D | E | 58) | A | B | C | D | E | 102) | A | B | C | D | E |
| 15) | A | B | C | D | E | 59) | A | B | C | D | E | 103) | 1 | 2 | 3 | 4 | |
| 16) | A | B | C | D | E | 60) | A | B | C | D | E | 104) | 1 | 2 | 3 | 4 | |
| 17) | A | B | C | D | E | 61) | A | B | C | D | E | 105) | 1 | 2 | 3 | 4 | |
| 18) | A | B | C | D | E | 62) | A | B | C | D | E | 106) | 1 | 2 | 3 | 4 | |
| 19) | A | B | C | D | E | 63) | A | B | C | D | E | 107) | 1 | 2 | 3 | 4 | |
| 20) | A | B | C | D | E | 64) | A | B | C | D | E | 108) | 1 | 2 | 3 | 4 | |
| 21) | A | B | C | D | E | 65) | A | B | C | D | E | 109) | 1 | 2 | 3 | 4 | |
| 22) | A | B | C | D | E | 66) | A | B | C | D | E | 110) | 1 | 2 | 3 | 4 | |
| 23) | A | B | C | D | E | 67) | A | B | C | D | E | 111) | 1 | 2 | 3 | 4 | |
| 24) | A | B | C | D | E | 68) | A | B | C | D | E | 112) | 1 | 2 | 3 | 4 | |
| 25) | A | B | C | D | E | 69) | A | B | C | D | E | 113) | 1 | 2 | 3 | 4 | |
| 26) | A | B | C | D | E | 70) | A | B | C | D | E | 114) | 1 | 2 | 3 | 4 | |
| 27) | A | B | C | D | E | 71) | A | B | C | D | E | 115) | 1 | 2 | 3 | 4 | |
| 28) | A | B | C | D | E | 72) | A | B | C | D | E | 116) | 1 | 2 | 3 | 4 | |
| 29) | A | B | C | D | E | 73) | A | B | C | D | E | 117) | 1 | 2 | 3 | 4 | |
| 30) | A | B | C | D | E | 74) | A | B | C | D | E | 118) | 1 | 2 | 3 | 4 | |
| 31) | A | B | C | D | E | 75) | A | B | C | D | E | 119) | 1 | 2 | 3 | 4 | |
| 32) | A | B | C | D | E | 76) | A | B | C | D | E | 120) | 1 | 2 | 3 | 4 | |
| 33) | A | B | C | D | E | 77) | A | B | C | D | E | 121) | 1 | 2 | 3 | 4 | |
| 34) | A | B | C | D | E | 78) | A | B | C | D | E | 122) | 1 | 2 | 3 | 4 | |
| 35) | A | B | C | D | E | 79) | A | B | C | D | E | 123) | 1 | 2 | 3 | 4 | |
| 36) | A | B | C | D | E | 80) | A | B | C | D | E | 124) | 1 | 2 | 3 | 4 | |
| 37) | A | B | C | D | E | 81) | A | B | C | D | E | 125) | 1 | 2 | 3 | 4 | |
| 38) | A | B | C | D | E | 82) | A | B | C | D | E | 126) | 1 | 2 | 3 | 4 | |
| 39) | A | B | C | D | E | 83) | A | B | C | D | E | 127) | 1 | 2 | 3 | 4 | |
| 40) | A | B | C | D | E | 84) | A | B | C | D | E | 128) | 1 | 2 | 3 | 4 | |
| 41) | A | B | C | D | E | 85) | A | B | C | D | E | 129) | 1 | 2 | 3 | 4 | |
| 42) | A | B | C | D | E | 86) | A | B | C | D | E | 130) | 1 | 2 | 3 | 4 | |
| 43) | A | B | C | D | E | 87) | A | B | C | D | E | 131) | 1 | 2 | 3 | 4 | |
| 44) | A | B | C | D | E | 88) | A | B | C | D | E | 132) | 1 | 2 | 3 | 4 | |

| 133) | 1 | 2 | 3 | 4 |
| 134) | 1 | 2 | 3 | 4 |
| 135) | 1 | 2 | 3 | 4 |
| 136) | 1 | 2 | 3 | 4 |
| 137) | 1 | 2 | 3 | 4 |
| 138) | 1 | 2 | 3 | 4 |
| 139) | 1 | 2 | 3 | 4 |
| 140) | 1 | 2 | 3 | 4 |
| 141) | 1 | 2 | 3 | 4 |
| 142) | 1 | 2 | 3 | 4 |
| 143) | 1 | 2 | 3 | 4 |
| 144) | 1 | 2 | 3 | 4 |
| 145) | 1 | 2 | 3 | 4 |
| 146) | 1 | 2 | 3 | 4 |
| 147) | 1 | 2 | 3 | 4 |
| 148) | 1 | 2 | 3 | 4 |
| 149) | 1 | 2 | 3 | 4 |
| 150) | 1 | 2 | 3 | 4 |
| 151) | 1 | 2 | 3 | 4 |
| 152) | 1 | 2 | 3 | 4 |
| 153) | 1 | 2 | 3 | 4 |
| 154) | 1 | 2 | 3 | 4 |
| 155) | 1 | 2 | 3 | 4 |
| 156) | 1 | 2 | 3 | 4 |
| 157) | 1 | 2 | 3 | 4 |
| 158) | 1 | 2 | 3 | 4 |
| 159) | 1 | 2 | 3 | 4 |
| 160) | 1 | 2 | 3 | 4 |
| 161) | 1 | 2 | 3 | 4 |
| 162) | 1 | 2 | 3 | 4 |
| 163) | 1 | 2 | 3 | 4 |
| 164) | 1 | 2 | 3 | 4 |
| 165) | 1 | 2 | 3 | 4 |
| 166) | 1 | 2 | 3 | 4 |
| 167) | 1 | 2 | 3 | 4 |
| 168) | 1 | 2 | 3 | 4 |
| 169) | 1 | 2 | 3 | 4 |
| 170) | 1 | 2 | 3 | 4 |
| 171) | 1 | 2 | 3 | 4 |
| 172) | 1 | 2 | 3 | 4 |
| 173) | 1 | 2 | 3 | 4 |
| 174) | 1 | 2 | 3 | 4 |

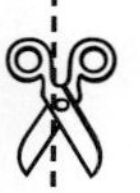

# Topic Indexed Answer Sheet

## ≡ BASIC SCIENCE ≡

### BOOK A

| | | | | | |
|---|---|---|---|---|---|
| 89) | A | B | C | D | E |
| 123) | A | B | C | D | E |
| 162) | A | B | C | D | E |
| 164) | A | B | C | D | E |
| 169) | A | B | C | D | E |

### BOOK B

| | | | | | |
|---|---|---|---|---|---|
| 12) | A | B | C | D | E |
| 46) | A | B | C | D | E |
| 82) | A | B | C | D | E |
| 84) | A | B | C | D | E |
| 86) | A | B | C | D | E |
| 157) | 1 | 2 | 3 | 4 | |

## ≡ EQUIPMENT/PHYSICS ≡

### BOOK A

| | | | | | |
|---|---|---|---|---|---|
| 1) | 1 | 2 | 3 | 4 | |
| 9) | 1 | 2 | 3 | 4 | |
| 11) | 1 | 2 | 3 | 4 | |
| 13) | 1 | 2 | 3 | 4 | |
| 29) | 1 | 2 | 3 | 4 | |
| 43) | 1 | 2 | 3 | 4 | |
| 45) | 1 | 2 | 3 | 4 | |
| 55) | 1 | 2 | 3 | 4 | |
| 65) | 1 | 2 | 3 | 4 | |
| 67) | 1 | 2 | 3 | 4 | |
| 96) | A | B | C | D | E |
| 102) | A | B | C | D | E |
| 107) | A | B | C | D | E |
| 111) | A | B | C | D | E |
| 113) | A | B | C | D | E |
| 128) | A | B | C | D | E |
| 129) | A | B | C | D | E |
| 133) | A | B | C | D | E |
| 141) | A | B | C | D | E |
| 151) | A | B | C | D | E |
| 153) | A | B | C | D | E |

### BOOK B

| | | | | | |
|---|---|---|---|---|---|
| 15) | A | B | C | D | E |
| 17) | A | B | C | D | E |
| 37) | A | B | C | D | E |
| 40) | A | B | C | D | E |
| 45) | A | B | C | D | E |
| 61) | A | B | C | D | E |
| 62) | A | B | C | D | E |
| 67) | A | B | C | D | E |
| 70) | A | B | C | D | E |
| 79) | A | B | C | D | E |
| 80) | A | B | C | D | E |
| 83) | A | B | C | D | E |
| 94) | A | B | C | D | E |
| 111) | 1 | 2 | 3 | 4 | |
| 143) | 1 | 2 | 3 | 4 | |
| 146) | 1 | 2 | 3 | 4 | |
| 167) | 1 | 2 | 3 | 4 | |
| 168) | 1 | 2 | 3 | 4 | |
| 169) | 1 | 2 | 3 | 4 | |

## ≡ CARDIOVASCULAR ≡

### BOOK A

| | | | | | |
|---|---|---|---|---|---|
| 16) | 1 | 2 | 3 | 4 | |
| 35) | 1 | 2 | 3 | 4 | |
| 39) | 1 | 2 | 3 | 4 | |
| 53) | 1 | 2 | 3 | 4 | |
| 66) | 1 | 2 | 3 | 4 | |
| 84) | A | B | C | D | E |
| 93) | A | B | C | D | E |
| 95) | A | B | C | D | E |
| 99) | A | B | C | D | E |
| 109) | A | B | C | D | E |
| 110) | A | B | C | D | E |
| 114) | A | B | C | D | E |
| 132) | A | B | C | D | E |
| 136) | A | B | C | D | E |
| 158) | A | B | C | D | E |

### BOOK B

| | | | | | |
|---|---|---|---|---|---|
| 20) | A | B | C | D | E |
| 27) | A | B | C | D | E |
| 32) | A | B | C | D | E |
| 39) | A | B | C | D | E |
| 53) | A | B | C | D | E |
| 55) | A | B | C | D | E |
| 59) | A | B | C | D | E |
| 64) | A | B | C | D | E |
| 73) | A | B | C | D | E |
| 74) | A | B | C | D | E |
| 123) | 1 | 2 | 3 | 4 | |
| 147) | 1 | 2 | 3 | 4 | |
| 161) | 1 | 2 | 3 | 4 | |

## ≡ CLINICAL ANESTHESIA ≡

### BOOK A

| | | | | | |
|---|---|---|---|---|---|
| 10) | 1 | 2 | 3 | 4 | |
| 15) | 1 | 2 | 3 | 4 | |
| 17) | 1 | 2 | 3 | 4 | |
| 18) | 1 | 2 | 3 | 4 | |
| 21) | 1 | 2 | 3 | 4 | |
| 23) | 1 | 2 | 3 | 4 | |
| 24) | 1 | 2 | 3 | 4 | |
| 28) | 1 | 2 | 3 | 4 | |
| 48) | 1 | 2 | 3 | 4 | |
| 63) | 1 | 2 | 3 | 4 | |
| 64) | 1 | 2 | 3 | 4 | |
| 68) | 1 | 2 | 3 | 4 | |
| 71) | 1 | 2 | 3 | 4 | |
| 75) | A | B | C | D | E |
| 81) | A | B | C | D | E |
| 88) | A | B | C | D | E |
| 90) | A | B | C | D | E |
| 94) | A | B | C | D | E |
| 97) | A | B | C | D | E |
| 115) | A | B | C | D | E |
| 118) | A | B | C | D | E |
| 119) | A | B | C | D | E |
| 120) | A | B | C | D | E |
| 121) | A | B | C | D | E |

127)   A   B   C   D   E
152)   A   B   C   D   E
155)   A   B   C   D   E
159)   A   B   C   D   E
160)   A   B   C   D   E
166)   A   B   C   D   E
167)   A   B   C   D   E
168)   A   B   C   D   E
174)   A   B   C   D   E

BOOK  B

  3)   A   B   C   D   E
  7)   A   B   C   D   E
 19)   A   B   C   D   E
 21)   A   B   C   D   E
 24)   A   B   C   D   E
 25)   A   B   C   D   E
 26)   A   B   C   D   E
 31)   A   B   C   D   E
 33)   A   B   C   D   E
 50)   A   B   C   D   E
 52)   A   B   C   D   E
 54)   A   B   C   D   E
 56)   A   B   C   D   E
 60)   A   B   C   D   E
 72)   A   B   C   D   E
 77)   A   B   C   D   E
 87)   A   B   C   D   E
 89)   A   B   C   D   E
 91)   A   B   C   D   E
 98)   1   2   3   4
116)   1   2   3   4
122)   1   2   3   4
129)   1   2   3   4
135)   1   2   3   4
137)   1   2   3   4
150)   1   2   3   4
151)   1   2   3   4
159)   1   2   3   4
164)   1   2   3   4
165)   1   2   3   4
170)   1   2   3   4

## ≡ NEUROANESTHESIA ≡

BOOK  A

 12)   1   2   3   4
 40)   1   2   3   4
142)   A   B   C   D   E
143)   A   B   C   D   E
154)   A   B   C   D   E

BOOK  B

 10)   A   B   C   D   E
 16)   A   B   C   D   E
 28)   A   B   C   D   E
 29)   A   B   C   D   E
 38)   A   B   C   D   E
 49)   A   B   C   D   E
 63)   A   B   C   D   E
 88)   A   B   C   D   E
 93)   A   B   C   D   E
101)   A   B   C   D   E
121)   1   2   3   4
139)   1   2   3   4
149)   1   2   3   4

## ≡ OBSTETRIC AND REGIONAL ANESTHESIA ≡

BOOK  A

 27)   1   2   3   4
 30)   1   2   3   4
 37)   1   2   3   4
 38)   1   2   3   4
 44)   1   2   3   4
 49)   1   2   3   4
 58)   1   2   3   4
 59)   1   2   3   4
 77)   A   B   C   D   E
 79)   A   B   C   D   E
 87)   A   B   C   D   E
116)   A   B   C   D   E
138)   A   B   C   D   E
145)   A   B   C   D   E
149)   A   B   C   D   E

150)   A   B   C   D   E
157)   A   B   C   D   E
170)   A   B   C   D   E
172)   A   B   C   D   E
173)   A   B   C   D   E

BOOK  B

  6)   A   B   C   D   E
 11)   A   B   C   D   E
 13)   A   B   C   D   E
 14)   A   B   C   D   E
 44)   A   B   C   D   E
 51)   A   B   C   D   E
 75)   A   B   C   D   E
 78)   A   B   C   D   E
 81)   A   B   C   D   E
 85)   A   B   C   D   E
 92)   A   B   C   D   E
102)   A   B   C   D   E
104)   1   2   3   4
114)   1   2   3   4
118)   1   2   3   4
119)   1   2   3   4
125)   1   2   3   4
126)   1   2   3   4
132)   1   2   3   4
134)   1   2   3   4
138)   1   2   3   4
141)   1   2   3   4
148)   1   2   3   4

## ≡ PAIN ≡

BOOK  A

 19)   1   2   3   4
 47)   1   2   3   4
 50)   1   2   3   4
 69)   1   2   3   4
105)   A   B   C   D   E

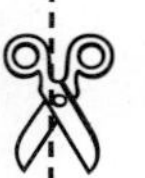

# Topic Indexed Answer Sheet

**BOOK B**

| | | | | | |
|---|---|---|---|---|---|
| 90) | A | B | C | D | E |
| 105) | 1 | 2 | 3 | 4 | |
| 106) | 1 | 2 | 3 | 4 | |
| 115) | 1 | 2 | 3 | 4 | |
| 127) | 1 | 2 | 3 | 4 | |
| 142) | 1 | 2 | 3 | 4 | |
| 174) | 1 | 2 | 3 | 4 | |

## ═══ PEDIATRICS ═══

**BOOK A**

| | | | | | |
|---|---|---|---|---|---|
| 6) | 1 | 2 | 3 | 4 | |
| 14) | 1 | 2 | 3 | 4 | |
| 26) | 1 | 2 | 3 | 4 | |
| 41) | 1 | 2 | 3 | 4 | |
| 56) | 1 | 2 | 3 | 4 | |
| 73) | A | B | C | D | E |
| 86) | A | B | C | D | E |
| 106) | A | B | C | D | E |
| 117) | A | B | C | D | E |
| 124) | A | B | C | D | E |
| 125) | A | B | C | D | E |
| 126) | A | B | C | D | E |
| 137) | A | B | C | D | E |

**BOOK B**

| | | | | | |
|---|---|---|---|---|---|
| 2) | A | B | C | D | E |
| 9) | A | B | C | D | E |
| 18) | A | B | C | D | E |
| 23) | A | B | C | D | E |
| 36) | A | B | C | D | E |
| 69) | A | B | C | D | E |
| 113) | 1 | 2 | 3 | 4 | |
| 117) | 1 | 2 | 3 | 4 | |
| 120) | 1 | 2 | 3 | 4 | |
| 124) | 1 | 2 | 3 | 4 | |
| 153) | 1 | 2 | 3 | 4 | |
| 163) | 1 | 2 | 3 | 4 | |

---

| 173) | 1 | 2 | 3 | 4 | |
|---|---|---|---|---|---|

## ═══ PHARMACOLOGY ═══

**BOOK A**

| | | | | | |
|---|---|---|---|---|---|
| 5) | 1 | 2 | 3 | 4 | |
| 22) | 1 | 2 | 3 | 4 | |
| 32) | 1 | 2 | 3 | 4 | |
| 33) | 1 | 2 | 3 | 4 | |
| 46) | 1 | 2 | 3 | 4 | |
| 52) | 1 | 2 | 3 | 4 | |
| 57) | 1 | 2 | 3 | 4 | |
| 62) | 1 | 2 | 3 | 4 | |
| 70) | 1 | 2 | 3 | 4 | |
| 74) | A | B | C | D | E |
| 78) | A | B | C | D | E |
| 83) | A | B | C | D | E |
| 85) | A | B | C | D | E |
| 92) | A | B | C | D | E |
| 100) | A | B | C | D | E |
| 104) | A | B | C | D | E |
| 108) | A | B | C | D | E |
| 112) | A | B | C | D | E |
| 134) | A | B | C | D | E |
| 135) | A | B | C | D | E |
| 140) | A | B | C | D | E |
| 148) | A | B | C | D | E |
| 161) | A | B | C | D | E |
| 163) | A | B | C | D | E |
| 165) | A | B | C | D | E |
| 171) | A | B | C | D | E |

**BOOK B**

| | | | | | |
|---|---|---|---|---|---|
| 1) | A | B | C | D | E |
| 4) | A | B | C | D | E |
| 5) | A | B | C | D | E |
| 8) | A | B | C | D | E |
| 30) | A | B | C | D | E |
| 35) | A | B | C | D | E |
| 41) | A | B | C | D | E |
| 42) | A | B | C | D | E |

---

| | | | | | |
|---|---|---|---|---|---|
| 43) | A | B | C | D | E |
| 47) | A | B | C | D | E |
| 48) | A | B | C | D | E |
| 57) | A | B | C | D | E |
| 65) | A | B | C | D | E |
| 68) | A | B | C | D | E |
| 95) | A | B | C | D | E |
| 97) | A | B | C | D | E |
| 100) | A | B | C | D | E |
| 107) | 1 | 2 | 3 | 4 | |
| 110) | 1 | 2 | 3 | 4 | |
| 112) | 1 | 2 | 3 | 4 | |
| 130) | 1 | 2 | 3 | 4 | |
| 144) | 1 | 2 | 3 | 4 | |
| 154) | 1 | 2 | 3 | 4 | |
| 156) | 1 | 2 | 3 | 4 | |
| 162) | 1 | 2 | 3 | 4 | |
| 166) | 1 | 2 | 3 | 4 | |
| 172) | 1 | 2 | 3 | 4 | |

## ═══ PHYSIOLOGY ═══

**BOOK A**

| | | | | | |
|---|---|---|---|---|---|
| 2) | 1 | 2 | 3 | 4 | |
| 3) | 1 | 2 | 3 | 4 | |
| 4) | 1 | 2 | 3 | 4 | |
| 7) | 1 | 2 | 3 | 4 | |
| 8) | 1 | 2 | 3 | 4 | |
| 20) | 1 | 2 | 3 | 4 | |
| 25) | 1 | 2 | 3 | 4 | |
| 31) | 1 | 2 | 3 | 4 | |
| 34) | 1 | 2 | 3 | 4 | |
| 36) | 1 | 2 | 3 | 4 | |
| 51) | 1 | 2 | 3 | 4 | |
| 54) | 1 | 2 | 3 | 4 | |
| 60) | 1 | 2 | 3 | 4 | |
| 61) | 1 | 2 | 3 | 4 | |
| 72) | 1 | 2 | 3 | 4 | |
| 76) | A | B | C | D | E |
| 80) | A | B | C | D | E |
| 82) | A | B | C | D | E |
| 91) | A | B | C | D | E |

| 98) | A | B | C | D | E |
| 101) | A | B | C | D | E |
| 103) | A | B | C | D | E |
| 122) | A | B | C | D | E |
| 130) | A | B | C | D | E |
| 131) | A | B | C | D | E |
| 139) | A | B | C | D | E |
| 144) | A | B | C | D | E |
| 146) | A | B | C | D | E |
| 147) | A | B | C | D | E |
| 175) | A | B | C | D | E |

## BOOK B

| 22) | A | B | C | D | E |
| 34) | A | B | C | D | E |
| 58) | A | B | C | D | E |
| 66) | A | B | C | D | E |
| 71) | A | B | C | D | E |
| 76) | A | B | C | D | E |
| 96) | A | B | C | D | E |
| 99) | A | B | C | D | E |
| 103) | 1 | 2 | 3 | 4 |
| 108) | 1 | 2 | 3 | 4 |
| 109) | 1 | 2 | 3 | 4 |
| 128) | 1 | 2 | 3 | 4 |
| 131) | 1 | 2 | 3 | 4 |
| 133) | 1 | 2 | 3 | 4 |
| 136) | 1 | 2 | 3 | 4 |
| 140) | 1 | 2 | 3 | 4 |
| 145) | 1 | 2 | 3 | 4 |
| 152) | 1 | 2 | 3 | 4 |
| 155) | 1 | 2 | 3 | 4 |
| 158) | 1 | 2 | 3 | 4 |
| 160) | 1 | 2 | 3 | 4 |
| 171) | 1 | 2 | 3 | 4 |

# ANSWERS TO
# BOOK A EXAMINATION

## Answer A

### Equipment/Physics

**QUESTION (K-type):**

During mechanical ventilation, factors that influence the correlation between set tidal volume and exhaled tidal volume include

(1) Inspiratory time.
(2) Fresh gas flow.
(3) Compliance of the breathing circuit.
(4) Addition of positive end-expiratory pressure to the circuit.

**CORRECT ANSWER: A (1, 2, and 3 are correct.)**

**SUMMARY:**

*A difference can exist between the set tidal volume of an anesthesia machine and the actual delivered tidal volume. This difference can be explained by several factors, including fresh gas flow rate, inspiratory time, and breathing circuit compliance. High flow rates can add additional volume to each inspired breath, thus resulting in increased delivered tidal volume. Prolonged inspiratory time provides an opportunity for more gas to enter the lungs for a given breath; this translates into an increase in the delivered tidal volume to the patient. The breathing circuit of an anesthesia machine can absorb some of the set tidal volume, which results in a decreased delivered tidal volume. Positive end-expiratory pressure (PEEP) does not alter the delivered tidal volume from the ventilator.*

**EXPLANATION:**

(1) ***Correct.*** Older ventilators added fresh gas to the inspired tidal volume only during the inspiratory phase. Therefore, an increase in the I:E ratio (ie, an increased inspiratory time) allows for a greater addition of fresh gas to the inspired tidal volume, and thus an increased tidal volume is delivered to the patient. Recent advances in ventilator technology have sought to eliminate this effect. For example, measurements of the inspired fresh gas flow can be coupled with compensatory changes in bellow excursion (fresh gas compensation). Another technique is to divert fresh gas into the reservoir bag during inspiration, thus preventing fresh gas from entering the breathing circuit during the inspiration phase (fresh gas decoupling).
(2) ***Correct.*** High fresh gas flows can increase the delivered tidal volume to the patient's lungs from the ventilator. Newer ventilators attempt to eliminate this effect with fresh gas compensation and fresh gas decoupling (see above).
(3) ***Correct.*** Compliance of the anesthesia breathing circuit can absorb tidal volume and result in a decrease in the delivered tidal volume (ie, pressure that was meant to contribute to the tidal volume delivered to the patient ends up expanding the circuit). More modern and advanced ventilators compensate for changes in compliance by changing the volume delivered; compliance assessments are performed during the machine checkout procedure. Other newer ventilators adjust ventilator excursion according to inspired volumes measured at the patient connection.
(4) ***Incorrect.*** PEEP is not considered to be an influencing factor in the correlation of set versus delivered tidal volume.

**REASONING:**

This question tests knowledge of the anesthesia machine ventilator and factors that influence delivered tidal volumes. The first three options (especially choices 2 and 3) usually are recognized as influencing factors. This knowledge makes the first option correct by default. The last option is not correct. Although there may be some evidence that PEEP influences the delivered tidal volume (in certain anesthesia machines), it generally is not regarded as a correlating factor.


**BIBLIOGRAPHY:**

Dorsch JA, Dorsch SE. *Understanding Anesthesia Equipment*. 5th ed. Philadelphia, PA: Lippincott Williams & Wilkins; 2008:314.

Gravenstein N, Banner MJ, McLaughlin G. Tidal volume changes due to the interaction of anesthesia machine and anesthesia ventilator. *J Clin Monit*. 1987;3:187-190.

Lancaster CT, Boyle PM, Kaczka DW. Delivered tidal volume from the Fabius GS depends upon breathing circuit configuration despite compliance compensation. *Anesthesiology*. 2005;103:A863.

Morgan GE, Mikhail MS, Murray MJ. *Clinical Anesthesiology*. 4th ed. New York, NY: McGraw-Hill; 2006:84.

Moynihan R, Cote CJ. Fresh gas flow changes during controlled mechanical ventilation with the circle system have significantly greater effects on the ventilatory parameters of toddlers compared with children. *Pediatric Anesthesia*. 1992;2:211-215.


---

| | |
|---|---|
| **BOOK A:** | **QUESTION 2** |

## *Answer E*

Physiology

**QUESTION (K-type):**

In a 45-year-old man with adult respiratory distress syndrome, which of the following will result from institution of mechanical ventilation with positive end-expiratory pressure?

(1) Decreased intrapulmonary shunt.
(2) Increased pulmonary compliance.
(3) Increased ventilation-perfusion ratio in the dependent portion of the lung.
(4) Decreased dead space to tidal volume ratio.

**CORRECT ANSWER: E (All are correct.)**

**SUMMARY:**

*Positive end-expiratory pressure (PEEP) is the alveolar pressure above atmospheric pressure that exists at the end of expiration. The main effect of PEEP is to prevent alveolar derecruitment and increase functional residual capacity (FRC). This results in decreased intrapulmonary shunting, which improves arterial oxygenation. Mechanical PEEP also serves to protect against injury caused by phasic opening and closing of alveolar units and to increase mean intrathoracic pressure. Excessive PEEP can overdistend alveoli, resulting in decreased lung compliance and increased dead space. Complications of PEEP include barotrauma and decreased cardiac output because of decreased venous return and/or decreased left ventricular filling pressure. Care must be made to adjust the amount of PEEP to an "optimal" level at which oxygen delivery to tissues is increased and dead space to tidal volume ratio is lowest. This is especially important in patients with acute respiratory distress syndrome (ARDS) where lung disease is heterogeneous and PEEP may not be distributed evenly.*

**EXPLANATION:**

(1) ***Correct.*** The addition of PEEP decreases intrapulmonary shunting and improves arterial oxygenation by increasing FRC and tidal ventilation above closing capacity, improving lung compliance, and correcting ventilation-perfusion abnormalities. This is accomplished by stabilization and recruitment of partially collapsed alveoli.

(2) **Correct.** PEEP improves, or increases, lung compliance by increasing transpulmonary distending pressure.

(3) **Correct.** Alveoli in dependent portions of the lung are at increased risk of atelectasis due to accumulation of interstitial edema fluid. PEEP can recruit these alveoli and improve the ventilation-perfusion ratio.

(4) **Correct.** Optimal PEEP provides maximal oxygen delivery and the lowest dead space to tidal volume ratio. Excessive PEEP can increase dead space by overdistending alveoli and lower cardiac output by decreasing venous return.

### REASONING:

Answering this question involves understanding key respiratory physiology and effects of PEEP. Choice 1 is true because recruited alveoli can participate in oxygen exchange, thereby decreasing intrapulmonary shunt. The same effect of PEEP also increases the ventilation-perfusion ratio in dependent portions of the lung (choice 3). Choices 2 and 4 are true for an optimal amount of PEEP, in which case pulmonary compliance is increased and dead space is decreased. If excessive levels of PEEP are used, pulmonary compliance can decrease and dead space can increase.

### BIBLIOGRAPHY:

Miller, 7th ed, pg. 2882-2884.
Morgan GE, Mikhail MS, Murray MJ. *Clinical Anesthesiology*. 4th ed. New York, NY: McGraw-Hill; 2006:1037-1039.

---

## BOOK A:

## Answer A

## Physiology

## QUESTION 3

### QUESTION (K-type):

A 58-year-old man with suspected carcinoma of the lung requires postoperative ventilation following general anesthesia for mediastinoscopy. Preoperatively, his shoulder muscles are weak bilaterally, but strength improves with exercise. This patient will show

(1) Inadequate reversal of neuromuscular block with an anticholinesterase drug.
(2) Increased sensitivity to both depolarizing and nondepolarizing muscle relaxants.
(3) Increased muscle strength following plasmapheresis.
(4) Resolution of symptoms following administration of hydrocortisone.

### CORRECT ANSWER: A (1, 2, and 3 are correct.)

### SUMMARY:

*Muscle weakness that improves with exercise and is associated with carcinoma of the lung is a hallmark of Lambert-Eaton myasthenic syndrome (LEMS). Antibodies to presynaptic voltage-gated calcium channels cause decreased release of acetylcholine (ACh) into the neuromuscular junction (NMJ). Both myasthenia gravis and LEMS are diseases of the NMJ. Fortunately, no neuronal damage occurs and functional recovery can be achieved. Treatment for LEMS includes immunosuppression and plasmapheresis. Anticholinesterases are less helpful in LEMS than myasthenia gravis. Curative procedures are directed toward the carcinoma. Patients with LEMS are sensitive to muscle relaxants.*

### EXPLANATION:

(1) **Correct.** Anticholinesterases do not appreciably increase the amount of ACh as it is not released in the first place in LEMS.

(2) *Correct.*

(3) *Correct.* Plasmapheresis will reduce the amount of circulating antibodies and reduce the symptoms of LEMS.

(4) *Incorrect.* Symptoms will improve but are not likely to resolve with immune suppression. The underlying malignancy needs to be treated.

**REASONING:**

This question is K-type. Choice 4 is the easiest to eliminate by knowing that immune suppression is not curative. However, it does improve symptoms, so statement 3 is correct. With decreased acetylcholine release into the NMJ, patients with LEMS are very sensitive to all types of muscle relaxants (choice 2). Anticholinesterases increase ACh by inhibiting the enzymes that degrade ACh. However, with very little ACh to begin with, the anticholinesterases are ineffective in LEMS (choice 1). Patients with myasthenia gravis are on chronic anticholinesterase therapy. Choices 1, 2, and 3 are correct, and therefore the answer is A.

**BIBLIOGRAPHY:**

Darnell RB, Posner JB. Paraneoplastic syndromes involving the nervous system. *New Engl J Med.* 2003;349(16):1543-1554.

Morgan GE, Mikhail MS, Murray MJ. *Clinical Anesthesiology.* 4th ed. New York, NY: McGraw-Hill; 2006:819.

---

**BOOK A:**      **QUESTION 4**

---

*Answer A*

Physiology

**QUESTION (K-type):**

Which of the following statements concerning postoperative shivering is true?

(1) It increases carbon dioxide production.

(2) It is suppressed by intravenous meperidine.

(3) It accentuates halothane-related tremors.

(4) It increases heat loss.

**CORRECT ANSWER: A (1, 2, and 3 are correct.)**

**SUMMARY:**

*Postoperative shivering is often more of a problem for patients than pain. The hypothermic patient shivers to generate heat. Unfortunately, shivering is an undesirable stress to the body. Shivering increases oxygen demand and carbon dioxide production several-fold. In the patient with marginal cardiac and pulmonary reserve, shivering is poorly tolerated. Shivering can be treated with warming and medications. Meperidine is the agent most commonly used in the recovery room for just this effect. Volatile agents decrease the vasoconstriction response to hypothermia but also lower the threshold for shivering.*

**EXPLANATION:**

(1) *Correct.* Shivering produces large amounts of carbon dioxide because of the increased activity of skeletal muscles.

(2) *Correct.* Meperidine is a first-line agent for treatment of shivering; other opioids can be used but are generally not as effective as meperidine.

(3) *Correct.* Shivering accentuates tremors associated with emergence from inhalational agents.

(4) *Incorrect.* Shivering generates heat and, in some instances, enough heat that the patient becomes hyperthermic.

**REASONING:**

This question is K-type. Shivering is the body's attempt to get warm (choice 4 is incorrect), but it is stressful (choice 1 is correct) and uncomfortable and probably should be suppressed (choice 2 is correct). The most difficult statement in this question is number 3. Halothane is rarely used in clinical practice in North America. However, inhalational agents, in general, are associated with emergence tremors. With logic on our side, if choices 1 and 2 are correct statements, choice 3 must also be correct.

**BIBLIOGRAPHY:**

Barash PG, Cullen BF, Stoelting RK, Cahalan MK, Stock MC. *Clinical Anesthesia.* 6th ed. Philadelphia, PA: Lippincott Williams & Wilkins; 2009:1439.

Morgan GE, Mikhail MS, Murray MJ. *Clinical Anesthesiology.* 4th ed. New York, NY: McGraw-Hill; 2006:148, 771-772.

---

| **BOOK A:** | **QUESTION 5** |
|---|---|

## *Answer B*

Pharmacology

**QUESTION (K-type):**

In which of the following conditions is the elimination half-life of an amide local anesthetic prolonged?

(1) Liver disease.
(2) Term pregnancy.
(3) Heart failure.
(4) Kidney disease.

**CORRECT ANSWER: B (1 and 3 are correct.)**

**SUMMARY:**

*Amide local anesthetics are metabolized by microsomal P-450 enzymes in the liver. Therefore, clearance of amide local anesthetics from plasma will be affected by liver disease and hepatic blood flow. The elimination half-life of these local anesthetics will be prolonged with liver dysfunction and decreases in hepatic blood flow. Less than 5% of amide local anesthetic is excreted by the kidneys; thus changes in kidney function will not appreciably affect their elimination half-life.*

**EXPLANATION:**

(1) *Correct.* Because amide local anesthetics are metabolized by microsomal enzymes in the liver, liver disease will reduce the metabolic rate and prolong the elimination half-life.
(2) *Incorrect.* During pregnancy, liver function and hepatic blood flow do not change.
(3) *Correct.* In patients with heart failure, cardiac output is reduced and thus blood flow to the liver is decreased. This will prolong the elimination half-life of amide local anesthetics as less drug is delivered to their site of metabolism.
(4) *Incorrect.* Amide local anesthetics are only minimally excreted by the kidneys.

**REASONING:**

This question tests knowledge of the metabolic elimination of amide local anesthetics. Knowing that amide local anesthetics are metabolized in the liver, we know choices 1 and 3 are correct. Because the kidney plays a small role in the elimination of amide local anesthetics, choice 4 can be eliminated. Choice 2 is incorrect because pregnancy does not affect liver function. Thus, the best answer is B, choices 1 and 3.


**BIBLIOGRAPHY:**

Barash PG, Cullen BF, Stoelting RK, Cahalan MK, Stock MC. *Clinical Anesthesia.* 6th ed. Philadelphia, PA: Lippincott Williams & Wilkins; 2009:539.

Morgan GE, Mikhail MS, Murray MJ. *Clinical Anesthesiology.* 4th ed. New York, NY: McGraw-Hill; 2006:269, 877.


**BOOK A:**

## QUESTION 6

*Answer A*

Pharmacology

**QUESTION (K-type):**

A 10-year-old child with asthma is undergoing anesthesia with nitrous oxide, oxygen, and halothane. Effects of the accidental injection of atropine 2 mg in this patient would include

(1) Postoperative delirium.
(2) Ventricular dysrhythmias.
(3) Increased body temperature.
(4) Bronchospasm.


**CORRECT ANSWER: A (1, 2, and 3 are correct.)**


**SUMMARY:**

*Atropine belongs to a class of drugs that are commonly referred to as anticholinergic agents. More accurately, they are drugs that block muscarinic acetylcholine receptors. These are to be differentiated from neuromuscular blocking agents that act at nicotinic acetylcholine receptors. Anticholinergic agents competitively block acetylcholine from activating the acetylcholine receptor. They can affect several organ systems, including cardiovascular, respiratory, central nervous, gastrointestinal, ophthalmic, genitourinary, and thermoregulatory. The recommended pediatric dose for atropine is 0.01 to 0.02 mg/ kg IV. An overdose of an anticholinergic agent may result in central nervous system (CNS) effects, tachycardia, dry mouth, hyperthermia, mydriasis, and cycloplegia. Physostigmine, an acetylcholinesterase inhibitor that can cross the blood-brain barrier, can rapidly reverse the toxic effects of atropine, but it must be administered with care because it causes potentially lethal nicotinic effects.*


**EXPLANATION:**

(1) ***Correct.*** Atropine is a tertiary amine that can cross the blood-brain barrier and can cause CNS effects of memory deficits and excitatory reactions, including hallucinations, agitation, delirium, and even loss of consciousness. This clinical presentation is also referred to as *central anticholinergic syndrome.*

(2) ***Correct.*** Effects of muscarinic blockade on the heart can result in tachycardia, shortening of the PR interval, and atrial and nodal dysrhythmias. Atropine does not typically cause ventricular dysrhythmias; however, there have been rare case reports of atropine causing ventricular fibrillation in susceptible patients.

(3) ***Correct.*** Blockade of sweat gland may lead to an inability to dissipate heat. This is also known as "atropine fever."

(4) ***Incorrect.*** Anticholinergic agents inhibit secretions of respiratory tract mucosa and cause relaxation of bronchial smooth muscle. Ipratropium bromide (Atrovent) is an atropine derivative commonly used for treatment of asthma.

**REASONING:**

This question tests knowledge of the pharmacology of atropine. Clearly, anticholinergic toxicity may cause delirium and hyperthermia. Ventricular dysrhythmias may result from tachycardia in patient with coronary artery disease, but healthy patients, including most children, will get only a transient sinus tachycardia. A case report of three children ages 7 to 9 years who were accidentally given massive doses of atropine (16-21 mg/kg orally) suffered CNS symptoms and tachycardia, but both of which resolved within 48 hours. Mydriasis, however, lasted for 1 week.

**BIBLIOGRAPHY:**

Arthurs GJ, Davies R. Atropine—a safe drug. *Anesthesia*. 1980 Nov;35(11):1077-1079.

Morgan GE, Mikhail MS, Murray MJ. *Clinical Anesthesiology*. 4th ed. New York, NY: McGraw-Hill; 2006:239-240, 928.

Prandota J, Iwanczak F. Long QT syndrome precipitated by atropine and hypokalemia. *Dev Pharmacol Ther*. 1983;6:356-364.

Santinelli V, Chiariello M, Condorelli M. Rapid increase of intraventricular conduction delay in the genesis of ventricular fibrillation after atropine. *Int J Cardiol*. 1983;3: 109-111.

---

| **BOOK A:** | **QUESTION 7** |
| --- | --- |

*Answer B*

Physiology

**QUESTION (K-type):**

True statements concerning the oculocardiac reflex include the following:

(1)  It is more likely to occur in a patient with hypercarbia than in a patient with normocarbia.
(2)  It is not seen during operative procedures on an empty orbit.
(3)  Its afferent limb is the trigeminal nerve.
(4)  It does not occur in the awake patient.

**CORRECT ANSWER: B (1 and 3 are correct.)**

**SUMMARY:**

*The oculocardiac reflex can be triggered by manipulation, pressure or pain of the eye or extraocular muscles and results in bradycardia and/or other dysrhythmias including ventricular fibrillation and sinus arrest. Most commonly seen in pediatric patients during strabismus surgery, this reflex can be evoked in all age grounds and during a range of ocular procedures. Hypercarbia can increase the incidence of the oculocardiac reflex, so prevention starts with normoventilation. Treatment includes discontinuation of instigating stimulus, adequate anesthetic depth, oxygen, Trendelenburg positioning, and intravenous anticholinergic medication, which may also be used for prophylaxis. Prophylactic administration of anticholinergics is not wholly effective, and some have argued that atropine may yield more serious and refractory dysrhythmias than the reflex itself. With repeated stimulation, the oculocardiac reflex fatigues.*

**EXPLANATION:**

(1)  ***Correct.*** The oculocardiac reflex is more likely to occur with hypercapnia or hypoxemia. Maintaining normocarbia can help reduce the incidence and severity of the oculocardiac reflex.
(2)  ***Incorrect.*** The oculocardiac reflex can be elicited by direct pressure on the tissue in the orbit after enucleation.

(3) **Correct.** Afferent impulses travel along the short and long ciliary nerves to the ciliary ganglion then to the gasserian ganglion via the ophthalmic division (V1) of the trigeminal nerve. The efferent limb is the vagal nerve.

(4) **Incorrect.** The oculocardiac reflex can be elicited by pressure on the eyeball, traction on extraocular muscles, orbital hematomas, eye trauma or pain, and retrobulbar blockade. All may occur in the awake patient who may experience somnolence and nausea instead of or in addition to bradycardia and dysrhythmias.

### REASONING:

This question hinges on understanding the occurrence and physiology of the oculocardiac reflex. The reader should be able to rule out choices 2 and 4 by knowing the various stimuli that can cause the oculocardiac reflex and that they can occur in the awake patient and in an enucleated patient. The reader is then left with answer B (choices 1 and 3) because there is no answer for all the choices to be incorrect.

### BIBLIOGRAPHY:

Barash PG, Cullen BF, Stoelting RK, Cahalan MK, Stock MC. *Clinical Anesthesia*. 6th ed. Philadelphia, PA: Lippincott Williams & Wilkins; 2009:1327.

Miller, 7th ed., pg 409, 2379.

Morgan GE, Mikhail MS, Murray MJ. *Clinical Anesthesiology*. 4th ed. New York, NY: McGraw-Hill; 2006:828.

---

| **BOOK A:** | **QUESTION 8** |
|---|---|

## *Answer E*

Physiology

### QUESTION (K-type):

Phase II succinylcholine block is characterized by

(1) A train-of-four ratio less than 0.7.
(2) Nonsustained response to tetanic stimulation.
(3) Post-tetanic facilitation.
(4) Improvement by edrophonium.

### CORRECT ANSWER: E (All are correct.)

### SUMMARY:

*Succinylcholine is a depolarizing muscle relaxant that can cause both phase I and II blocks. Phase I is the commonly recognized effect of succinylcholine: an acetylcholine receptor agonist causing motor end-plate depolarization (equally diminished train-of-four stimulation without fade). However, if enough succinylcholine is administered, a block that resembles a nondepolarizing block will develop (train-of-four stimulation with fade). This is thought to relate to conformational changes that accompany prolonged muscle membrane depolarization. Characteristics of phase II block include train-of-four fade, prolonged recovery, anticholinesterase antagonism, and fade with repeated tetanic stimulation.*

### EXPLANATION:

(1) **Correct.** Monitoring a patient receiving succinylcholine will show a decrease in the train of four to a ratio of less than 0.7 as the patient transitions from phase I to phase II block. Once the ratio is less than 0.4, the patient has a phase II block.

(2) **Correct.** Repeated tetanic stimulation has no effect on the patient with a normal phase I block, but phase II shows a reduced response with successive stimulations.

(3) **Correct.** A single tetanus will increase the ratio on train of four in phase II block.

(4) **Correct.** Phase II block can be improved with anticholinesterases. Phase I block is prolonged after administration of anticholinesterases.

## REASONING:

This question tests knowledge of types I and II neuromuscular blockade. Knowing that phase II block of succinylcholine has similar characteristics to nondepolarizing muscle relaxation makes answering this question much easier. Choices 2, 3, and 4 are clearly characteristics of phase II block. The first choice is a bit challenging because phase II is not formally established before a train-of-four ratio of less than 0.4. However, if choices 2, 3, and 4 are true, choice 1 must be as well. All choices are correct, and E is the best answer.

## BIBLIOGRAPHY:

Miller RD, Miller ED, Reves JG, et al. *Anesthesia.* 7th ed. Philadelphia, PA: Churchill Livingstone; 2010:1526-1527.

Morgan GE, Mikhail MS, Murray MJ. *Clinical Anesthesiology.* 3rd ed. New York, NY: McGraw-Hill; 2002:182.

---

| **BOOK A:** | **QUESTION 9** |
|---|---|

---

## *Answer C*

### Equipment/Physics

### QUESTION (K-type):

Advantages of closed-circuit anesthesia over a semiclosed anesthesia system include the ability to

(1) More quickly alter the inspired anesthetic concentration.
(2) Decrease the total amount of inhalational anesthetic used.
(3) More easily increase $Pa_{CO_2}$ during emergence.
(4) Decrease heat loss to a greater extent.

### CORRECT ANSWER: C (2 and 4 are correct.)

### SUMMARY:

*With closed-circuit anesthesia, all exhaled gases, except $CO_2$, are rebreathed and the inflow of gas exactly matches that being consumed. A semiclosed anesthesia system allows for high fresh gas flows to eliminate rebreathing of gases. The advantages of closed-circuit anesthesia include maximal humidification and warming of inhaled gases, less pollution of gases into the surrounding atmosphere, and less use of volatile anesthetics. A disadvantage of closed-circuit anesthesia is the inability to rapidly change concentrations of gases, including oxygen and volatile anesthetics, because of low fresh gas flows.*

### EXPLANATION:

(1) **Incorrect.** Closed-circuit anesthesia uses low fresh gas flows, which makes it difficult to quickly alter inspired anesthetic concentration.

(2) **Correct.** Because the inflow of gas exactly matches that being consumed, the total amount of inhalational anesthetic used is minimized.

(3) **Incorrect.** Both closed-circuit and semiclosed anesthesia systems do not allow rebreathing of $CO_2$, which is removed from the circuit by the $CO_2$ absorber. Thus, neither system will affect the rate of rise of $Pa_{CO_2}$ during emergence.

(4) **Correct.** An advantage of the closed-circuit anesthesia is humidification and warming of inhaled gases that decrease heat loss.

**REASONING:**
Knowing the differences between closed-circuit and semiclosed anesthesia systems will allow you to answer this question correctly. Choices 2 and 4 are correct because advantages of the closed-circuit anesthesia system are the ability to conserve heat and minimize use of anesthetics through low flows. Choices 1 and 3 are either both correct or both incorrect based on the answer choices. In this question, both choices 1 and 3 are incorrect. Knowing that either closed-circuit anesthesia systems slow the rate of rise of inspired anesthetic concentrations or does not affect the rise of $Paco_2$ during emergence will lead you to the best answer, choice C.


**BIBLIOGRAPHY:**
Stoelting RK, Miller RD. *Basics of Anesthesia*. 5th ed. Philadelphia, PA: Churchill Livingstone; 2007:194-196.

---

| **BOOK A:** | **QUESTION 10** |
| --- | --- |

*Answer C*

**Clinical Anesthesia**

**QUESTION (K-type):**

Chronic hyperglycemia from excessive glucose administration during parenteral hyperalimentation causes

(1) Retinal degeneration.
(2) Depression of granulocyte function.
(3) Inhibition of platelet aggregation.
(4) Hypercarbia.


**CORRECT ANSWER: C (2 and 4 are correct.)**


**SUMMARY:**
*The term "chronic" in the question is misleading and not entirely applicable to total parenteral nutrition (TPN) therapy. If TPN is stopped, the glucose level will normalize, provided that the patient does not have diabetes. This question also mixes the acute and chronic effects of hyperglycemia, even though the two conditions have different implications. Total parenteral nutrition therapy frequently leads to acute hyperglycemia, which has a number of adverse effects. Some of the undesirable effects of hyperglycemia are as follows:*
- *Increased rate of wound infection due to inhibition of neutrophilic granulocyte function as well as suppression of complement fixation.*
- *Hypercapnia and respiratory acidosis due to increased $CO_2$ production.*
- *Hypovolemia secondary to osmotic diuresis.*
- *Hyperglycemia increases the platelet aggregation. Retinal degeneration describes retinal pathology of different etiologies. It is usually not associated with TPN-induced acute hyperglycemia.*


**EXPLANATION:**
(1) ***Incorrect.*** Short-term excessive glucose administration with TPN will not cause retinal degeneration.
(2) ***Correct.*** High and uncontrolled blood glucose levels during TPN cause a depression of granulocyte function.
(3) ***Incorrect.*** Platelet aggregation may be enhanced but not diminished in patients receiving hyperalimentation.
(4) ***Correct.*** Hypercarbia is a side effect of hyperalimentation and TPN with high glucose content.

## REASONING:

Long-term hyperglycemia due to diabetes mellitus can cause microvascular disease and retinal scaring. There is no association between hyperalimentation-induced short-term hyperglycemia and retinal degeneration. TPN can be a risk factor for the retinopathy of prematurity. The rate of wound infection is increased with elevated levels of blood glucose. This can be due to reduction in chemotaxis, opsonization and phagocytosis capability of neutrophils. In addition, the complement fixation is inhibited, additionally attenuating the immune defense. Hyperglycemia can enhance platelet aggregation in vivo and in vitro, potentially causing adverse events such as myocardial infarction and deep venous thrombosis.

Hyperalimentation and TPN can cause excess $CO_2$ production moving the respiratory quotient ($RQ = V_{CO_2}/V_{O_2}$) toward 1.0, which means more ventilatory effort to exhale the additional $CO_2$. Patients with compromised respiratory function such as chronic obstructive pulmonary disease (COPD), asthma, pulmonary edema, etc may not tolerate the extra $CO_2$ load and develop respiratory insufficiency.

## BIBLIOGRAPHY:


Darlow B, Hutchinson JL, Henderson-Smart DJ, et al. Prenatal risk factors for severe retinopathy of prematurity among very preterm infants of the Australian and New Zealand Neonatal Network [abstract/free full text]. *Pediatrics.* 2005;115:990-996.

Miller RD, Eriksson LI, Fleisher LA, et al. *Miller's Anesthesia.* 7th ed. Philadelphia, PA: Churchill Livingstone; 2009:1069-1073.

Porta I, Planas M, Padro JB, Pico M, Valls M, Schwartz S. Effect of two lipid emulsions on platelet function. *Infusionsther Transfusionsmed.* 1994 Oct;21(5):316-321.

Sheean PM, Freels SA, Helton WS, Braunschweig CA. Adverse clinical consequences of hyperglycemia from total parenteral nutrition exposure during hematopoietic stem cell transplantation. *Biol Blood Marrow Transplant.* 2006;12(6):656-664.

Skibowska A, Raszeja-Specht A, Szutowicz A. Platelet function and acetyl-coenzyme A metabolism in type 1 diabetes mellitus. *Clin Chem Lab Med.* 2003 Sep;41(9): 1136-1143.

Worthley MI, Holmes AS, Willoughby SR, Kucia AM, Heresztyn T. The deleterious effects of hyperglycemia on platelet function in diabetic patients with acute coronary syndromes mediation by superoxide production, resolution with intensive insulin administration. *J Am Coll Cardiol.* 2007;49:304-310.


---

| **BOOK A:** | **QUESTION 11** |
| --- | --- |

*Answer B*

Clinical Anesthesia

### QUESTION (K-type):

Which of the following produces effective transtracheal jet ventilation through a 14-gauge intravenous catheter?

(1)  Oxygen through a 50-psi pressure regulator.
(2)  An Ambu bag with oxygen flow at 15 L/min.
(3)  Oxygen flush from the fresh gas outlet of the anesthesia machine.
(4)  The reservoir bag from the anesthesia circle system.

### CORRECT ANSWER: B (1 and 3 are correct.)

### SUMMARY:

*Transtracheal jet ventilation is reserved for the rare "cannot intubate, cannot ventilate" situation. A high-pressure oxygen source must be attached via noncompliant tubing to a 14-gauge intravenous catheter placed through the cricothyroid membrane. Sources of oxygen through a 50-psi regulator or from the oxygen flush valve (which is really the same thing) are both adequate. Unfortunately an Ambu bag and the reservoir bag from the circle system, while possibly providing oxygenation, are too compliant to effectively produce adequate transtracheal ventilation.*

**EXPLANATION:**

Transtracheal jet ventilation is a lifesaving maneuver that is reserved for patients who cannot be ventilated or intubated. Its purpose is to temporize until a more definitive airway can be established. Some specifically designed catheters (> 14 gauges) can be used with a circle system or Ambu bag (ie, the Nu-Trake). A 14-gauge catheter requires a driving force of 50 psi for effective ventilation. This can be provided both by an oxygen source (cylinder, etc) connected to a regulator to drop the pressure to 50 psi and by the anesthesia machine through the oxygen flush valve. The tubing from the circle system, the reservoir bag from the circuit, and Ambu bags are too compliant to be used during transtracheal ventilation. Special noncompliant tubing must be used between the oxygen source and the 14-gauge catheter. Remember that adequate exhalation must be carefully observed, by noting adequate chest rise and fall, noting phonation during exhalation and, if possible, $ETCO_2$ return, to avoid gas entrapment and barotrauma. It is also critical to avoid subcutaneous extravasation of gas during insufflation as neck anatomy will become obscured, the transtracheal catheter may dislodge, and the airway may further collapse from peritracheal gas.

**REASONING:**

As outlined above, choices 1 and 3 are correct: Oxygen must be provided at 50 psi either through the oxygen flush valve or through another source connected to a regulator. Choices 2 and 4 are incorrect: An Ambu bag and the reservoir bag are too compliant for effective transtracheal ventilation. Therefore, the correct answer is B.

**BIBLIOGRAPHY:**

Barash PG, Cullen BF, Stoelting RK, Cahalan MK, Stock MC. *Clinical Anesthesia.* 6th ed. Philadelphia, PA: Lippincott Williams & Wilkins; 2009:787-788.

Dorsch JA, Dorsch SE. *Understanding Anesthesia Equipment.* 5th ed. Philadelphia, PA: Lippincott Williams & Wilkins; 2008:668-669.

Morgan GE, Mikhail MS, Murray MJ. *Clinical Anesthesiology.* 4th ed. New York, NY: McGraw-Hill; 2006:839.

---

| **BOOK A:** | **QUESTION 12** |
|---|---|

*Answer A*

Neuroanesthesia

**QUESTION (K-type):**

During intraoperative mapping of a seizure focus under general anesthesia, electroencephalogram (EEG) activation may be enhanced or seizures induced by the use of

(1) Ketamine.
(2) Methohexital.
(3) Enflurane.
(4) Thiopental.

**CORRECT ANSWER: A (1, 2, and 3 are correct.)**

**SUMMARY:**

*Several commonly used anesthetics can induce seizures either directly or through their metabolites in susceptible individuals. These include enflurane, methohexital, ketamine, etomidate, and meperidine. Both thiopental and propofol suppress seizure activity and would not help elicit seizure foci during intraoperative mapping.*

### EXPLANATION:

(1) **Correct.** Ketamine has been reported to enhance EEG signals in patients with epilepsy.
(2) **Correct.** Methohexital, unlike the other barbiturates, has well-established epileptogenic effects in patients with epilepsy and is often used to activate cortical EEG seizure discharges.
(3) **Correct.** Deep enflurane anesthesia causes spike-and-wave pattern on EEG, which can progress to tonic-clonic seizures.
(4) **Incorrect.** Barbiturates, with the exception of methohexital, possess potent anticonvulsant activity and would not be effective in inducing seizures.

### REASONING:

This question tests knowledge of CNS effects of several anesthetics. Knowing that thiopental suppresses seizure activity and is often used to induce anesthesia in patients with seizures helps eliminate choice 4, making answers C, D, and E incorrect. Thus, you are left to decide on whether choice 2 is correct or incorrect. Methohexital is the preferred IV anesthetic for electroconvulsive therapy because it helps induce seizures, which may help you determine that choice 2 is correct and A is the best answer.

### BIBLIOGRAPHY:


Barash PG, Cullen BF, Stoelting RK, Cahalan MK, Stock MC. *Clinical Anesthesia.* 6th ed. Philadelphia, PA: Lippincott Williams & Wilkins; 2009:453-456.

Morgan GE, Mikhail MS, Murray MJ. *Clinical Anesthesiology.* 4th ed. New York, NY: McGraw-Hill; 2006:186-187, 202.


---

**BOOK A:**      **QUESTION 13**

## *Answer E*

Equipment/Physics

### QUESTION (K-type):

Transthoracic resistance to DC defibrillation is decreased by

(1) Use of conductive gel.
(2) Multiple attempts at defibrillation.
(3) Defibrillation during expiration.
(4) Larger electrodes.

### CORRECT ANSWER: E (All are correct.)

### SUMMARY:

*Proper defibrillation during cardiac arrest depends on appropriate flow of current through the heart. Based on Ohm's law, current flow (amperes) equals potential (volts) divided by impedance or resistance (ohms). Therefore, current flow during defibrillation depends on the transthoracic impedance or resistance. Increased resistance results in the dissipation of energy due to shunting to the lungs, thoracic cage, and other elements of the chest. Several factors can decrease transthoracic resistance, including larger electrode size, use of electrode-skin coupling material (gel pads, electrodes paste, or self-adhesive defibrillation/monitor pads), increased number of shocks, decreased time interval between shocks, and end-expiratory phase of ventilation.*

## EXPLANATION:

(1) **Correct.** Conductive gel or paste used between the defibrillators and skin decreases transthoracic resistance.
(2) **Correct.** Transthoracic resistance decreases with repeated shocks, increasing current flow to the heart
(3) **Correct.** Defibrillation during end expiration results in the least resistance to flow. This is so because the chest diameter and therefore distance the current must flow to the heart are at a minimum.
(4) **Correct.** The larger the electrodes, the greater is the area of contact for current flow and the lesser is the impedance.

## REASONING:

This question tests knowledge of the effect of transthoracic resistance on electric current flow during defibrillation. Choice 1 is correct because conductive gel should be used to decrease resistance during defibrillation. Because choice 1 is correct, answers C and D can be eliminated. Choice 4 is correct because a larger electrode decreases resistance to flow. Because choices 1 and 4 are correct, the only possible answer choice is E, all choices are correct.

## BIBLIOGRAPHY:


Barash PG, Cullen BF, Stoelting RK, Cahalan MK, Stock MC. *Clinical Anesthesia.* 6th ed. Philadelphia, PA: Lippincott Williams & Wilkins; 2009:1545-1546.
Cummens RO. *Advanced Cardiac Life Support.* Dallas, TX: American Heart Association; 1997:secs. 4.3-4.6.
Morgan GE, Mikhail MS, Murray MJ. *Clinical Anesthesiology.* 4th ed. New York, NY: McGraw-Hill; 2006:987-988.


---

## BOOK A:     QUESTION 14

*Answer A*

Pediatrics

### QUESTION (K-type):

Compared with a healthy 20-year-old, respiratory function in a healthy 1-year-old is characterized by

(1) Greater chest wall compliance.
(2) Lesser lung compliance.
(3) Greater small airway resistance.
(4) Similar functional residual capacity/total lung volume (FRC/TLC) ratio.

### CORRECT ANSWER: A (1, 2, and 3 are correct.)

### SUMMARY:

*The anatomy and physiology of the lungs and chest wall are different and evolving in a neonate and infant compared to an older child and adult. Neonates and infants have less efficient ventilation because of weak intercostal and diaphragmatic musculature (due to a paucity of type I fibers), horizontal and more pliable ribs, and a protuberant abdomen. Accessory respiratory muscles are less effective due to the rib orientation. This improves when the ribs gradually slant downward after the child learns to stand and walk. The chest wall of a neonate is floppy due to high cartilage content, poor musculature development, and incomplete calcification of the ribs. Paradoxical chest movement commonly occurs in children whenever there is an increase in respiratory effort. Prior to 37 weeks' gestational age, diaphragmatic muscles have less than 10% of type I (slow twitch, high oxidative capacity) muscle fibers compared to about 50% in an adult. Along with a higher rate of oxygen consumption, this leads to earlier fatigue.*

**EXPLANATION:**

(1) **Correct.** Neonates and infants have greater chest wall compliance due to weaker intercostal and diaphragmatic muscles, more horizontal rib orientation, pliable ribs, and greater proportion of cartilage versus bone in the ribs.

(2) **Correct.** The small and limited number of alveoli in neonates and infants reduces lung compliance. For the first 3 years of life, alveoli increase in number, but not size. At about 8 years of age, alveolar maturation is complete.

(3) **Correct.** Neonates and infants have less developed small airways, which leads to greater small airways resistance. Resistance in the larger "central airways" is constant in all ages, but resistance in the smaller airways decreases with age. Airway resistance declines markedly with growth from 19 to 28 $cmH_2O/L/s$ in newborns to less than 2 $cmH_2O/L/s$ in adults.

(4) **Incorrect.** FRC per kilogram, about 30 mL/kg, is similar for all ages. The healthy adult has a TLC of 82 mL/kg, while the healthy infant has a TLC of 63 mL/kg. Therefore, the ratio of FRC/TLC is not similar between a 20-year and a 1-year-old. Respiratory parameters that are not age dependent include tidal volume (6-8 cc/kg), dead space to tidal volume ratio (0.3), and FRC.

**REASONING:**

Key concepts for answering this question include understanding respiratory physiology and how it changes with age. Choices 1, 2, and 3 are clearly true because of the anatomy and physiology of the infant lung. Choice 4 can then be eliminated by understanding that adults have a greater volume per kilo of lung capacity. All of the above reasons explain why children desaturate and tire more quickly and have less tolerance for upper and lower respiratory illnesses.

**BIBLIOGRAPHY:**

Cote CJ. *A Practice of Anesthesia for Infants and Children.* 4th ed. Philadelphia, PA: Saunders; 2009:12-15.

Morgan GE, Mikhail MS, Murray MJ. *Clinical Anesthesiology.* 4th ed. New York, NY: McGraw-Hill; 2006:923.

---

**BOOK A:**

*Answer C*

Clinical Anesthesia

**QUESTION 15**

**QUESTION (K-type):**

True statements concerning insertion of a total hip prosthesis with methylmethacrylate cement include the following:

(1) Hypotension is more likely with placement in the acetabulum than with insertion in the femoral shaft.
(2) Absorbed volatile monomer causes vasodilation.
(3) A deliberate hypotensive technique is contraindicated.
(4) Arterial hemoglobin desaturation may result from fat embolization.

**CORRECT ANSWER: C (2 and 4 are correct.)**

**SUMMARY:**

*Methylmethacrylate cement is used to bind prosthetic devices to bone. Mixing the liquid and powder methylmethacrylate together causes an exothermic reaction that results in cement hardening. As it hardens, the cement expands against the prosthesis and within the bone, resulting in intramedullary hypertension (> 500 mm Hg) that may cause embolization of fat, bone marrow, cement, or air into the venous system. This bone cement implantation syndrome manifests clinically as hypoxemia, dysrhythmias, pulmonary hypertension, or decreased cardiac output. The monomer can also cause vasodilation and hypotension. Regional anesthesia and postoperative analgesia is preferred by many to decrease blood loss, risk of thromboembolism, and increase mobility. Controlled hypotension can decrease intraoperative blood loss and can be useful, especially in revision arthroplasty that may be associated with greater blood loss.*

**EXPLANATION:**

(1) ***Incorrect.*** Hypotension due to fat or bone marrow embolization is more likely with insertion in the femoral shaft than the acetabulum presumably because there is more marrow in the former.

(2) ***Correct.*** Residual methylmethacrylate monomer can cause vasodilation and decreased systemic vascular resistance (SVR).

(3) ***Incorrect.*** Controlled hypotensive anesthetic technique is indicated because it reduces blood loss by 30% to 50%. Controlled epidural anesthesia with a mean MAP of 50 to 60 mm Hg decreases blood loss to about 200 mL, improves prosthetic cementing, and decreases the duration of surgery.

(4) ***Correct.*** Arterial desaturation can result from fat or bone marrow embolization at the time of cementing and has been reported up to 5 days postoperatively.

**REASONING:**

Key concepts for answering this question are understanding the surgical issues with total hip arthroplasty and the potential problems using methylmethacrylate. Understanding the bone cement implantation syndrome, the reader should be able to verify that choices 2 and 4 are correct. Understanding the indications and advantages of a deliberate hypotensive anesthetic technique, the reader should be able to eliminate choice 3. Choice 1 can therefore be eliminated along with choice 3 even if the reader does not know whether hypotension is more likely with acetabulum placement or femoral shaft insertion.

**BIBLIOGRAPHY:**
Miller, 7th ed, pg 2251-2252.
Morgan GE, Mikhail MS, Murray MJ. *Clinical Anesthesiology.* 4th ed. New York, NY: McGraw-Hill; 2006:848-856.

---

**BOOK A:**      **QUESTION 16 (OPTIONAL)**

*Answer B*

Cardiovascular

**QUESTION (K-type):**

True statements concerning *direct* ventricular defibrillation during cardiopulmonary bypass include the following:

(1) Shocks greater than 30 J are associated with myocardial damage.
(2) Hypokalemia increases the chance of defibrillation.
(3) Myocardial impedance decreases after a single shock.
(4) Thin-walled ventricles defibrillate more easily than hypertrophied ventricles.

**CORRECT ANSWER: B (1 and 3 are correct.)**

**SUMMARY:**

*Direct ventricular defibrillation usually can be achieved with 5 to 10 J. Up to 60 J can be used, but higher and repeated defibrillations can be associated with myocardial injury.*

*Success with defibrillation can be improved by correcting any pH, blood gas, or electro-
lyte abnormalities and by ensuring adequate myocardial rewarming. Potassium at a high-
normal level favors defibrillation.*

### EXPLANATION:

(1) ***Correct.*** The higher energy levels used for direct defibrillation can lead to myocardial injury.
(2) ***Incorrect.*** Hypokalemia decreases the likelihood of defibrillation.
(3) ***Correct.*** Resistance to the electric current flow is decreased after the initial shock.
(4) ***Incorrect.*** Lake and colleagues studied energy dose and other variables that affect direct ventricular fibrillation during open-heart surgery in a cohort of 150 adult cardiac patients. They found that heart weight and thickness of ventricular myocardium appeared to be less important factors in direct defibrillation. The only exception was during low (1 J) shocks, where thinner-walled ventricles appeared to defibrillate more easily. Given that most delivered shocks are greater than 1 J and that choices 1 and 3 are correct, this statement must be incorrect.

### REASONING:

This is a somewhat challenging question that tests knowledge of direct ventricular defibrillation. It may not be entirely clear to the reader that thin-walled ventricles do not defibrillate more easily than hypertrophied ventricles. Indeed, there are some data in the literature to suggest that thin-walled ventricles defibrillate more easily when 1-J shocks are delivered. However, choice 1 is correct, and choice 2 is clearly incorrect. By the process of elimination, B (choices 1 and 3) is the best answer.

### BIBLIOGRAPHY:

Barash PG, Cullen BF, Stoelting RK, Cahalan MK, Stock MC. *Clinical Anesthesia*. 6th ed. Philadelphia, PA: Lippincott Williams & Wilkins; 2009:1095-1097.

Kaplan, JA, Reich DL, Konstadt SN. Cardiac Anesthesia. 6th ed. Philadelphia, PA: Saunders; 2011:1617, chap 32.

Lake CL, Sellers TD, Nolan SP, et al. Energy dose and other variables possibly affecting ventricular defibrillation during cardiac surgery. *Anesth Analg*. 1984;63:743-751.

---

| **BOOK A:** | **QUESTION 17** |
| --- | --- |

## *Answer C*

## Clinical Anesthesia

### QUESTION (K-type):

The indications for administration of fresh frozen plasma include

(1) Acute volume expansion in a hypovolemic patient.
(2) Bleeding in a patient with a normal activated clotting time after cardiopulmonary bypass.
(3) Transfusion of 6 units of red blood cells in a 70-kg patient.
(4) Bleeding in a patient with a prolonged bleeding time and abnormal factor VIII.

### CORRECT ANSWER: C (2 and 4 are correct.)

### SUMMARY:

*Fresh frozen plasma (FFP) contains all plasma proteins, which includes all the clotting
factors. The American Society of Anesthesiologist Task Force in 2006 recommended that
FFP be indicated for (1) correction of excessive microvascular bleeding in the presence*

### EXPLANATION:

(1) *Incorrect.* FFP is not indicated for acute volume expansion in a hypovolemic patient. FFP carries the same infectious risk as a unit of whole blood and can cause transfusion reactions.
(2) *Correct.* Routine prophylactic administration of FFP is not indicated for patients after cardiopulmonary bypass. However, FFP should be administered in a patient actively bleeding with a normal activated clotting time after cardiopulmonary bypass.
(3) *Incorrect.* Transfusion of 6 units of red blood cells in a 70-kg patient would not be considered a massive transfusion that would be 5 L or more in this patient.
(4) *Correct.* FFP is indicated in treatment of clotting factor deficiencies and prolonged bleeding time because it contains all clotting factors.

### REASONING:

This question tests knowledge of the criteria for transfusion of FFP. Choice 1 is incorrect because FFP is not used for volume expansion, eliminating answers A, B, and E. Because FFP contains clotting factors, choice 4 is obviously correct. FFP is indicated in a patient who is persistently bleeding after cardiopulmonary bypass despite heparin neutralization, making C the best answer.

### BIBLIOGRAPHY:

Barash PG, Cullen BF, Stoelting RK, Cahalan MK, Stock MC. *Clinical Anesthesia.* 6th ed. Philadelphia, PA: Lippincott Williams & Wilkins; 2009:380-381.
Kaplan JA, Reich DL, Savino JS. *Cardiac Anesthesia.* 6th ed. St. Louis, MO: Elsevier Saunders; 2011:983-984.

---

**BOOK A:**        **QUESTION 18**

---

*Answer E*

Neuroanesthesia

### QUESTION (K-type):

Immediately after sustaining a traumatic cord transection with a T4 level, a patient requires emergency laparotomy. Disease-related factors affecting anesthetic management include

(1) Venous pooling.
(2) Hypothermia.
(3) Decreased peripheral vascular resistance.
(4) Decreased alveolar ventilation.

### CORRECT ANSWER: E (All are correct.)

### SUMMARY:

*Spinal cord injury after trauma affects approximately 10,000 Americans per year and has significant bearing on the acute and chronic anesthetic management of patients. Acute injury at the T4 level can influence the respiratory, cardiovascular, and thermoregulatory* *systems markedly. Many of the hemodynamic changes that result from spinal cord injury can be explained by damage to the T1-L2 region of the sympathetic nervous system. T1-T4 lesions will eliminate sympathetic innervations of the heart leading to bradycardia. Loss of sympathetic tone from this area of the cord results in loss of vascular tone with venous pooling, loss of peripheral vascular resistance, and hypotension. Lesions at or above the T7 level often cause hypoventilation and hypoxia secondary to reduction in vital capacity (VC), forced expiratory volume in 1 second (FEV$_1$), expiratory reserve volume (ERV), and paralysis or impairment of intercostal muscle function. Thermoregulatory function is also impaired because of injured sympathetic pathways to the hypothalamic center.*

### EXPLANATION:

(1) ***Correct.*** Venous pooling is a likely result of injury to segments between T1-L2. This is secondary to loss of sympathetic tone and vasodilation.

(2) ***Correct.*** Hypothermia results secondary to loss of sympathetic relay to the hypothalamic regulatory center.

(3) ***Correct.*** Loss of sympathetic tone to the vasculature results in loss of peripheral vascular resistance and orthostatic hypotension.

(4) ***Correct.*** A lesion at T7 or higher can cause significant alteration in respiratory function with decreased alveolar ventilation.

### REASONING:

Knowledge of physiologic changes that occur during acute spinal cord injury is required to answer this question correctly. Knowing that loss of sympathetic outflow to the vasculature occurs with a lesion at this level makes choices 1 and 3 correct. Also, remembering that these patients become hypothermic in the operating room (OR) due to poor thermoregulation and that we must take measures to prevent this makes choice 2 correct. Significant respiratory compromise occurs at lesions above T7 that can lead to alveolar hypoventilation and hypoxia.

### BIBLIOGRAPHY:

Miller RD, Miller ED, Reves JG, et al. *Anesthesia.* 7th ed. New York, NY: Churchill Livingstone; 2009:297-298, 2299.

Morgan GE, Mikhail MS, Murray MJ. *Clinical Anesthesiology.* 4th ed. New York, NY: McGraw-Hill; 2006:867.

---

**BOOK A:**  **QUESTION 19**

---

*Answer B*

Pain

### QUESTION (K-type):

Trigeminal neuralgia is characterized by

(1) Unilateral, intense, paroxysmal pain of sudden onset.
(2) Diminished sensation in the distribution of the maxillary division of the trigeminal nerve.
(3) Normal function of the glossopharyngeal nerve.
(4) Resolution of symptoms by injection of local anesthetic at trigger points.

### CORRECT ANSWER: B (1 and 3 are correct.)

### SUMMARY:

*Trigeminal neuralgia (tic douloureux) is a chronic disorder characterized as a sudden, severe, usually unilateral, brief, stabbing, recurrent pain in the distribution of one or more branches of the fifth cranial nerve. Glossopharyngeal nerve function is typically normal. Examination shows that over 50% of patients may have at least one abnormal measure of sensation, not only in the trigger zone division but also in the adjacent division. Trigger point injections are not used for trigeminal neuralgia.*

### EXPLANATION:

Patients with trigeminal neuralgia suffer from chronic recurrent paroxysmal unilateral lancinating pains. Some patients complain of a constant, burning, gnawing pain in the same distribution. This is referred to by some as atypical or nonclassic trigeminal neuralgia. Once radiologic and surgical investigations have excluded causes such as multiple sclerosis and other structural abnormalities, the cause is thought to be due to arterial cross-compression of the trigeminal nerve at its exit from the brain stem. Glossopharyngeal neuralgia is an uncommon cause of facial pain. Injection of trigger points is not done for trigeminal neuralgia, but some patients have defined "trigger zones." These are areas that are not painful, but when touched, they will trigger the patient's typical pain.

### REASONING:

Choice 1 is correct as trigeminal neuralgia is characterized by "unilateral, intense, paroxysmal pain of sudden onset." Diminished sensation in the distribution of the maxillary division can occur but certainly does not characterize trigeminal neuralgia and so choice 2 is incorrect. Glossopharyngeal function is characteristically normal and therefore choice 3 is correct. Choice 4 is incorrect; trigger point injections are not used in trigeminal neuralgia.

### BIBLIOGRAPHY:

McMahon SB, Koltzenburg M. *Wall and Melzack's Textbook of Pain.* 5th ed. Philadelphia, PA: Churchill Livingstone; 2006:1001-1008.

Morgan GE, Mikhail MS, Murray MJ. *Clinical Anesthesiology.* 4th ed. New York, NY: McGraw-Hill; 2006:408-409.

---

**BOOK A:**      **QUESTION 20**

---

*Answer E*

Physiology

### QUESTION (K-type):

During general anesthesia in a healthy patient, hypothermia to 33°C results in

(1) Prolongation of vecuronium action.
(2) Protection against cerebral ischemia.
(3) Potentiation of isoflurane.
(4) Increased risk for ventricular dysrhythmias.

### CORRECT ANSWER: E (All are correct.)

### SUMMARY:

*Mild hypothermia is associated with many adverse and few positive effects. Hypothermia causes (1) coagulopathy, increasing the need for transfusions, (2) increased susceptibility to surgical wound infections, (3) prolonged recovery from anesthesia, (4) increased incidence of ventricular dysrhythmias and cardiac events, and (5) decreased metabolism of most drugs, including anesthetic agents and muscle relaxants. On the positive side, hypothermia provides a measure of protection against cerebral and cardiac ischemia and may help in recovery from ARDS.*

**EXPLANATION:**

(1) ***Correct.*** Hypothermia prolongs the action of muscle relaxants by decreasing metabolism and excretion.

(2) ***Correct.*** Hypothermia protects against cerebral ischemia by lowering $CMRO_2$. The potential protection afforded by mild hypothermia is so great that reduced core temperature (ie, ≈34°C) is increasingly being used during neurosurgery and other procedures in which tissue ischemia can be anticipated. The difficulty is that there are currently few outcome data substantiating an extrapolation from animal data to clinical practice. Furthermore, the appropriate target temperature for therapeutic hypothermia has yet to be established.

(3) ***Correct.*** Hypothermia decreases minimum alveolar concentration (MAC) requirements for all potent inhalational agents.

(4) ***Correct.*** Even mild hypothermia triples the incidence of ventricular dysrhythmias and cardiac events.


**REASONING:**

This question tests knowledge of the physiologic effects of hypothermia. Hypothermia can cause multisystem physiologic derangements and contribute to perioperative morbidity. The reader should review these effects carefully. All the choices are well-known effects of hypothermia; therefore, E is the correct answer.


**BIBLIOGRAPHY:**


Miller RD, Miller ED, Reves JG, et al. *Anesthesia.* 7th ed. Philadelphia, PA: Churchill Livingstone; 2010:1542-1544.

Morgan GE, Mikhail MS, Murray MJ. *Clinical Anesthesiology.* 3rd ed. New York, NY: McGraw-Hill; 2002:117, 136, 189.

Sessler DI. Mild perioperative hypothermia. *N Engl J Med.* 1997;24:1730-1737.


---

| **BOOK A:** | **QUESTION 21** |
| --- | --- |

*Answer B*

OB/Regional

**QUESTION (K-type):**

Factors that decrease the incidence of deep vein thrombosis (DVT) following total hip replacement include

(1) External compression of the lower extremities.
(2) Epidural anesthesia intraoperatively.
(3) Prophylactic aspirin.
(4) Deliberate hypotension intraoperatively.


**CORRECT ANSWER: B (1 and 3 are correct.)**


**SUMMARY:**

*Several studies have looked at the use of external compression devices on the rate of DVT after hip surgery with conflicting results. A recent literature review supports the significant, but small, effect of mechanical compression in DVT prevention, but does not advocate their use alone for this purpose. Also, a recent meta-analysis of available studies demonstrated that these devices augment the thromboprophylactic effect of pharmacologic agents. Meta-analysis of all available data seems to indicate that regional anesthesia does reduce the rate of DVT after hip surgery, but many of these studies were done before chemical prophylaxis was routine, and studies comparing intraoperative epidural, as opposed to all regional techniques, with general anesthesia for hip surgery have found no significant decrease in the rate of postoperative DVT formation. Hoek and colleagues found a post-operative DVT rate of 37% for the epidural group and 36% for general anesthesia. Another prospective, randomized trial also confirmed their observation. The largest clinical trial to date, the Pulmonary Embolism Prevention (PEP) trial, found that aspirin prophylaxis reduced the risk of pulmonary embolism (PE) and DVT by almost one-third in patients undergoing hip replacement surgery, although the difference was only true for those also given low-molecular-weight heparin (LMWH), but not against placebo when given alone.*

### EXPLANATION:

(1) **Correct.** External compression devices of the lower extremities have been shown to reduce the incidence of DVT following total hip replacement surgery, both when compared to placebo and when used in combination with chemical thromboprophylaxis.

(2) **Incorrect.** While regional techniques have been shown to decrease DVT incidence after hip surgery, the evidence supporting epidural anesthesia for DVT prevention is lacking. A prospective, randomized trial comparing general anesthesia with general anesthesia plus intraoperative epidural found no statistical difference in the rate of postoperative DVT following hip replacement surgery. These results corroborate previous findings.

(3) **Correct.** The Sixth ACCP Consensus Conference on Anticoagulation did not recommend aspirin as the sole therapy for DVT prophylaxis following hip replacement surgery (grade 1A recommendation). However, a recent meta-analysis of over 17,000 patients found that patients who received perioperative aspirin prophylaxis (160 mg for up to 35 days postoperatively) had at least one-third reduction in risk of PE and DVT, a difference that was significant only for those also given LMWH.

(4) **Incorrect.** A prospective, randomized trial comparing intraoperative hypotension, not using neuraxial techniques, versus normotensive anesthesia showed no difference in the incidence of DVT following hip replacement surgery.

### REASONING:

This question is challenging because there are conflicting data in the literature regarding the effects of prophylactic aspirin and incidence of DVT. Most people would have confidence in choice 1, and thus choice 3 also must be correct, regardless of the conflicting data. The best answer is B.

### BIBLIOGRAPHY:


Dauphin A, Raymer KE, Stanton EB, Fuller HD. Comparison of general anesthesia with and without lumbar epidural for total hip arthroplasty: effects of epidural block on hip arthroplasty. *J Clin Anesth*. 1997;9:200-203.

Fredin H, Gustafson C, Rosberg B. Hypotensive anesthesia, thromboprophylaxis and postoperative thromboembolism in total hip arthroplasty. *Acta Anaesthesiol Scand*. 1984;28:503-507.

Hoek JA, Henny CP, Knipscheer HC, et al. The effect of different anaesthetic techniques on the incidence of thrombosis following total hip replacement. *Thromb Haemost*. 1991;65(2):122-125.

Hu S, Zhang ZY, Hua YQ, et al. A comparison of regional and general anaesthesia for total replacement of the hip or knee. *J Bone Joint Surg Br*. 2009;91-B:935-942.

Kakkos, SK, Warwick D, Nicolaides AN, et al. Combined (mechanical and pharmacological) modalities for the prevention of venous thromboembolism in joint replacement surgery. *J Bone Joint Surg Br*. 2012;94-B:729-734.

Marsland D, Mears SC, Kates L. Venous thromboembolic prophylaxis for hip fractures. *Osteoporos Int*. 2010;21(suppl 4):S593-S604.

Parker MJ, Handoll HHG, Griffiths R. Anaesthesia for hip fracture surgery in adults. *Cochrane Database Syst Rev*. 2004;(4):CD000521. doi: 10.1002/14651858.CD000521.pub2.

Prevention of pulmonary embolism and deep vein thrombosis with low dose aspirin: Pulmonary Embolism Prevention (PEP) trial. *Lancet*. 2000;355:1295-1302.

*Answer B*

Pharmacology

**QUESTION (K-type):**

Ketamine administered in anesthetic doses

(1) Increases intracranial pressure.
(2) Does not cause respiratory depression.
(3) Is eliminated by hepatic metabolism.
(4) Increases bronchomotor tone.

**CORRECT ANSWER: B (1 and 3 are correct)**

**SUMMARY:**

*Ketamine is a unique nonopioid analgesic/hypnotic/amnestic agent. It induces a state of dissociative anesthesia and is unique because of its minimal effects on respiration. It is also the only intravenous induction agent that has stimulatory effects on the cardiovascular system.*

**EXPLANATION:**

(1) *Correct.* Ketamine is well known to increase cerebral blood flow and subsequently increase intracranial and cerebrospinal fluid (CSF) pressures. There are conflicting reports on the effect of ketamine on intraocular pressure, but it generally should be avoided for penetrating eye injuries.
(2) *Incorrect.* Although the customary induction dose of ketamine does not minimally affect ventilator drive, rapid IV bolus administration or pretreatment with opioids occasionally produces apnea.
(3) *Correct.* Ketamine is converted to norketamine through hydroxylation and demethylation by the liver. Factors that reduce hepatic blood flow, such as halothane, also prolong the effects of ketamine by impairing elimination.
(4) *Incorrect.* Ketamine has well-documented bronchodilatory properties and has been used to induce anesthesia in patients with reactive airways diseases such as asthma. Bronchodilatory effects of ketamine reflect a decrease in bronchomotor tone.

**REASONING:**

This question tests knowledge of the pharmacology of ketamine. Most readers will recognize immediately that choice 1 is true. Choice 2 is often considered true although review of textbooks shows that respiratory effects may occur, leading them to conclude that choice 3 is also true even if the reader is unsure of the elimination mechanism. Choice 4 is obviously false if the reader is familiar with the meaning of *bronchomotor tone (bronchoconstriction).*

**BIBLIOGRAPHY:**

Barash PG, Cullen BF, Stoelting RK. *Clinical Anesthesia.* 4th ed. Philadelphia, PA: Lippincott Williams & Wilkins; 2001:327-328.
Morgan GE, Mikhail MS, Murray MJ. *Clinical Anesthesiology.* 4th ed. New York, NY: McGraw-Hill; 2006:197-199.

*Answer A*

Clinical Anesthesia

**QUESTION (K-type):**

During laser excision of a sublaryngeal tumor, the risk of airway ignition would be decreased by using

(1)  Water-based lubricants.
(2)  Jet ventilation without an endotracheal tube.
(3)  Saline solution in the endotracheal tube cuff.
(4)  Nitrous oxide.

**CORRECT ANSWER: A (1, 2, and 3 are correct.)**

**SUMMARY:**

*A major hazard of laser airway surgery is fire. Endotracheal tubes (ETTs) can burn, particularly in the oxygen-enriched environment of the operating field. Nitrous also supports combustion. Thus it is imperative to reduce the amount of oxygen as much as possible, ideally under 30%, and to avoid the use of $N_2O$. Other methods to reduce the risk of airway fire include nonintubation techniques such as jet ventilation; periods of apnea and spontaneous breathing; conventional tubes with protection such as metallic tape wrapping and saline in the cuff; and laser-resistant tubes. Other measures include using saline-soaked pledgets and limiting laser use and power.*

**EXPLANATION:**

(1)  ***Correct.*** Lubricants should be water-based to reduce risk of ignition.
(2)  ***Correct.*** Attached to the operating laryngoscope is a device that allows jet ventilation during breaks from laser operation.
(3)  ***Correct.*** If laser or fire should break the cuff, the water will help douse the flames.
(4)  ***Incorrect.*** Nitrous supports combustion and should not be used.

**REASONING:**

This question is K-type. Choice 4 is clearly incorrect as nitrous increases the risk of airway fire. Choice 2 is one of several techniques that can be used to ventilate the patient having laser airway surgery. If choice 2 is true and 4 has been eliminated, 1 and 3 must also be true. The addition of water to the field helps reduce the risk of ignition.

**BIBLIOGRAPHY:**

Morgan GE, Mikhail MS, Murray MJ. *Clinical Anesthesiology.* 4th ed. New York, NY: McGraw-Hill; 2006:839-840.
Upper airway management guide provided for laser airway surgery. Anesthesia Patient Safety Foundation Newsletter. 8(2), Summer 1993.

## Answer D

## Physiology

**QUESTION (K-type):**

A 24-year-old patient with hypertension and hypercalcemia is scheduled for a parathyroidectomy. Serum calcium concentration may be decreased by the administration of

(1)  A calcium channel blocker.
(2)  Magnesium sulfate.
(3)  Sodium bicarbonate.
(4)  Vigorous volume expansion.

**CORRECT ANSWER: D (4 only is correct.)**

**SUMMARY:**

*This question is testing your knowledge of the treatment of hypercalcemia. Treatment of hypercalcemia consists of establishing a diuresis with volume expansion and a loop diuretic, bisphosphonate, calcitonin, and, in certain cases, plicamycin or corticosteroids.*

**EXPLANATION:**

(1)  *Incorrect.* The addition of calcium channel blocker is not only not advocated for hypercalcemia but would do nothing to the serum calcium concentration.
(2)  *Incorrect.* Magnesium would not reduce serum calcium concentration. This is a distracter answer to catch your attention based on the often-antagonistic effects of calcium and magnesium. For example, hypermagnesemia can temporarily be treated with IV calcium.
(3)  *Incorrect.* Hyperventilation will cause a respiratory alkalosis. This may result in a decrease in ionized calcium as serum proteins bind more calcium. However, the total serum calcium remains unchanged. Only the fraction of calcium that is bound changes.
(4)  *Correct.* Vigorous volume expansion with saline dilutes serum calcium and the sodium increases renal calcium clearance by inhibiting renal tubular calcium absorption. Patients with severe hypercalcemia are often profoundly dehydrated and in need of aggressive rehydration, if concomitant renal or heart failure present consider urgent dialysis.

**REASONING:**

This question is an example of a question with a variety of "distracter" answers. Calcium channel blockers and magnesium administration do nothing to serum calcium. However, they sound like they might have some vague "anticalcium effect." Similarly, hyperventilation can induce signs of hypocalcemia such as tetany by lowering ionized calcium, but it does not affect total serum calcium. The only choice that reduces calcium levels is vigorous volume expansion, by diluting serum calcium and increasing renal calcium clearance.

**BIBLIOGRAPHY:**

Hines RL, Marschall KE. Stoelting's Anesthesia and Co-existing Disease. 5th ed. Philadelphia, PA: Churchill Livingstone; 2008:399-400.

Morgan GE, Mikhail MS, Murray MJ. *Clinical Anesthesiology*. 4th ed. New York, NY: McGraw-Hill; 2006:684.

*Answer A*

Physiology

## QUESTION (K-type):

Effects of open cholecystectomy under general anesthesia with mechanical ventilation include

(1)  Increased intrapulmonary shunting.
(2)  Decreased lung volumes up to 48 hours postoperatively.
(3)  Decreased FRC.
(4)  Decreased dead space.

## CORRECT ANSWER: A (1, 2, and 3 are correct.)

## SUMMARY:

*Positive-pressure ventilation, supine positioning, and general anesthesia have a number of adverse effects on pulmonary mechanics. These include increased intrapulmonary shunting, decreased vital capacity, decreased FRC, and increased dead space. These changes are accentuated by upper abdominal surgery and may persist for days. These changes are offset in the OR by increased delivered $F_{IO_2}$ and increased minute ventilation.*

## EXPLANATION:

Spontaneous ventilation in the supine position decreases FRC by 10% to 15%, while general anesthesia produces a further 5% to 10% decrease in FRC, and this in turn results in increased intrapulmonary shunting as blood continues to perfuse unventilated regions. This is augmented by the impairment in hypoxic pulmonary vasoconstriction (HPV) that accompanies general anesthesia. Decreased lung volumes including vital capacity and FRC remain depressed for 10 to 14 days following upper abdominal surgery with general anesthesia. PEEP or continuous positive airway pressure (CPAP) in the postoperative period will reverse these anesthesia-induced decreases in lung volumes, but as soon as PEEP or CPAP is stopped, these lung volumes will promptly decrease again. Positive-pressure ventilation increases dead space by increasing alveolar dead space. This change occurs because ventilation increases relative to perfusion of nondependent alveoli under general anesthesia.

## REASONING:

Choice 4 is incorrect as dead space increases rather than decreases, as outlined above. Choices 1, 2, and 3 are correct. Therefore, choice A is correct.

## BIBLIOGRAPHY:

Barash PG, Cullen BF, Stoelting RK, Cahalan MK, Stock MC. *Clinical Anesthesia*. 6th ed. Philadelphia, PA: Lippincott Williams & Wilkins; 2009:252.

Morgan GE, Mikhail MS, Murray MJ. *Clinical Anesthesiology*. 4th ed. New York, NY: McGraw-Hill; 2006:551-557.

Stoelting RK, Dierdorf SF. *Anesthesia and Co-existing Disease*. 3rd ed. New York, NY: Churchill Livingstone; 1993:142.

*Answer C*

Pediatrics

**QUESTION (K-type):**

Features of the neonate's prompt adjustment to extrauterine life include

(1) Lung expansion resulting in increased pulmonary vascular resistance.
(2) Nonshivering thermogenesis as a response to cold stress.
(3) Anatomic closure of the ductus arteriosus.
(4) Initial expansion of airless collapsed lungs by creation of negative pressures of 40 to 80 cmH$_2$O.

**CORRECT ANSWER: C (2 and 4 are correct.)**

**SUMMARY:**

*Many physiologic changes occur at birth to allow the neonate to adapt to extrauterine life. In utero, the fetal lungs contain 90 mL of plasma ultrafiltrate that is normally squeezed out during vaginal birth. This is not absolutely necessary for normal respirations after birth as evidenced by successful births after cesarean deliveries. Fluid that remains is normally absorbed by the pulmonary capillaries and lymphatics. Transient tachypnea of the newborn is the self-limiting condition in which there is residual fluid in the lungs for 24 to 72 hours. This is manifested by tachypnea and chest x-ray findings of perihilar markings, fluid in the fissures, and streaky linear opacities in the parenchyma. Increased arterial oxygen content from expanded lungs decreases pulmonary vascular resistance (PVR) that leads to increased pulmonary blood flow and increased blood return to the left atrium. Elevated left atrial pressures (LAPs) help close the foramen ovale. Decreased PVR along with increased oxygen tensions functionally closes the ductus arteriosus resulting in adult circulation. Hypoxia or acidosis during the first few days of life can prevent or reverse these physiological changes, resulting in persistence of (or return to) the fetal circulation, or persistent pulmonary hypertension of the newborn (PPHN).*

**EXPLANATION:**

(1) *Incorrect.* Lung expansion at birth increases both alveolar and arterial oxygen tension and results in decreased PVR. The increase in oxygen tension is a potent pulmonary arterial vasodilator. The rapid drop in PVR starts from the first 5 minutes of life and takes 3 to 4 days to decrease to normal levels.
(2) *Correct.* The neonate has a large body surface area to weight ratio and is at risk for significant heat loss. They also do not shiver or sweat effectively to maintain body temperature. During the first 3 months of life, nonshivering thermogenesis (metabolism of brown fat) is the primary mechanism of heat production. However, metabolism of brown fat is severely limited in premature infants and in sick neonates who are deficient in fat stores.
(3) *Incorrect.* The ductus arteriosus functionally closes when pulmonary arterial pressure decreases to less than systemic arterial pressure, and there is increased arterial oxygen content. The ductus may not anatomically close until the full-term neonate is 2 to 3 weeks old.
(4) *Correct.* The initial expansion of airless collapsed lungs requires a gasp that generates negative pressures of 40 to 80 cmH$_2$O. This is how much transpulmonary pressure that is required to distend the lungs that have up till then been filled with lung fluid.

**REASONING:**

Key concepts for answering this question include understanding the physiologic and anatomic changes with the fetus during and after birth. One should be able to recognize that choices 1 and 3 are incorrect. Both attempt to deceive, but the reader should know that PVR decreases at birth. The reader may be deceived by the term anatomic closure versus functional closure but should remember that sometimes patients require surgery to ligate a patent ductus arteriosus. Choices 2 and 4 are reasonable and logical.

**BIBLIOGRAPHY:**

Barash PG, Cullen BF, Stoelting RK, Cahalan MK, Stock MC. *Clinical Anesthesia.* 6th ed. Philadelphia, PA: Lippincott Williams & Wilkins; 2009:1183.

Cote CJ. A *Practice of Anesthesia for Infants and Children.* 4th ed. Philadelphia, PA: Saunders; 2009:13, 751.

Morgan GE, Mikhail MS, Murray MJ. *Clinical Anesthesiology.* 4th ed. New York, NY: McGraw-Hill; 2006:885-887.

---

**BOOK A:**
**QUESTION 27**

---

*Answer D*

OB/Regional

**QUESTION (K-type):**

Landmarks used in performing a superior laryngeal nerve block include the

(1)  Transverse process of C6.
(2)  Cricoid cartilage.
(3)  Angle of the mandible.
(4)  Greater cornu of the hyoid cartilage.

**CORRECT ANSWER: D (4 only is correct.)**

**SUMMARY:**

*Superior laryngeal nerve block is used to anesthetize the airway for awake intubations. The superior laryngeal nerve is a branch of the vagus (CN X) nerve and divides into an external (motor) branch and internal (sensory) branch, which provides motor innervation to the cricothyroid muscle and sensory innervation to the larynx from the epiglottis to the level of the vocal cords. After it branches off the vagus nerve, the superior laryngeal nerve courses through the neck, passes caudal to the greater cornu of the hyoid cartilage, and enters the thyrohyoid membrane. The block is performed by finding the greater cornu of the hyoid cartilage with your needle and walking caudad until it just slips off the bone, penetrating the thyrohyoid membrane.*

**EXPLANATION:**

(1)  *Incorrect.* The transverse process of C6, the cricoid cartilage, and the angle of the mandible are not used as landmarks for the superior laryngeal nerve block.
(2)  *Incorrect.* See above.
(3)  *Incorrect.* See above.
(4)  *Correct.* The greater cornu of the hyoid bone is the only landmark used for the superior laryngeal nerve block.

**REASONING:**

This question tests knowledge of the upper airway nerves and performing a superior laryngeal nerve block. Knowing that the superior laryngeal nerve block is used for awake intubations and that the nerve supplies sensory innervation to the larynx from the epiglottis to the vocal cords should allow you to eliminate choices 1 and 2 as those landmarks are too caudal. Answer D is the only possibility.

**BIBLIOGRAPHY:**

Brown DL. *Atlas of Regional Anesthesia.* 3rd ed. Philadelphia, PA; Elsevier Saunders, 2006, pp. 221-222.

Morgan GE, Mikhail MS, Murray MJ. *Clinical Anesthesiology.* 4th ed. New York, NY: McGraw-Hill; 2006:269, 877.

---

**BOOK A:**

*Answer E*

Clinical Anesthesia

## QUESTION 28

**QUESTION (K-type):**

Blood products that transmit viruses include

(1)  Factor IX concentrate.
(2)  Plasma protein fraction.
(3)  Cryoprecipitate.
(4)  Albumin.

**CORRECT ANSWER: E (All are correct.)**

**SUMMARY:**

*Despite improvements in routine testing and pasteurization of certain blood products, transfusion of products derived from human plasma carries the risk of transmitting infectious diseases such as viruses or prions. All products transferred from one person to another carry the risk of transmitting infection.*

**EXPLANATION:**

(1)  **Correct.** Factor IX concentrate is used to treat patients with deficiencies in factor IX such as hemophilia B. It is derived from human plasma and has potential for infection.
(2)  **Correct.** Plasma protein fraction is used for plasma volume expansion and is also derived from human plasma. It contains albumin plus $\alpha$ and $\beta$ globulins.
(3)  **Correct.** Cryoprecipitate is derived from plasma and contains factor VIII, the von Willebrand factor, fibrinogen, fibronectin, and factor XIII.
(4)  **Correct.** Albumin and plasma protein fraction are pasteurized, heated at 60°C for 10 hours to minimize the risk of transmission of viruses. They have an excellent safety record in the United States with only one reported case of hepatitis B virus transmission after albumin transfusion and no cases of hepatitis C or human immunodeficiency virus. However, the risk of transmission of other viruses such as parvovirus B19 is still present.

**REASONING:**

The key to answering this question is knowing that any blood product from one person that is given to another can transmit infectious diseases despite improvement in testing and treatment. All the above answer choices are derived from human blood and thus carry a risk of transmitting infectious disease, however minuscule, as in the case of albumin and plasma protein fraction.

**BIBLIOGRAPHY:**

Barash PG, Cullen BF, Stoelting RK, Cahalan MK, Stock MC. *Clinical Anesthesia*. 6th ed. Philadelphia, PA: Lippincott Williams & Wilkins; 2009:370-372, 379-381.

Guertler LG. Virus safety of human blood, plasma, and derived products. *Thromb Res.* 2002;107:S39-S45.

Laub R, Strengers P. Parvoviruses and blood products. *Pathol Biol.* 2002;50:339-348.

---

| **BOOK A:** | **QUESTION 29** |
| --- | --- |

*Answer A*

Clinical Anesthesia

**QUESTION (K-type):**

Compared with heated cascade-type humidifiers, heated nebulizers used for humidification are associated with a greater risk for

(1) Bacterial transmission.
(2) Increased airway resistance.
(3) Water intoxication.
(4) Inspissated secretions in large airways.

**CORRECT ANSWER: A (1, 2, and 3 are correct.)**

**SUMMARY:**

*Heated nebulizers work by passing a jet of gas over water which subsequently entrains some water droplets via the Bernoulli effect. The gas subsequently contains both water vapor and unlike cascade-type humidifiers small droplets. This may result in large quantities of water being delivered with subsequent increased airway resistance (as secretion volume increases), water intoxication, and atelectasis. In addition, these droplets are large enough to suspend microorganisms while the units themselves are difficult to sterilize. Inspissation of secretions is not a significant problem as the devices transfer large amounts of water to the respiratory tract. Heated cascade-type nebulizers have been criticized for some of the same failings, but to a much lesser extent, as they merely add water vapor to respiratory gases to a maximum of 100% humidity at their set temperature, thus attempting to mimic the normal nasal respiratory tract.*

**EXPLANATION:**

(1) **Correct.** Bacterial transmission while a problem with both is considered more serious for the nebulizers.
(2) **Correct.** Increased airway resistance can be a problem with nebulizers through increasing secretion volume.
(3) **Correct.** Water intoxication is more of a problem for nebulizers as more water can be delivered, in the form of added water droplets.
(4) **Incorrect.** Inspissation of secretions is not a problem with the nebulizers. Therefore choice A is correct.

**REASONING:**

A heated cascade-type humidifier works by creating small bubbles from gas to be inspired and passing them through heated water to become fully saturated with water vapor. Risks of use include misconnection as these have one-way check valves, inconsistent efficiency, overheating of gases, and contamination of the unit particularly with *Pseudomonas*. Nonetheless, the nebulizer that delivers not only water vapor but also actual droplets, by creating an aerosolized mist, is considered more likely to transmit bacteria. The nebulizers are so efficient that water overload has been reported, and the large volume of water delivered can increase secretion volume beyond the ability of mucociliary clearance system to clear. This causes increased airway resistance. Inspissation of secretions in the large airways has not been a consistent problem with these devices. Because of their problems, nebulizers have fallen out of favor, and the use of heated cascade-type humidifiers is currently measured against heat and moisture exchangers (HMEs or "artificial nose").

**BIBLIOGRAPHY:**

Ballard K. Cheeseman W. Ripiner T. Wells S. Humidification for ventilated patients. *Intensive Crit Care Nurs.* 1992 Mar;8(1):2-9.

Chamney AR. Humidification requirements and techniques. Including a review of the performance of equipment in current use. *Anaesthesia.* 1969 Oct;24(4):602-617.

Dorsch JA, Dorsch SE. *Understanding Anesthesia Equipment.* 5th ed. Philadelphia, PA: Lippincott Wilkins & Williams; 2008:302-305.

Morgan GE, Mikhail MS, Murray MJ. *Clinical Anesthesiology.* 4th ed. New York, NY: McGraw-Hill; 2006:75-76.

Shelly MP. Lloyd GM. Park GR. A review of the mechanisms and methods of humidification of inspired gases. *Intensive Care Med.* 1988;14(1):1-9.

---

## BOOK A:    QUESTION 30

*Answer C*

OB/Regional

**QUESTION (K-type):**

Landmarks for caudal block include the

(1)  Sciatic notch.
(2)  Posterior-superior iliac spines.
(3)  Iliac crests.
(4)  Sacral cornu.

**CORRECT ANSWER: C (2 and 4 are correct.)**

**SUMMARY:**

*Caudal anesthesia is a commonly used regional technique for pediatric surgery, especially urologic, rectal, and inguinal procedures. It can also be performed in adults and has historical significance in obstetric anesthesia, where it can be especially useful in the second stage of labor. The caudal space is the sacral portion of the epidural space. The procedure is performed with the patient in the prone or lateral position by inserting a needle through the sacral hiatus at a 45-degree angle. A characteristic 'pop" is felt as the needle punctures the sacrococcygeal ligament (a distal extension of the ligamentum flavum) and the angle of the needle is flattened and then advanced. Aspiration for CSF and blood is mandatory. Local anesthetic is injected as a single shot, or a catheter is placed. The technique overall is very safe, but complications can include arrhythmias or seizures from inadvertent intravascular injection, total spinal, intraosseous injection, or damage to the fetal head or maternal rectum when used for obstetrics. The risk of dural puncture is highest in infants and neonates because the dural sac extends to S3 in this population and to S1 in adults.*

**EXPLANATION:**

(1)  *Incorrect.* The greater and lesser sciatic notches are located on the ileum and ischium, respectively. The sciatic nerve exits the pelvis through the greater sciatic notch. Both these notches are located below the gluteus maximus muscle and are not identified easily from the surface because of their depth in the pelvis.

(2) **Correct.** The sacral hiatus can best be identified by palpating the posterior-superior iliac spines, drawing a line between these two points and forming an equilateral triangle. The tip of the triangle will rest on the sacral hiatus. The midpoint between the posterior-superior iliac spines is a useful way to identify the midline of the sacral hiatus.

(3) **Incorrect.** The iliac crests are too superior to be useful landmarks for a caudal block.

(4) **Correct.** The sacral cornua are the lateral borders of the sacral hiatus.

### REASONING:

Determining the correct answer to this question requires knowledge of how a caudal block is performed and the anatomy of the sacrum. The major landmark for this block is the sacral hiatus, so choice 4 is correct. Choice 3 can be eliminated because the iliac crests are too high in the pelvis to serve as effective landmarks for a caudal block. Choice 1 is eliminated because the sciatic notch is not an easily palpable landmark. Choice 2 is correct because identifying the posterosuperior iliac spines can be useful in finding the sacral hiatus. Therefore, C is the best answer.

### BIBLIOGRAPHY:

Chu L, Fuller A. *Manual of Clinical Anesthesia*. Philadelphia, PA: Lippincott Williams and Wilkins. 2011:867-872 (Figure 125-2 Technique for Caudal Block).

Morgan GE, Mikhail MS, Murray MJ. *Clinical Anesthesiology*. 4th ed. New York, NY: McGraw-Hill; 2006:314-316.

Netter FH. *Atlas of Human Anatomy*. Summit, NJ: Ciba-Geigy Corporation; 1994, plates 457, 465.

---

| **BOOK A:** | **QUESTION 31** |
|---|---|

## *Answer C*

Physiology

### QUESTION (K-type):

Changes in pulmonary function associated with advanced age include

(1) Decreased lung compliance.
(2) Increased alveolar dead space.
(3) Decreased FRC.
(4) Decreased maximum voluntary ventilation.

**CORRECT ANSWER: C (2 and 4 are correct.)**

### SUMMARY:

*Reduced lung elasticity and recoil secondary to a decrease of elastin in lung tissue is the most profound effect of age on lung physiology, causing premature closure of small airways on expiration. Elderly lung tissue is more compliant (stretches more easily with volume expansion) yet exhibits decreased alveolar surface area available for effective gas exchange. These changes result in an increase in alveolar dead space, as well as FRC. Maximum voluntary ventilation (MVV) or forced vital capacity is decreased in patients owing to the loss of elastic recoil.*

### EXPLANATION:

(1) **Incorrect.** Elderly patients exhibit calcific chest walls leading to decreased thoracic (not lung) compliance. Structural changes in the lung with aging include the loss of elastic recoil after reorganization of collagen and elastin in lung parenchyma.

This loss of elastic recoil combined with altered surfactant production leads to an increase in lung compliance.

(2) **Correct.** Lung parenchyma in elderly patients exhibits decreased alveolar surface area available for effective gas exchange, leading to increased alveolar dead space.
(3) **Incorrect.** FRC is slightly increased in elderly patients secondary to the loss of elastic recoil that results in increased residual volume (FRC = ERV − RV).
(4) **Correct.** MVV or forced vital capacity is decreased in patients owing to the loss of elastic recoil.

### REASONING:

This is a difficult K-type question that challenges inherent assumptions concerning changes in respiratory physiology with age. The key to this question lies with the understanding that elastic recoil and alveolar surface area are most affected by age. The choices can be reasonably differentiated with this basic understanding.

### BIBLIOGRAPHY:


Miller RD, Miller ED, Reves JG, et al. *Anesthesia.* 7th ed. Philadelphia, PA: Churchill Livingstone; 2010:2151 (Figures 61-6 and 61-8),2263-2264.
Morgan GE, Mikhail MS, Murray MJ. *Clinical Anesthesiology.* 3rd ed. New York, NY: McGraw-Hill; 2002:876-878.


---

| **BOOK A:** | **QUESTION 32** |
| --- | --- |

*Answer D*

Pharmacology

### QUESTION (K-type):

The minimum alveolar concentration (MAC) of isoflurane is decreased by

(1) Ethanol-induced enzyme induction.
(2) Hyperventilation to a $Paco_2$ of 25 mm Hg.
(3) Chronic anemia to a hematocrit of 20%.
(4) Decreased body temperature to 34°C.

### CORRECT ANSWER: D (4 only is correct.)

### SUMMARY:

*Minimum alveolar concentration (MAC) is defined as the alveolar concentration of volatile anesthetic that will prevent movement following surgical incision in 50% of patients. Factors that decrease MAC include hypothermia, additional sedative medications, pregnancy, acute alcohol intoxication, chronic amphetamine abuse, advanced age, neonates, hyponatremia, hypercalcemia, hematocrit less than 10%, $Paco_2$ less than 15 mm Hg or greater than 95 mm Hg, $Pao_2$ less than 40 mm Hg, and hypotension with an MAP less than 40 mm Hg.*

### EXPLANATION:

(1) **Incorrect.** Ethanol-induced enzyme induction from chronic alcohol abuse most likely will increase MAC. Acute alcohol intoxication tends to decrease MAC.
(2) **Incorrect.** $Paco_2$ in the range of 15 to 95 mm Hg has no effect on MAC. Therefore, hyperventilation to a $Paco_2$ of 25 mm Hg will have no effect.
(3) **Incorrect.** Chronic anemia with a hematocrit of 20% will have no effect on MAC. Only anemia to a hematocrit of less than 10% will decrease MAC.
(4) **Correct.** Hypothermia will decrease MAC.

This commonly used question tests knowledge of factors that influence MAC. Choice 1 is incorrect because hepatic enzyme induction caused by ethanol should increase MAC. Because choice 1 is incorrect, choice 3 also must be incorrect. Hypothermia definitely decreases MAC, so choice 4 is correct. Choice 2 is not obvious, but the reader may recall that very high $Pa_{CO_2}$ values can cause narcosis. The easiest way to answer this question correctly is to memorize a table of factors affecting MAC found in commonly used texts.

**BIBLIOGRAPHY:**

Morgan GE, Mikhail MS, Murray MJ. *Clinical Anesthesiology*. 3rd ed. New York, NY: McGraw-Hill; 2002:135-137, 136 (Table 7-4 Factors Affecting MAC).

Stoelting RK, Miller RD. *Basics of Anesthesia*. 4th ed. New York, NY: Churchill Livingstone; 2000:32.

---

**BOOK A:**

*Answer B*

Pharmacology

## QUESTION 33

**QUESTION (K-type):**

Compared with fentanyl, characteristics of alfentanil include

(1) Greater protein binding.
(2) More rapid clearance.
(3) Shorter elimination half-life.
(4) Greater volume of distribution.

**CORRECT ANSWER: B (1 and 3 are correct.)**

**SUMMARY:**

*Parenteral opioids differ greatly in their pharmacokinetic and pharmacodynamic profiles. Fentanyl and alfentanil differ in their extent of protein binding, their context-sensitive half-lives (based on a multicompartment model that includes two distribution half-lives and a terminal elimination half-life), their volume of distribution, their rate of clearance, and their extent of hepatic metabolism. Alfentanil is slightly more protein bound and has a shorter elimination half-life and a smaller volume of distribution compared with fentanyl. These properties cause alfentanil to have a relatively short duration of action compared with fentanyl despite its lower rate of clearance. Alfentanil is used commonly in clinical settings in which rapid onset and short duration of action are desired (such as in placement of ocular blocks for ophthalmic surgery).*

**EXPLANATION:**

(1) ***Correct.*** Alfentanil is more protein bound than fentanyl.
(2) ***Incorrect.*** Alfentanil has a slower rate of clearance than fentanyl.
(3) ***Correct.*** Alfentanil has a shorter elimination half-life (in terms of both terminal half-life and distribution or central compartment half-life).
(4) ***Incorrect.*** Alfentanil has a lower volume of distribution than fentanyl.

**REASONING:**

This K-type question asks you to identify the pharmacokinetic properties of alfentanil compared with fentanyl. You should know that the volume of distribution of alfentanil is lower than that of fentanyl because this is one of the primary reasons alfentanil's clinical effect is so short. You can eliminate answers C and D based on this knowledge.

The challenging part of this question is not being tempted to select answer A, which includes the item "more rapid clearance." It would seem rational that a drug with a shorter duration of action would have a more rapid rate of clearance, but this is not the case with respect to alfentanil. Alfentanil's clinical effect is so short because it has so little volume of distribution, not because of its clearance. B is the best answer.

**BIBLIOGRAPHY:**

Miller RD, Miller ED, Reves JG, et al. *Anesthesia*. 5th ed. New York, NY: Churchill Livingstone; 2000:312-315.

Morgan GE, Mikhail MS, Murray MJ. *Clinical Anesthesiology*. 3rd ed. New York, NY: McGraw-Hill; 2002:152-155, 164-167.

---

**BOOK A:**  **QUESTION 34**

---

## Answer B

### Physiology

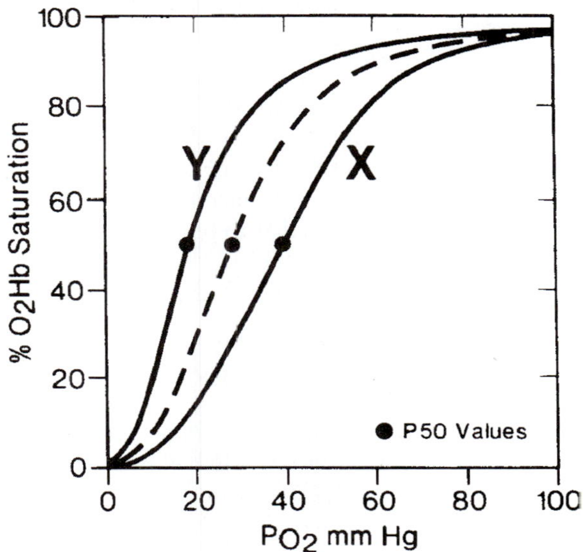


**QUESTION (K-type):**

The oxygen-dissociation curve in the center of the graph represents normal adult hemoglobin. True statements concerning curves X and Y include the following:

(1)  Curve Y represents hemoglobin characteristic of a normal neonate.
(2)  Curve X represents hemoglobin characteristic of 3-week-old banked blood.
(3)  Curve Y represents hemoglobin characteristic of an alkalotic patient.
(4)  Curve X represents hemoglobin characteristic of a hypothermic patient.

**CORRECT ANSWER: B (1 and 3 are correct.)**

**SUMMARY:**

*The hemoglobin-oxygen dissociation curve describes how avidly hemoglobin binds to oxygen as a function of $P_{O_2}$. Up to four oxygen molecules can bind one hemoglobin molecule. Many factors alter this curve, such as pH, body temperature, different forms of hemoglobin molecules, and levels of 2,3-diphosphoglycerate (2,3-DPG). When the curve shifts to the right, less oxygen is bound to hemoglobin at any given $Pa_{O_2}$, and the opposite is true when the curve is shifted to the left. Shifting to the right favors oxygen delivery to tissue, which occurs during hyperthermia, acidosis, and increased levels of 2,3-DPG.*

*Increased oxygen delivery is important during tissue hypoxia, when acidosis and increased 2,3-DPG occur. Increased temperature can result in increased cellular metabolism, a situation that also demands increased oxygen delivery. Conversely, hypothermia, alkalosis, and decreased 2,3-DPG suggest decreased oxygen demand and shift the curve leftward.*

**EXPLANATION:**

(1) ***Correct.*** Fetal hemoglobin has a higher affinity for oxygen because it relies on this to extract oxygen from their mother's adult hemoglobin. Neonatal hemoglobin is composed primarily of fetal hemoglobin, which has a greater affinity for oxygen, demonstrated by a shift to the left in the oxygen-hemoglobin dissociation curve.

(2) ***Incorrect.*** The longer blood is stored, the lower are the levels of 2,3-DPG, which shifts the oxygen-hemoglobin curve to the left, not right.

(3) ***Correct.*** Alkalosis shifts the oxygen-hemoglobin curve to the left because hemoglobin binds oxygen more avidly.

(4) ***Incorrect.*** Hypothermia shifts the curve to the left because hemoglobin binds oxygen more avidly.

**REASONING:**

This commonly used question asks for knowledge of the oxyhemoglobin dissociation curve and factors that can affect oxygen loading and unloading from hemoglobin. Choice 4 is obviously incorrect because alkalosis shifts the curve to the left. This allows answers C, D, and E to be eliminated, leaving choices 1 and 3 as correct. The only question is whether choice 2 is correct or incorrect. It is actually incorrect because banked blood causes a shift in the oxyhemoglobin dissociation curve to the left. B is correct.

**BIBLIOGRAPHY:**

Miller RD, Miller ED, Reves JG, et al. *Anesthesia.* 5th ed. New York, NY: Churchill Livingstone; 2000:1618-1621.

Morgan GE, Mikhail MS, Murray MJ. *Clinical Anesthesiology.* 3rd ed. New York, NY: McGraw-Hill; 2002:501-502.

---

| **BOOK A:** | **QUESTION 35** |

## *Answer C*

### Cardiovascular

**QUESTION (K-type):**

A 45-year-old man who is scheduled for coronary artery bypass grafting is receiving heparin and nitroglycerin infusions for preinfarction angina. True statements concerning the use of heparin during coronary revascularization in this patient include the following:

(1) The anticoagulant effect is enhanced by the nitroglycerin.
(2) Platelet count should be determined before the operation.
(3) Activated coagulation time is unreliable after prolonged administration of heparin.
(4) The dose of heparin necessary to provide adequate systemic anticoagulation is likely to be increased.

**CORRECT ANSWER: C (2 and 4 are correct.)**

**SUMMARY:**

*This patient is at risk for heparin resistance. There are various clinical factors and drugs that can influence the anticoagulant effect of heparin. Both heparin and nitroglycerine can cause heparin resistance, necessitating higher doses of heparin to achieve the required level of anticoagulation during cardiopulmonary bypass. Reported risk factors for altered heparin responsiveness include AT III levels less than 60% of normal, preoperative heparin therapy, a platelet count less than 300,000/mm³, and age younger than 65 years.*

### EXPLANATION:

(1) ***Incorrect.*** Heparin's anticoagulant effect is decreased by nitroglycerine.

(2) ***Correct.*** A heparin infusion can affect platelet count. Heparin-induced thrombocytopenia (HIT) can cause a decrease in platelet count and hypercoagulable state. The time frame usually is within 2 to 5 days in type I HIT, which is characterized by mild thrombocytopenia without thrombosis (proaggregatory effect on platelets). Type II HIT is a more serious and severe immune-mediated effect seen on average after 7 to 9 days of heparin infusion. This disorder produces clots in various arteries with significant morbidity and mortality.

(3) ***Incorrect.*** The reliability of ACT is not affected.

(4) ***Correct.*** Heparin's anticoagulant effect is decreased by nitroglycerine and an increased dose may be necessary. Antithrombin III deficiency should also be considered in the setting of heparin resistance. Antithrombin III binds to and inactivates thrombin and other activated clotting factors. Antithrombin III thrombin binding is accelerated several fold by the presence of heparin, which binds to a separate binding site on antithrombin III. Thus heparin's anticoagulation effect is mediated via antithrombin III. Antithrombin III deficiency can be treated with transfusion of FFP.

### REASONING:

This is an often-seen board question requiring knowledge of heparin resistance. Because choice 1 is clearly incorrect, answers A, B, and E can be eliminated. That leaves answers C and D. The pharmacologic effect of a heparin infusion includes an aggregatory effect on platelets (type I HIT and the more severe and serious type II HIT). C is the best answer.

### BIBLIOGRAPHY:

Barash PG, Cullen BF, Stoelting RK, Cahalan MK, Stock MC. *Clinical Anesthesia.* 6th ed. Philadelphia, PA: Lippincott Williams & Wilkins; 2009:400-402.

Hensley F, Martin DE, Gravlee FP. *Practical Approach to Cardiac Anesthesia.* 3rd ed. Philadelphia, PA: Lippincott Williams & Wilkins; 2002:498-499.

Miller RD, Miller ED, Reves JG, et al. *Anesthesia.* 7th ed. Philadelphia, PA: Churchill Livingstone; 2010:1898-1899.

Morgan GE, Mikhail MS, Murray MJ. *Clinical Anesthesiology.* 3rd ed. New York, NY: McGraw-Hill; 2002:450.

---

| **BOOK A:** | **QUESTION 36** |
|---|---|

## *Answer B*

Physiology

### QUESTION (K-type):

True statements concerning negative-pressure pulmonary edema include the following:

(1) It is associated with airway obstruction.
(2) It responds to diuretic therapy.
(3) Resolution occurs within 24 hours.
(4) Debilitated adults are predisposed to it.

### CORRECT ANSWER: B (1 and 3 are correct.)

### SUMMARY:

*Postobstructive or negative-pressure pulmonary edema (NPPE) is the development of sudden pulmonary edema following upper airway obstruction such as laryngospasm, ETT* *obstruction, or foreign body aspiration. The starling equation states that $Q = K[(P_{mv} - P_{imv}) - (\pi_{mv} - \pi_{imv})$ where $K$ = permeability coefficient, $Q$ = net transvascular flow of fluid, $P\,mv$ = pressure of microvasculature, $P\,imv$ = pressure of interstitium, $\pi_{mv}$ = oncotic pressure of microvasculature, and $\pi_{imv}$ = oncotic pressure of interstitium. The greater the negative pressure created, the worse is the pulmonary edema, explaining why young athletic men have an increased susceptibility to NPPE.*

### EXPLANATION:

(1) **Correct.** Forceful inspiration against a closed airway or airway obstruction causes NPPE.
(2) **Incorrect.** Current consensus therapy for NPPE involves oxygen and intubation. Diuretics have been used in the past, but their use is controversial and potentially even harmful. Total body volume may actually be decreased in these patients and diuretics could exacerbate hypovolemia.
(3) **Correct.** Resolution of NPPE is rapid, typically occurring within 24 hours.
(4) **Incorrect.** Young ASA 1 and 2 patients are predisposed to NPPE because they can generate the largest negative intrathoracic pressure.

### REASONING:

This question tests knowledge of NPPE. Clearly, choices 1 and 3 are correct. Choice 4 is incorrect because high negative intrathoracic pressure needs to be created to cause NPPE that occurs with upper airway obstruction in young athletes. This leaves only a question as to whether or not choice 2 is correct. It is incorrect because diuretics potentially can be harmful to patients with NPPE. B is correct.

### BIBLIOGRAPHY:

Barash P, Cullen BF, Stoelting RK, Cahalan MK, Stock MC. *Clinical Anesthesia*. 6th ed. Philadelphia, PA: Lippincott Williams & Wilkins; 2009:1308-1309.
Krodel D, Bittner EA, Abdulnour R, Brown R, Eikermann M. Case scenario: acute postoperative negative pressure pulmonary edema. *Anesthesiology*. 2010;113(1):200-207.
Maxwell B, Mihm F. Questioning diuretic use in negative pressure pulmonary edema. *Anesthesiology*. 2011;114(2):461.

---

**BOOK A:**   **QUESTION 37**

---

*Answer B*

OB/Regional

### QUESTION (K-type):

Landmarks for the sciatic nerve via a posterior approach include the

(1) Posterior-superior iliac spine.
(2) Coccyx.
(3) Greater trochanter of the femur.
(4) Iliac crest.

### CORRECT ANSWER: B (1 and 3 are correct.)

### SUMMARY:

*The sciatic nerve is composed of fibers from L4 to S3. It exits the pelvis below the piriformis muscle in the sciatic notch and passes distally dorsal to the lesser trochanter of the femur. At the superior portion of the popliteal fossa the sciatic nerve divides into the common peroneal and tibial nerves, which when combined with the saphenous nerve provide sensory and motor innervation to the lower leg and foot. A saphenous nerve block is appropriate for surgery on the lower leg, foot, and ankle but most often must be combined with femoral and other nerve blocks to provide complete anesthesia.*

### EXPLANATION:
(1) **Correct.** To perform a sciatic nerve block via the posterior approach a line is drawn between the greater trochanter of the femur and the posterosuperior iliac spine with the patient in the lateral position with the hip flexed. A second line 4 to 5 cm in length is drawn perpendicular and caudomedially to the midpoint of the first. The sciatic nerve is located at the terminus of this second line.
(2) **Incorrect.** The coccyx is the distal end of the vertebral column and is not a landmark for the sciatic nerve block.
(3) **Correct.** As discussed earlier, the greater trochanter of the femur is an important landmark for sciatic nerve block via the posterior approach.
(4) **Incorrect.** The iliac crest is not a landmark for the sciatic nerve block.

### REASONING:
Knowledge of the anatomy of the lower extremity and course of the sciatic nerve is essential to perform an effective sciatic nerve block. This question is one of many commonly tested regional procedures the reader should memorize in preparation for the written examination. Other important blocks for the examination include the axillary, ankle, interscalene, caudal, and stellate ganglion blocks. Choices 1 and 3 are used consistently to locate the sciatic nerve from the posterior approach. Therefore, B is correct.

### BIBLIOGRAPHY:

Chu L, Fuller A. *Manual of Clinical Anesthesia.* Philadelphia, PA: Lippincott Williams & Wilkins; 2011:1215-1216.
Morgan GE, Mikhail MS, Murray MJ. *Clinical Anesthesiology.* 4th ed. New York, NY: McGraw-Hill; 2006:348-350.


---

| **BOOK A:** | **QUESTION 38** |
|---|---|

*Answer A*

OB/Regional

### QUESTION (K-type):
Epidural anesthesia for cesarean delivery is planned for a 30-year-old woman in labor. She has preeclampsia and takes propranolol for mitral valve prolapse. A test dose of 3 mL of 2% lidocaine containing 15 µg of epinephrine is administered, and no change in heart rate is noted by palpation of the pulse. Before injection of more local anesthetic, blood is freely aspirated from the catheter. Explanations for failure of the intravenous test dose include the following:

(1) The pain of labor masked the change usually seen with the test dose
(2) Preexisting β-adrenergic blockade blunted the tachycardia from the intravenous epinephrine.
(3) Changes in pulse rate were too brief to be noted by palpation of the pulse.
(4) Preeclampsia decreased the sensitivity to exogenously administered catecholamines.

### CORRECT ANSWER: A (1, 2, and 3 are correct.)

### SUMMARY:
*The administration of epinephrine containing epidural test doses in laboring women is controversial because detection of an intravascular catheter in parturients can be hindered*

### EXPLANATION:

(1) **Correct.** The patient in the question is in labor, and it is possible that the heart rate response from the clearly intravascular catheter was masked by pain associated with labor.
(2) **Correct.** Propranolol is a β-antagonist and can prevent the tachycardic response to intravascular epinephrine.
(3) **Correct.** The average increased time to tachycardia with intravenous epinephrine is approximately 60 seconds, and the duration is approximately 60 seconds. Experts recommend a pulse oximeter or electrocardiogram (ECG) to detect this response because palpitation of the pulse or measurement of blood pressure can be unreliable.
(4) **Incorrect.** Preeclampsia increases sensitivity to exogenously administered catecholamines.

### REASONING:

This question tests knowledge of epidural catheter management and test dose administration to parturients. Choice 2 is clearly correct because the patient is on β-blocking medication. The next step is to examine choice 4, which is clearly incorrect because preeclamptic patients are more sensitive to catecholamines. These two steps eliminate B, C, D, and E as answers and make the only possible correct answer A. However, it is best to check yourself and verify that choices 1 and 3 are indeed correct before choosing A as the answer. Because the patient is in labor and you know that this can mask the tachycardia associated with test doses, choice 1 is clearly correct. Choice 3 is slightly more difficult to prove but makes intuitive sense and is proven correct on further review of the literature.

### BIBLIOGRAPHY:

Bucklin B, Gambling DR, Wlody DJ. *A Practical Approach to Obstetric Anesthesia.* Philadelphia, PA: Lippincott, Williams and Wilkins; 2009:156-157.
Chestnut DH, Polley LS, Lawrence CT, Wong CA. *Chestnut's Obstetric Anesthesia Principles and Practice.* 4th ed. St. Louis, MO: Mosby; 2009:239-240, 983.
Morgan GE, Mikhail MS, Murray MJ. *Clinical Anesthesiology.* 4th ed. New York, NY: McGraw-Hill; 2006:899.

---

**BOOK A:**     **QUESTION 39**

*Answer E*

Cardiovascular

### QUESTION (K-type):

A 76-year-old man with a history of angina, dyspnea on exertion, and syncope attributable to aortic stenosis is brought to the operating room for open reduction of an ankle fracture. An electrocardiogram (ECG) shows sinus rhythm. Anesthetic considerations include the following:

(1) Nitroglycerin is contraindicated.
(2) Atrial fibrillation should be treated with synchronized cardioversion.
(3) The risk for cardiac complications is the same as that in patients with coronary artery stenosis.
(4) Spinal anesthesia is relatively contraindicated.

**CORRECT ANSWER: E (All are correct.)**

## SUMMARY:

*The patient's symptoms are indicative of severe aortic stenosis (AS). Anesthetic considerations include maintaining adequate preload, good myocardial contractility and perfusion pressure, sinus rhythm, and normal rate. Myocardial supply and demand are impaired. Myocardial $O_2$ demand is increased by a hypertrophic ventricle. Increased intraventricular pressure compromises oxygen supply while increasing the demand. For these reasons, these patients do not tolerate even mild vasodilation and hypotension.*

## EXPLANATION:

(1) **Correct.** Venodilation, decreased preload, and possible hypotension make nitroglycerine unsafe.

(2) **Correct.** The hypertrophic noncompliant ventricle in AS develops diastolic dysfunction, which increases left ventricular end-diastolic pressure (LVEDP), thus decreasing the LA-to-LV pressure gradient in diastole, compromising passive filling. Atrial contraction assumes a greater role in maintaining cardiac output.

(3) **Correct.** Pathophysiology in AS leads to increased left ventricular (LV) afterload, resulting in ventricular hypertrophy and increased myocardial oxygen requirements. Supply also can be impaired in AS because aortic diastolic pressure can be decreased and ventricular filling pressures are increased owing to the noncompliant ventricle. This supply-demand imbalance places these patients at increased risk for myocardial ischemia.

(4) **Correct.** Spinal anesthesia can decrease afterload, leading to decreased coronary perfusion during diastole and possible myocardial ischemia.

## REASONING:

Aortic stenosis (AS) is a cardiac lesion that is tested frequently on board examinations. The key to the anesthetic management of AS is understanding that the pathophysiology stems from the fixed afterload increase in the stenotic valve. Normal aortic valve area is about 3 cm$^2$, and symptoms of AS appear when the valve narrows to less than 0.8 cm$^2$. Patients with AS need well-timed atrial contractions to augment left ventricular filling. These contractions can account for up to 30% to 40% of left ventricular end-diastolic volume. Adequate preload is also important to help offset decreased LV compliance from LV hypertrophy. Decreases in afterload should be avoided because they do not significantly offset the fixed afterload increase from the stenotic valve. Heart rates should be kept normal (60-70 bpm [beats per minute]) to allow adequate time for coronary perfusion during diastole while avoiding bradycardia (decreased cardiac output) and tachycardia (myocardial $O_2$ supply-demand imbalance and ischemia). The fact that choices 1, 2, and 4 are correct makes E the only possibility.

## BIBLIOGRAPHY:

Barash PG, Cullen BF, Stoelting RK, Cahalan MK, Stock MC. *Clinical Anesthesia*. 6th ed. Philadelphia, PA: Lippincott Williams & Wilkins; 2009:1078-1080.

Miller RD, Miller ED, Reves JG, et al. *Anesthesia*. 7th ed. New York, NY: Churchill Livingstone; 2010:1932-1933.

Morgan GE, Mikhail MS, Murray MJ. *Clinical Anesthesiology*. 3rd ed. New York, NY: McGraw-Hill; 2002:416-418.

*Answer A*

Physiology

**QUESTION (K-type):**

Use of hyperventilation to decrease brain swelling also decreases

(1) $P_{50}$ of hemoglobin.
(2) Serum-ionized calcium concentration.
(3) Serum potassium concentration.
(4) Cerebral metabolic rate.

**CORRECT ANSWER: A (1, 2, and 3 are correct.)**

**SUMMARY:**

*Hyperventilation causes a variety of physiologic changes, such as respiratory alkalosis. Sequelae of an acute respiratory alkalosis include leftward shift in the oxyhemoglobin curve, which lowers the $P_{50}$, decreased ionized serum calcium, and decreased serum potassium (secondary to an intracellular shift). Hyperventilation does not decrease the cerebral metabolic rate, although it will decrease regional and global cerebral blood flow.*

**EXPLANATION:**

(1) *Correct.* Respiratory alkalosis shifts the oxygen dissociation curve to the left, causing decreased hemoglobin $P_{50}$.
(2) *Correct.* Alkalemia secondary to hyperventilation can acutely decrease serum-ionized calcium concentration.
(3) *Correct.* Respiratory acidosis leads to hypokalemia.
(4) *Incorrect.* Hyperventilation does not decrease the cerebral metabolic rate.

**REASONING:**

This question tests knowledge of the physiologic effects of hyperventilation, specifically those changes related to the induced alkalemia and alkalosis. The oxygen dissociation shifts leftward with alkalosis. Changes in blood pH alter the fraction of calcium bound to albumin, thus changing the level of ionized calcium without changing the total calcium measured; acute alkalemia decreases the serum concentration of ionized calcium. Alkalosis-induced shifts of potassium from extracellular to intracellular fluid causes a decrease in serum potassium. The best answer is A.

**BIBLIOGRAPHY:**

Barash PG, Cullen BF, Stoelting RK, Cahalan MK, Stock MC. *Clinical Anesthesia*. 6th ed. Philadelphia, PA: Lippincott Williams & Wilkins; 2009:312, 317.
Miller RD, Eriksson LI, Fleisher LA, Wiener-Kronish JP, Young WL. *Miller's Anesthesia*. 7th ed. Philadelphia, PA: Churchill Livingstone; 2010:1710, 1712, 1746.
Morgan GE, Mikhail MS, Murray MJ. *Clinical Anesthesiology*. 4th ed. New York, NY: McGraw-Hill; 2006:616.

*Answer D*

Pediatrics

**QUESTION (K-type):**

A neonate born at 32 weeks' gestation has cyanosis, tachypnea, a scaphoid abdomen, and a cardiac impulse on the right. Immediate management of this child should include

(1)  Insertion of a chest tube.
(2)  Limiting inspired oxygen concentration to 50%.
(3)  Administration of rapid positive-pressure ventilation by mask.
(4)  Insertion of a nasogastric tube.

**CORRECT ANSWER: D (4 only is correct.)**

**SUMMARY:**

*Congenital diaphragmatic hernia (CDH) occurs in about 1 in 5000 live births. Around the eighth week of gestation, portions of the bowel, stomach, and abdominal viscera can herniate into the thorax through either the left or right posterolateral foramen of Bochdalek, or the anterior foramen of Morgagni. Ninety percent of herniations are through the posterolateral foramen of Bochdalek and 90% of the herniations occur on the left side. Clinical signs include cyanosis, hypoxia, respiratory distress, scaphoid abdomen, bowel obstruction, and auscultation of bowel sounds in the chest. Chest radiograph shows bowel in the left hemithorax with deviation of the heart and mediastinum to the right and compression of the right lung. The mass effect of the herniated abdominal contents leads to pulmonary hypoplasia and pulmonary hypertension. Despite modern therapies of extracorporeal membrane oxygenation (ECMO), nitric oxide, surfactant, and high-frequency ventilation morbidity, it is still associated with 40% to 50% mortality.*

**EXPLANATION:**

(1)  *Incorrect.* Chest tube insertion may be necessary at some point as these patients are at risk for pneumothoraces, but there is no evidence that the patient currently has a pneumothorax. A high index of suspicion for pneumothorax should be maintained for these patients, and signs of a contralateral pneumothorax include sudden fall in lung compliance, blood pressure, or oxygenation.
(2)  *Incorrect.* Limiting concentration of inspired oxygen in a premature infant may prevent retinopathy of prematurity, but it is a low priority in a patient who is cyanotic and tachypneic. Patients with CDH are often hypoxic due to pulmonary hypoplasia and are at increased risk of pulmonary hypertension. Treatment of pulmonary hypertension can include oxygen, along with hyperventilation, alkalosis, sedation, paralysis, pulmonary vasodilators such as inhaled nitric oxide.
(3)  *Incorrect.* Mask ventilation in patients with CDH is generally avoided to limit gastric insufflation and increase intrathoracic size of the herniated bowel. Patients with severe respiratory compromise may require positive-pressure mask ventilation, but this must be administered carefully.
(4)  *Correct.* Insertion of a nasogastric or orogastric tube serves to decompress the stomach of gas and fluids.

**REASONING:**

This is a tricky question because all of the choices sound reasonable, and in fact may be used at some point in the treatment. Choice 1 is not necessary for immediate management, so it can be ruled out. Choice 2 does not make good clinical sense, so it can also be ruled out. Choice 3, like 1, may be necessary in extreme situations, but that is not justified with the current clinical description. Choice 4 is the most reasonable immediate intervention.

BIBLIOGRAPHY:
Cote CJ. *A Practice of Anesthesia for Infants and Children.* 4th ed. Philadelphia, PA: Saunders; 2009:226-229, 757-758.
Morgan GE, Mikhail MS, Murray MJ. *Clinical Anesthesiology.* 4th ed. New York, NY: McGraw-Hill; 2006:940-941.

---

**BOOK A:**

*None of the choices are correct*

Basic Science

## QUESTION 42 (OPTIONAL)

**QUESTION (K-type):**

The principle underlying diffusion hypoxia also explains

(1)  Apneic oxygenation.
(2)  The concentration effect.
(3)  The solubility effect.
(4)  The second-gas effect.

**CORRECT ANSWER:** None of the choices are correct.

**SUMMARY:**

*After extensive discussion and research regarding this question, we have concluded that none of the choices can be correct. Diffusion hypoxia occurs when a patient who has been receiving nitrous oxide is placed on room air at the conclusion of an anesthetic. The nitrous oxide diffuses rapidly from the blood into the lungs, decreasing the alveolar concentration of oxygen and carbon dioxide. This is a dilutional effect on oxygen and carbon dioxide by nitrous oxide. The resulting hypocarbia can depress the respiratory drive, and the decreased alveolar oxygen concentration can lead to hypoxemia. Administration of 100% oxygen can help to prevent this phenomenon.*

**EXPLANATION:**

(1)  *Incorrect.* Apneic oxygenation is based on the augmented gas inflow effect that is a component of the concentration effect. With this technique, ventilation can be stopped for brief periods of time if 100% oxygen is insufflated—usually via a small catheter—into the airway. When oxygen is taken up from the alveoli into the blood, more gas (100% oxygen) is drawn in. Although adequate oxygenation often can be maintained effectively, development of hypercarbia and respiratory acidosis limits this technique. Arterial $P_{CO_2}$ increases 6 mm Hg in the first minute of apnea and 3 to 4 mm Hg each minute thereafter. Diffusion hypoxia is a *dilutional* effect that is not explained by apneic oxygenation.

(2)  *Incorrect.* The concentration effect is composed of two effects: (a) the augmented gas inflow effect (see choice 1) and (b) the concentrating effect. The concentrating effect occurs when an anesthetic is taken up from the lungs into the bloodstream. For example, if an anesthetic is at 10% of total gas inflow (10 parts per 100) and 50% or 5 parts are taken up into the bloodstream, the remaining anesthetic is at a concentration of 5.3% (5 per 95 remaining parts). In contrast, if an anesthetic is at 50% of total gas inflow (50 parts per 100) and 50% or 25 parts are taken up into the bloodstream, the remaining concentration is at a concentration of 33% (25 per 75 remaining parts. In the second case, we gave five times the amount of anesthetic. However, the remaining alveolar concentration is 33/5.2 or 6.2 times greater. The concentrating effect has the greatest effect at high concentrations of inspired anesthetic. The augmented gas inflow effect occurs when taking into account new gas coming in to replace that absorbed by the body. Based on the previous example, if anesthetic comprises 10% of gas inflow with 50% absorption, 5/95 parts remaining are anesthetic. With gas inflow of the same composition, 0.5 parts anesthetic would enter with 4.5 parts inert

gas to replace that which was absorbed. The final concentration of anesthetic is 5.5/100 or 5.5%, as compared to 5.3% without taking into account gas inflow. In contrast, if anesthetic comprises 50% of gas inflow with the same 50% absorption, 25/75 remaining parts are anesthetic. To replace this, inflow would comprise 12.5 parts anesthetic and 12.5 parts inert gas for a total of 37.5/100 parts anesthetic. This is compared to the value of 33% without gas inflow, and 37.5/5.5 is 6.8 times greater as opposed to the previous value of 6.2% without taking into account new gas inflow. Diffusion hypoxia is a *dilutional* effect that is not explained by the concentration effect.

(3) *Incorrect.* A review of standard anesthesia texts and experts within our department failed to find a definition or description of the "solubility effect." This is unfortunate wording because the solubility of nitrous oxide does explain the phenomenon of diffusion hypoxia. The speed at which a gas diffuses across the alveclar capillary membrane down a concentration gradient (eg, from areas of high gas concentration to low) is determined not only by the molecular weight of the gas but also by its solubility. The Graham law states that the rate at which gases diffuse is inversely proportional to the square root of their molecular weight, where

$$D_{N_2O} \alpha \ \frac{1}{\sqrt{MW_{N_2O}}} \qquad D_{O_2} \alpha \ \frac{1}{\sqrt{MW_{O_2}}} \qquad \frac{D_{N_2O}}{D_{O_2}} = 0.85 \qquad \frac{D_{O_2}}{D_{N_2O}} = 1.2$$

By this measure, alveolar oxygen diffuses 1.2 times faster than nitrous oxide. However, solubility of gas in blood also plays a factor in determining the speed of diffusion across the alveolar capillary membrane.

$$\frac{\sqrt{MW_{O_2}}}{\sqrt{MW_{N_2O}}} \times \frac{Sol\ N_2O}{Sol\ O_2} = \frac{\sqrt{32}}{\sqrt{44}} \times \frac{0.47}{0.024} = 16.7$$

When the solubility of nitrous oxide is taken into consideration, we see that it diffuses 17 times more rapidly across the alveolar capillary membrane compared with oxygen. Thus the rapid washout of nitrous oxide at the end of an anesthetic that causes diffusion hypoxia is due to rapid diffusion across the alveolar concentration gradient, which is related to its solubility. However, there is no such thing as a "solubility effect," and thus this choice is incorrect.

(4) *Incorrect.* The second-gas effect occurs when one gas, nitrous oxide, speeds the uptake of a potent anesthetic. For example, if a patient breathes 50% nitrous oxide (50 parts per 100) and 4% sevoflurane (4 parts per 100), and all the nitrous is taken up, the remaining 4 parts of sevoflurane is in only 50 parts of total gas. Its concentration is now 4/50 = 8%. The overall effect is concentration of the second gas, in this case sevoflurane. As we have already discussed, diffusion hypoxia is caused by a *dilutional* effect on alveolar oxygen and carbon dioxide.


## REASONING:

This is a challenging question because none of the choices reflects a clearly correct answer. The likely intent of this question is to test knowledge of the concentration effect, the second-gas effect, and diffusion hypoxia. It is important to understand the determinants of diffusion rates across the alveolar-capillary membrane. Blood/gas solubility is a major determinant of diffusion rates across the alveolar-capillary membrane and is the best reason that explains why nitrous oxide diffuses rapidly from blood and can lead to dilution of alveolar oxygen and carbon dioxide at the end of an anesthetic. Unfortunately, the choice "solubility effect" is not a widely known or conventional anesthetic term. None of the choices is correct.


## BIBLIOGRAPHY:

Barash PG, Cullen BF, Stoelting RK, Cahalan MK, Stock MC. *Clinical Anesthesia.* 6th ed. Philadelphia, PA: Lippincott Williams & Wilkins; 2009:419-420.
Fink BR. Diffusion anoxia. *Anesthesiology.* 1955;16:511-519.

Morgan GE, Mikhail MS, Murray MJ. *Clinical Anesthesiology*. 3rd ed. New York, NY: McGraw-Hill; 2002:132, 539.

Stoelting RK, Miller RD. *Basics of Anesthesia*. 4th ed. New York, NY: Churchill Livingstone; 2000:26-27.

---

**BOOK A:**        **QUESTION 43**

---

## *Answer D*

### Equipment/Physics

**QUESTION (K-type):**

True statements concerning carbon dioxide absorption in breathing-system canisters include the following:

(1) The major reactant of baralyme is barium hydroxide.
(2) Baralyme contains silica to minimize dust.
(3) The major component of soda lime is sodium hydroxide.
(4) Both baralyme and soda lime contain calcium hydroxide.

**CORRECT ANSWER: D (4 only is correct.)**

**SUMMARY:**

*Carbon dioxide is eliminated from semiclosed and closed breathing circuits through the use of $CO_2$ absorbers that chemically neutralize $CO_2$, such as soda lime and baralyme. The $CO_2$ reacts with water and hydroxides to form carbonates, water, and heat. In soda lime, the hydroxides are sodium hydroxide, potassium hydroxide, and calcium hydroxide. In baralyme, the hydroxides are barium hydroxide and calcium hydroxide. With both soda lime and baralyme, the sodium hydroxide and barium hydroxide are present as activators for the reaction, and calcium hydroxide comprises the majority of the absorber. Soda lime has silica added to prevent dust formation, whereas baralyme has harder granules and does not need silica because of water bound to the octahydrate salt of barium hydroxide.*

**EXPLANATION:**

(1) *Incorrect.* The major reactant of baralyme is calcium hydroxide, which comprises 80% of the absorbent.
(2) *Incorrect.* Baralyme does not contain silica to minimize dust, as does soda lime.
(3) *Incorrect.* 80% of soda lime is calcium hydroxide.
(4) *Correct.* The major reactant of both soda lime and baralyme is calcium hydroxide.

**REASONING:**

This question tests knowledge of similarities and differences in soda lime and baralyme components of $CO_2$-absorbing systems. Choice 4 is obviously correct, which allows answers A and B to be eliminated. Choice 2 is not correct because one of the differences between soda lime and baralyme is that soda lime contains silica, whereas baralyme does not. Answers C and E both contain choice 2 and can be eliminated. Only D remains and it is the best answer.

**BIBLIOGRAPHY:**

Morgan GE, Mikhail MS, Murray MJ. *Clinical Anesthesiology*. 3rd ed. New York, NY: McGraw-Hill; 2002:33-34.

Stoelting RK, Miller RD. *Basics of Anesthesia*. 4th ed. New York, NY: Churchill Livingstone; 2000:143-144.

## *Answer A*

## OB/Regional

**QUESTION (K-type):**

Factors that decrease local anesthetic concentration in the fetus include

(1)  Maternal hypotension.
(2)  Maternal acidemia.
(3)  Maternal serum alpha acid glycoprotein concentration.
(4)  Fetal acidosis.

**CORRECT ANSWER: A (1, 2, and 3 are correct.)**

**SUMMARY:**

*Fetal plasma drug concentration depends on the size and delivery of drug to the placenta via the uterine artery, transfer of drug across the placenta, and fetal uptake. Compounds less than 500 Da can cross the placenta, and local anesthetics are less than 300 Da. If blood flow to the uterine artery is compromised, as in the case of maternal hypotension or other conditions associated with uterine hypoperfusion (supine hypotension syndrome, administration of vasoconstrictors), delivery of drug to the placenta will be decreased. Transfer of drug across the placenta depends on many factors, including the concentration of free drug (non–protein-bound) and lipid solubility. Local anesthetics such as lidocaine are weak bases (the pKa of lidocaine is 7.8) and therefore are primarily in the nonionized form with higher pH and in the ionized form in conditions associated with low pH such as acidosis. If fetal acidosis is present, this can result in the drug crossing the placenta in the lipid-soluble form while circulating in maternal blood and then becoming ionized when exposed to the acidotic environment within the fetus. This can result in high fetal concentrations of local anesthetic and has been termed ion trapping.*

**EXPLANATION:**

(1)  *Correct.* Maternal hypotension decreases drug delivery to the placenta, which decreases drug concentration in the fetus.
(2)  *Correct.* Lidocaine is a weak base. When the pH is below the pKa, more of the drug is in the ionized form, which will impede placental transfer.
(3)  *Correct.* Alpha acid glycoprotein binds basic drugs like local anesthetics. A higher serum alpha acid concentration will cause more protein binding and less placental transfer. Fetal concentrations of alpha acid glycoprotein are lower than maternal.
(4)  *Incorrect.* Fetal pH has the same effect on a drug as maternal pH. If the pH is less than the pKa of a drug with weakly basic properties such as lidocaine, most of the drug will be in the ionized form and will not cross the placenta. When the fetus is acidotic and there is a significant difference in the maternal and fetal pH, this can result in a much higher concentration of local anesthetic in the fetus and has been termed *ion trapping.*

**REASONING:**

This question requires knowledge that lidocaine and most other local anesthetics are weak bases and therefore are in the nonionized form at high pH and in the ionized form at low pH. One must also know the factors that favor placental transfer, keeping in mind that the ionized form of the drug will tend not to cross the placenta. With this knowledge, one can identify choice 2 as correct and choice 4 as incorrect. With the K-type question, this means that the answer must be A (1, 2, and 3 are correct).

**BIBLIOGRAPHY:**

Bucklin B, Gambling DR, Wlody DJ. *A Practical Approach to Obstetric Anesthesia.* Philadelphia, PA: Lippincott, Williams and Wilkins; 2009:32.

Chestnut DH, Polley LS, Lawrence CT, Wong CA. *Chestnut's Obstetric Anesthesia Principles and Practice.* 4th ed. St. Louis, MO: Mosby; 2009:257-259.

---

**BOOK A:**  |  **QUESTION 45**

---

## *Answer D*

### Equipment/Physics

**QUESTION (K-type):**

An oxygen analyzer sensor placed in the inspiratory limb of a circle system

(1) Is useful as a disconnect alarm if placed near the patient.
(2) Will increase dead space.
(3) Will be more pressure sensitive than one placed in the expiratory limb.
(4) Should not be placed distal to an in-circuit humidifier.

**CORRECT ANSWER: D (4 only is correct.)**

**SUMMARY:**

*General anesthesia should never be administered without an oxygen analyzer. The oxygen analyzer is the only device on the anesthesia machine to monitor the integrity of the low-pressure circuit. Oxygen concentration in the circuit can be measured electrochemically or by paramagnetic analysis. The oxygen analyzer sensor can be placed in the inspiratory or expiratory limb of the circle system. It should not be placed in the fresh gas line, which would monitor the concentration of oxygen entering the circuit rather than the true delivered concentration. Placement of the sensor close to the patient may help detect a disconnection, but if placed distal to the Y connection, the analyzer will increase dead space.*

**EXPLANATION:**

(1) *Incorrect.* The oxygen analyzer placed near the patient will not reliably detect all disconnections because they may occur at locations far from the analyzer, and high fresh gas flow rates may prevent the oxygen concentration from dropping low enough to set off the alarm.

(2) *Incorrect.* Placement of the oxygen analyzer in the inspiratory limb of the circle system will not increase dead space. Only placing the analyzer between the Y piece and the ETT will increase dead space.

(3) *Incorrect.* The expiratory limb has a slightly lower partial pressure of oxygen compared to the inspiratory limb because of the patient's oxygen consumption. However, it is equally sensitive on either side.

(4) *Correct.* While increased humidity does not affect most modern oxygen analyzers, it is advisable to minimize the exposure to excessive humidity that may affect the sensor.

**REASONING:**

An understanding of the circle system and the purpose of the oxygen analyzer are necessary. While the analyzer alarm can detect a disconnection under some circumstances, Choice 1 can be ruled out because the sensor should not be relied on to do so. Choice 2 can also be eliminated because placement in the inspiratory limb does not affect dead space. Choice 3 is more obscure, but the location of the analyzer does not affect the overall sensitivity. Finally, while most modern analyzers are not affected by humidity, it is still recommended to minimize exposure to humidity.

**BIBLIOGRAPHY:**

Barash PG, Cullen BF, Stoelting RK, Cahalan MK, Stock MC. *Clinical Anesthesia.* 6th ed. Philadelphia, PA: Lippincott Williams & Wilkins; 2009:647.

Dorsch, JA, Dorsch, SE. *Understanding Anesthesia Equipment.* 5th ed. Philadelphia, PA: Williams & Wilkins; 2008:244-245.

Morgan GE, Mikhail MS, Murray MJ. *Clinical Anesthesiology.* 4th ed. New York, NY: McGraw-Hill; 2006:70.

---

**BOOK A:**

*Answer E*

Physiology

## QUESTION 46

**QUESTION (K-type):**

Agents that produce an acute withdrawal response in patients addicted to heroin include

(1) Pentazocine.
(2) Nalbuphine.
(3) Buprenorphine.
(4) Naloxone.

**CORRECT ANSWER: E (All are correct.)**

**SUMMARY:**

*Withdrawal from opioids can occur within 3 to 4 hours after the last dose. Patients may initially exhibit restlessness, diaphoresis, nausea, nasal congestion, lacrimation, stomach cramps, and drug-seeking behavior. Later symptoms include piloerection (hence the term "cold turkey"), muscle spasms ("kicking the habit"), fever, chills, hypertension, and tachycardia. Acute withdrawal may be produced by pure opioid antagonists such as naloxone, or opioid agonist-antagonists such as pentazocine and nalbuphine. The agonists-antagonists may have opposite effects at different opiate receptors and are used for both analgesia and treating side effects of opiate use.*

**EXPLANATION:**

(1) *Correct.* Pentazocine is an opioid agonist-antagonist (primarily κ receptor stimulation) that is one-fourth to one-half as potent as morphine. It can cause an acute withdrawal response in addicts.

(2) *Correct.* Nalbuphine is an opioid agonist-antagonist structurally related to oxymorphone and naloxone that acts as an agonist at κ receptors and as an antagonist at μ receptors. Nalbuphine can cause acute withdrawal symptoms in addicts.

(3) *Correct.* Buprenorphine is an opioid agonist-antagonist with high κ receptor affinity and partial μ receptor agonism. Use in persons physically dependent on full opioid agonists can precipitate acute withdrawal. However, cessation of buprenorphine has been associated with withdrawal symptoms itself.

(4) *Correct.* Naloxone is a pure opioid antagonist (μ >> δ or κ) that can produce an acute withdrawal response in patients addicted to heroin. Because naloxone has a relatively short duration of action (30-45 minutes) compared to longer-acting opioids, repeated doses or continuous infusion may be required to treat opioid-induced respiratory depression.

**REASONING:**

Key concepts for answering this question include understanding opioid and opioid antagonist pharmacology. Choices 1, 2, and 4 are well known for causing acute withdrawal responses in patients addicted to heroin. Choice 3, buprenorphine, is described as having minimal effects on methadone users and causes withdrawal symptoms itself. However, buprenorphine can also cause precipitated withdrawal, making E the correct answer.

BIBLIOGRAPHY:
Miller, 7th ed, pg 808-810.
Morgan GE, Mikhail MS, Murray MJ. *Clinical Anesthesiology*. 4th ed. New York, NY:
McGraw-Hill; 2006:285.

| BOOK A: | QUESTION 47 |
|---|---|

## *Answer B*

### Pain

**QUESTION (K-type):**

A 68-year-old man has had severe, constant burning and aching in the right forehead and anterior scalp for 6 weeks after an episode of herpes zoster. True statements concerning this patient's condition include the following:

(1) It is more common in elderly patients.
(2) The neuralgia involves the supraorbital branches of the ophthalmic division of the facial nerve.
(3) Tricyclic antidepressants often provide effective pain relief.
(4) Opioid analgesics are the first-line treatment.

**CORRECT ANSWER: B (1 and 3 are correct.)**

**SUMMARY:**

*Postherpetic neuralgia (PHN) more often afflicts the elderly, following the distribution of a particular sensory nerve. Motor nerves are not affected. Antineuropathic pain medicines such as tricyclic antidepressants and gabapentin are effective. Opioid analgesics may be effective but have been controversial*

**EXPLANATION:**

(1) *Correct.* Choice 1 is correct. The elderly are more at risk.
(2) *Incorrect.* Choice 2 is incorrect. The facial nerve (cranial nerve VII) is a motor nerve. The question describes an affliction of the supraorbital branch of the ophthalmic division of cranial nerve V (the trigeminal nerve).
(3) *Correct.* Choice 3 is correct. Tricyclic antidepressants are first-line treatment of PHN.
(4) *Incorrect.* Choice 4 is incorrect. Opioids may be helpful to some but their use in PHN is controversial.

**REASONING:**

More than half of those who develop shingles are over 60 years old. Ten to 15% of patients with herpes zoster will go on to develop PHN and this may reach 28% in people over 70 years old. Only sensory nerves are affected as the varicella virus reactivates in sensory ganglia either in the dorsal root ganglia or the gasserian ganglia of the trigeminal nerve. The commonest sites for herpes zoster and PHN are the midthoracic dermatomes and the ophthalmic division of the trigeminal nerve, but they may occur in any dermatome. Treatment often involves tricyclic antidepressants (amitriptyline), anticonvulsants (carbamazepine, gabapentin, and sodium valproate), Lidoderm patches, or capsaicin cream, but use of opioids has been controversial. Answer B is the correct answer as 1 and 3 are correct.

**BIBLIOGRAPHY:**
McMahon SB, Koltzenburg M. *Wall and Melzack's Textbook of Pain*. 5th ed. Philadelphia, PA: Churchill Livingstone; 2006:992-994.

Morgan GE, Mikhail MS, Murray MJ. *Clinical Anesthesiology*. 4th ed. New York, NY: McGraw-Hill; 2006:407.

Pickering G, Leplege A. Review article. Herpes zoster pain, postherpetic neuralgia, and quality of life in the elderly. *Pain Pract*. 2010 Dec;29. doi: 10.1111/j.1533-2500.2010.00432.x. [Epub ahead of print]

Warfield CA, Bajwa ZH. *Principles & Practice of Pain Medicine*. 2nd ed. New York, NY: McGraw-Hill; 2004:424-428.

---

## BOOK A:

*Answer E*

Pharmacology

## QUESTION 48

### QUESTION (K-type):

Three weeks after exposure to toxic levels of an organophosphate insecticide, a farm worker is scheduled for inguinal herniorrhaphy. Which of the following should be avoided?

(1)  Spinal anesthesia with tetracaine.
(2)  Epidural anesthesia with 2-chloroprocaine.
(3)  Atracurium neuromuscular block.
(4)  Succinylcholine infusion.

### CORRECT ANSWER: E (All are correct.)

### SUMMARY:

*Ester-linked local anesthetics such as 2-chloroprocaine and tetracaine are metabolized by pseudocholinesterase. Succinylcholine is as well. Atracurium is largely degraded by enzymatic degradation of nonspecific plasma esterases. Organophosphates irreversibly inhibit a number of enzymes, including pseudocholinesterase, acetylcholinesterase, as well as other nonspecific plasma esterases. Thus, following exposure to organophosphates the above drugs are best avoided.*

### EXPLANATION:

Organophosphate insecticides are irreversible inhibitors of cholinesterases affecting pseudocholinesterase, acetylcholinesterase, and nonspecific plasma cholinesterases. Their effects may last weeks. Pseudocholinesterase is involved in the metabolism of succinylcholine and ester-linked local anesthetics such as tetracaine and 2-chloroprocaine. Nonetheless, delayed metabolism of these local anesthetics in people with pseudocholinesterase deficiency has rarely been documented. Atracurium undergoes both ester hydrolysis by nonspecific plasma esterases, and by nonenzymatic degradation (Hofmann reaction). It has been estimated that two-thirds of the degradation of atracurium occurs via enzymatic ester hydrolysis. *cis*-Atracurium, on the other hand, does not undergo significant enzymatic hydrolysis. Therefore, all of the above should be avoided in a patient exposed to an organophosphate insecticide.

### REASONING:

All of the choices are best avoided in a patient exposed to organophosphates; thus answer E is the correct answer.

### BIBLIOGRAPHY:

Barash PG, Cullen BF, Stoelting RK, Cahalan MK, Stock MC. *Clinical Anesthesia*. 6th ed. Philadelphia, PA: Lippincott Williams & Wilkins; 2009:506, 509, 539.

Morgan GE, Mikhail MS, Murray MJ. *Clinical Anesthesiology*. 4th ed. New York, NY: McGraw-Hill; 2006:228.

*Answer D*

OB/Regional

**QUESTION (K-type):**

The addition of halothane 0.5% to nitrous oxide and oxygen 50% each for cesarean delivery

(1) Increases the incidence of low Apgar scores.
(2) Increases operative blood loss.
(3) Increases the incidence of maternal hypotension.
(4) Decreases the incidence of maternal awareness.

**CORRECT ANSWER: D (4 only is correct.)**

**SUMMARY:**

*The addition of a low-dose volatile agent such as halothane or isoflurane is common practice during general anesthesia for cesarean section. When compared with a technique using 50% nitrous oxide and 50% oxygen and no volatile agent, many clinically significant differences are observed. A deeper level of anesthesia is achieved, which results in decreased circulating catecholamine levels and a significantly reduced incidence of maternal awareness. High maternal catecholamine levels have been shown to cause uterine artery vasoconstriction and decreased uterine blood flow, which is ablated with the use of volatile agents. While intraoperative blood loss is greater in patients who receive general anesthesia for cesarean section, it is not increased with the addition of a volatile agent in low doses (< 1 MAC).* Note that parturients have approximately a 30% decrease in MAC. *Adverse neonatal effects have not been observed.*

**EXPLANATION:**

(1) *Incorrect.* Volatile agents have not been shown to cause low Apgar scores. In fact, the addition of volatile agents allows the anesthesiologist to give the mother higher inhaled oxygen concentrations for a given level of anesthesia, which has been shown to improve the condition of the newborn.
(2) *Incorrect.* Halogenated agents produce a dose-related decrease in uterine tone. However, addition of low doses of these agents during cesarean section has not been shown to increase operative blood loss when compared with a technique using 50% nitrous oxide and 50% oxygen and no volatile agent.
(3) *Incorrect.* Patients given a volatile agent in addition to nitrous oxide and oxygen have lower blood pressures than those without volatile agents. However, in the *hemodynamically stable* patient, the incidence of true maternal hypotension is not increased significantly.
(4) *Correct.* Cesarean section is associated with a high incidence of awareness, especially in emergency cases. Compared with a technique with no volatile agent, the incidence of awareness is virtually eliminated by using a volatile agent (at close to 1 MAC).

**REASONING:**

For K-type questions, it is best to first determine which statements are true. Once this is done, some answers can be eliminated just because of their location on the list. In this question, choice 4 is definitely true, which eliminates A and B as possible answers. Then one must decide if all the statements are true. Choice 1 is definitely not true owing to the low dose of halothane given, which eliminates E as a possible answer. Then one must decide if choice 2 is true to choose between C and D as answers. While it is true that halogenated agents cause decreased uterine tone, low doses have not been associated with increased operative blood loss (< 1 MAC). The key here is the low dose, which eliminates choice 2 and makes D the correct answer.

**BIBLIOGRAPHY:**
Bucklin B, Gambling DR, Wlody DJ. *A Practical Approach to Obstetric Anesthesia.* Philadelphia, PA: Lippincott, Williams and Wilkins; 2009:202-203.
Chestnut DH, Polley LS, Lawrence CT, Wong CA. *Chestnut's. Obstetric Anesthesia Principles and Practice.* 4th ed. St. Louis, MO: Mosby; 2009:543-549.
Morgan GE, Mikhail MS, Murray MJ. *Clinical Anesthesiology.* 4th ed. New York, NY: McGraw-Hill; 2006:901-906.

---

**BOOK A:**

## QUESTION 50

*Answer D*

Pain

**QUESTION (K-type):**

Stellate ganglion block is associated with ipsilateral

(1) Mydriasis.
(2) Diaphoresis.
(3) Exophthalmos.
(4) Scleral hyperemia.

**CORRECT ANSWER: D (4 only is correct.)**

**SUMMARY:**

*Stellate ganglion block is performed by injection of local anesthetic in the neck to block the sympathetic innervation of the ipsilateral head, face, and arm. Interruption of the sympathetic tone leads to Horner syndrome. Horner syndrome is characterized by ptosis, miosis, anhidrosis, and enophthalmos. In addition, interruption of sympathetic tone results in vasodilation of the affected areas. This yields an increase in temperature of the skin, hyperemia of the ipsilateral sclera, and nasal congestion.*

**EXPLANATION:**

(1) *Incorrect.* Mydriasis (pupil enlargement) is the opposite of what is seen following successful stellate block.
(2) *Incorrect.* Diaphoresis (sweating) is blocked by successful stellate block.
(3) *Incorrect.* Exophthalmos (protruding eye) is the opposite of what is seen following successful stellate.
(4) *Correct.* Scleral hyperemia caused by vasodilation is seen following successful stellate block.

**REASONING:**

The stellate ganglion is composed of the fusion of the inferior cervical ganglion and the first thoracic ganglion. However, the sympathetic innervation of the head, face, and upper extremity does not all pass through the stellate ganglion. Thus, when stellate ganglion block is performed, 15 to 20 mL of solution is used with the hope that it will spread along the prevertebral fascia superiorly and inferiorly down to T4. When this is accomplished, interruption of sympathetic tone will result in ipsilateral ptosis (lid droop) by blocking sympathetic innervation to the superior tarsal muscle (Mueller's third), anhidrosis (lack of facial sweating), miosis (small pupil), and enophthalmos (recession of the eyeball into the orbit). Slight enophthalmos results from interruption of sympathetic tone to the orbitalis muscle (Mueller's first), which spans the inferior orbital fissure. Release of vasoconstrictive tone results in nasal congestion, scleral hyperemia, facial flushing, and upper extremity temperature increase. The best answer is D.

BIBLIOGRAPHY:
Cousins M, Bridenbaugh P. *Neural Blockade in Clinical Anesthesia and Management of Pain*. 3rd ed. Philadelphia, PA: Lippincott Williams & Wilkins; 1998:428-429.
Morgan GE, Mikhail MS, Murray MJ. *Clinical Anesthesiology*. 4th ed. New York, NY: McGraw-Hill; 2006:383.

---

## BOOK A:   QUESTION 51

*Answer A*

Pharmacology

**QUESTION (K-type):**

A 22-year-old man is unconscious after free-basing "crack." Likely findings include

(1) Depressed ST segments.
(2) Hyperthermia.
(3) Premature ventricular contractions.
(4) Pinpoint pupils.

**CORRECT ANSWER: A (1, 2, and 3 are correct.)**

**SUMMARY:**

*Crack is cocaine. Signs of cocaine overdose relate to its actions both as a local anesthetic and its inhibition of norepinephrine reuptake. Complications include coronary vasospasm, myocardial ischemia or infarction, serious and sudden dysrhythmias, high-output congestive heart failure, rhabdomyolysis, acute renal failure, seizures, hyperpyrexia, thrombocytopenia, and respiratory depression. The increased sympathetic tone associated with cocaine use leads to enlarged pupils, agitation, heightened reflexes, hypertension, and tachycardia.*

**EXPLANATION:**

(1) **Correct.** Crack cocaine may cause ischemia-related ST-segment depression.
(2) **Correct.** Cocaine is associated with life-threatening hyperthermia.
(3) **Correct.** PVCs are often seen in cocaine overdose.
(4) **Incorrect.** Pupils would likely be large following cocaine use. Therefore, answer A is the best choice.

**REASONING:**

Through its sympathomimetic effects, cocaine increases heart rate, blood pressure, and myocardial work, while decreasing coronary blood flow by inducing coronary vasospasm. Myocardial ischemia is not infrequent and can manifest as ST depression. Hyperthermia is also commonly seen resulting from the increased metabolic rate driven by the sympathetic nervous system. Ventricular dysrhythmias both with and without ischemia can be seen including premature ventricular contractions (PVCs). The increased sympathetic tone leads to the look of "wide-eyed surprise" associated with increased sympathetic tone. Pupil size is increased. Pinpoint pupils are associated with opiate overdose rather than crack. When an opiate is mixed with cocaine or an amphetamine, this is referred to as "speed-balling." The pupil size may then be hard to predict.

**BIBLIOGRAPHY:**

Haim DY, Lippmann ML, Goldberg SK, Walkenstein MD. The pulmonary complications of crack cocaine. A comprehensive review. Chest. 1995;107(1):233-240.
Hines RL, Marschall KE. *Stoeling's Anesthesia and Co-existing Disease*. 5th ed. Philadelphia, PA: Churchill Livingstone; 2008:543-544.

Lange RA, Hillis LD. Medical progress: cardiovascular complications of cocaine use. *N Engl J Med.* 2001 Aug 2;345:351-358.

Traub SJ, Hoffman RS, Nelson LS. Current concepts: body packing—the internal concealment of illicit drugs. *N Engl J Med.* 2003 Dec 25;349:2519-2526.

---

**BOOK A:** | **QUESTION 52**

---

## *Answer A*

## Pharmacology

**QUESTION (K-type):**

Administration of halothane to a healthy patient causes

(1) Decreased myocardial contractility.
(2) Depressed baroreceptor response.
(3) Increased venous capacitance.
(4) Decreased systemic vascular resistance.

**CORRECT ANSWER: A (1, 2, and 3 are correct.)**

**SUMMARY:**

*Halothane is a halogenated alkane volatile anesthetic that has many cardiovascular effects. It causes a decrease in mean arterial pressure (MAP) through direct myocardial depression. Halothane blunts the baroreceptor response because an elevated heart rate would be expected with a decreased MAP, but heart rate does not increase with halothane. Vasodilation does occur with halothane, but systemic vascular resistance (SVR) does not change because cardiac output also decreases.*

**EXPLANATION:**

(1) *Correct.* Halothane depresses the heart and cardiac output in a dose-dependent manner. This effect occurs because halothane interferes with intracellular calcium utilization.
(2) *Correct.* Halothane is thought to blunt the carotid baroreceptor response to decreases in MAP via inhibition of central sympathetic efferents to the baroreceptors.
(3) *Correct.* Halothane causes an increase in venous capacitance.
(4) *Incorrect.* Halothane minimally affects SVR when compared to other inhalational agents. The decrease in MAP with halothane is primarily due to decreased CO from myocardial depression.

**REASONING:**

Choice 1 is clearly correct because one of the unique properties of halothane is its depression on myocardium. This allows answers C and D to be eliminated. Choice 2 is correct because an increase in heart rate is not seen when using halothane, leaving only answers A and E as possibilities. Answer A is correct because choice 4 is incorrect. When deciding whether or not choice 4 is correct, it is helpful to write out the equation for SVR. In examining the equation, it becomes obvious that not only MAP affects SVR, but CO does as well, and because both decrease equally, SVR is unchanged. The best answer is A.

**BIBLIOGRAPHY:**

Benia R, Koushanpour E. Local versus central effect of halothane on carotid sinus baroreceptor function. *Anesthesiology.* 1984;61:161-168.

Morgan GE, Mikhail MS, Murray MJ. *Clinical Anesthesiology.* 3rd ed. New York, NY: McGraw-Hill; 2002:139-140.

Stoelting RK, Miller RD. *Basics of Anesthesia.* 4th ed. New York, NY: Churchill Livingstone; 2000:46-49.

## Answer A

### Cardiovascular

**QUESTION (K-type):**

Indications for administration of calcium chloride during cardiopulmonary resuscitation include

(1)  Acute hyperkalemia.
(2)  Electromechanical dissociation.
(3)  Verapamil toxicity.
(4)  Digoxin toxicity.

**CORRECT ANSWER: A (1, 2, and 3 are correct.)**

**SUMMARY:**

*Calcium chloride is indicated during cardiopulmonary resuscitation (CPR) under specific conditions such as hyperkalemia, hypocalcemia, calcium channel blocker toxicity, and hypermagnesemia. Electromechanical dissociation (EMD) or the newer term pulseless electrical activity (PEA) is a generic diagnosis where the patient has electrical cardiac activity without perfusion. It includes the above-mentioned conditions in addition to other causes such as hypoxia, hypovolemia, acidosis, hypothermia, drug overdose, tamponade, tension pneumothorax, and massive pulmonary embolus.*

**EXPLANATION:**

(1)  *Correct.* Calcium chloride is indicated in the treatment of hyperkalemia. It antagonizes the effect of high potassium levels on the heart.
(2)  *Correct.* Pulseless electrical activity includes many conditions, among which are hyperkalemia, hypermagnesemia, and calcium channel blocker toxicity that can be treated with calcium chloride.
(3)  *Correct.* Calcium chloride can be used to treat verapamil overdose.
(4)  *Incorrect.* Hyperkalemia and hypokalemia worsen the digoxin toxicity. Therefore, calcium chloride is contraindicated.

**REASONING:**

This question tests knowledge of the indications for calcium administration during CPR. Specific pathology such as hyperkalemia, hypermagnesemia, and calcium channel blocker toxicity all can be treated with administration of calcium chloride. Choices 1, 2, and 3 are correct. Therefore, A is the best answer.

**BIBLIOGRAPHY:**

Barash PG, Cullen BF, Stoelting RK, Cahalan MK, Stock MC. *Clinical Anesthesia.* 6th ed. Philadelphia, PA: Lippincott Williams & Wilkins; 2009:1544-1545.
Miller RD, Miller ED, Reves JG, et al. *Anesthesia.* 7th ed. New York, NY: Churchill Livingstone; 2010:2988.
Morgan GE, Mikhail MS, Murray MJ. *Clinical Anesthesiology.* 3rd ed. New York, NY: McGraw-Hill; 2002:924.

## *Answer D*

### Physiology

**QUESTION (K-type):**

A 27-year-old man is undergoing emergency bronchoscopy with propofol-vecuronium anesthesia after aspirating a peanut. Intervals of apneic oxygenation are used to facilitate the procedure. Initial blood gas values while breathing pure oxygen are $Pa_{O_2}$ = 400 mm Hg and $Pa_{CO_2}$ = 30 mm Hg. Effects of 10 minutes of apneic oxygenation at a flow rate of 10 L/min include

(1) Decreased heart rate.
(2) Decreased $Pa_{O_2}$ to 50 mm Hg.
(3) Cutaneous vasoconstriction.
(4) Increased $Pa_{CO_2}$ to 60 mm Hg.

**CORRECT ANSWER: D (4 only is correct.)**

**SUMMARY:**

*Apneic oxygenation is a technique used to maintain oxygenation without maintaining ventilation. A catheter supplying oxygen is placed above the carina to replace oxygen absorbed by the lungs. This technique can provide adequate oxygenation for more than 30 minutes, but it is limited by the development of hypercapnia. Without ventilation, hypercapnia occurs as a function of the duration of apnea. Hypercapnia leads to signs of increased sympathetic tone, including tachycardia and hypertension, as well as dilation of conjunctival and superficial facial vessels leading to flushing.*

**EXPLANATION:**

(1) *Incorrect.* Not only is a decreased heart rate not expected, but the apnea-induced hypercapnia would cause tachycardia.
(2) *Incorrect.* $Pa_{O_2}$ would be better maintained after only 10 minutes.
(3) *Incorrect.* Cutaneous vasodilation is expected due to hypercarbia.
(4) *Correct.* $Pa_{CO_2}$ would be predicted to rise at least to 60 mm Hg. Therefore, answer D is correct and is the best answer.

**REASONING:**

An increased heart rate rather than a decreased heart rate would be expected due to the development of hypercapnia and its associated increase in sympathetic tone. Hypercapnia also leads to facial flushing and cutaneous vasodilation rather than vasoconstriction despite the increase in sympathetic tone. Apneic oxygenation can maintain adequate levels of oxygen despite a lack of ventilation for up to a half an hour and the $pa_{O_2}$ would be expected to be significantly higher than 50 mm Hg after an apneic period of only 10 minutes. During apnea carbon dioxide is not eliminated and its partial pressure will rise. In the apneic anesthetized patient, the partial pressure of carbon dioxide typically rises by approximately 12 mm Hg/min for the first minute and by 3.5 mm Hg/min every minute thereafter. The expected rise after 10 minutes would be approximately 12.5 + (3.5 × 9) = 44 mm Hg. With a staring $Pa_{CO_2}$ of 30, the total $Pa_{CO_2}$ would be approximately 74. Therefore, an increase in $Pa_{CO_2}$ to at least 60 mm Hg would be expected.

**BIBLIOGRAPHY:**

Barash PG, Cullen BF, Stoelting RK, Cahalan MK, Stock MC. *Clinical Anesthesia*. 6th ed. Philadelphia, PA: Lippincott Williams & Wilkins; 2009:241.
Morgan GE, Mikhail MS, Murray MJ. *Clinical Anesthesiology*. 4th ed. New York, NY: McGraw-Hill; 2006:838-839.

*Answer B*

Equipment/Physics

**QUESTION (K-type):**

In a patient with normal hemodynamics, systemic blood pressure is measured using a radial artery catheter and a noninvasive oscillometric blood pressure (NIBP) monitor on the same arm. Compared with the readings from the NIBP monitor, the indwelling catheter would show

(1)  The same or higher systolic blood pressure.
(2)  Lower diastolic pressure if the transducer is damped.
(3)  The same mean blood pressure.
(4)  Lower blood pressure values if the catheter is replaced by one with a larger diameter.

**CORRECT ANSWER: B (1 and 3 are correct.)**

**SUMMARY:**

*The "gold standard" for blood pressure monitoring is intra-arterial monitoring. Overdamping by lengthy tubing, extra stopcocks, air bubbles, and increased blood viscosity would reduce the arterial waveform and therefore systolic pressure. Underdamping by decreasing tubing size or increasing catheter size would raise the blood pressure artifactually. Compared with the noninvasive blood pressure cuff, the catheter-transducer system usually gives a higher blood pressure value owing to underdamping and resonance. (See also question 153, Book A for an explanation of pulse-wave amplification.)*

**EXPLANATION:**

(1)  *Correct.* An old study comparing automated auscultatory and oscillometric pressure against direct invasive measurements of arterial pressure showed that indirect methods underestimated the systolic and overestimated diastolic pressure. One way to remember this is that the catheter-transducer system includes extra components such as tubing and stopcocks that contribute to underdamping and resonance. This results in direct systolic arterial pressure often exceeding indirect noninvasive pressure.
(2)  *Incorrect.* A dampened system would result in lowered systolic but not diastolic pressure. This occurs when the frequency of the system is too low to faithfully reproduce the arterial waveform, producing a more protracted or smaller wave.
(3)  *Correct.* Mean arterial pressure (MAP) is the most accurate value measured by oscillometry and is taken at the cuff pressure at which maximal oscillation of the arterial pulse occurs. In the catheter-transducer system, the MAP is calculated by integrating the area under the arterial waveform. Although studies have reported slight differences between the invasive and noninvasive MAP, this is questionably significant. Overthinking would lead one to eliminate this choice. However, simply understanding that the MAP is one of the more accurate values measured in oscillometry and less subjected to a dampening or overshooting in the catheter-transducer system would make this choice correct.
(4)  *Incorrect.* Larger catheters create greater ringing or resonance in the system. This would result in higher systolic pressure.

**REASONING:**

This is a challenging question that demands a thorough understanding of noninvasive and catheter-transducer methods for measuring arterial blood pressure. It is important for the reader to review the principles of oscillometric methods as well as factors that affect damping of catheter-transducer systems. Understanding the physics behind intraarterial monitoring helps eliminate choices 2 and 4. Whether or not one knows that choice 3 is correct; the only logical choice left is answer B (1 and 3).

**BIBLIOGRAPHY:**

Barash PG, Cullen BF, Stoelting RK, Cahalan MK, Stock MC. *Clinical Anesthesia.* 6th ed. Philadelphia, PA: Lippincott Williams & Wilkins; 2009:703-705.

Davis RF. Clinical comparison of automated auscultatory and oscillometric and catheter-transducer measurements of arterial pressure. *J Clin Monit.* 1985;1:114.

Miller RD, Miller ED, Reves JG, et al. *Anesthesia.* 7th ed. Philadelphia, PA: Churchill Livingstone; 2010:1274-1276.

Morgan GE, Mikhail MS, Murray MJ. *Clinical Anesthesiology.* 4th ed. New York, NY: McGraw-Hill; 2006:127-128.

---

| **BOOK A:** | **QUESTION 56** |

*Answer D*

Pharmacology

**QUESTION (K-type):**

A 20-kg, 4-year-old boy receives atropine 0.3 mg intramuscularly 1 hour before inguinal herniorrhaphy under general anesthesia. Forty minutes later while still in the preoperative preparation room, his temperature is 38.6°C. Likely causes of the temperature elevation include

(1)  Malignant hyperthermia.
(2)  Alteration of central temperature regulation.
(3)  Release of catecholamines.
(4)  Suppression of sweating.

**CORRECT ANSWER: D (4 only is correct.)**

**SUMMARY:**

*Anticholinergic agents are used in anesthesia for various purposes. Understanding the pharmacology of these agents is important as there are many side effects, including atrial dysrhythmias, CNS effects of both stimulation and depression, decreased peristalsis, mydriasis, cycloplegia, and urinary retention. Atropine is a tertiary amine that can be administered intravenously, intramuscularly, and into the trachea. It is particularly effective on the heart (treating bradycardia) and the bronchial smooth muscle (bronchodilation). Scopolamine is also a tertiary amine with greater antisialagogue properties than atropine. It also has greater CNS effects as evidenced by the use of the agent as a sedative, and for prevention of motion sickness. Glycopyrrolate is a quaternary agent that does not cross the blood-brain barrier. It causes a mild increase in heart rate, has antisialagogue effects, and has little or no CNS effects. Glycopyrrolate is often given to counter the bradycardia of neostigmine when reversing neuromuscular blockade. (Also see question 6A.)*

**EXPLANATION:**

(1)  *Incorrect.* While malignant hyperthermia (MH) should always be a concern in the presence of hyperthermia, there is no other clinical indication that the patient is at risk for MH or that the patient has signs of MH other than the elevated temperature.

(2)  *Incorrect.* While atropine, a tertiary amine, does cross the blood-brain barrier, the CNS effects are behavioral, including memory deficits, restlessness, unconsciousness, and hallucinations. This is known as *central anticholinergic syndrome.* There is no known alteration of central temperature regulation.

(3)  *Incorrect.* Anticholinergic agents blocks acetylcholine from binding to the muscarinic cholinergic receptor. Blockade of the receptors in the sinoatrial node results in tachycardia, but this is due to inhibition of vagal tone, not release of catecholamines.

(4)  *Correct.* Suppression of sweating is a known effect of anticholinergic agents, and is the likely mechanism of the patient's elevated temperature (atropine fever).

This question is testing whether the reader understands the pharmacology of anticholinergics. Choice 1 is possible, but without further information, is not likely. If there is any uncertainty about choice 1, the reader should know that choice 3 is not the mechanism of anticholinergic agents. This should narrow the choices to 2 and 4. The reader should know that the mechanism of hyperthermia with anticholinergic agents is suppression of sweating, and not central alterations.

**BIBLIOGRAPHY:**

Morgan GE, Mikhail MS, Murray MJ. *Clinical Anesthesiology*. 4th ed. New York, NY: McGraw-Hill; 2006:237-241.

---

## BOOK A:

*Answer B*

Pharmacology

## QUESTION 57

**QUESTION (K-type):**

If ketorolac 30 mg were substituted for meperidine 100 mg after an outpatient inguinal herniorrhaphy, the patient would experience less

(1) Respiratory depression.
(2) Analgesia.
(3) Nausea.
(4) Bleeding.

**CORRECT ANSWER: B (1 and 3 are correct.)**

**SUMMARY:**

*Ketorolac is a nonsteroidal anti-inflammatory drug (NSAID) that is administered either intravenously or intramuscularly. It is used for short-term management of acute pain and works by blocking prostaglandin synthesis. Ketorolac is mainly a peripherally acting drug and causes minimal, if any, central side effects associated with opiates such as nausea and vomiting, sedation, and respiratory depression. Disadvantages of ketorolac include inhibition of platelet aggregation, renal toxicity, gastrointestinal ulcerations, and a ceiling effect to the amount of analgesia produced by increasing the dose of ketorolac. In addition, patients with asthma, nasal polyps, and aspirin allergies have a higher incidence of allergic reactions to ketorolac.*

**EXPLANATION:**

(1) *Correct.* Ketorolac primarily acts peripherally, with no respiratory depressive effects and minimal nausea in comparison with opiates, which act centrally and can cause both side effects.
(2) *Incorrect.* Ketorolac 30 mg and meperidine 100 mg are equivalent analgesic doses.
(3) *Correct.* See above.
(4) *Incorrect.* Ketorolac produces more bleeding when compared with opiates because ketorolac inhibits platelet aggregation. This occurs because ketorolac inhibits cyclooxygenase, preventing thromboxane synthesis, which is necessary for platelet aggregation.

**REASONING:**

Clearly, choices 1 and 3 are correct because nausea and respiratory depression are well-known opiate side effects not usually associated with ketorolac. Choice 4 is incorrect because one of the principal concerns with using ketorolac is the increased bleeding postoperatively caused by platelet inhibition. This allows answers C, D, and E to be eliminated. Only choice 2 remains, which is incorrect because the doses listed provide roughly equivalent analgesia. B is the best answer.

**BIBLIOGRAPHY:**

Morgan GE, Mikhail MS, Murray MJ. *Clinical Anesthesiology.* 3rd ed. New York, NY: McGraw-Hill; 2002:248.

Stoelting RK. *Pharmacology and Physiology in Anesthetic Practice.* 3rd ed. Philadelphia, PA: Lippincott Raven Publishers; 1999:255-256.

---

| BOOK A: | QUESTION 58 |
|---|---|

## *Answer D*

### OB/Regional

**QUESTION (K-type):**

An asymptomatic 32-year-old man with asthma undergoes herniorrhaphy under 1.5% lidocaine epidural anesthesia to a sensory level of T2-3. Which of the following will occur with this level of anesthesia?

(1)  The ability to cough will be normal.
(2)  Vital capacity will be unchanged.
(3)  Intraoperative bronchospasm will be prevented.
(4)  Tidal volume will be unchanged.

**CORRECT ANSWER: D (4 only is correct.)**

**SUMMARY:**

*Epidural anesthesia with high sensory levels can cause paralysis of abdominal and intercostal muscles, leading to decreased ERV, peak expiratory flow, and maximum minute ventilation. Vital capacity is reduced in these patients as a result of the decrease in ERV. Abdominal and intercostal muscle paralysis with high sensory levels is also associated with decreased ability to cough, which can be problematic in patients with lung disease and/or copious secretions. While the sympathectomy associated with high sensory epidural anesthesia theoretically could increase bronchomotor tone owing to unopposed parasympathetic innervation of the airways, this is not a clinically significant problem in asthmatic patients.*

**EXPLANATION:**

(1)  *Incorrect.* The ability to cough in these patients is abnormal owing to paralysis of abdominal and intercostal muscles.
(2)  *Incorrect.* Vital capacity is reduced owing to the reduction in ERV.
(3)  *Incorrect.* Intraoperative bronchospasm will not be prevented in this patient because the airways will have primarily parasympathetic tone due to the sympathectomy associated with a T2 epidural sensory level.
(4)  *Correct.* Tidal volume is unchanged in patients with high sensory levels from neuraxial anesthesia.

**REASONING:**

The question tests the reader's knowledge of the effects of a high sensory level of anesthesia associated with neuraxial blockade. Choice 1 is incorrect because cough is impaired in this situation. Because ERV is a component of vital capacity and is reduced, vital capacity must be reduced, making choice 2 incorrect. Choice 3 can be eliminated because choice 1 is incorrect. However, bronchospasm in an asthmatic patient will not be prevented by a sympathectomy because increased sympathetic tone favors bronchodilation. Choice 4 is correct because lung volumes do not change considerably with high sensory levels. This makes D the best answer.

**BIBLIOGRAPHY:**

Barash PG, Cullen BF, Stoelting RK, Cahalan M, Stock M. *Clinical Anesthesia*. 6th ed. Philadelphia, PA: Lippincott Williams & Wilkins; 2010:947.

Miller RD, Eriksson LI, Fleisher LA, Wiener-Kronish JP, William YL. *Miller's Anesthesia*. 7th ed. Philadelphia, PA: Churchill Livingstone; 2010:1618.

Morgan GE, Mikhail MS, Murray MJ. *Clinical Anesthesiology*. 4th ed. New York, NY: McGraw-Hill; 2006:297, 545 (Figure 22-4).

---

| **BOOK A:** | **QUESTION 59** |
| --- | --- |

## *Answer D*

### OB/Regional

**QUESTION (K-type):**

True statements concerning epidurally administered morphine include the following:

(1) The long duration of analgesia results from high lipid solubility.
(2) Pruritus is completely reversed by naloxone.
(3) Plasma morphine levels are lower than those seen after intramuscular administration.
(4) Analgesia is inadequate for the pain of labor.

**CORRECT ANSWER: D (4 only is correct.)**

**SUMMARY:**

*Morphine is a hydrophilic opiate. With epidural administration, a small amount diffuses into the intrathecal space and acts on spinal opiate receptors. Its water solubility allows it to remain in the intrathecal space, resulting in a duration of action of approximately 12 to 16 hours. Side effects of epidural morphine include pruritus, urinary retention, sedation, and respiratory depression. While epidural narcotics alone are inadequate for the pain of labor, they can be used to minimize local anesthetic concentration and the motor blockade associated with local anesthetics.*

**EXPLANATION:**

(1) *Incorrect.* Morphine is a water-soluble narcotic.
(2) *Incorrect.* The pruritus associated with epidural morphine is reduced significantly by naloxone but not completely eliminated. A study in 2000 that looked at 80 patients showed that high-dose naloxone infusions could significantly reduce the incidence of pruritus, in those patients receiving epidural morphine, but not eliminate it.
(3) *Incorrect.* When compared, plasma levels of morphine were similar when intravenous and epidural doses were given. Plasma levels tend to fluctuate more with intramuscular bolus administration but have similar pharmacokinetics to intravenous dosing. Therefore, plasma morphine levels are similar to those seen after intramuscular administration.
(4) *Correct.* Intrathecal morphine can provide adequate analgesia for labor. When epidural morphine was studied, it had a slow onset and required high doses associated with unacceptable side effects to be used as a sole analgesic in labor.

A good general rule when taking tests is that if an answer is absolute (such as choice 2), it is usually not true. Very few things are absolute in medicine. Naloxone is an effective agent for pruritus but will not completely reverse this side effect. This question requires knowledge that morphine is hydrophilic, which eliminates choice 1. Because choices 1 and 2 are wrong, the correct answer must be D.

**BIBLIOGRAPHY:**

Barash PG, Cullen BF, Stoelting RK, Cahalan MK, Stock MC. *Clinical Anesthesia*. 6th ed. Philadelphia, PA: Lippincott Williams & Wilkins; 2010:598-600.
Bucklin B, Gambling DR, Wlody DJ. *A Practical Approach to Obstetric Anesthesia*. Philadelphia, PA: Lippincott, Williams and Wilkins; 2009:198-199.
Choi JH, Lee J, Bishop MJ. Epidural naloxone reduces pruritus and nausea without effecting analgesia by epidural morphine in bupivacaine. *Can J Anaesth*. 2000;47(1):33-37.

---

**BOOK A:**

## QUESTION 60

*Answer B*

Clinical Anesthesia

**QUESTION (K-type):**

A 36-year-old woman is scheduled for cholecystectomy. She is 65 in tall and weighs 180 kg. Compared with a patient of the same height who weighs 60 kg, this patient is at increased risk for

(1) Hypoxemia in the supine position.
(2) Fasting hypoglycemia.
(3) Acid aspiration syndrome.
(4) Difficult reversal of neuromuscular block.

**CORRECT ANSWER: B (1 and 3 are correct.)**

**SUMMARY:**

*Obese patients have a higher incidence of many diseases, including type 2 diabetes, coronary artery disease, gastroesophageal reflux, and hypertension. In addition, increased abdominal mass leads to restrictive lung disease, reduced FRC, and arterial hypoxemia. Morbid obesity is defined as a body mass index (BMI) of greater than 35 $kg/m^2$. Lipid-soluble drugs have a higher volume of distribution and may require higher loading doses to achieve clinical effect, whereas water-soluble drugs such as neuromuscular blockers have a decreased volume of distribution and should be dosed according to ideal body weight.*

**EXPLANATION:**

(1) ***Correct.*** Obese patients develop restrictive lung disease owing to compression of the diaphragm by abdominal adipose tissue. This results in decreased FRC that may fall below closing capacity. The supine position further reduces FRC, leading to atelectasis and ventilation-perfusion mismatch.
(2) ***Incorrect.*** Obese patients are at risk for developing type 2 diabetes mellitus that is characterized by insulin resistance and hyperglycemia. These patients should not develop fasting hypoglycemia secondary to insulin resistance.
(3) ***Correct.*** Hiatal hernia and gastroesophageal reflux disease are more common in the obese. In addition, delayed gastric emptying and hyperacidic gastric fluid place obese patients at higher risk for acid aspiration syndrome.
(4) ***Incorrect.*** Water-soluble drugs such as neuromuscular blockers can have a decreased volume of distribution in obese patients. Following an appropriate dose of muscle

relaxant based on ideal body weight, obese patients should respond to anticholinesterase reversal agents normally.

### REASONING:

There are several challenging aspects to this question. Although choice 2 may sound good, obese patients with diabetes mellitus type 2 should not develop fasting hypoglycemia owing to their disease alone. Patients using exogenous insulin for glycemic control may be at risk for hypoglycemia when fasting. Choice 4 is incorrect because obese patients should respond to neuromuscular blocking drugs appropriately. B is the best answer.

### BIBLIOGRAPHY:


Barash PG, Cullen BF, Stoelting RK. *Clinical Anesthesia*. 4th ed. Philadelphia, PA: Lippincott Williams & Wilkins; 2001;975, 1035-1041.

Morgan GE, Mikhail MS, Murray MJ. *Clinical Anesthesiology*. 3rd ed. New York, NY: McGraw-Hill; 2002:748-749.

Stoelting RK, Miller RD. *Basics of Anesthesia*. 4th ed. New York, NY: Churchill Livingstone; 2000:316-318.


---

## BOOK A:

*Answer D*

Physiology

## QUESTION 61

### QUESTION (K-type):

Radiologic findings in advanced emphysema include

(1)  Ground-glass appearance of lung fields.
(2)  Increased cardiothoracic ratio.
(3)  Increased bronchial markings.
(4)  Flattening of the hemidiaphragms.

### CORRECT ANSWER: D (None are correct; 3 and 4 are correct.)

### SUMMARY:

*Emphysema is one of the chronic obstructive pulmonary disease, characterized by destruction of alveolar septa, which may result in cystic cavities known as* bullae. *Destruction of alveoli decreases elastic recoil, causing premature airway collapse during exhalation. Macroscopically, emphysema is characterized by lung hyperinflation, leading to increased residual volume, increased functional residual capacity, and increased total lung capacity. Emphysema is characterized on chest x-ray as more radiolucent or darker, hyperinflated lungs, diaphragmatic depression, a small narrowly oriented cardiac silhouette in the setting of a low diaphragm, and dilation of pulmonary arteries with rapid tapering secondary to pulmonary hypertension.*

### EXPLANATION:

(1)  *Incorrect.* Ground-glass appearance of the lung fields is not associated with emphysema. This has a wide differential, including interstitial lung disease and ARDS.
(2)  *Incorrect.* Increased cardiothoracic ratio occurs with either an increase in heart size or decrease in lung size. Despite the fact that many patients with emphysema have cardiac disease and a potentially enlarged heart, cardiothoracic ratio is decreased in emphysematous patients as lung size increases significantly.
(3)  *Correct.* Increased bronchial markings are found in association primarily with chronic bronchitis, because of peribronchial fibrosis. This pattern may also be associated with emphysema because many patients manifest both processes.
(4)  *Correct.* The hemidiaphragms are flattened as the lungs are hyperinflated, pushing downward on the hemidiaphragms.

**REASONING:**

This is a difficult question, because bronchial markings are more typically associated with chronic bronchitis than with emphysema. However, the two-disease processes manifest together commonly. Thus choice 3 is correct. Choice 4 is clearly correct, as the enlarged lungs in emphysematous patients flatten the diaphragm. Thus none of the choices are correct.

**BIBLIOGRAPHY:**

Goodman LR. *Felson's Principles of Chest Roentgenology*. 2nd ed. Philadelphia, PA: Saunders; 1999:159, 239-240.

Lange S, Walsh G. *Radiology of Chest Diseases*. 3rd ed. New York, NY: Thieme; 2007:101-104.

Morgan GE, Mikhail MS, Murray MJ. *Clinical Anesthesiology*. 3rd ed. New York, NY: McGraw-Hill; 2002:516-517.

---

| **BOOK A:** | **QUESTION 62** |
| --- | --- |

*Answer A*

Pharmacology

**QUESTION (K-type):**

Anesthetic agents that are safe for use in a patient with acute intermittent porphyria include

(1) Ketamine.
(2) Isoflurane.
(3) Pancuronium.
(4) Etomidate.

**CORRECT ANSWER: A (1, 2, and 3 are correct.)**

**SUMMARY:**

*This is a classic boards question that tests knowledge of an interesting but rare condition that can affect anesthetic care. The porphyrias are a group of enzymatic disorders in the production of heme from δ-aminolevulinic acid (δ-ALA). The heme formed by these enzymatic reactions is used in the synthesis of hemoglobin and cytochrome P-450s. Importantly, anything inducing the formation of hemoglobin, myoglobin, or cytochrome P-450s will induce δ-ALA synthetase, causing the buildup of harmful porphyrin precursors. The subset of porphyrias that can be induced by drug exposure include intermittent porphyria, variegate porphyria, and hereditary coproporphyria. Acute intermittent porphyria occurs when the enzyme porphobilinogen deaminase is defective, leading to the buildup of porphobilinogen when δ-ALA synthetase is induced. Porphobilinogen is neurotoxic and can cause autonomic dysfunction, electrolyte abnormalities (hypokalemia, hyponatremia, and hypomagnesemia), neuropsychiatric disturbances, cranial nerve palsies, and muscle weakness severe enough to progress to respiratory failure. Attacks are precipitated by drugs or physiologic factors such as menstruation, fasting, dehydration, infection, and stress that can induce heme synthesis. Drugs that may induce a crisis include barbiturates, sedative such as chlordiazepoxide and diazepam, lidocaine, and phenytoin. Etomidate has also been implicated in animal models. Importantly, the stress of surgery and anesthesia can precipitate an attack in the absence of triggering agents.*

**EXPLANATION:**

(1) ***Correct.*** The following drugs have been used safely in patients with porphyria or are unlikely to provoke an attack: inhaled anesthetics, propofol, ketamine, neuromuscular blockers, anticholinergics, acetylcholinesterase inhibitors, local anesthetics, benzodiazepines, $H_2$ blockers, α- and β-agonists, epinephrine, and diltiazem.

(2) **Correct.** See above.

(3) **Correct.** See above.

(4) **Incorrect.** Possible triggering agents include all barbiturates (thiopental, thiamylal, and methohexital), etomidate, chlordiazepoxide, lidocaine, pentazocine, phenytoin, sulfonamides, and methyldopa. Etomidate is the only choice listed that can precipitate an attack, and choice 4 is incorrect.

### REASONING:

This is a difficult question to answer because the well-known triggering agents, barbiturates, are not listed as one of the answer choices. Nonetheless, knowledge that anything inducing cytochrome P-450s can incite acute intermittent porphyria allows choices 2 and 3 to be chosen as correct answers because neither isoflurane nor pancuronium induces cytochrome P-450s. Thus answers B, C, and D can be eliminated. This allows a 50% chance at obtaining the correct answer if you are not sure about etomidate, which can induce liver enzymes and precipitate an attack. A is the best answer.

### BIBLIOGRAPHY:


Barash PG, Cullen BF, Stoelting RK, Cahalan MK, Stock MC. *Clinical Anesthesia*. 6th ed. Philadelphia, PA: Lippincott Williams & Wilkins; 2009:615-616.

Morgan GE, Mikhail MS, Murray MJ. *Clinical Anesthesiology*. 3rd ed. New York, NY: McGraw-Hill; 2002:159.

Stoelting RK, Dierdorf SF. *Anesthesia and Co-existing Disease*. 4th ed. New York, NY: Churchill Livingston; 2002:455-460.


---

## BOOK A:   QUESTION 63

*Answer E*

Physiology

### QUESTION (K-type):

Recurrent laryngeal nerve paralysis is a recognized complication of which of the following procedures?

(1) Ligation of a patent ductus arteriosus.

(2) Stellate ganglion block.

(3) Mediastinoscopy.

(4) Use of topical ice slush during heart surgery.

### CORRECT ANSWER: E (All are correct.)

### SUMMARY:

*The recurrent laryngeal nerve, which is a branch of the vagus nerve, innervates all the muscles of the larynx except the cricothyroid muscle, which is innervated by the superior laryngeal branch of the vagus nerve. Unilateral injury to the recurrent laryngeal nerve may result in paralysis of the ipsilateral vocal cord, which may present as hoarseness. Acute bilateral injury to the nerve may result in stridor or respiratory distress because of unopposed adduction of the vocal cord by the cricothyroid muscle. Bilateral complete palsy affecting abductor and adductor fibers results in both cords adopting a paramedian position, while incomplete palsy may affect only the more sensitive abductor fibers and cause serious airflow compromise. Chronic bilateral injury may result in aphonia and become less severe, as the vocal cord eventually is positioned more medially due to atrophy. The vagus nerve or any of its branches may be injured during many different types of cardiothoracic surgery or nonthoracic surgery due to endotracheal intubation, positioning, central line placement, or surgical dissection.*

### EXPLANATION:

(1) **Correct.** Recurrent laryngeal nerve paralysis is a reported complication of ligation of patent ductus arteriosus, along with inadvertent ligation of the left pulmonary artery or descending aorta and bleeding from PDA disruption.

(2) **Correct.** Recurrent laryngeal nerve paralysis is a reported complication of stellate ganglion block.

(3) **Correct.** Recurrent laryngeal nerve paralysis is a reported complication of mediastinoscopy, along with cerebral ischemia from compression innominate artery, pneumothorax, air embolism, and phrenic nerve injury.

(4) **Correct.** Recurrent laryngeal nerve paralysis is a reported complication of use of topical ice slush during heart surgery, along with phrenic nerve injury.

### REASONING:

Answering this question necessitates understanding the anatomy of the recurrent laryngeal nerve and the brachial plexus, as well as the factors that contribute to nerve injuries. Each choice listed is a procedure in proximity to the course of the recurrent laryngeal nerve. Paralysis is a recognized complication of each of the procedures.

### BIBLIOGRAPHY:

Miller, 7th ed, pg 2358, 2637.

Morgan GE, Mikhail MS, Murray MJ. *Clinical Anesthesiology*. 4th ed. New York, NY: McGraw-Hill; 2006:92, 383-384, 607.

Sharma AD, Parmley CL, Sreeram G, Grocott H. Peripheral nerve injuries during cardiac surgery: risk factors, diagnosis, prognosis, and prevention. *Anesth Analg*. 2000 Dec; 91(6):1358-1369.

---

## BOOK A:                    QUESTION 64

*Answer A*

Physiology

### QUESTION (K-type):

Clinical situations associated with an increase in parasympathetic activity include

(1) Manipulation of the carotid sinus.
(2) Intestinal insufflation during colonoscopy.
(3) Traction on the superior oblique muscle during strabismus surgery.
(4) Caudal anesthesia for excision of a pilonidal cyst.

### CORRECT ANSWER: A (1, 2, and 3 are correct.)

### SUMMARY:

*Manipulation of the carotid sinus often will increase parasympathetic tone and in fact is known as a "vagal maneuver." Intestinal insufflation during colonoscopy can also provoke increases in parasympathetic tone and so called "vasovagal reactions." Strabismus surgery also may provoke bradycardia as a result of increased parasympathetic tone due to traction on the ocular musculature. This has been termed the* oculocardiac *reflex. Caudal anesthesia is not typically associated with increases in parasympathetic tone.*

### EXPLANATION:

Manipulation of the carotid sinus is often deliberately done during paroxysmal supraventricular tachycardia and may end AV junctional tachyarrhythmias by increasing parasympathetic tone to the AV node. Approximately 17% of patients undergoing colonoscopy experience some type of vasovagal reaction during colonoscopy often associated with insufflation of the colon. The oculocardiac reflex is mediated by afferent impulses traveling via V1 and efferent parasympathetic impulses mediated by the vagus. It may be seen in association with retrobulbar block, pressure on the eyeball, or traction of the extraocular muscles. It is most common in pediatric patients undergoing strabismus surgery. The severity of the oculocardiac reflex is variable ranging from bradycardia to sinus arrest or ventricular fibrillation. Management of the oculocardiac reflex involves cessation of the surgical stimulation, IV atropine, and possible infiltration of local anesthetic. Adequate depth of anesthesia should also be confirmed. Typical complications of caudal anesthesia do not include vasovagal reactions and caudal anesthesia is contraindicated for pilonidal cyst excisions.

### REASONING:

(1) *Correct.* Carotid sinus massage increases parasympathetic tone.
(2) *Correct.* Intestinal insufflation often provokes an increase in sympathetic tone.
(3) *Correct.* Extraocular muscle traction can elicit an increase in parasympathetic tone via the oculocardiac reflex.
(4) *Incorrect.* This choice is a bit of a trick question as caudal anesthesia is contraindicated for a pilonidal cyst excision, as anatomically the access point to the caudal space underlies the area of the pilonidal cyst itself. Further, caudal anesthesia is not associated with increases in parasympathetic activity. Therefore, answer A is correct.

### BIBLIOGRAPHY:


Herman LL, Kurtz RC, McKee KJ, Sun M, Thaler HT, Winawer SJ. Risk factors associated with vasovagal reactions during colonoscopy. *Gastrointest Endosc.* 1993 May-Jun;39(3): 388-391.

Morgan GE, Mikhail MS, Murray MJ. *Clinical Anesthesiology.* 4th ed. New York, NY: McGraw-Hill; 2006:316, 828.


---

**BOOK A:**  **QUESTION 65**

---

*Answer A*

Physiology

**QUESTION (K-type):**

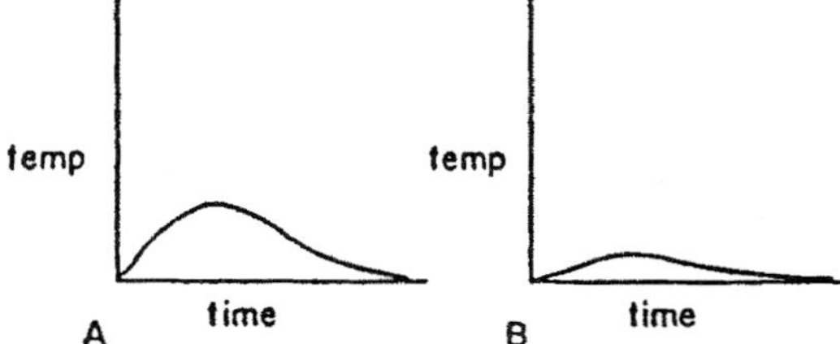


Curve A shown here is an accurate thermodilution curve from a patient with a cardiac output of 4 L/min. Curve B was obtained at the same time from the same patient. Curve B is consistent with

(1) An opening at the syringe-catheter junction that allows some injectate to leak out of the system.
(2) Use of room-temperature injectate when the computer is programmed for iced injectate.
(3) Injection of cold indicator solution through a long extension tube rather than directly into the correct catheter lumen.
(4) Use of 10 mL of cold indicator solution when the cardiac output computer is programmed for 5 mL of injectate.

**CORRECT ANSWER: A (1, 2, and 3 are correct.)**

## SUMMARY:

*Thermodilution cardiac output determination involves the injection of a known quantity of fluid of a known temperature at a proximal site and measuring the change in temperature of blood at a thermistor distal to the injection site; temperature change is inversely proportional to cardiac output. Accurate measurements are dependent on: cardiac anatomy (eg, presents of intracardiac shunts, valvular pathology), phase of respiratory cycle at time of measurement, proper delivery of thermal indicator (eg, absence of leaks in system, use of correct injection sites, volumes, and temperatures of injectate), stable pulmonary artery blood temperatures, and a properly functioning thermistor.*

## EXPLANATION:

(1) ***Correct.*** A leak at the syringe-catheter junction, with a resultant decreased quantity of injectate reaching the thermistor, would produce less of a change in measured temperature. This would be interpreted as a falsely lower calculated cardiac output.

(2) ***Correct.*** When room-temperature injectate is injected into a system programmed for iced injectate, the measured temperature change will be smaller, resulting in an erroneously low calculated cardiac output.

(3) ***Correct.*** Injectate injected through a long extension tube would undergo a change in temperature change in the extension tube, thus resulting in a decreased measured temperature change at the distal thermistor.

(4) ***Incorrect.*** Excess volume of injectate would result in a greater measured temperature change, and thus be interpreted as a falsely high calculated cardiac output.

## REASONING:

Understanding the mechanism by which a thermodilution technique is used to calculate the cardiac output is the key to answering this question correctly. Choices 1 through 3 correctly predict curve B; these scenarios result in less predicted (volume or temperature of) injectate reaching the thermistor, and thus result in a lower calculated cardiac output (the calculation is based on the area under the curve). Choice 4 is incorrect because a greater volume of cold injected would result in a greater measured temperature change, and thus a falsely high calculated cardiac output.

## BIBLIOGRAPHY:

Barash PG, Cullen BF, Stoelting RK, Cahalan MK, Stock MC. *Clinical Anesthesia.* 6th ed. Philadelphia, PA: Lippincott Williams & Wilkins; 2009:709.

Fegler G. Measurement of cardiac output in anesthetized animals by thermodilution method. *Exp Physiol.* 1954;39:153-64.

Miller RD, Eriksson LI, Fleisher LA, Wiener-Kronish JP, Young WL. *Miller's Anesthesia.* 7th ed. Philadelphia, PA: Churchill Livingstone; 2010:1314-1315.

Morgan GE, Mikhail MS, Murray MJ. *Clinical Anesthesiology.* 4th ed. New York, NY: McGraw-Hill; 2006:137-138.

Pearl RG, Rosenthal MH, Nielson L, Ashton J, Brown BW. Effect of injectate volume and temperature on thermodilution cardiac output determination. *Anesthesiology.* 1986;64:798-801.

*Answer C*

Cardiovascular

**QUESTION (K-type):**

While oliguria is evaluated after operative repair of an aortic aneurysm, large "V" waves are noted in a pulmonary artery occlusion pressure trace. This finding is consistent with which of the following disorders?

(1) Tricuspid regurgitation.
(2) Mitral regurgitation.
(3) Aortic regurgitation.
(4) Coronary artery disease.

**CORRECT ANSWER: C (2 and 4 are correct.)**

**SUMMARY:**

*Large "V" waves are seen in any condition that can produce acute mitral regurgitation. This can be seen with rupture of chordae tendineae or papillary muscle dysfunction secondary to ischemia. The height of the "V" wave correlates with the regurgitant volume and pulmonary blood flow and is indicative of the severity. It is inversely related to compliance of the atrium and pulmonary vasculature. The "V" wave may not be very prominent in chronic mitral regurgitation (MR). Prominent wedge pressure "V" waves may exist in the absence of mitral regurgitation when LAP is high, as might occur when the left atrium is compressed. Tall "V" waves are also seen commonly in patients with hypervolemia, congestive heart failure, and ventricular septal defects (VSDs).*

**EXPLANATION:**

(1) *Incorrect.* Tricuspid regurgitation does not produce large "V" waves. Most often it may be challenging to pass the pulmonary artery (PA) catheter.
(2) *Correct.* Acute MR of any etiology, including ischemia, endocarditis, and trauma, is associated with large "V" waves.
(3) *Incorrect.* Aortic regurgitation does not produce large "V" waves.
(4) *Correct.* Coronary artery disease can produce MR from various mechanisms. It can produce papillary muscle dysfunction from ischemia causing restriction of leaflet motion, chordal rupture, and papillary muscle rupture from infarction.

**REASONING:**

This question tests knowledge of pulmonary artery catheter interpretation and causes of "V" waves. It is important to understand the mechanism of normal and abnormal waveforms during invasive monitoring. The important points to remember include the association of "V" waves on pulmonary artery catheter tracing with mitral regurgitation and the causes of acute MR. The best answer is C.

**BIBLIOGRAPHY:**

Barash PG, Cullen BF, Stoelting RK, Cahalan MK, Stock MC. *Clinical Anesthesia.* 6th ed. Philadelphia, PA: Lippincott Williams & Wilkins; 2009:1076.

Miller RD, Miller ED, Reves JG, et al. *Anesthesia.* 7th ed. New York, NY: Churchill Livingstone; 2010:1281-1282.

Morgan GE, Mikhail MS, Murray MJ. *Clinical Anesthesiology.* 3rd ed. New York, NY: McGraw-Hill; 2002:412-415.

## *Answer B*

### Equipment/Physics

**QUESTION (K-type):**

Under which of the following conditions is the output of an agent-specific vaporizer is higher than the dial setting?

(1)  The vaporizer is filled with an agent of higher vapor pressure.
(2)  Ambient temperature increases from 20°C to 24°C.
(3)  The vaporizer is used at an elevation of 5000 ft.
(4)  The inspiratory valve is incompetent.

**CORRECT ANSWER: B (1 and 3 are correct.)**

**SUMMARY:**

*Agent-specific vaporizers are properly classified as "variable-bypass, flow-over, temperature-compensated, agent-specific, out-of-breathing circuit vaporizers." As the classification suggests, these vaporizers are designed to deliver a constant output over a large range of temperatures and flow rates; they are also calibrated for specific agents and most vaporizers are calibrated at sea level. The ratio of flow from the flowmeters that enters through the bypass chamber compared to that through the vaporizing chamber is determined by the concentration control dial setting. The gas mixture that exits the vaporizer outlet is the combination of flow through the vaporizing chamber with entrained anesthetic vapor and flow through the bypass chamber. The amount of vapor output for an anesthetic is determined by the following equation:*

$$\text{Vapor output} = \frac{\text{carrier gas} \times \text{vapor pressure}}{(\text{barometric pressure} - \text{vapor pressure})}$$

**EXPLANATION:**

(1)  ***Correct.*** Using this equation, assume that a sevoflurane vaporizer is used for both sevoflurane (vapor pressure = 160 mm Hg) and isoflurane (vapor pressure = 240 mm Hg). The same amount of carrier gas will be used for each because the vaporizer is set for sevoflurane. For simplicity, we will use 100 mL of carrier gas. Based on the preceding equation, this would yield

$$\text{For sevoflurane: Vapor output} = \frac{100 \text{ mL} \times 160 \text{ mm Hg}}{(760 \text{ mm Hg} - 240 \text{ mm Hg})} = 27 \text{ mL}$$

$$\text{For isoflurane: Vapor output} = \frac{100 \text{ mL} \times 240 \text{ mm Hg}}{(760 \text{ mm Hg} - 240 \text{ mm Hg})} = 46 \text{ mL}$$

Clearly, the vaporizer filled with an agent of higher vapor pressure has a higher output.

(2)  ***Incorrect.*** Agent-specific vaporizers are not affected by changes in ambient temperature. The vaporizers contain a metallic strip composed of two metals welded together; the strips expand or contract with changes in ambient temperature. The differential contraction causes the strip to bend such that the proportion of gas flowing through the bypass chamber is adjusted to maintain a constant vaporizer output.

(3)  ***Correct.*** At an elevation of 5000 ft, the barometric pressure decreases to roughly 700 mm Hg. Based on the preceding equation and the same example as in answer choice 1, the sevoflurane vaporizer with 100 mL of carrier gas, the following numbers are obtained:

$$\text{Vapor output} = \frac{100 \text{ mL} \times 160 \text{ mm Hg}}{(700 \text{ mm Hg} - 160 \text{ mm Hg})} = 30 \text{ mL}$$

which is greater than the 27 mL of output at sea level.

(4) **Incorrect.** An incompetent inspiratory valve would not change the output of a variable-bypass vaporizer because typically there is a valve located after the vaporizers and prior to the common gas outlet to prevent backflow of gases into the anesthesia machine.

### REASONING:

This question tests knowledge of variable bypass vaporizers and calculation of vapor output. Choice 2 is clearly incorrect because ambient temperature does not affect vaporizer output. Knowledge of the equation for vapor output allows simple calculations to ascertain that choices 1 and 3 are correct. Choice 4 is incorrect because an incompetent inspiratory valve does not change vaporizer output.

### BIBLIOGRAPHY:


Barash PG, Cullen BF, Stoelting RK, Cahalan MK, Stock MC. *Clinical Anesthesia*. 6th ed. Philadelphia, PA: Lippincott Williams & Wilkins; 2009:663-664.

Dorsch JA, Dorsch SE. *Understanding Anesthesia Equipment*. 5th ed. Philadelphia, PA: Lippincott Williams & Wilkins; 2008:124-128.

Miller RD, Eriksson LI, Fleisher LA, Wiener-Kronish JP, Young WL. *Miller's Anesthesia*. 7th ed. Philadelphia, PA: Churchill Livingstone; 2010:690.

Morgan GE, Mikhail MS, Murray MJ. *Clinical Anesthesiology*. 4th ed. New York, NY: McGraw-Hill; 2006:61-66.

Shafer S. Shafer's online lectures [Internet]. Stanford, CA: Stanford University, Department of Anesthesia; 2006. Equipment: How Vaporizers Work; 2008 Jul 15 [cited 2011 Jul 1]. http://anesthesia.stanford.edu/onlinelectures/Equipment/Forms/AllItems.aspx.


---

**BOOK A:**  **QUESTION 68 (OPTIONAL)**

*No Answer*

Clinical Anesthesia

### QUESTION (K-type):

The advantages of colloid over crystalloid for massive volume replacement include

(1) Lower incidence of pulmonary edema.
(2) Greater urine output.
(3) Less disruption of hemostasis.
(4) Greater potency in restoring circulatory homeostasis.

### CORRECT ANSWER: No answer (1 and 4 are correct.)

### SUMMARY:

*An ongoing controversy exists over whether crystalloid or colloid solutions should be used in fluid replacement therapy. Crystalloids such as normal saline or lactated Ringer are cheaper, more ubiquitous, and lack the risk of exposure to infectious agents, coagulopathy, or transfusion reactions. However, three to four times the volume as compared to colloid solutions must be given to obtain the equivalent intravascular replacement. Also, normal saline given in large amounts can cause a dilutional hyperchloremic metabolic acidosis. Colloid solutions such as blood-derived albumin or synthetic hetastarch maintain plasma oncotic pressure better and have an intravascular half-life of 3 to 6 hours compared to the 20 to 30 minute half-life of crystalloids. Whether crystalloid or colloid is used, the practitioner also must be cognizant of the appropriate indications for blood product transfusion in massive volume replacement.*

### EXPLANATION:

(1) *Correct.* There is a greater risk of developing pulmonary edema with massive crystalloid infusions because the dilution of plasma proteins results in reduction of plasma oncotic pressure and subsequent movement of fluid from the intravascular into the interstitial compartment.

(2) *Incorrect.* When given in sufficient amounts, crystalloids are just as effective in restoring intravascular volume, which is the main determinant in preserving urine output.

(3) *Incorrect.* While there is a wide range of colloid products available, many are known for their disruption of hemostasis. Infusion of the synthetic colloid dextran has been associated with prolonged bleeding time and antiplatelet effects. Hetastarch generally does not affect coagulation studies when less than 1 L is administered but can reduce clotting factors, prolong partial thromboplastin time, and interfere with platelet adhesion.

(4) *Correct.* Three to four times the volume of crystalloids as compared to colloids is usually required to replace the equivalent intravascular volume. Thus, colloids are more potent in restoring circulatory homeostasis. Less volume is required to achieve the same intravascular replacement.

### REASONING:

This question requires understanding crystalloid and colloid solutions and their clinical applications, made difficult by the ongoing debates over resuscitation fluids. Choice 4 is clearly correct based on the criteria of potency. Choice 3 is incorrect because certain colloids have been directly associated with coagulopathies, although hemodilution with crystalloids can also cause relative factor deficiencies. Choice 2 is also incorrect because adequate fluid resuscitation with either solution should preserve renal function. Finally, in K-type questions, choices 1 and 3 are tied together. For this question, the evidence that choice 1 is correct is at least as convincing as the evidence that choice 3 is incorrect. This leaves the question unanswerable in its current incarnation.

### BIBLIOGRAPHY:

Miller, 7th ed, pg 1725-1727.
Morgan GE, Mikhail MS, Murray MJ. *Clinical Anesthesiology.* 4th ed. New York, NY: McGraw-Hill; 2006:692-694.

---

**BOOK A:**  **QUESTION 69**

---

*Answer E*

Pain

### QUESTION (K-type):

A 24-year-old man has constant burning pain 3 months after sustaining a crush injury to the arm. The injured muscles and joints are healed. Findings consistent with a diagnosis of causalgia include

(1) Beads of perspiration on the skin.
(2) Skin discoloration.
(3) Hypersensitivity to touch.
(4) Warm extremity.

### CORRECT ANSWER: E (All are correct.)

### SUMMARY:

*Causalgia is now known as complex regional pain syndrome type II (CRPS type II). Reflex sympathetic dystrophy is now known as complex regional pain syndrome type I (CRPS type I). Both are characterized by chronic pain disproportionate to an initial inciting event, with symptoms not confined to the distribution of a single nerve and associated with signs of sympathetic dysfunction such as edema, color changes, sweating changes, or skin and hair changes that cannot be explained by another disease process. Both diseases may be accompanied by allodynia (pain to a nonnoxious stimuli), hyperalgesia (exaggerated pain response to a noxious stimuli), and hyperpathia (progressively more intense and longer pain caused by repetitive stimulation). CRPS type II differs from CRPS type I in that CRPS type II, or causalgia, should be diagnosed only in the presence of a known injury to a distinct nerve.*

### EXPLANATION:

(1) ***Correct.*** Sudomotor dysfunction is consistent with causalgia.
(2) ***Correct.*** Skin discoloration is consistent with the vasomotor dysfunction of causalgia.
(3) ***Correct.*** Allodynia is seen often in causalgia.
(4) ***Correct.*** In causalgia, the affected extremity may be warm or cold as a function of vasomotor dysfunction. This is not confined to an acute or chronic phase.

### REASONING:

This question tests knowledge of the findings associated with CRPS (types I and II). Signs of sympathetic dysfunction can be thought of as vasomotor, sudomotor, and pilomotor signs referring to aberrant blood vessel tone, sweat activity, and cutaneous hair activity (goosebumps), respectively. Beads of perspiration on the skin clearly can be a sign of sudomotor dysfunction, especially when seen only in the distribution of the pain. Skin discoloration and a warm extremity both may be caused by changes in cutaneous blood vessel diameter as a result of sympathetic dysfunction. Hypersensitivity to the touch (allodynia) is also frequently, though not necessarily, seen in CRPS type II (causalgia). Given the history provided in the question, a diagnosis of CRPS type I (reflex sympathetic dystrophy) is more appropriate than CRPS type II (causalgia) because a single nerve injury is not identified.

### BIBLIOGRAPHY:

Benzon R, Borsook M, Strichartz. *Essentials of Pain Medicine and Regional Anesthesia.* New York, NY: Churchill Livingstone;1999:245-246.

Morgan GE, Mikhail MS, Murray MJ. *Clinical Anesthesiology.* 4th ed. New York, NY: McGraw-Hill; 2006:406.

---

## BOOK A:

## QUESTION 70

*Answer B*

Pharmacology

### QUESTION (K-type):

A 45-year-old patient who takes tranylcypromine (Parnate), a monoamine oxidase (MAO) inhibitor, is scheduled for elective surgery under general anesthesia. True statements include the following:

(1) Meperidine can produce hyperthermia.
(2) Surgery must be delayed for 2 weeks after discontinuation of MAO inhibitor therapy.
(3) An exaggerated response to ephedrine should be expected.
(4) A decrease in pressor response to phenylephrine should be expected.

### CORRECT ANSWER: B (1 and 3 are correct.)

### SUMMARY:

*MAO inhibitors are used for the treatment of depression and panic disorder. There are two types of MAOs, A and B, that oxidatively deaminate naturally occurring monoamines such as dopamine, serotonin, norepinephrine, and epinephrine. The MAO inhibitors phenelzine (Nardil) and tranylcypromine block MAO irreversibly, causing an increase in monoamines.* Accumulation of norepinephrine causes an exaggerated response to ephedrine administration. In addition, meperidine can precipitate a hypertensive crisis, seizures, and coma.

### EXPLANATION:

(1) **Correct.** Meperidine and other opiates can precipitate either an excitatory response characterized by agitation, headache, skeletal muscle rigidity, and hyperthermia or a depressive response characterized by hypotension, depressed ventilation, and coma. Meperidine causes the excitatory response by blocking neuronal uptake of serotonin. MAO inhibitors slow the breakdown of meperidine, causing the depressive response.

(2) **Incorrect.** Previously, in an attempt to prevent possibly life-threatening cardiovascular and neurologic instability, elective surgery was delayed for 2 weeks after discontinuation of MAO inhibitors to allow sufficient time for MAO regeneration. However, adverse drug reactions are very uncommon in patients receiving MAOIs who undergo anesthesia. In addition, these patients may be at risk of suicide with cessation of MAOIs. Therefore, current clinical opinion supports continuing MAOI therapy up to the time of surgery, with preoperative monitoring of LFTs and close intraoperative monitoring of hemodynamics with an arterial cannula.

(3) **Correct.** Ephedrine acts indirectly at $\alpha$ and $\beta$ receptors by causing the release of catecholamines. Because MAO inhibitors decrease the breakdown of catecholamines, concomitant administration of ephedrine will cause an exaggerated response.

(4) **Incorrect.** An exaggerated response to phenylephrine would be expected, and lower doses should be used.

### REASONING:

This question tests knowledge of drug interactions associated with MAO inhibitor therapy. Choice 3 obviously is correct because ephedrine causes an exaggerated response. This allows answers C and D to be eliminated. Choice 4 is incorrect because any sympathomimetic agents should be used in small doses owing to the potential for an exaggerated response. This leaves only answers A and B as possibilities. B is correct because surgery need not be delayed for patients taking MAO inhibitors.

### BIBLIOGRAPHY:

Barash PG, Cullen BF, Stoelting RK, Cahalan MK, Stock MC. *Clinical Anesthesia.* 6th ed. Philadelphia, PA: Lippincott Williams & Wilkins; 2009:357-358.

Morgan GE, Mikhail MS, Murray MJ. *Clinical Anesthesiology.* 3rd ed. New York, NY: McGraw-Hill; 2002:591-593.

Stoelting RK. *Pharmacology and Physiology in Anesthetic Practice.* 3rd ed. Philadelphia, PA: Lippincott Raven Publishers; 1999:364-367.

Yao FF, Fontes ML, Malhotra V. *Yao and Artusio's Anesthesiology: Problem-Oriented Patient Management.* 6th ed. Philadelphia, PA: Lippincott, Williams & Wilkins; 2008:644-645.

---

**BOOK A:**      **QUESTION 71**

*Answer C*

Clinical Anesthesia

### QUESTION (K-type):

A 52-year-old man with a chronic cough associated with a long history of smoking is scheduled for elective cholecystectomy. Cessation of smoking for 48 hours will result in

(1) Decreased bronchial secretions.
(2) Shift of the oxyhemoglobin dissociation curve to the right.
(3) Decreased airway irritability.
(4) Decreased carboxyhemoglobin level.

**CORRECT ANSWER: C (2 and 4 are correct.)**

### SUMMARY:

*Cigarette smoking causes many potentially reversible adverse effects on respiratory function and oxygen delivery such as decreased mucociliary clearance, increased mucous production, and increased carboxyhemoglobin levels. Smoking cessation at least 8 weeks before surgery has been shown to decrease the risk of postoperative pulmonary complications. However, patients who quit smoking less than 8 weeks before surgery actually have an increased rate of pulmonary complications, likely because of increased bronchial secretions and airway irritability. Acute smoking cessation does have benefits, including return of carboxyhemoglobin levels to near normal within 12 to 24 hours.*

### EXPLANATION:

(1) *Incorrect.* Mucociliary clearance requires 2 to 3 weeks to normalize after smoking cessation. In the interim, bronchial secretions and airway irritability (bronchospasticity) increase, leading to potential respiratory problems during anesthesia.

(2) *Correct.* Decreased carboxyhemoglobin levels improve both oxygen-carrying capacity and oxygen delivery to tissues because hemoglobin has a 200-fold greater affinity for carbon monoxide than oxygen, and carbon monoxide interferes with oxygen release from hemoglobin. Therefore, decreasing levels of carbon monoxide shift the oxyhemoglobin curve to the right.

(3) *Incorrect.* See above.

(4) *Correct.* Carboxyhemoglobin levels decrease within 12 to 48 hours after smoking cessation.

### REASONING:

This question tests knowledge of the physiologic effects of acute smoking cessation. Choice 4 is obviously correct because carboxyhemoglobin levels decrease rapidly with smoking cessation. This allows answers A and B to be eliminated. Choices 1 and 3 are both incorrect because airway irritability and bronchial secretions both increase 2 days after smoking cessation. Answer B can be eliminated. The only question is whether or not choice 2 is correct. Choice 2 is correct because carboxyhemoglobin worsens oxygen delivery, shifting the oxyhemoglobin dissociation curve to the left. C is the best answer.

### BIBLIOGRAPHY:

Barash PG, Cullen BF, Stoelting RK, Cahalan MK, Stock MC. *Clinical Anesthesia.* 6th ed. Philadelphia, PA: Lippincott Williams & Wilkins; 2009:252.

Miller RD, Miller ED, Reves JG, et al. *Anesthesia.* 5th ed. New York, NY: Churchill Livingstone; 2000:1673.

---

**BOOK A:**  **QUESTION 72**

---

*Answer B*

Physiology

### QUESTION (K-type):

A 55-year-old woman has a urine output of 15 mL during the first 2 hours following a radical hysterectomy. Findings consistent with a prerenal cause include

(1) Urine osmolality of 590 mOsm/L.
(2) Plasma creatinine concentration of 1.1 mg/dL.
(3) Urine-specific gravity of 1.025.
(4) Urine sodium concentration of 40 mEq/L.

CORRECT ANSWER: B (1 and 3 are correct.)

**SUMMARY:**

*Azotemia can be defined as either prerenal, intrarenal, or postrenal. The most common cause of prerenal azotemia is decreased renal perfusion. A fall in arterial pressure, an increase in venous pressure, or an increase in renal vascular tone can lead to decreased renal perfusion. Laboratory tests can be useful in differentiating prerenal from other forms of azotemia. Specific gravity and osmolality are high, and the amount of sodium being excreted by the kidney is low, reflecting the kidney's attempt to maintain intravascular volume.*

**EXPLANATION:**

(1) *Correct.* The osmolality in prerenal azotemia is greater than 500 mmol/kg. This is in contrast to renal azotemia, where the osmolality is less than 350 mmol/kg.

(2) *Incorrect.* The plasma creatinine concentration may be elevated from baseline in prerenal azotemia, but a single number does not help differentiate prerenal from other forms of azotemia. A trend, not an isolated number, is important for monitoring renal function. In addition, creatinine can be elevated in all forms of azotemia.

(3) *Correct.* The urine-specific gravity is increased greater than 1.018 in prerenal azotemia. It is less than 0.012 in renal azotemia.

(4) *Incorrect.* The urine sodium concentration in prerenal azotemia is less than 10 mEq/L as the kidney attempts to hold onto sodium to maintain intravascular volume.

**REASONING:**

This question tests knowledge of oliguria and the laboratory values associated with various etiologies. It is clear that in a prerenal state the kidney will attempt to maintain intravascular volume through sodium retention and concentrating urinary output. However, the specific numbers for each test need to be memorized. B is the best answer.

| | Urine Na$^+$ | Urine Osmolality | FENa$^+$ | Urine-Specific Gravity |
|---|---|---|---|---|
| Prerenal | < 10 | > 500 | < 1% | > 1.018 |
| Renal | > 40 | < 350 | > 3% | < 1.012 |
| Postrenal | Variable | Variable | Variable | Variable |

**BIBLIOGRAPHY:**

Barash PG, Cullen BF, Stoelting RK, Calahan M, Stock MC. *Clinical Anesthesia.* 6th ed. Philadelphia, PA: Lippincott Williams & Wilkins; 2009:303, 1354, 1459.
Morgan GE, Mikhail MS, Murray MJ. *Clinical Anesthesiology.* 4th ed. New York, NY: McGraw-Hill; 2006:1047 (Table 49-8 Urinary Indices in Azotemia).

---

**BOOK A:**　　　　　**QUESTION 73**

*Answer B*

Pediatrics

**QUESTION (Choose single best answer):**

An 8-kg, 1-year-old child has a measured blood loss of 50 mL during the first 2 hours of a rectal pull-through operation. Preoperative hematocrit was 31%. Balanced saline solution 150 mL has been administered for replacement. Urine output has been 2 mL for the last hour, heart rate is 160 bpm, and blood pressure is 40/15 mm Hg. The most appropriate fluid therapy is

(A) 25% albumin.
(B) Balanced salt solution.
(C) Balanced salt solution and mannitol.
(D) 5% dextrose in 0.45% saline solution.
(E) Packed red blood cells.

**CORRECT ANSWER: B**

**SUMMARY:**

*In estimating maximal allowable blood loss (MABL) before needing to transfuse red blood cells (RBCs), multiple factors must be taking into consideration including the patient's age, weight, cardiovascular status, metabolic needs, and potential for ongoing blood loss. The following formula may be used to estimate MABL:*

$$MABL = \frac{[EBV \times (starting\ Hct - minimum\ acceptable\ Hct)]}{starting\ Hct}$$

*where Hct = hematocrit and EBV = estimated blood volume. EBV varies with age ranging from 95 cc/kg for a premature infant to 65 cc/kg for an adult woman. For infants it is approximately 80 cc/kg. Blood loss may be replaced with crystalloid or colloid solution initially, but neither can replace the oxygen-carrying ability of RBCs. Most healthy children can tolerate hematocrit levels in the 20% to 25% range. However, premature infants, patients with cyanotic heart disease or severe pulmonary disease may require higher baseline hematocrits. The most common hazards of transfusion include hemolytic transfusion reaction, bacterial infection, and transfusion-related acute lung injury. Therefore, the administration of blood products must be clearly indicated.*

**EXPLANATION:**

(A) *Incorrect.* 25% albumin is a hypertonic solution that is used to treat hypoalbuminemia. 5% albumin is an isotonic colloid solution that may be used as replacement fluid.

(B) *Correct.* Balanced salt solution such as lactated Ringer or normal saline is appropriate initial fluid replacement for hypovolemia. Because of equilibration into the extravascular space, crystalloid should be administered 3 mL per mL of blood lost. Because the hematocrit is adequate, an initial fluid bolus of 10 mL/kg should be given for treatment of hypovolemia in an otherwise healthy child.

(C) *Incorrect.* Mannitol is a six-carbon sugar used to treat raised intracranial pressure and as an osmotic diuretic. In a patient who is oliguric, it will increase urinary output but may worsen hypovolemia.

(D) *Incorrect.* Dextrose-containing solutions may be used as maintenance fluids in neonates and children, but they should not be used as replacement fluids as they are hypotonic and may result in hyperglycemia.

(E) *Incorrect.* Healthy children can tolerate hematocrit levels in the 20% to 25% range. This child has lost less than 10% of blood volume and therefore his hematocrit should be adequate. However, if the patient continues to show evidence of shock (hypotension, tachycardia, oliguria) after volume expansion with crystalloids, transfusion of RBCs should be considered.

**REASONING:**

This question is challenging because it tests clinical judgment rather than scientific fact. Choices A, C and D can be ruled out because they are not appropriate choices for isotonic fluid resuscitation. The question that remains is whether the clinical situation warrants the risk of blood transfusion. Based on calculation of MABL and fluid replaced, the answer would be no. Choice E is appropriate if the patient did not respond to other initial therapies, but not as the first step.

**BIBLIOGRAPHY:**

Cote CJ. *A Practice of Anesthesia for Infants and Children.* 4th ed. Philadelphia, PA: Saunders; 2009:196-197, 1015-1016.

Morgan GE, Mikhail MS, Murray MJ. *Clinical Anesthesiology.* 4th ed. New York, NY: McGraw-Hill; 2006:736-737.

## *Answer C*

### Pharmacology

**QUESTION (Choose single best answer):**

An increased initial dose and a decreased maintenance dose of pancuronium are required in patients with

(A) Advanced age.
(B) Burns.
(C) Cirrhosis.
(D) Chronic renal failure.
(E) Fever.

**CORRECT ANSWER: C**

**SUMMARY:**

*Pancuronium is a long-acting nondepolarizing neuromuscular blocking agent that is (up to 80%) eliminated primarily unchanged by the kidneys. The liver metabolizes 10% to 40% of pancuronium into several metabolites. One has about 50% of the activity of pancuronium at the NMJ, and the other has only minimal activity. Renal and liver functions primarily govern the clearance and appropriate initial and maintenance dosages of pancuronium. Cirrhotic patients with decreased liver function require greater initial doses of pancuronium because of their greater volume of distribution but decreased maintenance doses because clearance is slightly decreased. In contrast, patients with chronic renal failure should receive smaller initial and maintenance doses because clearance is severely affected.*

**EXPLANATION:**

(A) *Incorrect.* Advanced age does not alter the receptor affinity for pancuronium, so the initial dose is unchanged; however, the maintenance dose is decreased because renal function worsens with aging.
(B) *Incorrect.* Burn patients are resistant to nondepolarizing agents and require increased doses. This is so because burn patients have altered protein binding and an increased number of extrajunctional acetylcholine receptors that bind nondepolarizing neuromuscular blocking drugs.
(C) *Correct.* Cirrhotic patients have an increased volume of distribution for neuromuscular blocking drugs, increasing the initial dose required. Cirrhotics also have decreased maintenance requirement for pancuronium because of impaired hepatic clearance.
(D) *Incorrect.* Patients with chronic renal failure require decreased initial and maintenance doses of pancuronium because the kidneys are primarily responsible for its excretion.
(E) *Incorrect.* Fever does not decrease the maintenance requirements of pancuronium.

**REASONING:**

This question requires knowledge of the elimination pathways of pancuronium. It is important to understand that pancuronium is eliminated primarily through the kidney, with a small amount of hepatic elimination. Knowledge of the pharmacokinetic and pharmacodynamic differences associated with aging and different physiologic states is also important. The best answer is C.

**BIBLIOGRAPHY:**

Dulvadestin P, Agoston S, Henzel D, Kersten UW, Desmonts JM. Pancuronium pharmacokinetics in patients with liver cirrhosis. *Br J Anaesth.* 1978;50(11):1131-1136.

Morgan GE, Mikhail MS, Murray MJ. *Clinical Anesthesiology*. 3rd ed. New York, NY: McGraw-Hill; 2002:194-195, 687-688, 802.

Stoelting RK. *Pharmacology and Physiology in Anesthetic Practice*. 3rd ed. Philadelphia, PA: Lippincott Raven Publishers; 1999:202-204.

---

**BOOK A:**  **QUESTION 75**

---

## Answer C

### Clinical Anesthesia

**QUESTION (Choose single best answer):**

Which of the following statements concerning banked blood is true?

(A) Red blood cells preserved with CPDA-1 (citrate phosphate dextrose adenine 1) have a shelf life of approximately 21 days.
(B) Packed red blood cells deliver oxygen normally immediately after administration.
(C) Packed red blood cells contain most of the leukocytes present in the donated unit.
(D) Citrate is used as a source of energy for whole blood.
(E) Stored whole blood contains all coagulation factors except II and VIII.

**CORRECT ANSWER: C**

**SUMMARY:**

*Whole blood is collected in solutions containing CDPA which has (1) citrate to chelate calcium and prevent clotting, (2) phosphate buffer, (3) dextrose as a fuel source, and (4) adenine as a substrate for ATP synthesis. Whole blood is then separated into its components. Packed red blood cells (PRBCs) in CDPA-1 have a shelf life of 42 days. The longer blood is stored, the lower are the levels of 2,3-DPG, shifting the oxyhemoglobin dissociation curve to the left, which impairs oxygen delivery. PRBCs are derived from whole blood from which the plasma has been removed. PRBCs contain leukocytes unless they have been specifically leukoreduced.*

**EXPLANATION:**

(A) *Incorrect.* RBCs stored with CPDA-1 can be stored for 35 days, not 21.
(B) *Incorrect.* RBCs deliver oxygen abnormally because 2,3-DPG levels are depleted in stored blood, shifting the oxyhemoglobin dissociation curve to the left.
(C) *Correct.* PRBCs, unless leukodepleted, contain most of the leukocytes found in a donated unit. Platelets contain the remainder.
(D) *Incorrect.* Citrate is used as an anticoagulant, and dextrose is used as an energy source.
(E) *Incorrect.* Stored whole blood initially contains all coagulation factors, but factor V and VIII activities decline rapidly with storage as they are labile at room temperature.

**REASONING:**

This question tests knowledge of blood banking and transfusion practices. Answers B, D, and E are obviously incorrect because stored RBCs do not deliver oxygen normally, citrate is an anticoagulant, and whole blood contains all clotting factors, albeit some with decreased activity. Answer A is incorrect because stored blood with CPD is good for 21 days, but stored blood with CPDA-1 is good for 35 days. C is the best choice because RBCs contain leukocytes unless specifically leukodepleted.

**BIBLIOGRAPHY:**

Barash PG, Cullen BF, Stoelting RK, Cahalan MK, Stock MC. *Clinical Anesthesia*. 6th ed. Philadelphia, PA: Lippincott Williams & Wilkins; 2009:383.

Miller RD, Miller ED, Reves JG, et al. *Anesthesia*. 5th ed. New York, NY: Churchill Livingstone; 2000:1618-1621.

Morgan GE, Mikhail MS, Murray MJ. *Clinical Anesthesiology*. 3rd ed. New York, NY: McGraw-Hill; 2002:634-635.

## *Answer C*

### Physiology

**QUESTION (Choose single best answer):**

A 73-year-old woman with a preoperative serum creatinine concentration of 2.1 mg/dL develops oliguria during enflurane anesthesia. Urine sodium concentration is 10 mEq/L, and urine osmolality is 450 mOsm/L. The most likely cause of these findings is

(A) Acute renal failure.
(B) Chronic renal insufficiency.
(C) Decreased renal perfusion.
(D) Fluoride nephrotoxicity.
(E) Intraoperative administration of furosemide.

**CORRECT ANSWER: C**

**SUMMARY:**

*Inhalational agents decrease renal blood flow, which can also decrease urinary output. The accumulation of fluoride is more pronounced in patients with renal failure but this does not necessarily translate into increased renal impairment. Decreased urine production with laboratory values indicating a prerenal cause (low urine sodium and concentrated urine) is an appropriate physiologic response to low renal perfusion.*

**EXPLANATION:**

(A) *Incorrect.* The low sodium level combined with increased osmolality points to a kidney able to scavenge sodium and concentrate urine, not a failing kidney.
(B) *Incorrect.* Chronic renal insufficiency predisposes to acute renal failure but should not, in itself, lead to oliguria.
(C) *Correct.* Inhalational anesthetics decrease renal blood flow, glomerular filtration rate, and urinary output.
(D) *Incorrect.* Fluoride toxicity manifests as polyuric failure.
(E) *Incorrect.* Furosemide increases sodium excretion and urinary output.

**REASONING:**

This question is tricky in that the patient has existing renal impairment, is given an inhalational agent that is associated with fluoride nephrotoxicity, and develops signs of renal impairment during anesthesia! There are multiple factors at work. Fortunately, we can eliminate choices D and E easily. ARF may be caused by prolonged hypoperfusion of the kidneys, but we do not yet have evidence of this. The most likely cause of oliguria, to which all patients are susceptible, is hypoperfusion secondary to inhalational agents.

**BIBLIOGRAPHY:**
Barash PG, Cullen BF, Stoelting RK, Cahalan MK, Stock MC. *Clinical Anesthesia.* 6th ed. Philadelphia, PA: Lippincott Williams & Wilkins; 2009:1356.
Morgan GE, Mikhail MS, Murray MJ. *Clinical Anesthesiology.* 4th ed. New York, NY: McGraw-Hill; 2006:734, 735, 737, 739.

*Answer C*

OB/Regional

**QUESTION (Choose single best answer):**

During active labor, 10 mL bupivacaine 0.5% with epinephrine 1:200,000 is administered epidurally. Fifteen minutes later, maternal blood pressure is 70/50 mm Hg, and heart rate is 70 bpm; fetal heart rate is 90 bpm for 45 seconds, with loss of beat-to-beat variability. The most likely explanation for the fetal vital signs is

(A) Fetal bupivacaine cardiotoxicity.
(B) Maternal bupivacaine cardiotoxicity.
(C) Maternal hypotension.
(C) Uterine artery vasoconstriction.
(D) Umbilical cord compression.

**CORRECT ANSWER: C**

**SUMMARY:**

*Complications associated with epidural anesthesia with local anesthetics include hypotension and bradycardia from sympathectomy, unintended dural puncture, catheter migration into the intrathecal or intravascular space, epidural abscess or hematoma, and failed block. In obstetric practice, hypotension associated with epidural anesthesia can decrease placental perfusion and oxygen delivery to the fetus, as the placenta has limited autoregulation. Fetal heart rate monitoring is the best means of assessing fetal well-being. Changes in fetal oxygen delivery would be manifested by heart rate decelerations, loss of beat-to-beat variability, and changes in the fetal baseline heart rate.*

**EXPLANATION:**

(A) *Incorrect.* The question states that the bupivacaine was injected epidurally. Owing to the high protein binding of bupivacaine, maternal bupivacaine toxicity (from an intravenous injection) would manifest as cardiac arrest before fetal effects are seen.

(B) *Incorrect.* Maternal bupivacaine toxicity would result from intravenous injection, and the question states that the medication was administered epidurally. The absence of tachycardia in the presence of an epinephrine-containing injection is further evidence that the injection was not intravascular.

(C) *Correct.* A known side effect of epidural analgesia is hypotension. The onset of the hypotension is 15 minutes, which is consistent with the onset of epidural bupivacaine. Low maternal blood pressure can cause decreased oxygen delivery to the fetus, leading to bradycardia and loss of beat-to-beat variability.

(D) *Incorrect.* Although uterine artery vasoconstriction can occur with the administration of intravascular epinephrine, this is an epidural injection.

(E) *Incorrect.* While fetal bradycardia can result from umbilical cord compression, the temporal nature of the change in fetal status suggests that it is related to the hypotension. Furthermore, umbilical cord compression usually is associated with variable decelerations and likely would not have such a long duration (45 seconds) until after a long period of fetal compromise.

**REASONING:**

The key to answering this question is the temporal nature of the hypotension and fetal bradycardia. Think as if you had just placed this epidural catheter. Rule out an intravascular injection. The onset of hypotension is 15 minutes, and there is no increase in blood pressure or heart rate with the epinephrine-containing solution. Most likely this is not intravascular, and the solution is epidural. This eliminates answers A, B, and D. The fact that the bradycardia coincides with the hypotension makes C the best answer.

**BIBLIOGRAPHY:**

Bucklin B, Gambling DR, Wlody DJ. *A Practical Approach to Obstetric Anesthesia.* Philadelphia, PA: Lippincott, Williams and Wilkins; 2009:95-101.

Chestnut DH, Polley LS, Lawrence CT, Wong CA. *Chestnut's Obstetric Anesthesia Principles and Practice.* 4th ed. St. Louis, MO: Mosby; 2009:95-96, 143-147.

---

**BOOK A:**  **QUESTION 78**

---

*Answer D*

Pharmacology

**QUESTION (Choose single best answer):**

Compared with diazepam, midazolam

(A) Is more lipid-soluble.
(B) Has a longer elimination half-life.
(C) Has a larger volume of distribution.
(D) Has a greater clearance.
(E) Undergoes slower hepatic metabolism.

**CORRECT ANSWER: D**

**SUMMARY:**

*Both midazolam and diazepam are benzodiazepines that act by binding to γ-aminobutyric acid (GABA) receptors, facilitating the action of GABA. These drugs cause anxiolysis, sedation, and anterograde amnesia. Although both midazolam and diazepam are used in anesthetic practice, midazolam is administered much more commonly. Midazolam has an imidazole ring in its structure that is open at acidic pH, allowing it to be available as an aqueous solution with a pH of 3.5 that is painless on injection. The ring closes at physiological pH, making it more lipid-soluble. Diazepam is more lipid-soluble, requiring a propylene glycol solubilizer that causes venoirritation on injection. Both drugs are metabolized by the liver via oxidation and glucuronide conjugation. Midazolam is metabolized much more quickly than diazepam, accounting for its greater clearance and shorter-elimination half-life.*

**EXPLANATION:**

(A) *Incorrect.* Diazepam is more lipid-soluble than midazolam.
(B) *Incorrect.* Diazepam has a longer-elimination half-life.
(C) *Incorrect.* Diazepam and midazolam have similar volumes of distribution.
(D) *Correct.* Midazolam has a greater clearance than diazepam.
(E) *Incorrect.* Diazepam undergoes slower hepatic metabolism.

**REASONING:**

This commonly asked question tests knowledge of the similarities and differences between midazolam and diazepam. Answers B and E can be eliminated because diazepam has a longer-elimination half-life and undergoes slower hepatic metabolism. Answer D is the opposite of these and is correct because midazolam is cleared more rapidly than diazepam. Answer A is incorrect because midazolam is less lipid-soluble and more soluble in aqueous solutions. Answer C is incorrect because the two drugs have similar volumes of distribution. The best answer is D.

**BIBLIOGRAPHY:**

Miller RD, Eriksson LI, Fleisher LA, Wiener-Kronish JP, Young WL. *Miller's Anesthesia.* 7th ed. Philadelphia, PA: Churchill Livingston; 2009:734-736.

Morgan GE, Mikhail MS, Murray MJ. *Clinical Anesthesiology.* 3rd ed. New York, NY: McGraw-Hill; 2002:160-164.

Stoelting RK. *Pharmacology and Physiology in Anesthetic Practice.* 3rd ed. Philadelphia, PA: Lippincott Raven Publishers; 1999:126-136.

---

| **BOOK A:** | **QUESTION 79** |
|---|---|

## *Answer E*

### OB/Regional

**QUESTION (Choose single best answer):**

A 30-year-old woman has difficulty talking 15 minutes after initiation of interscalene block for closed reduction of a dislocated shoulder. The most likely cause is

(A) Cervical sympathetic block.
(B) Delayed systemic toxic reaction.
(C) Phrenic nerve paralysis.
(D) Pneumothorax.
(E) Recurrent laryngeal nerve block.

**CORRECT ANSWER: E**

**SUMMARY:**

*Interscalene blocks are used for shoulder, arm, and forearm procedures and block the nerves of the brachial plexus. The brachial trunks are located between the anterior and middle scalene muscles at the level of the cricoid cartilage. Complications related to placement of this block include (1) inadvertent blockade of the recurrent laryngeal nerve (hoarseness), phrenic nerve (dyspnea), or stellate ganglion (Horner syndrome), (2) intra-arterial injection (seizure), (3) epidural or spinal injection (neuraxial block or total spinal), and more rarely, (4) pneumothorax.*

**EXPLANATION:**

(A) *Incorrect.* This is also known as a *stellate ganglion block.* It causes increased temperature of the ipsilateral arm, nasal congestion, and Horner syndrome: ipsilateral ptosis, miosis, and facial anhidrosis.

(B) *Incorrect.* Local anesthetic toxicity usually presents as CNS complaints: tinnitus, blurred vision, circumoral numbness, and dizziness.

(C) *Incorrect.* Phrenic nerve paralysis is usually asymptomatic (except in patients with limited pulmonary function at baseline) and occurs in 100% of interscalene nerve blocks and is associated with a 25% reduction in pulmonary function. Patients with preexisting pulmonary disease are more likely to complain of dyspnea following phrenic nerve blockade.

(D) *Incorrect.* Pneumothorax is a rare complication of interscalene block.

(E) *Correct.* Almost all laryngeal muscles are innervated by the recurrent laryngeal nerve. Unilateral nerve blockade leads to paralysis of the ipsilateral vocal cord, causing hoarseness.

**REASONING:**

While all choices are possible complications of the interscalene block, some are less probable, namely, pneumothorax (based on frequency) and toxicity (based on presentation). Knowing the complications involved with blockade of the remaining nerves leads to phrenic versus recurrent laryngeal nerve paralysis. The difficulty talking is most likely vocal cord dysfunction and not dyspnea. E is the single best answer.

**BIBLIOGRAPHY:**

Barash PG, Cullen BF, Stoelting RK, Cahalan M, Stock M. *Clinical Anesthesia*. 6th ed. Philadelphia, PA: Lippincott Williams & Wilkins; 2010;1490-1493.

Miller RD, Eriksson LI, Fleisher LA, Wiener-Kronish JP, William YL. *Miller's Anesthesia*. 7th ed. Philadelphia, PA: Churchill Livingstone; 2010:1640-1643.

Morgan GE, Mikhail MS, Murray MJ. *Clinical Anesthesiology*. 4th ed. New York, NY: McGraw-Hill; 2006:331-332.

---

## BOOK A: QUESTION 80

*Answer C*

Physiology

**QUESTION (Choose single best answer):**

An acutely ill 65-year-old-man with sepsis has severe hypophosphatemia. Which of the following is most likely to result from this electrolyte disorder?

(A) Bronchospasm.
(B) Diarrhea.
(C) Muscle weakness.
(D) Seizures.
(E) Ventricular ectopy.

**CORRECT ANSWER: C**

**SUMMARY:**

*To answer this question, you must understand how phosphate is used in the body. The energy in adenosine triphosphate (ATP) and adenosine diphosphate (ADP) phosphate bonds is harnessed to make nucleic acids (DNA, RNA), oxygen-release facilitators such as 2,3-DPG, and other energy stores (NADPH). Hypophosphatemia causes several sequelae, the most common from the choices given being C, muscle weakness, with skeletal myopathy and respiratory failure. In addition, a low phosphorus level (< 0.3 mmol/dL or < 1.0 mg/dL) can also cause a cardiomyopathy with impaired oxygen delivery (decreased levels of 2,3 DPG, hemolysis, impaired leukocyte and platelet function, encephalopathy, rhabdomyolysis, hepatic dysfunction, and metabolic acidosis).*

**EXPLANATION:**

(A) *Incorrect.* Patients with hypocalcemia tend to go into laryngospasm or laryngeal stridor.

(B) *Incorrect.* Diarrhea frequently results from the abuse of phosphorus containing laxatives, and thus the patient becomes hyperphosphatemic and not the reverse.

(C) *Correct.* Patients with low phosphorus levels suffer from weakness and subsequent respiratory failure and skeletal myopathies. Hypophosphatemia of clinical consequence is often seen in ICU patients who have a total-body phosphate deficiency. The range of clinical manifestations includes respiratory insufficiency from muscle weakness, cardiomyopathy, metabolic acidosis, red and white blood cell dysfunction, and CNS dysfunction.

(D) *Incorrect.* Hypophosphatemia leads to muscle weakness before anything else, whereas other electrolyte imbalances, such as those with sodium, produce seizures more frequently.

(E) *Incorrect.* Phosphorus does not produce ventricular ectopy principally, as do the other electrolytes, mainly calcium and potassium.

Of the choices given, phosphorus is most clearly related to muscle weakness. Frequently, patients on prolonged TPN are difficult to wean from mechanical ventilation because of inadequate phosphorus supplementation and, subsequently, develop weakness of respiratory muscles. Recent carbohydrate or insulin administration shifts phosphorus intracellularly. Other circumstances that may cause low phosphorus levels include diabetic ketoacidosis, aluminum or magnesium containing antacids, severe burns, alcohol withdrawal, and prolonged respiratory alkalosis. With respiratory alkalosis, there is an intracellular shift of phosphorus to counteract the decrease in bicarbonate.

**BIBLIOGRAPHY:**

Miller RD, Eriksson LI, Fleisher LA, Wiener-Kronish JP, Young WL. *Miller's Anesthesia.* 7th ed. Philadelphia, PA: Churchill Livingstone; 2010:1715.

Morgan GE, Mikhail MS, Murray MJ. *Clinical Anesthesiology.* 4th ed. New York, NY: McGraw-Hill; 2006:685-686.

---

## BOOK A:      QUESTION 81

*Answer E*

Clinical Anesthesia

**QUESTION (Choose single best answer):**

During a right lower lobe resection, $Spo_2$ decreases from 99 to 70% after institution of one-lung ventilation. $Fio_2$ is 1.0. The most appropriate management is to

(A) Administer an inhaled bronchodilator.
(B) Apply continuous positive airway pressure to the right lung.
(C) Apply positive end-expiratory pressure to the left lung.
(D) Increase tidal volume.
(E) Reinflate the right lung.

**CORRECT ANSWER: E**

**SUMMARY:**

*The correct answer is E. With an acute drop in oxygen saturation of this magnitude, first reinflate the lung and keep the patient on 100% $Fio_2$. This patient was already on 100% $Fio_2$. The next step is to check the position of the double-lumen tube (DLT) with a fiberoptic scope and listen for breath sounds upon clamping each side of the tube. If hypoxemia occurs during one-lung ventilation, it is a result of inadequate $Fio_2$, alveolar hypoventilation, or a large alveolar to arterial oxygen tension gradient. In addition to ruling out malposition of the tube, check for mechanical problems (ie, obstruction or bronchospasm) and hemodynamic stability (ie, no arrhythmias or hypotension).*

**EXPLANATION:**

(A) *Incorrect.* An inhaled bronchodilator may help somewhat with a sudden onset of wheezing and worsening asthma, however, with such an acute drop in $Spo_2$ to 70%, the next best thing to do is to reinflate the right lung and then start to rule out other causes of hypoxemia.

(B) *Incorrect.* Continuous positive airway pressure (CPAP) (5-10 mm Hg) to the nondependent lung is one of the maneuvers that consistently reduces the risk of hypoxemia during one-lung ventilation. CPAP allows for some oxygenation of the blood perfusing the collapsed lung and can also increase PVR in this lung, thereby shunting more blood to the dependent, ventilated lung. Unfortunately, CPAP is most efficacious when the nondependent lung has been partially reexpanded. However, with such an acute drop in saturation upon starting one-lung ventilation, you must first fix the hypoxemia by reinflating the lung and rule out malposition of the ETT (check for changes in peak pressures, tidal volumes, and repeat fiberoptic bronchoscopy) before instituting CPAP.

(C) *Incorrect.* A low level of PEEP to the ventilated, dependent lung can help improve arterial oxygenation somewhat; however, this can also increase pulmonary resistance and shunt more blood to the collapsed, nondependent lung. PEEP to the ventilated lung should be attempted if there is persistent hypoxemia even after CPAP to the nondependent lung has been instituted. However, in the setting of acute desaturation, reinflating the lung should be done first.

(D) *Incorrect.* With one-lung ventilation, try to keep tidal volumes the same as prior to clamping the ETT. Monitor peak pressure carefully, as they should rise 3 to 5 $cmH_2O$ with the initiation of one-lung ventilation. If peak inspiratory pressures are within normal limits (ie, below 35-40), small adjustments in tidal volumes can be made, but this will not correct such a rapid desaturation to 70%.

(E) *Correct.* Upon initiating one-lung ventilation, with a sudden drop in $Spo_2$, first reexpand the nondependent lung and rule out malposition and mechanical problems (ie, obstruction, bronchospasm, hemodynamic instability). After maximizing oxygen delivery with both lungs inflated, attempt one-lung ventilation again, possibly using CPAP or PEEP if necessary.

## REASONING:

E is correct with a rapid desaturation to 70% upon the initiation of one-lung ventilation. Again, it is important to rule out malposition of the DLT with a fiberoptic scope and a stethoscope. If positioning is not a problem, rule out any possible bronchospasm and hemodynamic instability. Only then can you attempt one-lung ventilation again and possibly use CPAP on the nondependent, collapsed lung, and PEEP on the dependent, ventilated lung to help maintain higher saturations. If a patient cannot tolerate one-lung ventilation despite these maneuvers and surgeons are unwillingly to reinflate the lung, the surgeons can ultimately ligate the ipsilateral pulmonary artery to shunt all blood to the ventilated lung.

## BIBLIOGRAPHY:
Morgan GE, Mikhail MS, Murray MJ. *Clinical Anesthesiology.* 4th ed. New York, NY: McGraw-Hill; 2006:588-593.

---

| **BOOK A:** | **QUESTION 82 (OPTIONAL)** |
| --- | --- |

*Answer Unknown*

Physiology

### QUESTION (Choose single best answer):

Carbon dioxide retention first occurs when the ratio of forced expiratory volume in 1 second to vital capacity ($FEV_1/VC$) decreases below

(A) 15%.
(B) 35%.
(C) 50%.
(D) 65%.
(E) 75%.

**CORRECT ANSWER: The answer to this question is unknown.**

## SUMMARY:

*Chronic obstructive pulmonary disease (COPD) is characterized by progressive limitation of airflow that is not fully reversible. Pulmonary function testing provides valuable information on the severity of disease in COPD. FEV₁ is a measure of the volume of gas expired during the first second of forced expiration from total lung capacity (TLC). Vital capacity (VC) is the volume change in the lung between maximal inspiration (TLC) and maximal expiration (RV). An FEV₁ of less than 80% of predicted and an FEV₁/FVC ratio of less than 70% are consistent with a diagnosis of COPD.*

## EXPLANATION:

(A) ***Unknown.*** The degree of airflow obstruction measured by the $FEV_1$/FVC ratio that is associated with the first onset of clinically significant $CO_2$ retention is unknown.

(B) ***Unknown.*** See below.

(C) ***Unknown.*** See below.

(D) ***Unknown.*** See below.

(E) ***Unknown.*** The reader might assume that any degree of obstruction will lead to some "theoretical" amount of hypoventilation and $CO_2$ retention (even if it is not clinically significant). Because this is a normal ratio, the reader might assume that $CO_2$ retention might "first occur" when the ratio decreases below this value. However, there is no scientific evidence to support this assumption.

## REASONING:

This question is extremely challenging because it is not clear whether the examiners are referring to the first onset of any amount of $CO_2$ retention or to clinically significant retention. There are no data in the literature to support either hypothesis.

In general, carbon dioxide retention is caused by impairment of pulmonary gas exchange. There are four major processes that can impair pulmonary gas exchange: hypoventilation, diffusion limitation, shunt, and ventilation-perfusion inequality. Hypoventilation has many etiologies, including obstructive lung disease. The severity of obstruction can be measured by pulmonary function testing, with a normal $FEV_1$/FVC ratio that is greater than or equal to 75%. This question asks us to determine what $FEV_1$/VC ratio (ie, degree of obstruction/hypoventilation) corresponds to the first onset of carbon dioxide retention. We presume that the only cause of $CO_2$ retention in this patient stems from airway obstruction/hypoventilation owing to COPD. The severity of the associated obstruction can be quantified by the $FEV_1$/FVC ratio.

No clinical studies, however, have correlated $FEV_1$/FVC with $Paco_2$. Indeed, Montes de Oca and Celli studied a cohort of 33 patients with COPD and stratified them into eucapneic ($Paco_2 < 44$ mm Hg) and hypercapnic ($Paco_2 > 45$ mm Hg) patients. They found that the $FEV_1$ and FVC measurements were significantly lower for the hypercapnic group compared with the eucapneic group ($FEV_1$ was 0.9 vs 0.6; FVC was 2.6 vs 1.7). However, their $FEV_1$/FVC ratios were virtually identical (0.346 vs 0.353). This evidence suggests that the $FEV_1$/FVC ratio is a poor predictor of $Paco_2$ in patients with COPD. Interestingly, the authors found that ventilatory drive in response to $CO_2$ was significantly lower in the hypercapneic cohort. This is an important feature of the disease that is independent of level of obstruction (although the two components clearly can combine to make hypercapnia more likely).

The reader should not be discouraged by the difficulty of this question. Critical care faculty in the department of anesthesia and expert pulmonologists from the faculty of medicine at Stanford agree that the answer to this question is unknown.

## BIBLIOGRAPHY:

Barash PG, Cullen BF, Stoelting RK, Calahan M, Stock MC. *Clinical Anesthesia.* 6th ed. Philadelphia, PA: Lippincott Williams & Wilkins; 2009:1034-1035.

Ibid.

Montes de Oca M, Celli BR. Mouth occlusion pressure, $CO_2$ response and hypercapnia in severe chronic obstructive pulmonary disease. *Eur Respir J.* 1998;12:666-671.

Morgan GE, Mikhail MS, Murray MJ. *Clinical Anesthesiology*. 4th ed. New York, NY: McGraw-Hill; 2006:576-578.

Murray JF, Nadel JA. *Textbook of Respiratory Medicine*. 3rd ed. Philadelphia, PA: Saunders; 2000:71.

| **BOOK A:** | **QUESTION 83 (OPTIONAL)** |

## *Answer D*

### Pharmacology

**QUESTION (Choose single best answer):**

During recovery from halothane anesthesia, an alveolar concentration of 0.1% will have the greatest effect on

(A) Myocardial contractility.
(B) Ventilatory response to hypercarbia.
(C) Atrioventricular conduction.
(D) Ventilatory response to hypoxia.
(E) Neuromuscular transmission.

**CORRECT ANSWER: D**

**SUMMARY:**

*Residual alveolar volatile anesthetic is important in the differential diagnosis of hypoxia in the recovery room. Volatile anesthetics cause ventilatory depression by decreasing both tidal volume and minute ventilation despite an increase in respiratory rate. Volatiles result in a dose-dependent decrease in the response to both hypercapnia and hypoxia, but at subanesthetic levels (< 0.2 MAC), only the ventilatory response to hypoxia is attenuated (with halothane > isoflurane > sevoflurane > desflurane). The mechanism for this is unknown. Halothane directly depresses myocardial contractility and can render the heart susceptible to junctional rhythms, but these effects would not be the most prominent during recovery.*

**EXPLANATION:**

(A) *Incorrect.* Although halothane causes direct depression of myocardial contractility, cardiac output, and blood pressure, with no effect on SVR, this effect would not be the greatest of those listed during recovery at subanesthetic concentrations.

(B) *Incorrect.* This was the correct ABA answer in 1993. However, published reviews have since suggested a lack of significant effect at 0.2 MAC. While surgical MAC levels of volatile anesthetics show dose-dependent ventilatory depression in response to hypercapnia (with equal effect on both peripheral and central chemoreceptors, it is less clear whether low concentration (< 0.2 MAC) depresses this same response.

(C) *Incorrect.* While it is true that halothane can cause junctional rhythms and bradycardia in addition to sensitizing the myocardium to the proarrhythmic effects of epinephrine, it would not be significant during recovery.

(D) *Correct.* Hypoxic drive is blunted by levels of volatile agents, including halothane, as low as 0.1 MAC, which is mediated mostly by peripheral chemoreceptors. Pulmonary ciliary function and mucus clearance are also blunted, possibly leading to atelectasis and hypoxia in some patients.

(E) *Incorrect.* Although neuromuscular transmission is slowed by volatiles, this would not be the greatest effect seen during recovery. Halothane blunts both neuromuscular transmission and excitation-contraction coupling equally, while all other volatiles mostly affect transmission only.

**REASONING:**

Volatile anesthetics, including halothane, can have some effect on most of the listed parameters, making this question tricky. However, only at subanesthetic (< 0.2 MAC) levels will halothane have a blunting effect on the ventilatory response to hypoxia. Choices A, C, and E can be eliminated as they would not predominate during the recovery period with 0.1% halothane, while choice B has conflicting evidence, even suggesting no significant effect at subanesthetic levels.

**BIBLIOGRAPHY:**
Miller RD, Eriksson LI, Fleisher LA, Wiener-Kronish JP, Young WL. *Miller's Anesthesia.* 7th ed. Philadelphia, PA: Churchill Livingstone; 2010:577-586.
Morgan GE, Mikhail MS, Murray MJ. *Clinical Anesthesiology.* 4th ed. New York, NY: McGraw-Hill; 2006:167-168 (Table 7-6 Clinical Pharmacology of Inhalational Anesthetics).

## BOOK A:    QUESTION 84

*Answer B*

Cardiovascular

**QUESTION (Choose single best answer):**

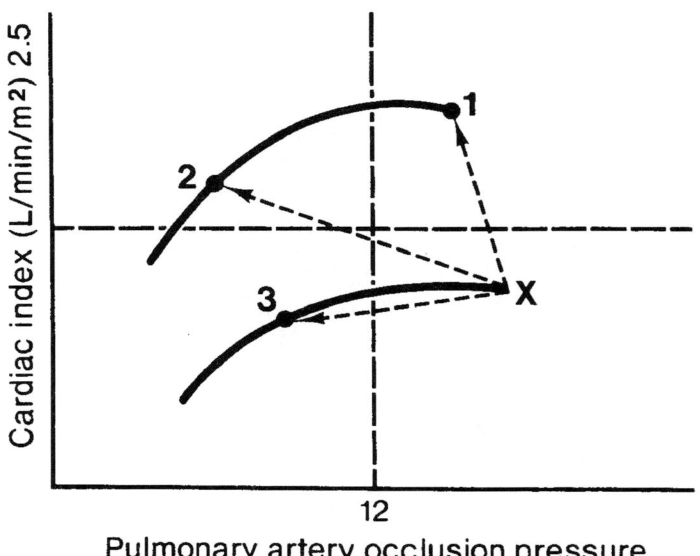


In this diagram, point *X* represents a patient with severe left ventricular dysfunction. The points labeled 1, 2, and 3 each represent the results of a different therapeutic intervention. Which of the following represents the most likely intervention at each point?

|  | **Point 1** | **Point 2** | **Point 3** |
|---|---|---|---|
| (A) | Dopamine | Furosemide | Nitroprusside |
| (B) | Dopamine | Nitroprusside | Furosemide |
| (C) | Furosemide | Dopamine | Nitroprusside |
| (D) | Nitroprusside | Dopamine | Furosemide |
| (E) | Nitroprusside | Furosemide | Dopamine |

**CORRECT ANSWER: B**

**SUMMARY:**
*The graph represents a patient with severe left ventricular (LV) dysfunction with a pulmonary artery occlusion pressure (PAOP) of approximately 18 mm Hg and a cardiac index*

*of less than 2 L/min/m². Dopamine is an adrenergic agent with dose-dependent β and α activity that increases cardiac output and cardiac index and slightly decreases PAOP. Furosemide is a loop diuretic that produces diuresis and reduces preload. This results in decreased PAOP. Sodium nitroprusside causes both arteriolar and venodilation. This decreases both preload and afterload. The decrease in afterload improves LV stroke volume, cardiac output, renal perfusion, and diuresis. The net effect is a decrease in PAOP and an increase in cardiac output (CO).*

### EXPLANATION:
(A) *Incorrect.*
(B) *Correct.* Point 1 on the graph illustrates an increase in cardiac index from point $X$ and a small reduction in PAOP. This effect can be seen after treatment with an inotropic agent such as dopamine. Point 2 on the graph shows greater reduction in PAOP and improvement in cardiac index seen with sodium nitroprusside. Point 3 on graph shows a large reduction in PAOP and even a very small decrease in cardiac index. This is produced by furosemide, which reduces preload by diuresis.
(C) *Incorrect.*
(D) *Incorrect.*
(E) *Incorrect.*

### REASONING:
This complex question tests knowledge of the pathophysiology of LV dysfunction and the associated hemodynamic responses to pharmacologic therapy. It is important to understand the pathophysiology of congestive heart failure with its attendant maladaptive changes, such as increased activity in the sympathetic and renin-angiotensin systems leading to excess sodium and thus water accumulation and vasoconstriction leading to increased afterload on a failing heart. The pharmacologic therapy in heart failure is directed toward correcting these changes. The best answer is B.

The ABA answer D is incorrect, because point 2 on the graph represents increase in cardiac index and significant reduction in PAOP. The increase in cardiac index is secondary to afterload reduction by arteriolar dilation and reduced PAOP due to venodilation. This can be seen with nitroprusside therapy. Diuresis produced by furosemide will merely reduce preload, thus PAOP and by extension slight reduction in cardiac index, set point 3. Set point 1 shows greater rise in cardiac output and very small decrease in PAOP, produced by dopamine.

### BIBLIOGRAPHY:
Stoelting R. *Anesthesia and Co-existing Diseases*. 3rd ed. New York, NY: Churchill Livingstone; 1993:91-95.

---

| **BOOK A:** | **QUESTION 85** |
|---|---|

## *Answer A*

### Pharmacology

### QUESTION (Choose single best answer):

With long-term administration, which of the following drugs produces the most prolonged sedative effect of diazepam?

(A) Cimetidine.
(B) Famotidine.
(C) Metoclopramide.
(D) Ranitidine.
(E) Warfarin.

**CORRECT ANSWER: A**

**SUMMARY:**

*Diazepam is considered a long-acting benzodiazepine and it is metabolized via the hepatic microsomal oxidation (cytochrome P-450 enzyme) pathway in the liver. This matters because unlike the glucuronide conjugation pathway in the liver, oxidation reduction (Phase I reaction) is subject to inhibition by the coadministration of other drugs (cimetidine). The oxidation of diazepam may also be impaired by age (reduced clearance) and race (mutations in the genes that code for CYP2C19 in Asians may explain the slowed biotransformation of diazepam in this population). Diazepam's protein binding and volume of distribution is not significantly different from that of midazolam, but its slow hepatic oxidation results in a slower clearance and longer-elimination half-life (0.2-0.5 mL/kg/ min vs 6-11 mL/kg/min, respectively). Cimetidine binds and inhibits the cytochrome P-450 and reduces hepatic blood flow, thereby producing a more prolonged sedative effect with diazepam. Cimetidine has no effect on the clearance of lorazepam.*

**EXPLANATION:**

(A) *Correct.* Cimetidine is an $H_2$-receptor antagonist and binds to the cytochrome P-450 system, thereby reducing the metabolism of diazepam. Approximately 30% is slowly inactivated by the liver's microsomal, oxygenase system, while the other 70% is excreted unchanged in the urine.

(B) *Incorrect.* Famotidine is also an $H_2$-receptor antagonist; however, it does not inhibit the P-450 system in the liver. It is more similar to ranitidine in its pharmacologic action. However, it is 3 to 20 times more potent than ranitidine.

(C) *Incorrect.* Metoclopramide binds dopaminergic receptors both peripherally and centrally and increases LES tone, gastric motility, and decreases gastric fluid volume. Because of its antagonism at the dopaminergic receptors, metoclopramide may cause some sedation and extrapyramidal side effects. It does not interact with the P-450 system.

(D) *Incorrect.* Ranitidine is also an $H_2$-receptor antagonist; however, like famotidine, it does not bind the P-540 cytochrome system. It is 5 to 10 times more potent than cimetidine and has fewer side effects as well.

(E) *Incorrect.* Warfarin uses the P-450 system for metabolism, and with concurrent administration of diazepam, it acts as an enzyme inducer to the speed the catabolism of diazepam rather than prolonging its effects.

**REASONING:**

Cimetidine reduces hepatic blood flow and binds to the cytochrome P-450 mixed-function oxidases. Thus, this drug potentiates the action of several drugs by slowing their metabolism, including diazepam, warfarin, phenytoin, quinidine, carbamazepine, theophylline, and imipramine. Phase I reactions in the liver convert the parent drug to a metabolite via different reactions (ie, hydrolysis, oxidation, or reduction). It is these phase I reactions that occur on the heme protein known as *cytochrome P-450*. Such phase I reactions are under genetic control and are highly sensitive to induction or inhibition by such things as drugs, insecticides, herbicides, smoking, and caffeine. Once the phase I reactions occur, phase II reactions follow to bind the metabolite to an endogenous substrate (ie, glucuronide or sulfate) so that the drug can be excreted.

**BIBLIOGRAPHY:**

Miller RD, Eriksson LI, Fleisher LA, Wiener-Kronish JP, Young WL. *Miller's Anesthesia.* 7th ed. Philadelphia, PA: Churchill Livingstone; 2010:735-736.

Morgan GE, Mikhail MS, Murray MJ. *Clinical Anesthesiology.* 4th ed. New York, NY: McGraw-Hill; 2006:188, 192.

*Answer B*

Pediatrics

**QUESTION (Choose single best answer):**

During uncomplicated mask induction with halothane and 50% nitrous oxide in oxygen in a 6-month-old infant with a large ventricular septal defect and valvular pulmonic stenosis, $SpO_2$ decreases from 85% (room air) to 60%, heart rate is 100 bpm, and blood pressure is 62/40 mm Hg. The most appropriate management is to

(A) Administer atropine.
(B) Administer phenylephrine.
(C) Administer propranolol.
(D) Increase anesthetic depth.
(E) Intubate the trachea.

**CORRECT ANSWER: B**

**SUMMARY:**

*Ventricular septal defects (VSDs) are the most common congenital heart lesions encompassing up to 25% to 35% of all defects. The balance between PVR and SVR determines the direction of shunting and therefore whether the blood is oxygenated in the lungs prior to circulation to the rest of the body. Blood always flows down the path of least resistance. Beyond the first few days to weeks of life, the resistance in the pulmonary bed drops so that shunting in most VSD occurs left to right. Valvular pulmonic stenosis causes obstruction to pulmonary arterial flow. In the presence of an intracardiac communication, right-to-left shunting may also occur. With right-to-left shunting, abrupt increases in PVR or decreases in SVR are poorly tolerated and lead to hypoxia.*

**EXPLANATION:**

(A) *Incorrect.* There is no need to administer an anticholinergic agent. Mean heart rate for a 6-month-old infant is 90 to 120 bpm. The patient is not bradycardic and there is no reason to make him tachycardic.

(B) *Correct.* Phenylephrine is the drug of choice to raise the SVR. This selective $\alpha_1$-adrenergic agonist will increase SVR relative to PVR, decreasing the right-to-left shunting through the VSD, and cause some blood to go to the lungs to be oxygenated. Alternatively, one could put the patient's knees to chest or press on the femoral arteries.

(C) *Incorrect.* Propranolol, a $\beta$-adrenergic antagonist, has been used in the past to relieve dynamic infundibular spasm in hypercyanotic spells in patients with tetralogy of Fallot, but is unlikely to be effective in relieving a fixed valvular pulmonic stenosis.

(D) *Incorrect.* Increasing anesthetic depth may be effective in treating dynamic infundibular spasm, but it will not affect a fixed pulmonic stenosis. Also, increasing anesthetic depth will lower SVR, which could worsen shunting.

(E) *Incorrect.* Intubating the trachea alone without increasing the $FIO_2$ delivered will not help especially if little blood is reaching the pulmonary circulation to be oxygenated. Increasing the $FIO_2$ to 100% will maximize oxygen in the lungs to be absorbed once pulmonary circulation has been reestablished.

**REASONING:**

The clinical situation described is similar to that of a patient with tetralogy of Fallot—a congenital heart defect consisting of VSD, right ventricular outflow tract obstruction (pulmonic stenosis), right ventricular hypertrophy, and overriding aorta. The first two lesions are primarily responsible for the hypercyanotic (or "Tet") spells that may occur in these patients. During a hypercyanotic spell, deoxygenated blood from the right side of the heart preferentially is shunted through the VSD out the aorta because of obstruction along the right ventricular outflow tract. In other words, PVR is greater than SVR. Immediate interventions aim to raise SVR relative to PVR. The goals of anesthetic management in these patients are to maintain intravascular volume and SVR and avoid increases in PVR. Choice B is the only answer that will raise SVR. The others have no direct effect or an undesirable effect on SVR.

**BIBLIOGRAPHY:**

Cote CJ. *A Practice of Anesthesia for Infants and Children*. 4th ed. Philadelphia, PA: Saunders; 2009:18.

Morgan GE, Mikhail MS, Murray MJ. *Clinical Anesthesiology*. 4th ed. New York, NY: McGraw-Hill; 2006:247, 480-482.

---

**BOOK A:**

*Answer A*

OB/Regional

**QUESTION 87**

**QUESTION (Choose single best answer):**

Which of the following statements concerning variable decelerations of fetal heart rate is true?

(A) It indicates compression of the umbilical cord.
(B) It indicates compression of the fetal head.
(C) It indicates prematurity.
(D) It is obliterated by atropine.
(E) It occurs normally following epidural anesthesia.

**CORRECT ANSWER: A**

**SUMMARY:**

*Monitoring of the fetal heart rate is currently the best indicator of fetal oxygenation and tolerance of labor. Heart rate decelerations are evaluated regarding uterine contractions. Early decelerations occur at the onset of the contraction, nadir at the peak of the contraction (usually < 20 bpm below baseline), and return to baseline at the end. They are due to a vagal response to fetal head compression. Late decelerations begin 10 to 30 seconds after the onset of the contraction, nadir after the peak, and return to baseline 10 to 30 seconds after the contraction has terminated. Late decelerations are associated with uteroplacental insufficiency (response to hypoxemia). Variable contractions are variable in onset, duration, relationship to contractions, and often have abrupt onset and termination. Typically, this pattern is vagally mediated and due to umbilical cord compression, although repeated hypoxia due to cord compression can result in bradycardia owing to intrinsic myocardial depression. While early decelerations are not associated with fetal hypoxia, variable and late patterns can be associated with fetal hypoxia and acidosis, especially when associated with tachycardia and loss of beat-to-beat variability.*

**EXPLANATION:**

(A) ***Correct.*** Variable decelerations are thought to be a vagal response to the increased afterload associated with umbilical cord compression.
(B) ***Incorrect.*** Early decelerations are associated with fetal head compression.
(C) ***Incorrect.*** Variable decelerations may be more common in preterm fetuses, but preterm fetal heart tracings generally show decreased variability and a higher baseline heart rate.
(D) ***Incorrect.*** The efferent component of variable decelerations is vagally mediated and can be blocked by atropine. However, the variable decelerations also can occur due to intrinsic myocardial depression from prolonged hypoxia, and this response will not be blocked by atropine.

(E) *Incorrect.* Decelerations are not normal after epidural anesthesia. If fetal heart rate changes occur after institution of epidural anesthesia, causes include maternal hypotension or uterine hypertonus.

## REASONING:

Correctly answering this question requires knowledge of commonly occurring fetal heart rate patterns. Answer E can be eliminated because decelerations do not normally occur after epidural anesthesia. Answers B and D are associated with early decelerations. Answer C can be eliminated because variable decelerations are also seen in term fetuses. A is the single best answer.

## BIBLIOGRAPHY:


Chestnut DH, Polley LS, Lawrence CT, Wong CA. *Chestnut's Obstetric Anesthesia Principles and Practice.* 4th ed. St. Louis, MO: Mosby; 2009:144-147.

Itskovitz J, LaGamma EF, Rudolph AM. Heart rate and blood pressure responses to umbilical cord compression in fetal lambs with special reference to the mechanism of variable deceleration. *Am J Obstet Gynecol.* 1983 Oct 15;147(4):451-457.

Morgan GE, Mikhail MS, Murray MJ. *Clinical Anesthesiology.* 4th ed. New York, NY: McGraw-Hill; 2006:913-915.


---

**BOOK A:**

*Answer E*

Clinical Anesthesia

## QUESTION 88 (OPTIONAL)

### QUESTION (Choose single best answer):

During enflurane anesthesia for colectomy in a 75-year-old man with sepsis, urine output decreases to 10 mL/h. Heart rate is 120 bpm, blood pressure is 100/50 mm Hg, central venous pressure is 10 mm Hg, and pulmonary artery occlusion pressure is 15 mm Hg. The most appropriate management at this time is to

(A) Measure cardiac output.
(B) Increase fluid administration.
(C) Infuse dopamine.
(D) Administer propranolol.
(E) Switch from enflurane to isoflurane.

### CORRECT ANSWER: E

### SUMMARY:

*Sepsis and the associated intraoperative hypotension is a common occurrence. A patient with sepsis may demonstrate hypotension for several different reasons, including decreased SVR, intravascular volume depletion from third spacing, or from direct myocardial depression from toxins associated with the septic state. Treatment would involve maintaining adequate filling pressures with volume, maintaining SVR with medications/infusions, and avoiding myocardial depressants such as halothane and enflurane.*

### EXPLANATION:

(A) *Incorrect.* Although obtaining a cardiac output can help distinguish various causes of a shock state (cardiogenic versus hypovolemic for instance), clinical clues in this case indicate septic shock. Obtaining a cardiac output is not the most important or most appropriate next step in treating this patient's hypotension.

(B) **Incorrect.** Fluid administration is vitally important in maintaining an adequate preload in septic patients, but in this case the central venous pressure (CVP) is 10 indicating adequate preload. Therefore a different treatment choice would be warranted.

(C) **Incorrect.** Maintaining adequate oxygen delivery to the tissues is an important part of management of sepsis, and inotropes are indicated if evidence of inadequate tissue perfusion exists (elevated lactate or decreased mixed venous oxygen saturation). In this case, the patient's blood pressure appears to be adequate and adding an inotrope is not the best management strategy at this time.

(D) **Incorrect.** The patient's tachycardia is a direct result of the sepsis state and is needed to maintain perfusion. Giving a β-blocker at this point may precipitate cardiovascular collapse.

(E) **Correct.** Minimizing use of myocardial depressants to maintain adequate cardiac output is an important part of intraoperative management of sepsis. While all volatile anesthetics decrease SVR, enflurane and halothane also depress myocardial contractility. Changing from enflurane to isoflurane is the best immediate action to improve hemodynamics in this patient.

## REASONING:

This question is difficult. Many of the answer choices are appropriate therapy for management of sepsis. One could argue that the appropriate response would be to give additional fluid even with an adequate CVP secondary to the increased fluid requirements in septic patients. In addition, one could argue that despite the tachycardia, dopamine should be started to improve overall cardiac performance. However, it is reasonable to eliminate any detrimental factors such as myocardial depressants before initiating additional therapy.

## BIBLIOGRAPHY:

Morgan GE, Mikhail MS, Murray MJ. *Clinical Anesthesiology*. 4th ed. New York, NY: McGraw-Hill; 2006:142-143.

---

**BOOK A:**            **QUESTION 89**

*Answer B*

Pharmacology

## QUESTION (Choose single best answer):

The effect of neomycin at the neuromuscular junction is

(A) Decreased by depolarizing relaxants.
(B) Partially reversed by calcium.
(C) Potentiated by anticholinesterases.
(D) Prevented by pretreatment with magnesium.
(E) Primarily prejunctional.

## CORRECT ANSWER: B

## SUMMARY:

*Antibiotics, especially aminoglycosides such as neomycin, potentiate neuromuscular blockade. Neomycin impairs neuromuscular transmission and produces clinically significant weakness. The mechanism responsible is a decrease in both the release of acetylcholine from prejunctional nerve endings and the sensitivity of the postsynaptic site. Studies have also shown that neomycin preferentially interacts with the open state of the acetylcholine receptor ion channel complex. Cholinesterase inhibitors (ie, neostigmine), the infusion of calcium, and aminopyridines can partially reverse the weakness.*

**EXPLANATION:**

(A) *Incorrect.* Neomycin potentiates the effect of depolarizing agents, and its action at the neuromuscular junction (NMJ) is not decreased by the administration of paralytics.

(B) *Correct.* Calcium can partially reverse the effect of neomycin at the NMJ. Calcium gluconate or calcium chloride supplementation must be administered, especially because neomycin decreases the intestinal absorption of calcium in patients.

(C) *Incorrect.* Anticholinesterases can partially reverse the effect of neomycin at the NMJ like calcium rather than potentiating any muscle weakness.

(D) *Incorrect.* Magnesium will not prevent the effect of neomycin at the NMJ. Hypermagnesemia actually decreases the release of acetylcholine and can potentiate neuromuscular blockade. Similar to calcium, neomycin actually decreases intestinal absorption of magnesium in patients.

(E) *Incorrect.* Studies have proven that neomycin acts to decrease acetylcholine release at prejunctional sites, as well as to stabilize the effects on some functional components on postsynaptic membranes to decrease neuromuscular transmission.

**REASONING:**

Neomycin is an aminoglycoside that interferes with bacterial protein synthesis by binding the 30S subunit of bacterial ribosomes. It acts synergistically with both depolarizers and nondepolarizers to prolong paralysis by decreasing acetylcholine release presynaptically and stabilizing membranes postsynaptically. Such potentiation of neuromuscular blockade can be partially reversed with calcium supplementation or the administration of cholinesterase inhibitors such as neostigmine. Impaired neuromuscular transmission has been reported in those patients receiving concurrent paralytics, those with myasthenia gravis, those with other disorders that may alter pharmacokinetics, and in those with exposure to other drugs having an adverse effect of neuromuscular transmission.

**BIBLIOGRAPHY:**

Fiekers JF. Sites and mechanisms of antibiotic-induced neuromuscular block: a pharmacological analysis using quantal content, voltage clamped end-plate currents, and single channel analysis. *Acta Physiol Pharmacol Ther Latinoam.* 1999;49(4):242-250.

Karatas Y. Possible postsynaptic action of aminoglycosides in frog rectus abdominis. *Acta med Okayama.* 2000 Apr;54(2):49-56.

Morgan GE, Mikhail MS, Murray MJ. *Clinical Anesthesiology.* 4th ed. New York, NY: McGraw-Hill; 2006:212.

Mycek M, Harvey R, Champe P. *Pharmacology.* 2nd ed. Philadelphia, PA: Lippincott Raven; 1997:317.

Singh YN. Antibiotic induced paralysis of mouse phrenic nerve hemidiaphragm preparation and reversibility by calcium and by neostigmine. *Anesthesiology.* 1978;48:418-424.

---

**BOOK A:**        **QUESTION 90 (OPTIONAL)**

*Answer D*

Clinical Anesthesia

**QUESTION (Choose single best answer):**

A patient is bleeding excessively after routine transurethral resection of the prostate (TURP). Reexploration discloses diffuse oozing. The most appropriate management is administration of

(A) Platelets.
(B) Fresh frozen plasma.
(C) Desmopressin.
(D) $\varepsilon$-Aminocaproic acid.
(E) Cryoprecipitate.

**SUMMARY:**

*Abnormal bleeding is rare after TURP. Fewer than 1% of patients develop abnormal bleeding after TURP. Disseminated intravascular coagulation (DIC) has been reported and is thought to be secondary to release of thromboplastins from the prostate cancer tissue. Others believe that primary fibrinolysis can occur from prostatic tumors that excrete plasminogen activator, which converts plasminogen to plasmin. Treatment of DIC involves supportive care and repletion of coagulation factors and platelets. If primary fibrinolysis is suspected, administration of ε-aminocaproic acid and cryoprecipitate may be beneficial.*

**EXPLANATION:**

(A) *Incorrect.* A dilutional thrombocytopenia may be seen following TURP due to increased intravascular volume from absorption of the irrigating solution. However, this is not the most common cause of bleeding following TURP.

(B) *Incorrect.* In the absence of perioperative elevated international normalized ratio (INR), bleeding following TURP is unlikely to be related to an abnormal INR and FFP would not indicated.

(C) *Incorrect.* The use of desmopressin may be indicated for excessive postoperative bleeding due to platelet dysfunction. In this situation, epsilon aminocaproic acid is a better option.

(D) *Correct.* The use of epsilon-aminocaproic acid is indicated as therapy for primary fibrinolysis, which can occur following prostate surgery.

(E) *Incorrect.* The use of cryoprecipitate would be indicated if the patient's fibrinogen level was low. It is not likely the most common cause of this patient's coagulopathy.

**REASONING:**

This question is difficult because there is little information to help narrow down the cause of bleeding. Additional patient information and laboratory values would be helpful in narrowing the diagnosis, but in the absence of additional information, it is assumed that the bleeding is specific to the procedure. This question tests the anesthesiologists knowledge that primary fibrinolysis is associated with prostate surgery because of enzymes produced and released by the prostate and should be suspected when there is persistent postoperative bleeding.

**BIBLIOGRAPHY:**

American Society of Anesthesiologists Task Force on Perioperative Blood Transfusion and Adjuvant Therapies. Practice guidelines for perioperative blood transfusion and adjuvant therapies: an updated report by the American Society of Anesthesiologists Task Force on Perioperative Blood Transfusion and Adjuvant Therapies. *Anesthesiology.* 2006;105:198-208.
Miller, 7th ed, chap. 65

---

| **BOOK A:** | **QUESTION 91** |
|---|---|

*Answer B*

Physiology

**QUESTION (Choose single best answer):**

Which of the following statements concerning FRC is true?

(A) It decreases linearly during a 3-hour anesthetic.

(B) It decreases in pregnancy primarily because of a decrease in the expiratory reserve volume.

(C)  It increases in patients with a history of heavy smoking.

(D)  It increases with pulmonary contusions.

(E)  It is smaller (mL/kg) in children than in adults.


**CORRECT ANSWER: B**


**SUMMARY:**

*Functional residual capacity (FRC) is the lung's resting volume or the volume remaining at end exhalation. FRC is decreased in term parturients, obesity, supine and prone positions, restrictive lung disease, general anesthesia, upper abdominal surgery, and in neonates and infants, while FRC increases with increasing height, age, and COPD. Induction of anesthesia abruptly reduces FRC by up to 500 cc, resulting in altered V/Q relationships and predisposition to atelectasis and hypoxemia. A recent review found that the evidence for intraoperative PEEP to reduce postoperative respiratory complications and mortality is currently insufficient.*


**EXPLANATION:**

(A)  *Incorrect.* This was the correct ABA answer in 1993. However, it has been shown that the reduction in FRC occurs mostly on induction and not linearly during a general anesthetic. Assuming a supine position reduces FRC by up to 800 cc and induction by a further 400 to 500 cc. FRC is not significantly changed as the duration of the anesthetic increases or by the use of muscle paralysis or positive-pressure ventilation. FRC is reduced by both inhalation and IV agents, with the exception of ketamine.

(B)  *Correct.* The FRC reduction by 20% at term is due to diaphragmatic elevation and reduction in ERV (FRC = RV + ERV). Half of all supine term parturients will have a closing capacity higher than their FRC, and combined with their elevated rate of oxygen consumption, are susceptible to hypoxemia.

(C)  *Incorrect.* While it is true that COPD patients have an increased FRC and TLC, not all heavy smokers have COPD. Air trapping from expiratory obstruction elevates the residual volume (and hence the FRC) in COPD.

(D)  *Incorrect.* Pulmonary contusion or other trauma such as rib fracture or thoracotomy decreases chest expansion with a resultant decrease in lung volumes.

(E)  *Incorrect.* By age 8 (but not by infancy), alveolar development and lung compliance resemble those of adults with similar FRC values of 30 mL/kg.


**REASONING:**

This question is challenging as it requires knowledge of FRC changes across multiple patient types and pathophysiological processes. Choice A is false as the decreased FRC from anesthesia occurs immediately postinduction. Choice D is clearly wrong as lung contusion would decrease most lung volumes. For choice C one cannot assume that the smoker has COPD. Choice E would be true if it referred to the FRC of infants and neonates.


**BIBLIOGRAPHY:**

Barash PG, Cullen BF, Stoelting RK, Calahan M, Stock MC. *Clinical Anesthesia*. 6th ed. Philadelphia, PA: Lippincott Williams & Wilkins; 2009:1174.

Imberger G, McIlroy D, Pace NL, Wetterslev J, Brok J, Møller AM. Positive end-expiratory pressure (PEEP) during anaesthesia for the prevention of mortality and postoperative pulmonary complications. *Cochrane Database Syst Rev*. 2010 Sep 8;(9):CD007922.

Miller RD, Eriksson LI, Fleisher LA, Wiener-Kronish JP, Young WL. *Miller's Anesthesia*. 7th ed. Philadelphia, PA: Churchill Livingstone; 2010:377.

Morgan GE, Mikhail MS, Murray MJ. *Clinical Anesthesiology*. 4th ed. New York, NY: McGraw-Hill; 2006:544-546, 572-573, 876, 923.

## Answer A

### Pharmacology

**QUESTION (Choose single best answer):**

After 2 hours of anesthesia with halothane 1.2% and oxygen, nitrous oxide 75% is added to the inspired gas mixture. This addition would

(A) Increase the alveolar halothane and oxygen concentrations above inspired.
(B) Increase the alveolar halothane concentration only.
(C) Cause no change in alveolar gas concentrations compared with inspired.
(D) Decrease alveolar oxygen concentration compared with inspired.
(E) Decrease alveolar oxygen and halothane concentrations below inspired.

**CORRECT ANSWER: A**

**SUMMARY:**

*The rapid uptake of nitrous oxide augments the uptake of a concurrently administered potent anesthetic gas. This phenomenon is referred to as the* second-gas effect. *For example, if 75% (75 parts/100) nitrous is administered with 1.2% (1.2 parts/100) halothane and the remainder oxygen 23.8% (23.8 parts/100) and two-thirds of the nitrous is taken up (50 parts), the remaining 1.2 parts of halothane and 23.8 parts of oxygen are at a higher concentration. The gas mixture now becomes 1.2 parts halothane per 50 total parts or 2.4% halothane and 23.8 parts oxygen per 50 total parts or 47.6% oxygen. Therefore, when nitrous oxide is administered initially and taken up rapidly, it increases the alveolar partial pressure of the other agents.*

**EXPLANATION:**

(A) **Correct.** The second-gas effect causes an increase in alveolar concentration of both oxygen and halothane when it is added because of its rapid uptake.
(B) **Incorrect.** The alveolar partial pressures of both oxygen and halothane are increased because of the second-gas effect.
(C) **Incorrect.** See above.
(D) **Incorrect.** See above.
(E) **Incorrect.** See above.

**REASONING:**

Understanding the second-gas effect is the key to answering this question correctly. As nitrous oxide at a high concentration of 75% is added to the system, a large portion of the gas will be taken up, concentrating the remaining gases in the lungs in comparison with the inspired gases. Answer A describes the effect and is correct.

**BIBLIOGRAPHY:**

Barash PG, Cullen BF, Stoelting RK. *Clinical Anesthesia.* 4th ed. Philadelphia, PA: Lippincott Williams & Wilkins; 2001:384.
Morgan GE, Mikhail MS, Murray MJ. *Clinical Anesthesiology.* 3rd ed. New York, NY: McGraw-Hill; 2002:131-132.

## *Answer D*

### Basic Science

**QUESTION (Choose single best answer):**

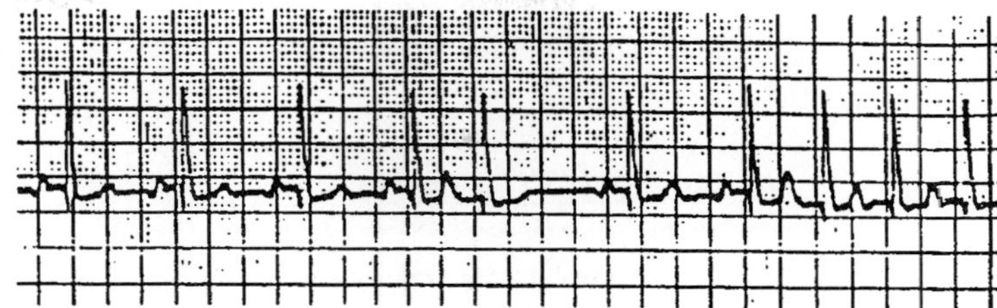

The ECG tracing shown here shows

(A) Aberrant intraventricular conduction.
(B) Acceleration of phase 4 depolarization of the sinus node.
(C) A compensatory pause.
(D) Initiation of reentrant supraventricular tachycardia (SVT).
(E) Paroxysmal atrial fibrillation.

**CORRECT ANSWER: D**


**SUMMARY:**

*The ECG shows a normal pattern in first half with normal PR interval and QRS complex and a rate of approximately 75 bpm. The midsection shows what looks like a junctional beat with a preceding unusual looking T wave, in which may be buried in the atrial premature beat, morphing the T wave to a different looking wave compared to other T waves. This is followed by a normal QRS complex without a P wave. The end segment shows a normal-looking QRS complex at the rate of 150 bpm without discernible P waves. SVT usually occurs at a rate of 130 to 220 bpm and often is initiated by a premature supraventricular beat (atrial or junctional).*


**EXPLANATION:**

(A) *Incorrect.* Aberrant intraventricular conduction has a widened, abnormal-looking QRS complex.
(B) *Incorrect.* Unlike cardiac ventricular muscle cells, pacemaker cells of the heart (SA and AV nodes) undergo a slow, spontaneous depolarization during phase 4 owing to pacemaker currents. The tracing shows a reentrant supraventricular tachycardia. The mechanism of the tachycardia is reentry, not increased rate of spontaneous depolarization of the SA node.
(C) *Incorrect.* A compensatory pause follows a premature ventricular beat.
(D) *Correct.* The ECG shows a narrow-complex tachycardia with a rate of 150 bpm.
(E) *Incorrect.* Atrial fibrillation occurs with an irregular heart rate without P waves.


**REASONING:**

There are several different causes of reentrant supraventricular tachycardias. Etiologies include Wolff-Parkinson-White (WPW) syndrome, AV reentrant tachycardia, AV nodal reentrant tachycardia (AVNRT), and SA node and atrial reentrant tachycardias. Reentry is usually triggered by a premature cardiac impulse. The salient features of this ECG are the triggering junctional beat followed by regular narrow-complex tachycardia at a rate of 150 to 180 bpm. D is the best answer. AVNRT is the most common cause of SVT (not atrial flutter or atrial fibrillation). The ECG shows a pause in the middle without a preceding PVC to qualify as compensatory pause.

**BIBLIOGRAPHY:**

Barash PG, Cullen BF, Stoelting RK. *Clinical Anesthesia.* 4th ed. Philadelphia, PA: Lippincott Williams & Wilkins; 2001:863.

Morgan GE, Mikhail MS, Murray MJ. *Clinical Anesthesiology.* 4th ed. New York, NY: McGraw-Hill; 2002:436-437.

Stoelting RK, Dierdorf SF. *Anesthesia and Co-existing Diseases.* 4th ed. New York, NY: Churchill Livingstone; 1993:81-82.

| BOOK A: | QUESTION 94 |
|---|---|

*Answer C*

Physiology

**QUESTION (Choose single best answer):**

One hour after an open cholecystectomy, a 42-year-old patient is hemodynamically stable and breathing spontaneously (rate 10 breaths/min and regular) at an $F_{IO_2}$ of 0.4. Fentanyl, isoflurane, nitrous oxide, and pancuronium were used during the procedure. Analysis of arterial blood gases is most likely to show the following:

|  | pH | $P_{CO_2}$ (mm Hg) | $P_{O_2}$ (mm Hg) |
|---|---|---|---|
| (A) | 7.18 | 40 | 100 |
| (B) | 7.18 | 60 | 140 |
| (C) | 7.28 | 50 | 85 |
| (D) | 7.40 | 26 | 220 |
| (E) | 7.40 | 40 | 40 |

**CORRECT ANSWER: C**

**SUMMARY:**

*General anesthesia and abdominal surgery have a number of adverse effects on pulmonary mechanics. These include increased shunting, decreased vital capacity, decreased functional residual capacity, and increased dead space. These changes are accentuated by upper abdominal surgery and may persist for days. These changes are offset in the OR by increased delivered $F_{IO_2}$ and increased minute ventilation. However, in the postoperative period they will be reflected by a mild respiratory acidosis and larger than normal arterial-alveolar oxygen gradient.*

**EXPLANATION:**

In a hemodynamically stable patient 1 hour following an open upper abdominal procedure, a mild respiratory acidosis would be expected due to the ventilatory depression of the opiates and lingering volatile anesthetics. In addition, diminished $Pa_{O_2}$ as a result of shunting caused by altered ventilatory mechanics and subsequent atelectasis would be observed. General anesthesia in the supine position consistently produces a decrease in functional residual capacity of 15% to 20%. This in turn results in increased intrapulmonary shunting as blood continues to perfuse unventilated regions. This may be augmented by the impairment in HPV that accompanies general anesthesia. Decreased lung volumes including vital capacity and functional residual capacity remain depressed for 10 to 14 days following upper abdominal surgery with general anesthesia. A mild nongap hyperchloremic metabolic acidosis may be present following administration of hyperchloremic intravenous fluids such as normal saline or lactated ringers.

A pH of 7.18 would be unusual in a spontaneous breathing patient who was hemodynamically stable following an open cholecystectomy. This degree of acidemia would tend to cause some hemodynamic instability, such as tachycardia and blood pressure instability, in addition to probable obtundation. A pH of 7.28, $P_{CO_2}$ of 50, and $P_{O_2}$ of 85 are consistent with the expected mild acute mixed respiratory and metabolic acidosis as well as decreased lung volumes and shunting.

Choices A and B are wrong due to the severity of the acidemia, which is not consistent with a hemodynamically stable patient breathing regularly at 10/min. Choice C is correct. One would expect a mild respiratory acidosis as a result of the lingering anesthetic and opioids. The $P_{CO_2}$ of 50 would alone decrease pH to approximately 7.32 and the lower pH would indicate a mild metabolic acidosis as well. The $P_{O_2}$ of 85 is consistent with the splinting, atelectasis, and intrapulmonary shunting expected following upper abdominal surgery, resulting in an increase in the A-a gradient. Choice D is incorrect. A pH of 7.4 with a $P_{CO_2}$ of 26 implies a significant respiratory alkalosis and equally matching significant metabolic acidosis, which would be unexpected, while the $P_{O_2}$ of 220 would imply virtually intact pulmonary mechanics. Choice E is incorrect. The patient demonstrates no respiratory acidosis and severe hypoxemia.

**BIBLIOGRAPHY:**

Hines RL, Marschall KE. *Stoelting's Anesthesia and Co-existing Disease*. 5th ed. Philadelphia, PA: Churchill Livingstone; 2008:360-361.

Morgan GE, Mikhail MS, Murray MJ. *Clinical Anesthesiology*. 4th ed. New York, NY: McGraw-Hill; 2006:558-561.

---

| **BOOK A:** | **QUESTION 95** |
|---|---|

*Answer B*

Pharmacology

**QUESTION (Choose single best answer):**

A 6-year-old child with asthma begins wheezing during anesthesia with halothane and nitrous oxide in oxygen. A loading dose of aminophylline is administered, followed by continuous infusion. Premature ventricular contractions appear on the ECG. The most appropriate management is to

(A) Administer fentanyl.
(B) Discontinue aminophylline.
(C) Increase exhalation time.
(D) Increase the inspired concentration of halothane.
(E) Switch the inhalational agent to isoflurane.

**CORRECT ANSWER: B**

**SUMMARY:**

*Aminophylline is an older intravenous drug used in the treatment of asthma. It is a methylxanthine that increases the level of cyclic adenosine monophosphate (cAMP), resulting in bronchodilation. Its major side effects, ventricular dysrhythmias and seizures, warrant close monitoring of blood level. Acute administration of aminophylline decreases the threshold of epinephrine to induce arrhythmias. Halothane also sensitizes the myocardium to arrhythmias from epinephrine. The inhaled β-agonists are considered the first line of therapy in the acute management of bronchospasm. They have much superior safety profile compared to aminophylline.*

**EXPLANATION:**

(A) ***Incorrect.*** Fentanyl will not affect the interaction between halothane and aminophylline. It may be appropriate to increase the depth of anesthesia if light level is suspected. However, the temporal relationship of aminophylline and premature ventricular contraction (PVC) is the suspect here.

(B) ***Correct.*** The onset of ventricular arrhythmias with administration of aminophylline should be scrutinized, especially given its narrow therapeutic window. In addition, studies suggest that aminophylline does not improve outcomes and can cause adverse effects in children with acute asthma. There are several other more effective treatments for bronchospasm, including sympathomimetic agents (aerosolized $\beta_2$-selective drugs such as albuterol) and parasympatholytics such as ipratropium. It would be best to terminate aminophylline therapy and initiate other safer and more efficacious treatments.

(C) ***Incorrect.*** Exhalation time has no effect on the PVCs. It is a reasonable maneuver in asthma with airway obstruction.

(D) ***Incorrect.*** This maneuver will further exacerbate the arrhythmogenic effect of halothane.

(E) ***Incorrect.*** Isoflurane does not sensitize the myocardium to catecholamines. Although switching from halothane to isoflurane theoretically might minimize arrhythmias, it does not address the primary concern—aminophylline toxicity. In reality, we probably also would discontinue halothane; however, the *most appropriate management* is to first address the potential aminophylline toxicity by terminating the infusion.


### REASONING:

The key elements to this question are the toxicity profile of aminophylline and the drug interaction between halothane and aminophylline. Aminophylline has a narrow therapeutic range and variable clearance, mandating close attention to drug interactions that can compound its toxicity. This question is made somewhat challenging by two seemingly plausible answers (B and E). However, the key is to recognize that the examination is asking for the "most appropriate management." In this case, addressing the potential aminophylline toxicity is the primary concern. The best answer is B.


### BIBLIOGRAPHY:

Barash PG, Cullen BF, Stoelting RK. *Clinical Anesthesia.* 4th ed. Philadelphia, PA: Lippincott Williams & Wilkins; 2001:817.

Stoelting RK, Dierdorf SF. *Anesthesia and Co-existing Diseases.* New York, NY: Churchill Livingstone; 1993.

Strauss RE, Wertheim DL, Bonagura VR, Valacer DJ. Aminophylline therapy does not improve outcome and increases adverse effects in children hospitalized with acute asthmatic exacerbations. *Pediatrics.* 1994;93:205-210.


## BOOK A: QUESTION 96

*Answer B*

Equipment/Physics

### QUESTION (Choose single best answer):

Oxygen 100 mL/min is bubbled through a vaporizer containing an anesthetic with a vapor pressure of 150 mm Hg, and this mixture is added to a fresh gas flow of 5 L/min. The delivered anesthetic concentration is

(A) 0.25%.
(B) 0.5%.
(C) 1%.
(D) 2.5%.
(E) 5%.


### CORRECT ANSWER: B

**SUMMARY:**

*The amount of vapor leaving a copper kettle–type vaporizer depends on the vapor pressure of the anesthetic agent, the flow rate of the carrier gas (ie, oxygen), and the barometric pressure at which the vaporizer is used. Thus, the equation needed to figure out the delivered anesthetic concentration is as follows:*

$$Vapor\ output = \frac{carrier\ gas\ flow\ rate \times vapor\ pressure\ of\ gas}{barometric\ pressure - vapor\ pressure\ of\ gas}$$

$$= \frac{100(cc/mL) \times 150(mm\ Hg)}{760(mm\ Hg) - 150(mm\ Hg)}$$

*This calculation equals 23 cc/min of anesthetic. This is the amount of gas picked up by the oxygen carrier gas. Thus, to get the final concentration, add 23 to 100 cc/min of carrier gas flow and to 5000 cc/min of fresh gas flow (5123 cc/min total). Finally, divide actual anesthetic gas flow by the total as follows:*

$$\frac{23\ cc/min}{5123\ cc/min} = 0.5\%$$


**EXPLANATION:**

(A) *Incorrect.* See above.

(B) *Correct.* To figure out this answer, four numbers must be defined: the barometric pressure, the vapor pressure of the anesthetic gas, the carrier flow rate, and the fresh gas flow. Frequently, the carrier gas number is 100 cc/min of oxygen and the barometric pressure at sea level is 760 mm Hg. With these numbers, one can determine the final anesthetic concentration of any anesthetic gas using the following equation:

$$Vapor\ output = \frac{carrier\ gas\ flow \times vapor\ pressure\ of\ gas}{barometric\ pressure - vapor\ pressure\ of\ gas}$$

$$\frac{Final\ anesthetic}{concentration} = \frac{vapor\ output}{carrier\ gas\ flow + vapor\ output + fresh\ gas\ flow}$$

(C) *Incorrect.* See above.

(D) *Incorrect.* See above.

(E) *Incorrect.* See above.

**REASONING:**

To figure out a copper kettle question, one must understand the mechanism of this particular type of vaporizer. A carrier gas, such as oxygen, is driven into a chamber of gas vapor that has its own, distinct vapor pressure. Dependent on the vapor pressure of the gas and the barometric pressure (760 mm Hg), this carrier gas will pick up a certain amount of gas, otherwise known as *vapor output*. The vapor output is calculated as follows:

$$\frac{100\ cc/min \times 150\ mm\ Hg}{760\ mm\ Hg - 150\ mm\ Hg} = 23\ cc/min\ of\ anesthetic\ output$$

The actual anesthetic concentration is calculated by dividing the vapor output by the total gas flow or

$$\frac{23\ cc/min}{5123\ cc/min\ (5000\ cc/min + 23\ cc/min + 100\ cc/min)} = 0.5\%$$

**BIBLIOGRAPHY:**

Morgan GE, Mikhail MS, Murray MJ. *Clinical Anesthesiology.* 4th ed. New York, NY: McGraw-Hill; 2006:59-65.

*Answer D*

Physiology

**QUESTION (Choose single best answer):**

A 50-year-old man who takes aspirin and nifedipine is scheduled for thoracotomy with one-lung ventilation. Which of the following is associated with the greatest risk for intra-operative hypoxemia?

(A) Preoperative withdrawal of nifedipine therapy.
(B) Intraoperative mild respiratory acidosis.
(C) Intraoperative administration of isoflurane.
(D) Intraoperative administration of nitroglycerin.
(E) Intraoperative thoracic epidural morphine.

**CORRECT ANSWER: D**

**SUMMARY:**

*During one-lung ventilation protection from hypoxemia arises from HPV. Factors that impair HPV will increase the risk of hypoxemia. Calcium channel blockers such as nifedipine impair HPV and their withdrawal preoperatively will reduce the risk of intraoperative hypoxemia. Hypocapnia (respiratory alkalosis), but not mild respiratory acidosis, can impair HPV increasing the risk of intraoperative hypoxemia. Intraoperative isoflurane at clinically useful doses (1 MAC and less) does not significantly impair HPV in human studies, but it might have a slight effect at higher doses. Nonspecific vasodilators such as nitroglycerin can significantly impair HPV and increase the risk of intraoperative hypoxia. Thoracic epidural morphine would not be expected to have an effect on intraoperative hypoxemia.*

**EXPLANATION:**

(A) *Incorrect.* Withdrawal of nifedipine will reduce the risk of intraoperative hypoxemia, as it normally interferes with HPV.
(B) *Incorrect.* While hypocapnia may impair HPV, mild respiratory acidosis does not.
(C) *Incorrect.* Isoflurane used at clinical concentrations appears to have a minimal effect on HPV.
(D) *Correct.* Nitroglycerin vasodilates the normally vasoconstricted pulmonary vasculature in poorly oxygenated regions, increasing the risk of shunt and hypoxemia.
(E) *Incorrect.* Epidural opiates have not been linked to impairments in HPV.

**REASONING:**

Hypoxic pulmonary vasoconstriction (HPV) shunts blood away from poorly oxygenated lung regions to regions of the lung where oxygenation is better maintained. This results in better matching of blood flow to well-oxygenated regions (better V/Q matching). This is especially important during one-lung ventilation. Much of the blood passing through the nonventilated lung will act as a shunt mixing with well-oxygenated blood traveling through the ventilated lung and thus reducing systemic $Pa_{O_2}$. This is minimized by HPV in the nonventilated lung, which preferentially reduces blood flow in the nonventilated lung. Factors known to inhibit HPV and increase the risk of hypoxemia during one-lung ventilation include hypocapnia from hyperventilation, extremes of mixed venous $P_{O_2}$, extremes of pulmonary artery pressure, systemic vasodilators such as calcium channel blockers, nitroglycerin, and sodium nitroprusside, infection, and at high doses some inhaled anesthetics particularly halothane. Nonetheless, studies in humans have either failed to demonstrate or have demonstrated very slight changes in $Pa_{O_2}$ during one-lung ventilation with up to 1 MAC of isoflurane. There is no clear link between epidural opiates and HPV.

**BIBLIOGRAPHY:**
Barash PG, Cullen BF, Stoelting RK, Calahan M, Stock MC. *Clinical Anesthesia*. 6th ed. Philadelphia, PA: Lippincott Williams & Wilkins; 2009:1054-1055.
Morgan GE, Mikhail MS, Murray MJ. *Clinical Anesthesiology*. 4th ed. New York, NY: McGraw-Hill; 2006:557.

---

| **BOOK A:** | **QUESTION 98** |
|---|---|

*Answer C*

Physiology

**QUESTION (Choose single best answer):**

A 35-year-old woman with severe myasthenia gravis is scheduled for thymectomy. Which of the following preoperative pulmonary function tests is most likely to be normal?

(A) Forced expiratory volume in 1 second ($FEV_1$).
(B) Forced vital capacity (FVC).
(C) $FEV_1$/FVC.
(D) Maximum voluntary ventilation.
(E) Peak inspiratory force.

**CORRECT ANSWER: C**

**SUMMARY:**

*Myasthenia gravis is an autoimmune skeletal muscle disease that causes weakness and fatigability by destruction of postsynaptic acetylcholine receptors at the NMJ. In approximately 80% of patients, the thymus gland is the origin of the antibodies to the acetylcholine receptors. Pulmonary function tests (PFTs) measure muscle strength and endurance and will be below normal in a patient with myasthenia gravis.*

**EXPLANATION:**

(A) *Incorrect.* A patient weak with myasthenia will have an impaired ability to forcefully exhale.
(B) *Incorrect.* Again, the severe myasthenic will not have a normal forced capacity.
(C) *Correct.* If both FEV1 and FVC are lowered, the ratio may be normal.
(D) *Incorrect.* Maximum voluntary ventilation (MVV) measures muscle endurance and is likely to be abnormal.
(E) *Incorrect.* Peak inspiratory flow (PIF) requires good muscle strength. This number has predictive value for postoperative respiratory complications and impending respiratory failure in the myasthenic patient.

**REASONING:**

This question tests knowledge of pulmonary function testing in the setting of myasthenia gravis. The answer to this question relies in part on your mathematical prowess. It does not take much knowledge of myasthenia and PFTs. Weak patients have below normal PFTs for effort-dependent assessments such as $FEV_1$, FVC, MVV, and PIF. However, answer C is a ratio that eliminates units (liters) and seemingly corrects for impaired patient effort. With both $FEV_1$ and FVC decrease in the myasthenic patient, the ratio may be normal.

**BIBLIOGRAPHY:**
Miller RD, Miller ED, Reves JG, et al. *Anesthesia*. 7th ed. Philadelphia, PA: Churchill Livingstone; 2010:1180.
Morgan GE, Mikhail MS, Murray MJ. *Clinical Anesthesiology*. 3rd ed. New York, NY: McGraw-Hill; 2002:753-754.

## Answer E

Physiology

**QUESTION (Choose single best answer):**

A 66-year-old man with aortic regurgitation is brought to the operating room for aortic valve replacement after having received morphine and scopolamine premedication. The $P_{O_2}$ is 40 mm Hg in a sample of pulmonary artery blood drawn 10 minutes after the patient started breathing pure oxygen. This finding is compatible with

(A) Wedging of the catheter tip.
(B) Left-to-right intracardiac shunting.
(C) Increased intrapulmonary shunting.
(D) Excessively depressed ventilation.
(E) Normal cardiac output.

**CORRECT ANSWER: E**

**SUMMARY:**

*Mixed venous saturation represents the global oxygen supply and demand balance and is useful in assessing overall blood supply and tissue demand. In the absence of increased oxygen demand, hypoxia, and anemia, a drop in mixed venous saturation is indicative of decreased blood flow in relation to tissue requirements. This results in increased extraction and a drop in mixed venous oxygen saturation. This relationship allows mixed venous saturation to be used as a surrogate measure of adequate cardiac output. Normal mixed venous saturation is 75% with a partial pressure of 40 mm Hg.*

**EXPLANATION:**
(A) *Incorrect.* Wedging of the catheter tip is diagnosed by PA catheter tracing.
(B) *Incorrect.* Left-to-right shunt would exhibit a higher $P_{O_2}$ and saturation.
(C) *Incorrect.* Intrapulmonary shunt would contribute toward hypoxia and thus further decrease mixed venous saturation and partial pressure.
(D) *Incorrect.* Excessively depressed ventilation would affect $CO_2$ elimination. Unless extreme, it would not affect oxygenation or $S_{VO_2}$.
(E) *Correct.* The $P_{O_2}$ of 40 mm Hg is normal and indicates a saturation near 75%. This is consistent with an adequate cardiac output.

**REASONING:**
The relationship between $S\bar{v}_{O_2}$, $\dot{V}_{O_2}$, and $\dot{D}_{O_2}$ is described by the equation

$$S\bar{v}O_2 = SaO_2 - \frac{\dot{V}O_2}{Hb \times 13.8 \times CO}$$

where $Sa_{O_2}$ is the arterial $O_2$ saturation, Hb is the hemoglobin concentration, $\dot{V}_{O_2}$ is the rate of oxygen consumption, 13.8 represents the volume of $O_2$ carried by 1 g Hb/L, and CO is the cardiac output. In clinical practice, $S\bar{v}_{O_2}$ can be measured continuously using reflectance spectrophotometry of blood at the tip of a pulmonary artery catheter. It is important to understand that $S\bar{v}_{O_2}$ represents global tissue oxygen extraction in the body, with a normal value of 75% indicating 25% tissue extraction. Various end organs, however, have different extraction ratios that can vary from 55% to 70% for myocardium to 7 to 10% for the kidney and skin. It is important for the reader to be familiar with the relationship of cardiac output and mixed venous oxygen saturation and the factors that influence mixed venous saturation. The best answer is E.

**BIBLIOGRAPHY:**
Barash PG, Cullen BF, Stoelting RK. *Clinical Anesthesia*. 6th ed. Philadelphia, PA: Lippincott Williams & Wilkins; 2001:201-202, 678. (Note that the equation is printed incorrectly in this text.)
Morgan GE, Mikhail MS, Murray MJ. *Clinical Anesthesiology*. 3rd ed. New York, NY: McGraw-Hill; 2002:499-502.
Ibid., 6th ed, pp 708-709.

---

**BOOK A:**  **QUESTION 100**

---

*Answer A*

Pharmacology

**QUESTION (Choose single best answer):**

Which of the following statements concerning metoclopramide is true?

(A) It is antagonized by concomitant administration of atropine.
(B) It decreases gastrointestinal motility.
(C) It decreases gastric secretion.
(D) It lacks antiemetic properties.
(E) It stimulates dopamine receptors.

**CORRECT ANSWER: A**

**SUMMARY:**

*Metoclopramide functions at both dopamine and acetylcholine receptors. Peripherally, its cholinomimetic activities include (1) increase smooth muscle tone at the lower esophageal sphincter and gastric fundus, (2) relax the pylorus and duodenum during gastric contraction, and (3) increase gastric and small intestinal motility; the net effect is accelerated gastric clearance and decreased transit time through the small intestine. Metoclopramide requires background cholinergic activity to be effective, and thus its effect on the proximal gastrointestinal tract can be antagonized by atropine. Gastric acid secretion is not affected by metoclopramide. Centrally, metoclopramide antagonizes dopamine receptors, especially in the chemoreceptor trigger zone, and this theoretically contributes to an antiemetic effect (in addition to antiemetic effects from increased lower esophageal sphincter tone and increased gastric emptying into the small intestine).*

**EXPLANATION:**
(A) *Correct.* Metoclopramide's peripheral cholinergic activity is dependent on the presence of background cholinergic activity and thus can be antagonized by an anticholinergic agent such as atropine.
(B) *Incorrect.* Metoclopramide increases proximal gastrointestinal motility.
(C) *Incorrect.* Metoclopramide does not change gastric acid secretion, but gastric fluid volume is decreased secondary to the resultant accelerated gastric clearance.
(D) *Incorrect.* Although metoclopramide's ability to prevent postoperative nausea and vomiting is equivocal, several of its mechanisms of action contribute to an antiemetic effect and it can blunt opioid-induced nausea and vomiting.
(E) *Incorrect.* Metoclopramide antagonizes both central and peripheral dopamine receptors, although its effects on dopamine-induced inhibition of gastrointestinal motility are not clinically significant.

**REASONING:**

This question tests knowledge of metoclopramide's mechanism of action, particularly its effects in the proximal gastrointestinal tract and the CNS. The best answer is A.

**BIBLIOGRAPHY:**

Brock-Utne JG, Dow TGB, Welman S, et al. The effect of metoclopramide on lower oesophageal sphincter tone in late pregnancy. *Anaesth Intensive Care*. 1978;6:26-29.

Cohen SE, Jasson J, Talafre ML, Chauvelot-Moachon L, Barrier G. Does metoclopramide decrease the volume of gastric contents in patients undergoing cesarean section? *Anesthesiology*. 1984;61:604-607.

Henszi I, Walder B, Tramer MR. Metoclopramide in the prevention of postoperative nausea and vomiting: a quantitative systematic review of randomized, placebo-controlled studies. *Br J Anaesth*. 1999;83:761-771.

Klinkenberg-Knol EC, Festen HPM, Meuwissen SGM. Pharmacological management of gastro-oesophageal reflux disease. *Drugs*. 1995;49:695-710.

Morgan GE, Mikhail MS, Murray MJ. *Clinical Anesthesiology*. 4th ed. New York, NY: McGraw-Hill;2006:280-281.

Schulze-Dlrieu L. Drug therapy: metoclopramide. *N Engl J Med*. 1981;305:28-33.

Stoelting RK, Hillier SC. *Pharmacology & Physiology in Anesthetic Practice*. 4th ed. Philadelphia, PA: Lippincott Williams & Wilkins; 2006:499-502.

Wyner J, Cohen SE. Gastric volume in early pregnancy: effect of metoclopramide. *Anesthesiology*. 1982;57:209-212.

---

## BOOK A:     QUESTION 101

*Answer C*

Physiology

**QUESTION (Choose single best answer):**

During halothane anesthesia with spontaneous ventilation, the most reliable sign of malignant hyperthermia is

(A) Hypertension.
(B) Increased temperature.
(C) Increased minute ventilation.
(D) Muscle rigidity.
(E) Tachycardia.

**CORRECT ANSWER: C**

**SUMMARY:**

*Malignant hyperthermia (MH) is a rare and potentially fatal complication of general anesthesia. It is a hypermetabolic state that results from abnormal calcium release from the sarcoplasmic reticulum in myocytes. The clinical signs of MH are the result of the associated hypermetabolism, increased sympathetic activity, muscle damage, and hyperthermia. Treatment includes stopping the triggering agent, supportive care, and administration of intravenous dantrolene.*

**EXPLANATION:**

(A) *Incorrect.* Although sympathetic activation is a sign of MH, it is not the most sensitive sign. Other signs of increased sympathetic activity associated with MH include tachycardia and arrhythmias.

(B) *Incorrect.* An elevated temperature is a late sign of MH. The temperature rise can be as much as 1°C every 5 minutes.

(C) *Correct.* Unexpected elevation of end-tidal carbon dioxide in the absence of equipment malfunction is the most sensitive and specific sign of MH. This is due to increased $CO_2$ production from the hypermetabolic state. In a patient who is breathing spontaneously, the increased $CO_2$ will result in increased minute ventilation.

(D) *Incorrect.* Muscle rigidity is a sign of MH, but it does not have to be present for the diagnosis of MH.

(E) *Incorrect.* Once again, sympathetic activation is a sign of MH, but tachycardia is not specific or sensitive for the diagnosis of MH.

**BIBLIOGRAPHY:**
Barash PG, Cullen BF, Stoelting RK, Calahan M, Stock MC. *Clinical Anesthesia*. 6th ed. Philadelphia, PA: Lippincott Williams & Wilkins; 2009:598-613.
Morgan GE, Mikhail MS, Murray MJ. *Clinical Anesthesiology*. 4th ed. New York, NY: McGraw-Hill; 2006:945-949.

---

**BOOK A:**

*Answer D*

Equipment/Physics

## QUESTION 102

**QUESTION (Choose single best answer):**

Which of the following is the most appropriate action after an anesthetic vaporizer is tipped?

(A) Return to the manufacturer for recalibration.
(B) Flush the vaporizer with oxygen at 5 L/min for 24 hours.
(C) Store the vaporizer for 24 hours at room temperature.
(D) Set the vaporizer at low concentration and flush with oxygen at 10 L/min for 30 minutes.
(E) Verify the vaporizer output with mass spectrography.

**CORRECT ANSWER: D**

**SUMMARY:**

*By tilting a vaporizer, the anesthetic agent may flood the bypass area of the vaporizer which is usually only crossed by the carrier gas (ie, oxygen). This is particularly common with older vaporizers (Tec 4, Tec 5) and can lead to a dangerously high concentration of vapor output, as the carrier gas picks up more of the agent as it crosses the bypass chamber. The appropriate action after the tipping of a vaporizer is to set it at a low concentration and flush the vaporizer with the carrier gas, or oxygen, at high flows (10 L/min).*

**EXPLANATION:**
(A) *Incorrect.* Returning the vaporizer to the manufacturer is not necessary. The problem is easily solved by flushing out any excess vapor from the bypass chamber and running the vaporizer at low concentrations to be reassured that equilibrium is reestablished. This is essentially the same as recalibrating the vaporizer because now one can be sure that the dialed concentration is the same as that amount of anesthetic vapor being delivered to the patient.
(B) *Incorrect.* Flushing the vaporizer with oxygen for 24 hours is unnecessary as it will not take that long to rid the bypass chamber of any excess vapor. Also, keeping a vaporizer on for this amount of time with medium to high flows will rid the vaporizer of all inhalational agent.

(C) *Incorrect.* Storing the vaporizer for 24 hours at room temperature does nothing to rid the vaporizer of potential agent in the bypass chamber. Thus, restarting the vaporizer after this time may put the patient in jeopardy of getting more vapor output than dialed on the vaporizer.

(D) *Correct.* By setting the vaporizer on a low concentration and flushing it with oxygen at 10 L/min for 30 minutes, any excess vapor is flushed through the ventilator and the bypass chamber reestablishes an equilibrium with the dialed concentration on the vaporizer. Only then can one be reassured that a patient receives the appropriate concentration of vapor output.

(E) *Incorrect.* Mass spectrography will probably identify an increased amount of vapor output going to the patient compared to that dialed into the vaporizer. However, this number will vary minute to minute until the bypass chamber is cleared of any excess anesthetic agent. Also, it is inconvenient to follow mass spectrography continuously until an equilibrium is reestablished.

## REASONING:

Vaporizers have two chambers through which gases pass before entering the inspiratory limb to the patient. The carrier gas, which is frequently oxygen, goes through the liquid anesthetic agent to pick up vapor as well as through a bypass chamber. Eventually, all the carrier gas and vapor output exit together. Thus, by tipping a vaporizer, there is potential for the agent to cross over into the bypass chamber and for the oxygen carrier gas to pick up more anesthetic than is dialed into the vaporizer. The first action that must be taken when this happens is to flush the vaporizer while turned on at low concentrations to clear that bypass chamber, while minimizing the waste of anesthetic agent. After approximately half an hour at high carrier flow rate, the vaporizer can once again be safely used without fear of delivering a dangerously high amount of vapor to the patient.

## BIBLIOGRAPHY:

Morgan GE, Mikhail MS, Murray MJ. *Clinical Anesthesiology.* 4th ed. New York, NY: McGraw-Hill; 2006:66.

---

## BOOK A:    QUESTION 103

*Answer A*

Physiology

### QUESTION (Choose single best answer):

Following pneumonectomy, a paralyzed patient being ventilated mechanically has the following arterial blood gas values: $Pao_2$ 71 mm Hg, $Paco_2$ 55 mm Hg, pH 7.29, and 45%. The most likely explanation for this is

(A) Decreased red cell mass.
(B) High cardiac output.
(C) Hypothermia.
(D) Peripheral left-to-right arteriovenous shunt.
(E) Ventilation-perfusion mismatch.

### CORRECT ANSWER: A

### SUMMARY:

*Mixed venous oxygen saturation ($S\bar{v}o_2$) is the percent saturation of venous blood before entering the lungs. A normal $S\bar{v}o_2$ typically is around 75%. Many factors can cause an* *alteration in the S$\overline{v}o_2$, as demonstrated by the following equation derived from the Fick relationship:*

$$S\overline{v}o_2 = Sao_2 - [\dot{V}o_2/(Hb \times 13.8 \times CO)]$$

*where Sao$_2$ is the arterial O$_2$ saturation, Hb is the hemoglobin concentration, S$\dot{v}o_2$ is the rate of oxygen consumption, 13.8 represents the volume of O$_2$ carried by 1 g Hb/L, and CO is the cardiac output. Based on this equation, it is easy to see how each variable can affect.*

### EXPLANATION:

(A) **Correct.** A decreased red cell mass, according to the preceding equation, will lead to a decreased S$\overline{v}o_2$. Because there is less hemoglobin to carry oxygen, more oxygen will be extracted from the hemoglobin by tissues, causing a decreased S$\overline{v}o_2$.

(B) **Incorrect.** A high cardiac output would deliver more oxygen to tissue, leading to less extraction and a greater S$\overline{v}o_2$.

(C) **Incorrect.** Hypothermia would decrease oxygen consumption, leading to less oxygen extraction and a greater S$\overline{v}o_2$.

(D) **Incorrect.** A left-to-right arteriovenous shunt would prevent the shunted blood from coming into contact with tissue, decreasing oxygen extraction for the shunted blood and leading to a greater S$vo_2$ and likely increased cardiac output.

(E) **Incorrect.** A $\dot{V}/\dot{Q}$ mismatch would cause hypoxemia and decrease Sao$_2$, causing a decrease in S$\overline{v}o_2$. However, a Pao$_2$ of 71 mm Hg is not sufficiently hypoxemic to explain the observed of 45%.

### REASONING:

This question tests knowledge of the factors that influence S$\overline{v}o_2$. Knowing that a decreased S$\overline{v}o_2$ can occur with either a decreased supply of oxygen or increased demand allows answers, B, C, and D to be eliminated because they either increase supply or decrease demand. Choice E is tempting, but it is hard to explain a very low with a Pao$_2$ of 71 mm Hg, which corresponds to a Sao$_2$ above 90% saturation. The only answer remaining is decreased red cell mass, which can be explained easily by bleeding during the procedure.

### BIBLIOGRAPHY:


Barash PG, Cullen BF, Stoelting RK, Calahan M, Stock MC. *Clinical Anesthesia*. 6th ed. Philadelphia, PA: Lippincott Williams & Wilkins; 2009:708-709.

Morgan GE, Mikhail MS, Murray MJ. *Clinical Anesthesiology*. 4th ed. New York, NY: McGraw-Hill; 2006:564.


---

**BOOK A:**

## QUESTION 104

*Answer C*

Pharmacology

### QUESTION (Choose single best answer):

Which of the following is a sign of cyclosporine toxicity?

(A) Abnormal hepatic enzyme activity.
(B) Decreased hemoglobin concentration.
(C) Increased serum creatinine concentration.
(D) Nodular density on radiograph of the chest.
(E) ST–T-wave changes on ECG.

**SUMMARY:**

*Cyclosporine is an immunosuppressant associated with multiple toxicities that include seizures, hypertension, elevated liver enzymes, gingival hyperplasia, and renal toxicity, resulting in elevated blood urea nitrogen (BUN) and creatinine concentrations. Nephrotoxicity can occur with either acute or chronic use and is due to renal fibrosis and tubular atrophy. Cyclosporine works by (1) inhibiting interleukin 1 (IL-1) production, (2) inhibiting IL-2 secretion, and (3) blocking activation of CD4 helper cells.*

**EXPLANATION:**

(A) *Incorrect.* Cyclosporine can result in elevated liver enzymes, not abnormal liver enzyme function.

(B) *Incorrect.* Unlike other immunosuppressant drugs, cyclosporine does not suppress bone marrow cellular production.

(C) *Correct.* Cyclosporine can elevate serum creatinine by causing interstitial renal fibrosis and tubular atrophy. Cyclosporine nephrotoxicity renders the kidney sensitive to acute insults such as radiographic dye and hypotension-induced nephropathy.

(D) *Incorrect.* This is not a toxicity of cyclosporine.

(E) *Incorrect.* This is not a toxicity of cyclosporine.

**REASONING:**

This question tests knowledge of cyclosporine toxicity. It is important for the reader to be familiar with the side effects of other antirejection medications as well. Tacrolimus has a similar side-effect and toxicity profile. Glucocorticoids can produce adrenal suppression, glucose intolerance, cushingoid appearance, and exacerbation of peptic ulcer disease. Azathioprine can produce anemia, thrombocytopenia, and hepatitis, and can increase the requirement for nondepolarizing muscle relaxants.

**BIBLIOGRAPHY:**

Barash PG, Cullen BF, Stoelting RK. *Clinical Anesthesia.* 4th ed. Philadelphia, PA: Lippincott Williams & Wilkins; 2001:1367 (Table 52-16).

---

| **BOOK A:** | **QUESTION 105** |
|---|---|

*Answer D*

Pain

**QUESTION (Choose single best answer):**

Myofascial pain is an example of

(A) A central pain state.
(B) Neuropathic pain.
(C) Psychogenic pain.
(D) Somatic pain.
(E) Visceral pain.

**CORRECT ANSWER: D**

**SUMMARY:**

*Myofascial pain originates from muscle. It is therefore a type of somatic pain that refers to all types of pain originating from the structures of the body wall (eg, muscle, tendon, ligament, and bone) rather than a type of visceral pain originating from internal organs (eg, the pain of pancreatitis). It is distinct from the pain caused by direct injury to the CNS (central pain states) and the peripheral nervous system (neuropathic pain). Psychogenic pain refers to pain caused by psychological conflict rather than pathology in the structure felt to be in pain.*

**EXPLANATION:**

(A) *Incorrect.* Central pain states and neuropathic pain are the result of pain caused by injury to nervous system tissue.
(B) *Incorrect.* See above.
(C) *Incorrect.* The term *psychogenic pain* specifically excludes pain caused by pathology in the muscles and only refers to pain stemming entirely from psychological factors.
(D) *Correct.* Myofascial pain is a subset of somatic pain that also includes pain from bones (fractures), joints (arthritis), tendons (tendonitis), and other structures of the body wall.
(E) *Incorrect.* Visceral pain comes from structures such as internal organs.

**REASONING:**

Myofascial pain is pain originating from a muscle group. It is often associated with trigger points. These trigger points are tender to palpation, and when stimulated, they refer pain along stereotypical distributions that are nondermatomal in nature. Trigger point injection with local anesthetic or without (dry-needling) in conjunction with physical therapy may provide relief. The cause of myofascial pain and trigger points is not clear but is not associated with overt central or peripheral nervous system injury, as in central pain states or neuropathic pain. Psychogenic pain is also different and refers to pain based purely on psychological factors such as a need to suffer because of extreme guilt or other psychological conflict. Visceral pain refers to pain arising from the internal organs. Myofascial pain is a type of somatic pain that refers to pain originating from structures in the body wall (as opposed to internal viscera) or skeletal structures such as muscle, bone, tendon, and joint.

**BIBLIOGRAPHY:**

Barash PG, Cullen BF, Stoelting RK, Calahan M, Stock MC. *Clinical Anesthesia*. 6th ed. Philadelphia, PA: Lippincott Williams & Wilkins; 2009:1515.
Morgan GE, Mikhail MS, Murray MJ. *Clinical Anesthesiology*. 4th ed. New York, NY: McGraw-Hill; 2006:400-401.

---

| **BOOK A:** | **QUESTION 106** |

*Answer B*

Pediatrics

**QUESTION (Choose single best answer):**

In children with preoperative upper respiratory tract infection, which of the following is associated with the greatest risk for postoperative airway obstruction?

(A) Age less than 1 year.
(B) Endotracheal intubation.
(C) Head and neck injury.
(D) Inadequate airway humidification.
(E) Surgery for more than 2 hours.

**CORRECT ANSWER: B**

**SUMMARY:**

*Children commonly present for elective surgery with symptoms of an active upper respiratory tract infection (URI) or with a recent history of one. Because children can develop 6 to 8 URIs a year, this places the clinician in a difficult situation regarding postponing surgery. Studies have documented that changes in pulmonary reactivity and spirometry can last as long as 6 to 8 weeks after a URI. A viral infection within 2 to 4 weeks before general anesthesia appears to place the child at increased risk of perioperative pulmonary complications such as wheezing, laryngospasm, hypoxemia, and atelectasis. Independent risk factors for adverse respiratory events in children with active URIs include use of an ETT (< 5 years of age), history of prematurity, history of reactive airway disease, parental smoking, surgery involving the airway, the presence of copious secretions, and nasal congestion. Elective surgery should be postponed for children with severe URI symptoms such as fever, mucopurulent secretions, productive cough, and lower airway involvement. There is no consensus on the exact duration of postponement, but duration of 3 to 4 weeks is suggested to be a prudent timeframe.*

**EXPLANATION:**

(A) *Incorrect.* Children younger than 5 years with active URI who received an ETT had a significantly increased risk of respiratory events. Age less than 1 year alone has not been shown to be associated with increased risk.

(B) *Correct.* Endotracheal intubation has been associated consistently with an increased risk of bronchospasm, laryngospasm, and desaturation events. Most of these events are not severe and are treated easily.

(C) *Incorrect.* Head and neck surgery in general is not associated with adverse respiratory events. Surgical procedures involving the airway, such as tonsillectomy and adenoidectomy, direct laryngoscopy, and bronchoscopy, however, are associated with an increased incidence of adverse respiratory events.

(D) *Incorrect.* Humidified air is used to treat croup, but its lack of use is not associated with increased risk of airway obstruction.

(E) *Incorrect.* Duration of surgery in and of itself is not associated with postoperative airway obstruction. Increased duration of endotracheal intubation, however, is directly correlated with an increased incidence of airway obstruction.

**REASONING:**

This is a challenging question because all the answers appear to be reasonable. The literature itself is inconclusive and often conflicting. The one factor that was most consistently associated with increased postoperative airway obstruction in previous studies was endotracheal intubation. The final decision whether to anesthetize a child should take into consideration factors that include other medical problems, severity of symptoms, urgency of surgery, availability of postoperative care, and the family wishes.

**BIBLIOGRAPHY:**

Cote CJ. *A Practice of Anesthesia for Infants and Children.* 4th ed. Philadelphia, PA: Saunders; 2009:226-229.

Koka BV, Jeon IS, Andre JM, et al. Postintubation croup in children. Anesth Analg. 1977;56:501-505.

Morgan GE, Mikhail MS, Murray MJ. *Clinical Anesthesiology.* 4th ed. New York, NY: McGraw-Hill; 2006:932.

Tait AR, Malviya S, Voepel-Lewis T, et al. Risk factors for perioperative adverse respiratory events in children with upper respiratory tract infections. *Anesthesiology.* 2001;95:299-306.

## *Answer B*

### Equipment/Physics

**QUESTION (Choose single best answer):**

In an anesthetized patient being ventilated mechanically, end-expired carbon dioxide is 58 mm Hg, and peak inspiratory airway pressure is 15 cmH$_2$O. Ventilator settings indicate a delivered tidal volume of 800 mL, but the expiratory flowmeter shows a tidal volume of 360 mL. Which of the following is the most likely cause of this discrepancy?

(A) Fresh gas flow of 0.5 L/min.
(B) Incompetence of the pressure-relief valve.
(C) Low ventilatory rate.
(D) Presence of a hole in the ventilator bellows.
(E) Prolongation of the inspiratory phase.

**CORRECT ANSWER: B**

**SUMMARY:**

*Discrepancies between set and actual tidal volumes received by the patient can be due to (1) compliance, (2) compression volumes, (3) fresh gas flow, (4) leaks, and (5) location of tidal volume sensor. Increased compliance of the breathing circuit results in a greater proportion of the inspiratory flow being expended to expand the circuit. Compression losses are due to gas compression within the bellows of the ventilator; these depend on the pressure during inspiration, as well as the volume of the breathing circuit. Compliance and compression losses will not be apparent unless the spirometer (tidal volume sensor) is placed at the Y connector in the breathing circuit. In older ventilators, the tidal volume delivered to the patient varied with changes in fresh gas flow, the I:E ratio, or respiratory rate; tidal volumes were proportional to fresh gas flow and prolonged inspiratory time; changes in tidal volume secondary to changes in fresh gas flow were attenuated as respiratory rate increased. Reengineering of modern ventilators has eliminated the fresh gas effect on delivered tidal volume. Leaks throughout the breathing circuit will also decrease the tidal volume delivered to the patient.*

*Most modern ventilators use an ascending bellows assembly. Delivered tidal volumes may be lower than set tidal volumes in the context of a disconnection or leak in the breathing system, or insufficient inspiratory flow (that is needed to fully compress the bellows or achieve or the set tidal volume). An ascending bellows will not fill if a total disconnection occurs.*

*Ventilators contain a pressure relief valve (also known as a spill valve) because the APL valve is isolated from the breathing system while the ventilator is in operation. During inspiration, this valve is closed. During expiration, this valve remains closed until the bellows are fully expanded; it then opens after its minimum opening pressure (usually 2-4 cmH$_2$O) is reached (allowing the bellows to fill during exhalation), and directs excess breathing system gases into the scavenging system. If the valve is incompetent, part of driving gas that is meant to enter the bellows chamber will escape into the scavenging system, resulting in a decreased delivered tidal volume.*

**EXPLANATION:**

(A) ***Incorrect.*** Modern ventilators are no longer susceptible to the fresh gas effect on delivered tidal volumes.

(B) ***Correct.*** An incompetent pressure relief valve allows part of the driving gas that is meant to enter the bellows chamber to escape into the scavenging system, resulting in a decreased delivered tidal volume.

(C) ***Incorrect.*** If a ventilator is susceptible to the fresh gas effect on delivered tidal volumes, changes in tidal volume secondary to changes in fresh gas flow are attenuated

as respiratory rate increases. However, most modern ventilators are no longer susceptible to the fresh gas effect on delivered tidal volumes.

(D) *Incorrect.* A hole in the ventilator bellows would cause a decrease in both the indicated delivered tidal volume, as well as the measured expiratory tidal volume.

(E) *Incorrect.* In older ventilators, changes in tidal volumes were proportional to prolongation of the inspiratory time.

## REASONING:

The key to answering this question is understanding the factors that can cause a discrepancy to occur between set tidal volumes and the delivered tidal volumes that the patient
actually receives. This question also assesses an understanding of modern ventilators, as
well as the pressure relief valves found in ventilators. The case describes a hypoventilated
patient with a low peak inspiratory airway pressure relative to the indicated delivered tidal
volume of 800 mL. Choices A, C, and D could lead to hypoventilation in older ventilators,
but the ventilator settings would show low tidal volumes equivalent to expired volumes
measured in the expiratory flowmeter. Choice E is incorrect because an increase in the
inspiratory time would increase the expired tidal volume relative to the ventilator settings.

## BIBLIOGRAPHY:


Barash PG, Cullen BF, Stoelting RK, Cahalan MK, Stock MC. *Clinical Anesthesia*. 6th
ed. Philadelphia, PA: Lippincott Williams & Wilkins; 2009:676.

Dorsch JA, Dorsch SE. *Understanding Anesthesia Equipment*. 5th ed. Philadelphia, PA:
Lippincott Williams & Wilkins; 2008:314-316.

Gravenstein JS, Nederstigt JA. Monitoring for disconnection: ventilators with bellows
rising on expiration can deliver tidal volumes after disconnection. *J Clin Monit*.
1990;6:207-210.

Gravenstein N, Banner MJ, McLaughlin G. Tidal volume changes due to the interaction
of anesthesia machine and anesthesia ventilator. *J Clin Monit*. 1987;3:187-190.

Lancaster CT, Boyle PM, Kaczka DW. Delivered tidal volume from the Fabius GS depends
upon breathing circuit configuration despite compliance compensation. *Anesthesiology*.
2005;103:A863.

Morgan GE, Mikhail MS, Murray MJ. *Clinical Anesthesiology*. 4th ed. New York, NY:
McGraw-Hill; 2006:81, 84.

Moynihan R, Cote CJ. Fresh gas flow changes during controlled mechanical ventilation
with the circle system have significantly greater effects on the ventilatory parameters
of toddlers compared with children. *Pediatr Anesth*. 1992;2:211-215.


---

**BOOK A:**

## QUESTION 108 (OPTIONAL)

---

*Answer D*

Pharmacology

### QUESTION (Choose single best answer):

Which of the following statements concerning pipecuronium is true?

(A) It has a faster onset than pancuronium.
(B) It increases systemic vascular resistance.
(C) It induces tachycardia.
(D) It is eliminated by the kidney.
(E) It induces histamine release.

### CORRECT ANSWER: D

### SUMMARY:

*Pipecuronium is a long-acting steroid-based bisquaternary nondepolarizing muscle relax-
ant that is similar to pancuronium. Like pancuronium, it is eliminated primarily unchanged*

*by the kidney. The two drugs also share a similar onset and duration of action. However, unlike pancuronium, pipecuronium does not release histamine and does not have any significant cardiovascular side effects (eg, tachycardia or altered systemic vascular resistance [SVR]).*

### EXPLANATION:

(A) *Incorrect.* The onset of pipecuronium (3-5 minutes) is similar to that of pancuronium (2-4 minutes).

(B) *Incorrect.* Pipecuronium is devoid of significant cardiovascular side effects due to lack of binding to cardiac muscarinic receptors.

(C) *Incorrect.* See above.

(D) *Correct.* Pipecuronium is excreted primarily unchanged by the kidney (70%) and has a small amount of biliary secretion (20%). The duration of action is increased in patients with renal failure but not with hepatic insufficiency.

(E) *Incorrect.* Unlike pancuronium, pipecuronium does not cause histamine release.

### REASONING:

This question tests knowledge of pipecuronium, an old and now uncommonly used non-depolarizing muscle relaxant. It has become obsolete because of the drawbacks of being a long-acting agent (difficult to reverse and potential for residual paralysis).

It is best answered by process of elimination. In general, pipecuronium and pancuronium have similar onset, duration, and metabolism but differ in their side-effect profiles. Like many board examination questions, the key is being able to compare one drug with another and knowing the specific differences between them.

### BIBLIOGRAPHY:

Barash PG, Cullen BF, Stoelting RK, Calahan M, Stock MC. *Clinical Anesthesia.* 6th ed. Philadelphia, PA: Lippincott Williams & Wilkins; 2009:504-512.

Morgan GE, Mikhail MS, Murray MJ. *Clinical Anesthesiology.* 4th ed. New York, NY: McGraw-Hill; 2006:215-218, 223.

---

| BOOK A: | QUESTION 109 |
|---|---|

## *Answer B*

Cardiovascular

### QUESTION (Choose single best answer):

Left ventricular end-diastolic volume is most likely to be underestimated by pulmonary artery occlusion pressure in patients with

(A) Acute myocardial ischemia.
(B) Aortic insufficiency.
(C) Mitral stenosis.
(D) Primary pulmonary hypertension.
(E) Tricuspid stenosis.

### CORRECT ANSWER: B

### SUMMARY:

*Left ventricular end-diastolic volumes (LVEDVs) rarely are measured directly in clinical practice. Instead, pulmonary artery catheters are used to measure a pulmonary artery occlusion pressure (PAOP) that provides an estimate of left ventricular end-diastolic pressure (LVEDP). Clinicians use LVEDP as a surrogate measure of LVEDV. This interpretation is*

**EXPLANATION:**

(A) *Incorrect.* Acute myocardial ischemia is associated with mitral regurgitation that can cause "V" waves on pulmonary artery occlusion tracing. Systolic "V" waves raise mean PAOP and can lead to an overestimation of PAOP.

(B) *Correct.* Aortic insufficiency is a classic example of PAOP underestimating LVEDV. Because of the incompetent aortic valve, diastolic ventricular filling begins before the mitral valve opens. More important, diastolic ventricular filling continues *after* atrial contraction and closure of the mitral valve. Because the mitral valve closes before diastolic filling is complete (and LVEDP is maximal), PAOP underestimates the true LVEDP/LVEDV.

(C) *Incorrect.* Mitral stenosis leads to an overestimate of LVEDP because the PAOP is greater than the LVEDP.

(D) *Incorrect.* Pulmonary hypertension increases PVR and pulmonary artery diastolic pressures. However, the PAOP should provide an accurate estimate of LVEDP.

(E) *Incorrect.* Tricuspid stenosis does not alter the relationship between PAOP and LVEDP.


**REASONING:**

It is important to remember that PAOP is an indirect surrogate measure of LVEDV. There are many factors that can challenge the validity of the assumptions used for the interpretation of PAOP as an estimate of LVEDV. The reader should review these carefully. Choice B is the best answer.


**BIBLIOGRAPHY:**

Mark JB. *Atlas of Cardiovascular Monitoring*. New York, PA: Churchill Livingstone; 1998:60-79, 248-259.

---

**BOOK A:**

**QUESTION 110**

---

*Answer A*

Pharmacology

**QUESTION (Choose single best answer):**

Which of the following statements concerning the cardiovascular effects of intravenous bupivacaine is true?

(A) Bretylium is effective in treating bupivacaine-induced ventricular arrhythmias.
(B) Cardiovascular toxicity is decreased during pregnancy.
(C) Cardiovascular toxicity occurs at lower blood levels than central nervous system toxicity.
(D) Systemic vascular resistance is unchanged.
(E) The rate of impulse conduction through the heart is increased.


**CORRECT ANSWER: A**

## SUMMARY:

*Bupivacaine is distinguished among local anesthetics for its pronounced cardiotoxicity. It has a high binding affinity for myocardial sodium and potassium channels, inhibits calcium channels and release of calcium from the sarcoplasmic reticulum, inhibits intracellular cAMP production, and may act centrally in the CNS to elicit dysrhythmias that are resistant to resuscitation. Bupivacaine toxicity also causes vasodilation and decreased myocardial contractility and can lead to cardiovascular collapse. Parturients are more prone to local anesthetic toxicity.*

*The local anesthetics block the sodium channels in the cardiac conduction system in a dose-dependent manner. Potent and more lipid-soluble bupivacaine differs from other local anesthetics such as lidocaine, in its greater affinity for binding to these channels and preventing conduction. Local anesthetics bind to sodium channels in phasic manner; that is, they bind during systole and release from the channel during diastole. Bupivacaine differs from lidocaine, in much slower release during diastole leading to cumulative block. With increased potency comes the greater direct myocardial depression. Bupivacaine also affects the calcium release, mitochondrial energy generation especially during hypoxia. All these multiple mechanisms lead to irresuscitable cardiovascular collapse.*

*Given the catastrophic nature of bupivacaine cardiac toxicity, the current management of suspected cardiac toxicity is with 20% lipid solution bolus of 100 cc followed by infusion. There are multiple case reports of successful resuscitation of patients in completely cardiovascular collapse with this treatment.*

*Therefore, given the current knowledge of bupivacaine toxicity and management, there is no role for bretylium in the management of cardiac toxicity of bupivacaine.*

## EXPLANATION:

(A) **Correct.** Bretylium is the drug of choice in the treatment of ventricular tachyarrhythmia in bupivacaine toxicity.

(B) **Incorrect.** Local anesthetic sensitivity is increased during pregnancy, including toxic reactions.

(C) **Incorrect.** Symptoms of CNS toxicity are first to appear in the awake patient.

(D) **Incorrect.** Arteriolar dilation occurs with intravenous bupivacaine, resulting in decreased SVR.

(E) **Incorrect.** The rate of impulse conduction is depressed owing to blocking of myocyte sodium channels.

## REASONING:

*None of the above are the right answer for the above-mentioned clinical scenario.* This question tests knowledge of the diagnosis and treatment of bupivacaine toxicity. Lidocaine is not a preferred drug for the management of bupivacaine-induced ventricular tachyarrhythmias. Treatment of bupivacaine-induced dysrhythmias may require aggressive treatment with large amounts of bretylium, epinephrine, and magnesium, and multiple attempts at electrical cardioversion. A is the best answer.

## BIBLIOGRAPHY:


Barash PG, Cullen BF, Stoelting RK. *Clinical Anesthesia.* 6th ed. Philadelphia, PA: Lippincott Williams & Wilkins; 2001:543-545.

Brull SJ. Lipid emulsion for the treatment of local anesthetic toxicity: patient safety implications. *Anesth Analg.* 2008;106:1337-1339.

Weinberg G. Treatment regimens. http://www.lipidrescue.org/. Accessed July 11, 2013.

Weinberg GL. Lipid infusion therapy: translation to clinical practice. *Anesth Analg.* 2008;106:1340-1342.

*Answer E*

Equipment/Physics

**QUESTION (Choose single best answer):**

Which of the following is indicated by an alarm condition in the line-isolation monitor?

(A)  An electric shock to the patient.
(B)  A power surge in the main hospital power supply.
(C)  Disconnection of the patient from an electrocautery grounding pad.
(D)  Overload of the operating room circuits.
(E)  The presence of a current leak between an operating room electrical device and ground.

**CORRECT ANSWER: E**

**SUMMARY:**

*For a patient to be electrocuted, current must flow from a live conductor from a grounded circuit, through the patient's body, and back to a ground. One way to prevent patient electrocution is to isolate the power system to the operating room (OR) from any grounds. Isolating or ungrounding the OR power supply is the function of the isolation transformer that divides the wiring to the OR into a primary (grounded) and secondary ungrounded circuit. The secondary circuit or wiring consists of two live ungrounded voltage lines. When a grounded individual touches one of the live lines, no current will flow through the body because there is no circuit back to the second live ungrounded wire. The isolation transformer, however, does not offer complete protection from electrocution for two reasons. Electrocution is still possible if a grounded individual touches both live wires or if a fault develops between either live wire and a ground and contact with the other wire occurs. The line isolation monitor (LIM) aims to prevent the second scenario by detecting faults between ground and either of the two isolated live voltage lines and by predicting the amount of current that could flow through the circuit in the setting of a second fault. The alarm is set to respond when high enough current flow to the ground becomes possible (usually 2-5 mA) and should prompt OR personnel to unplug one piece of equipment at a time (starting from the most recently plugged) until the alarm ceases to alarm. In other words, the LIM is activated when the isolated secondary wiring to the OR has reverted to a grounded system. The activation of the LIM alarm does not interrupt power to the OR as this could lead to catastrophic discontinuation of live-sustaining support machines. To interrupt OR power, a ground-leakage circuit breaker must also be activated.*

**EXPLANATION:**

(A)  *Incorrect.* The line-isolation monitor serves a warning and alarms when the secondary, ungrounded wiring of an isolation transformer becomes grounded. Once activated, try to postpone the procedure if not yet started or unplug each electric device in the OR (starting with whichever one was plugged in last). By catching one fault, hopefully a second fault will be prevented, as will any electrical hazard to the patient and OR personnel.
(B)  *Incorrect.* Each LIM is specific to one OR and does not reflect what is going on in the main hospital power supply. Every OR has electricity that is separate from the main supply by the isolation transformer. If a power surge were to occur, usually hospitals have main generators as backup power so emergency equipment can continue to function.
(C)  *Incorrect.* The electric circuit from such things as a Bovie must be complete and the current returned to the Bovie. An electrocautery grounding pad must be placed on a patient to provide a large surface area for this current to return to the Bovie and prevent burns to the patient (ie, through ECG leads). The LIM has nothing to do with such a grounding pad.

(D) *Incorrect.* LIMs do not alarm based on the amount of current within OR circuits or the amount of equipment utilized in one OR. They alarm only if the secondary, ungrounded circuit of the main isolation transformer becomes grounded and the maximum current that a short circuit could cause is 2 to 5 mA.

(E) *Correct.* If there is a leakage of current between OR devices and a ground, such that the secondary, ungrounded circuit becomes grounded, the LIM will be activated. Its main purpose is to advise the OR personnel that there is a potential to complete a circuit with a maximum amount of current from one more fault and surgery must be stopped and/or electric devices slowly unplugged to discover what is causing the problem.

### REASONING:

Every OR has a main isolation transformer to isolate its electricity from the hospital's main power supply. It has a primary circuit that is grounded and a secondary circuit that is not. Unfortunately, every electric device has a small amount of leakage current to ground and this has the potential to turn an ungrounded circuit into a grounded one. LIMs are activated when the secondary circuit of a main isolation transformer becomes grounded. This acts as a forewarning before one more fault occurs to complete a circuit and cause potential electrical hazard to OR personnel and the patient. Usually, 2 to 5 mA will activate the alarm so that if the circuit were to become complete with one more fault, such a macroshock would be perceptible but not harmful to someone.

### BIBLIOGRAPHY:

Morgan GE, Mikhail MS, Murray MJ. *Clinical Anesthesiology.* 4th ed. New York, NY: McGraw-Hill; 2006:23-27.

---

## BOOK A:

## QUESTION 112

*Answer E*

Pharmacology

### QUESTION (Choose single best answer):

Which of the following statements concerning ketorolac is true?

(A) It binds to opioid receptors.
(B) It causes dose-related thrombocytopenia.
(C) It decreases heart rate during isoflurane anesthesia.
(D) It is eliminated unchanged in urine.
(E) It reversibly inhibits cyclooxygenase.

### CORRECT ANSWER: E

### SUMMARY:

*Ketorolac is a nonsteroidal anti-inflammatory drug (NSAID) that works by reversibly inhibiting cyclooxygenase activity, nonspecifically, and inhibiting prostaglandin production. It is metabolized by hepatic enzymes and eliminated by the kidney (both unchanged and in the form of metabolites). Ketorolac is a known inhibitor of platelet function (not quantity) and can result in prolonged bleeding time.*

### EXPLANATION:

(A) *Incorrect.* Ketorolac binds to cyclooxygenase and blocks prostaglandin synthesis. It does not exert its analgesic effect by binding to opioid receptors.

(B) *Incorrect.* Ketorolac inhibits platelet function, not platelet quantity. Therefore, it does not result in thrombocytopenia.

(C) **Incorrect.** This is not a known effect of ketorolac. Ketorolac does not affect MAC and does not alter hemodynamics of anesthetized patients.

(D) **Incorrect.** Ketorolac is metabolized in the liver and then eliminated by the kidney. Although some ketorolac is eliminated renally as whole drug, most is metabolized by the liver.

(E) **Correct.** Ketorolac reversibly inhibits the cyclooxygenase enzyme, like most NSAIDs.

### REASONING:

Ketorolac was the first parental NSAID approved for use in 1990. Ketorolac is an effective analgesic that avoids respiratory depression, sedation, nausea, vomiting, and constipation associated with opioid analgesics. It has a 6 to 8 mg morphine equivalent analgesic potency. Ketorolac reversibly and nonspecifically inhibits the cyclooxygenase enzyme, blocking prostaglandin synthesis. Because of its inhibitory effects on platelet function, some surgeons prefer to avoid the use of ketorolac for postoperative pain control. It may also be inappropriate in patients with bleeding disorders. Potential adverse effects of NSAID use include exacerbation of bronchospasm in patients with a history of nasal polyps, asthma, and rhinitis. As with other NSAIDS, it should also be avoided in patients with preexisting nephropathies and the dose should be decreased in patients with renal insufficiency and the elderly. It can also cause GI tract ulceration. Although D is partly true, E is the single best answer.

### BIBLIOGRAPHY:


Barash PG, Cullen BF, Stoelting RK, Calahan M, Stock MC. *Clinical Anesthesia*. 6th ed. Philadelphia, PA: Lippincott Williams & Wilkins; 2009:16, 1484-1485.

Morgan GE, Mikhail MS, Murray MJ. *Clinical Anesthesiology*. 4th ed. New York, NY: McGraw-Hill; 2006:282-283.


---

## BOOK A:  QUESTION 113

*Answer D*

Equipment/Physics

### QUESTION (Choose single best answer):

Postoperatively, a patient is being ventilated mechanically by a constant-flow, pressure-cycled ventilator with the following initial settings: inspiratory–expiratory (I:E) ratio of 1:2, peak inspiratory pressure (PIP) of 25 cmH$_2$O, and rate of 10 breaths/min. One hour later, the I:E ratio is 1:4. Which of the following would ensure that the minute ventilation is the same as that set initially?

(A) Inflate the endotracheal tube cuff to prevent leakage.

(B) Double the respiratory rate.

(C) Decrease the expiratory pause until the I:E ratio is 1.0.

(D) Increase the PIP until the I:E ratio is 1:2.

(E) Increase the PIP to 50 cmH$_2$O.

### CORRECT ANSWER: D

### SUMMARY:

*Pressure-cycled ventilators, also referred to as* pressure-controlled ventilators, *use a ventilatory mode in which inspiratory pressure is set, as is respiratory rate and inspiratory time; tidal volume fluctuates and is determined by the set pressure and rise time (ie, once the set pressure is reached, the ventilator will not cycle until from inspiration to expiration until the present inspiration time has elapsed). Tidal volume can change in response to alterations in resistance and compliance; tidal volume can decrease due to either increased resistance or decreased compliance (set inspiratory pressure is reached sooner, and thus a smaller tidal volume is delivered). Given a set inspiratory time (ie, a preset I:E ratio), increases in respiratory rate shorten the inspiratory time and thus decrease the tidal volume.*

**EXPLANATION:**

(A) *Incorrect.* Assuming that a leak was not present when the ventilator was initially set and that a leak has not occurred in the breathing circuit over the past hour, inflating the ETT cuff will not change the parameters influencing the minute ventilation.

(B) *Incorrect.* Although doubling the respiratory rate would increase time in inspiration, dead-space ventilation would increase more than alveolar ventilation with smaller tidal volumes and higher respiratory rates.

(C) *Incorrect.* Decreasing the expiratory pause to obtain an I:E ratio of 1.0 likely will increase the minute ventilation because more time is spent in inspiration; however, the minute ventilation is unlikely to be the same as that attained with an I:E ratio of 1:2.

(D) *Correct.* Increasing the PIP until the I:E ratio is 1:2 will allow for the same tidal volumes to be delivered as before because it is a constant-flow ventilator. Because it is a constant flow ventilator, the same time in inspiration will yield the same total amount of flow and tidal volume.

(E) *Incorrect.* Increasing the PIP to 50 $cmH_2O$ will increase the tidal volume delivered and minute ventilation, but it likely will not be the same as set initially because we are not sure how much the compliance and/or airway resistance of the lungs has changed.

**REASONING:**

The key to answering this question is knowing how a pressure-cycled ventilator functions. Choice A can be eliminated easily because a cuff leak would increase the inspiratory time, not decrease it. Choices B, C, and E do increase the minute ventilation, but not to the same minute ventilation as the initial settings. Only choice D ensures the same minute ventilation as the previous setting. The best answer is D.

**BIBLIOGRAPHY:**
Botz GH, Sladen RN. Conventional modes of mechanical ventilation. *Int Anesthesiol Clin.* 1997;35(1):19-28.

Dorsch JA, Dorsch SE. *Understanding Anesthesia Equipment.* 5th ed. Philadelphia, PA: Lippincott Williams & Wilkins; 2008;317.

Morgan GE, Mikhail MS, Murray MJ. *Clinical Anesthesiology.* 4th ed. New York, NY: McGraw-Hill; 2006:1030-1031, 1033-1034.

Tung A, Drum ML, Morgan S. Effect of inspiratory time on tidal volume delivery in anesthesia and intensive care unit ventilators operating in pressure control mode. J Clin Anesth. 2005;17:8-15.

Tung A, Morgan SE. Modeling the effect of progressive endotracheal tube occlusion on tidal volume in pressure-control mode. Anesth Analg. 2002;95:192-7.

---

**BOOK A:**        **QUESTION 114**

---

*Answer B*

Physiology

**QUESTION (Choose single best answer):**

Left ventricular subendocardial perfusion pressure is best estimated by the difference between

(A) Mean arterial and central venous pressures.
(B) Diastolic arterial and pulmonary artery occlusion pressures.
(C) Mean arterial and pulmonary artery occlusion pressures.
(D) Systolic arterial and pulmonary artery occlusion pressures.
(E) Diastolic arterial and central venous pressures.

CORRECT ANSWER: B

**SUMMARY:**

*Myocardial perfusion is intermittent and occurs primarily during diastole for the left ventricle. Left ventricular cavity pressures during systole are high enough to occlude coronary vessels, preventing any flow during systole. Because right ventricular systolic pressures are lower, the right ventricle is perfused during both systole and diastole. The majority of right ventricular perfusion occurs during systole. Left ventricular subendocardial perfusion pressure is determined by the difference between aortic diastolic pressure and left ventricular end-diastolic pressure (or pulmonary artery occlusion pressure [PAOP] as an estimate of LVEDP).*

**EXPLANATION:**
(A) *Incorrect.* See above.
(B) *Correct.* Coronary flow occurs during diastole; thus the difference between diastolic and left ventricular end-diastolic pressure determines coronary perfusion pressure.
(C) *Incorrect.* See above.
(D) *Incorrect.* See above.
(E) *Incorrect.* Subendocardial perfusion pressure is determined by the difference between aortic diastolic pressure and left ventricular end-diastolic pressure or PAOP.

**REASONING:**

This question tests knowledge of the determinants of left ventricular coronary perfusion pressure. Left ventricular coronary perfusion occurs primarily during diastole, when the aortic valve closes and diastolic aortic pressures drive blood through the coronary ostia to perfuse myocardium. Coronary perfusion pressure for the left ventricle is defined as aortic diastolic pressure minus LVEDP (or PAOP as an estimate of LVEDP). The best answer is B.

**BIBLIOGRAPHY:**

Barash PG, Cullen BF, Stoelting RK. *Clinical Anesthesia.* 6th ed. Philadelphia, PA: Lippincott Williams & Wilkins; 2001:1074 (Figure 32-1).
Morgan GE, Mikhail MS, Murray MJ. *Clinical Anesthesiology.* 4th ed New York, NY: McGraw-Hill; 2002:431-432.

---

**BOOK A:**     **QUESTION 115**

---

*Answer C*

Clinical Anesthesia

**QUESTION (Choose single best answer):**

A 29-year-old man who has been nasotracheally intubated for 2 weeks following a motor vehicle accident has a fever (39°C) and a constant headache. Leukocyte count is 18,000/mm$^3$. The most likely cause is

(A) Fractured nasal septum.
(B) Retropharyngeal abscess.
(C) Maxillary sinusitis.
(D) Meningitis.
(E) Rhinovirus infection.

**CORRECT ANSWER: C**

**SUMMARY:**

*Endotracheal intubation may be accomplished via the oral or nasal routes. Nasal intubation is often considered more comfortable for the patient and more secure from accidental extubation. There are, however, complications associated with nasotracheal intubation, including nasal necrosis, bacteremia, epistaxis, sinusitis, submucosal dissection of the nasopharynx that can develop into retropharyngeal abscesses, or accidental insertion of the endotracheal tube into the cranial vault through a basilar skull fracture. The decision on the route of intubation should be based on the clinical situation, experience of the practitioner, and expected duration of ventilation.*

### EXPLANATION:

(A) *Incorrect.* There is inadequate evidence for a fractured nasal septum. One would not expect a fever and increased leukocyte count with a fracture.

(B) *Incorrect.* Retropharyngeal abscess is a reported complication with nasal intubations, but presents with a sore throat rather than headache.

(C) *Correct.* Sinusitis is a reported common complication from nasal intubation, and the signs and symptoms are consistent with this diagnosis.

(D) *Incorrect.* While all the symptoms listed are consistent with an ongoing infection, meningitis is not a reported common complication with nasotracheal intubation and is less likely to occur idiopathically.

(E) *Incorrect.* Rhinovirus infection, while a cause of common upper respiratory infections, is not associated with nasal intubations and is typically not contracted nosocomially. The most common organisms associated with nasal intubations are bacteria that colonize the nasopharynx, for example *Streptococcus viridans*.

### REASONING:

Key concepts for answering this question include an understanding of the complications of nasotracheal intubation and symptoms of infection. A fractured nasal septum, choice A, might occur after a motor vehicle accident but by itself would not explain the signs and symptoms of infection or time to onset. Meningitis, choice D, is not a common complication of motor vehicle accident or nasotracheal intubation. Rhinovirus infection, choice E, can also cause fever, headache, and increased leukocyte count, but it is not associated with motor vehicle accident or nasotracheal intubation. Choices B and C are both reported complications from nasotracheal intubation, and can cause fever and increased white count. Because a constant headache is more consistent with maxillary sinusitis than retropharyngeal abscess, choice C is the more likely correct answer.

### BIBLIOGRAPHY:

Benumof JL, Saidman LJ. *Anesthesia and Perioperative Complications*. 2nd ed. St. Louis, MO: Mosby; 1999:5-6.
Miller, 7th edition, pg 1586-1587.
Morgan GE, Mikhail MS, Murray MJ. *Clinical Anesthesiology*. 4th ed. New York, NY: McGraw-Hill; 2006:106-107, 110-111.

---

**BOOK A:**    **QUESTION 116**

---

*Answer D*

OB/Regional

### QUESTION (Choose single best answer):

Surgery is cancelled 10 minutes after initiation of intravenous regional anesthesia with 50 mL lidocaine 0.5%. To terminate anesthesia safely, what is the most appropriate timing for deflating the tourniquet?

(A) Immediately if benzodiazepines have been administered.
(B) Immediately after intravenous administration of ephedrine 10 mg.
(C) Immediately, followed by repeated reinflation and deflation.
(D) In no less than 20 minutes after initial injection.
(E) In no less than 45 minutes after initial injection.

**CORRECT ANSWER: D**

## SUMMARY:

*Intravenous regional anesthesia (Bier block) is an excellent anesthetic for short surgeries involving the forearm and hand. The block involves placing an intravenous catheter in the distal extremity, followed by exsanguination and inflation of a tourniquet placed on the upper arm. Once cessation of arterial inflow into the extremity has been established, 40 mL 0.5% lidocaine is injected through the distal intravenous catheter. The anesthesia is intense and develops within 10 minutes. The patient eventually starts to experience tourniquet pain, which is the limiting factor for the duration of the block. Once the surgery is complete, the tourniquet is deflated and the residual lidocaine is taken up into the systemic circulation. The principal risk of this type of anesthetic is local anesthetic toxicity from premature release of the tourniquet. The generally agreed-on minimal time that the tourniquet needs to remain inflated is 20 minutes regardless of the duration of surgery.*

## EXPLANATION:

(A) *Incorrect.* Signs of local anesthetic toxicity include circumoral numbness, tongue paresthesia, dizziness, tinnitus, blurred vision, central nervous system (CNS) excitation, CNS depression, and tonic-clonic seizures. Prior benzodiazepine administration does not decrease the risk of developing these complications significantly. It has only been 10 minutes, and no maneuver is safe at this point.

(B) *Incorrect.* The dangers of local anesthetic toxicity are not eliminated by administration of intravenous ephedrine. It has only been 10 minutes, and no maneuver is safe at this point.

(C) *Incorrect.* It has only been 10 minutes, and no maneuver is safe at this point.

(D) *Correct.* The minimal time that should transpire is at least 20 minutes before tourniquet release to minimize a large bolus of drug into the systemic circulation.

(E) *Incorrect.* Within the 20- to 40-minute period, one can slowly deflate the tourniquet or deflate the tourniquet and rapidly reinflate it followed by a second deflation to decrease the initial bolus of local anesthetic. After 40 minutes, the tourniquet simply can be released with little risk of toxicity.

## REASONING:

This question tests knowledge of local anesthetic toxicity and Bier block regional anesthesia. It is a classic example that illustrates the need to read choices carefully. On first pass, you might think that choice C could be correct, but it states *immediately*. Even though repeated deflation and reinflation is a correct strategy for early tourniquet release, it is still only safe after at least 20 minutes.

## BIBLIOGRAPHY:

Barash PG, Cullen BF, Stoelting RK, Cahalan M, Stock M. *Clinical Anesthesia.* 6th ed. Philadelphia, PA: Lippincott Williams & Wilkins; 2010:981.

Morgan GE, Mikhail MS, Murray MJ. *Clinical Anesthesiology.* 4th ed. New York, NY: McGraw-Hill; 2006:387.

## Answer D

### Pediatrics

**QUESTION (Choose single best answer):**

A 2500-g, 12-hour-old infant is tracheally intubated and mechanically ventilated at a rate of 20 breaths/min with an $F_{IO_2}$ of 0.4 and peak inspiratory pressure of 25 cmH$_2$O. At birth, amniotic fluid was meconium-stained, and Apgar scores were 2 and 7. The most recent arterial blood gas levels are $Pa_{O_2}$ 50 mm Hg, $Pa_{CO_2}$ 55 mm Hg, and pH 7.20. The most appropriate management is to

(A)  Administer sodium bicarbonate.
(B)  Begin intravenous infusion of prostaglandin E$_1$.
(C)  Increase $F_{IO_2}$.
(D)  Increase ventilation.
(E)  Perform bronchial lavage.


**CORRECT ANSWER: D**


**SUMMARY:**

*Meconium-stained amniotic fluid is a relatively common occurrence seen in 10% to 15% of deliveries and approximately 5% of these develop into true meconium aspiration syndrome. The passage of meconium in utero is correlated with advanced fetal maturity and fetal distress. When aspirated into the fetal lungs, the meconium particles cause mechanical obstruction of small airways and a chemical pneumonitis. The meconium aspiration syndrome is manifested in the newborn by respiratory compromise with tachypnea, cyanosis, and reduced pulmonary compliance. Persistent pulmonary hypertension due to increased pulmonary vascular resistance occurs in 15% to 20% of the infants. Newborns with meconium aspiration have an increased incidence of pneumothorax (10% compared with 1% for all vaginal deliveries). Prevention begins at delivery with immediate suctioning of oropharynx and continues with endotracheal intubation and suctioning of meconium from the lungs. With severe meconium aspiration pneumonia, surfactant therapy, inhaled nitric oxide, high-frequency ventilation, and even extracorporeal membrane oxygenation may be necessary.*


**EXPLANATION:**

(A)  *Incorrect.* Sodium bicarbonate may be used to treat metabolic acidosis, but it actually may worsen respiratory acidosis when the bicarbonate is converted to carbon dioxide and water. It also increases risk of intracranial hemorrhage.
(B)  *Incorrect.* Prostaglandin E$_1$ is used to maintain patency of the ductus arteriosus in ductal-dependent congenital cardiac lesions. It also may be used to decrease pulmonary vascular resistance in pulmonary hypertension. There is not enough evidence that either of these situations exists in this patient.
(C)  *Incorrect.* The fetus tolerates intrauterine $Pa_{O_2}$ levels in the high 20s owing to fetal hemoglobin, polycythemia, and a rightward shift of the hemoglobin-oxygen dissociation curve in response to increased amounts of 2,3-diphosphoglycerate (2,3-DPG). Increasing $F_{IO_2}$ in a neonate may not be desirable because hyperoxia may increase the risk of retinopathy of prematurity, especially in infants younger than 32 weeks' gestation.
(D)  *Correct.* A pH of 7.20 and a $Pa_{CO_2}$ of 55 mm Hg indicate respiratory acidosis. Treatment involves increasing the minute ventilation, which can be accomplished by increasing either respiratory rate or tidal volume.
(E)  *Incorrect.* Treatment of meconium aspiration includes chest physiotherapy and warmed humidified oxygen. Bronchial lavage is contraindicated because it may worsen lung function.

**REASONING:**

This is a difficult question that tests the reader's ability to analyze multiple clinical data and prioritize treatment. One can rule out choice B immediately because there is inadequate information supporting the presence of congenital cardiac disease. Choice A can also be ruled out because the blood gas indicates primarily respiratory acidosis. If the reader does not know that bronchial lavage may exacerbate lung function in meconium aspiration pneumonia, one should recognize that a rate of 20 breaths/min and a $Paco_2$ of 55 mm Hg demonstrate inadequate ventilation and that improving ventilation may also improve oxygenation. Thus choice D is the best answer.


**BIBLIOGRAPHY:**

Asad A, Bhat B. Pharmacotherapy for meconium aspiration. *J Perinatol.* 2008;28:S72-S78.

Cote CJ. *A Practice of Anesthesia for Infants and Children.* 4th ed. Philadelphia, PA: Saunders; 2009:790-791.

Morgan GE, Mikhail MS, Murray MJ. *Clinical Anesthesiology.* 4th ed. New York, NY: McGraw-Hill; 2006:915-917, 919.

Ross MG. Meconium aspiration syndrome—more than intrapartum meconium. *N Eng J Med.* 2005;353:946-948.


---

**BOOK A:**  **QUESTION 118**

*Answer C*

Clinical Anesthesia

**QUESTION (Choose single best answer):**

A 60-year-old woman who is taking propranolol for hypertension and is allergic to penicillins is anesthetized with thiopental and halothane for resection of an abdominal aortic aneurysm. Shortly after intubation, she is given vancomycin 500 mg intravenously, after which her blood pressure decreases from 140/80 to 70/50 mm Hg while her heart rate remains steady at 64 bpm. The most likely explanation for the decrease in blood pressure is

(A)  Cross-sensitivity of penicillin and vancomycin.
(B)  Interaction of vancomycin and propranolol.
(C)  Vancomycin-induced anaphylactoid reaction.
(D)  Interaction of halothane and propranolol.
(E)  Interaction of halothane and vancomycin.

**CORRECT ANSWER: C**

**SUMMARY:**

*Administration of vancomycin is commonly associated with "red man syndrome." This nonimmunologic, histamine-mediated, anaphylactoid-type reaction consists of flushing, pruritus, and hypotension. Alternatively, patients may develop isolated hypotension without the other symptoms. The rate of administration is a key factor in the development of these symptoms. Vancomycin should never be given by bolus administration. In a patient on chronic β-blocker therapy, tachycardia may not develop as a compensating response to hypotension.*

**EXPLANATION:**

(A)  *Incorrect.* Vancomycin is a glycopeptide antibiotic and is not cross-sensitive with the β-lactam antibiotics such as penicillin and cephalosporins.

(B)  *Incorrect.* Chronic β-blockade prevents an increase in heart rate but does not interact with vancomycin to produce hypotension.

(C)  *Correct.* This hypotension most likely is mediated by histamine release secondary to rapid administration of vancomycin.

(D) *Incorrect.* The myocardial depressant effects of halothane may be exacerbated by β-blockade. However, halothane has a slow uptake and would not cause such severe hypotension immediately after induction.

(E) *Incorrect.* The concentration of halothane immediately after induction would likely be negligible and would not interact with the vancomycin to cause hypotension.

**REASONING:**

The temporal relationship of the administration of vancomycin and the development of hypotension is incriminating. While the use of propranolol and halothane may cause hypotension, the rapid decrease in blood pressure points to a drug reaction. Patients can develop anaphylaxis to vancomycin, but they are far more likely to develop a nonimmunologic reaction, such as "red man syndrome" or simply hypotension from administration. Choice C is the best answer.

**BIBLIOGRAPHY:**

Barash PG, Cullen BF, Stoelting RK, Cahalan MK, Stock MC. *Clinical Anesthesia.* 6th ed. Philadelphia, PA: Lippincott Williams & Wilkins; 2009:263.

Levy JH, Kettlekamp N, Goertz P. Histamine release by vancomycin: a mechanism for hypotension in man. *Anesthesiology.* 1987;67:122.

Morgan GE, Mikhail MS, Murray MJ. *Clinical Anesthesiology.* 4th ed. New York, NY: McGraw-Hill; 2006:974.

---

**BOOK A:** | **QUESTION 119**

*Answer E*

Clinical Anesthesia

**QUESTION (Choose single best answer):**

During a reoperative total hip arthroplasty requiring transfusion of 8 units of packed red blood cells, blood begins to ooze from the operative field and intravenous catheter sites. The urine is pink. The most likely cause is

(A) Citrate intoxication.
(B) Factor V and VIII deficiencies.
(C) Rhabdomyolysis.
(D) Thrombocytopenia.
(E) Transfusion reaction.

**CORRECT ANSWER: E**

**SUMMARY:**

*Pink urine in the setting of a blood transfusion is indicative of an acute, hemolytic reaction and destruction of the transfused red blood cells by the recipient's antibodies. It can also occur with large transfusion of plasma-rich products such as platelets, fresh frozen plasma (FFP) or cryoprecipitate with anti-A or anti-B alloantibodies. In either case, an acute hemolytic reaction is due to ABO blood incompatibility and occurs in 1:38,000 transfusions. The risk of a fatal hemolytic reaction is 1 in 100,000 transfusions. The severity of the reaction directly correlates with the amount of blood product given. Awake patients present with fever, chills, nausea, and chest pain, whereas anesthetized patients present with fever, tachycardia, hypotension, hemoglobinuria, and diffuse oozing in the surgical field. Once such signs are detected, one should stop the transfusion immediately, recheck the blood (compare the blood slip with a patient bracelet), and send laboratory tests to identify hemoglobin in the plasma and full clotting studies due to the potential of disseminated intravascular coagulation (DIC).*

*Renal protection measures should be instituted rapidly by initiating an osmotic diuresis with mannitol, inserting a Foley catheter and administration of additional intravenous fluids to achieve adequate perfusion pressure. Pressors and additional blood products (FFP or cryoprecipitate) may be required to stabilize hemodynamics and prevent further blood loss.*

## EXPLANATION:

(A) ***Incorrect.*** The is a potential for citrate intoxication with a large amount of blood transfusions due to the citrate preservative that binds calcium. Usually, anesthetized patients would not reflect the signs of hypocalcemia unless the transfusion rate exceeded 1 unit every 5 minutes. Such things to watch for would be cardiac arrhythmias with a prolonged QT, hypotension, and a decreased cardiac output.

(B) ***Incorrect.*** Clinically significant dilution of procoagulant factors, such as factors V and VII, are unusual in otherwise healthy people and only become a possibility with massive transfusions of over 10 to 12 units. These two particular factors are not as stable as all others in stored, red blood, and, thus have the highest likelihood of being diluted out with massive transfusions.

(C) ***Incorrect.*** Rhabdomyolysis signals acute muscle breakdown due to such things as succinylcholine being given to patients with Duchenne muscular dystrophy. Such muscle deterioration would not cause generalized oozing or hematuria as with this patient. Instead, it can cause acute renal failure, with hyperphosphatemia and, subsequent, hypocalcemia.

(D) ***Incorrect.*** Thrombocytopenia is the most common cause of bleeding following massive transfusions, which usually exceed one to two times a patient's blood volume. Platelets are extremely sensitive to cold temperatures and become nonviable if stored at low temperatures. The answer is incorrect because only 8 units were transfused in this patient and, also, a dilutional thrombocytopenia would result in bleeding and oozing from the surgical site and probably not cause hematuria.

(E) ***Correct.*** An acute, hemolytic blood transfusion reaction is the cause of the hematuria and oozing in this patient. It is probably due to ABO incompatibility and the transfusion must be stopped immediately. The physician should attempt to prevent acute renal failure and support the patient amid developing DIC and potential cardiovascular collapse.

## REASONING:

With massive transfusions, usually considered to be one to two times a patient's blood volume or 10 to 20 units, there is a potential for coagulopathy from two sources: dilutional thrombocytopenia and dilution of procoagulants. Dilutional thrombocytopenia is most common, with generalized oozing from the surgical site as the main sign. It is quite rare for a normal individual to develop such oozing from an inadequate supply of factors V and VII, as one needs fewer than half of these factors for appropriate coagulation. In this patient, only 8 units were transfused, and intraoperatively the patient developed hematuria and oozing not only from the surgical site but from catheter sites as well. Because of the acuity of the presentation and the hematuria, an acute, hemolytic reaction is the most plausible cause due to ABO incompatibility and the patient's antibodies reacting with the donor blood. Citrate intoxication would cause hypocalcemia and subsequent cardiac depression instead. Likewise, rhabdomyolysis or muscle breakdown would not lead to these symptoms either. Besides the hematuria, the patient could become tachycardic, hypotensive, and febrile, necessitating cardiovascular support in the midst of developing acute renal failure and DIC. Laboratory tests should be drawn to check coagulation studies, identify hemoglobin in the plasma, and repeat compatibility testing. Also, urine should be sent to identify hemoglobin as well.

## BIBLIOGRAPHY:

Morgan GE, Mikhail MS, Murray MJ. *Clinical Anesthesiology*. 4th ed. New York, NY: McGraw-Hill; 2006:698-703.

*Answer C*

OB/Regional

**QUESTION (Choose single best answer):**

Eight hours after abdominal surgery, a 51-year-old patient becomes increasingly somnolent. Epidural morphine 5 mg was administered immediately following the procedure. Postoperatively, respiratory rate has not decreased below 12 breaths/min, and $SpO_2$ has remained greater than 92%. Arterial blood gas (ABG) analysis shows a $PaO_2$ of 80 mm Hg, a $PaCO_2$ of 82 mm Hg, and a pH of 7.1. Which of the following is the most appropriate conclusion?

(A) Analysis of the blood sample was delayed.
(B) The blood sample was venous rather than arterial.
(C) The patient is receiving supplemental oxygen.
(D) The pulse oximeter readings are falsely high.
(E) No treatment is required at this time.

**CORRECT ANSWER: C**

**SUMMARY:**

*The patient is hypercarbic with a respiratory acidosis caused by opioid-induced respiratory depression. Her $CO_2$ response curve has shifted to the right. $SpO_2$ is a measure of oxygenation not ventilation, and appears to be in the low normal range despite hypoventilation, suggesting that the patient is receiving supplemental oxygen. An $SpO_2$ of 92% is consistent with a $PaO_2$ of 80 mm Hg. Despite titration of epidural morphine to a respiratory rate above 12, this patient is experiencing respiratory acidosis and $CO_2$ narcosis with CNS depression, and must be treated.*

**EXPLANATION:**

(A) *Incorrect.* The ABG suggests respiratory acidosis secondary to hypoventilation consistent with her current state. There is nothing in the question to suggest a delayed analysis of the blood sample.
(B) *Incorrect.* Normal mixed venous oxygen tension ($PvO_2$) and carbon dioxide tension ($PvCO_2$) are 40 and 46, respectively. The $SpO_2$ would be 100% with a $PvO_2$ value of 80 mm Hg.
(C) *Correct.* Despite hypoventilation secondary to a reduced hypercarbic and hypoxic respiratory drive, this patient is being adequately oxygenated. She must be receiving supplemental oxygen.
(D) *Incorrect.* There is nothing to suggest that the $SpO_2$ reading is inaccurate as it correlates with the $PaO_2$ of 80 mm Hg. There is no suggestion of anything, that is, carbon monoxide poisoning that may falsely elevate oximeter readings.
(E) *Incorrect.* This patient is acidotic and experiencing CNS depression from $CO_2$ narcosis. Acidosis causes a rightward shift in the hemoglobin-$O_2$ binding curve, as well as cardiac, smooth muscle and CNS depression. The patient should be treated with an opioid antagonist or mechanically ventilated to correct respiratory acidosis.

**REASONING:**

The key to answering this question is recognizing that the patient is experiencing $CO_2$ narcosis and respiratory acidosis secondary to opioid administration. Because the $SpO_2$ and $PaO_2$ correlate, there is nothing in the question to suggest that the analysis was delayed, that a venous sample was erroneously analyzed, or that the pulse oximeter was reading falsely high. The severe respiratory acidosis with $CO_2$ narcosis must be treated.

**BIBLIOGRAPHY:**

Morgan GE, Mikhail MS, Murray MJ. *Clinical Anesthesiology*. 4th ed. New York, NY: McGraw-Hill; 2006:195, 397,397f, 715.

*Answer B*

Clinical Anesthesia

**QUESTION (Choose single best answer):**

A 76-year-old patient is restless and hallucinating in the preoperative holding area. He received morphine 5 mg and scopolamine 0.4 mg intramuscularly as premedication and is now breathing oxygen 2 L/min through nasal prongs. The $SpO_2$ is 98%. Which of the following is the most appropriate next step?

(A) Administration of naloxone.
(B) Administration of physostigmine.
(C) Induction of general anesthesia.
(D) Determination of serum electrolyte concentrations.
(E) Computed tomographic (CT) scan of the head.

**CORRECT ANSWER: B**

**SUMMARY:**

*Recognizing central anticholinergic syndrome as a diagnosis of exclusion is the target of this question. Elderly patients and children are sensitive to medications given in the preoperative setting. The most probable cause for hallucination, agitation, and restlessness in this scenario is central anticholinergic syndrome. Scopolamine had a comeback and is recently often used as a dermal patch for prevention of nausea. It is the most probable cause for central anticholinergic syndrome in this case because it easily passes the blood-brain barrier.*

**EXPLANATION:**

(A) *Incorrect.* Morphine causes mostly sedation with hypoventilation and consequent hypercapnia that affects the oxygenation of the patient ($SpO_2$ is here 98%). This answer can easily confuse the reader, especially when one reads the answers quickly.
(B) *Correct.* Given the scenario, the most plausible cause is central anticholinergic syndrome and the best treatment would be IV-physostigmine application.
(C) *Incorrect.* If a patient behaves abnormally and has no good explanation for it, it is not wise to "quiet" the patient with general anesthesia.
(D) *Incorrect.* Even though it is reasonable to check for electrolyte abnormalities, the intention of the question is central anticholinergic syndrome and the treatment with physostigmine.
(E) *Incorrect.* After all the other causes are ruled out, a head-CT can be reasonable. However, the scenario does not give enough clues for a stroke.

**REASONING:**

Even though central anticholinergic syndrome is an uncommon phenomenon, it should be part of the differential diagnosis of the mental status assessment, especially in connection with a variety of lipophilic medications, capable of passing the blood-brain barrier. A 67-year-old patient is chosen here because this age group has diminished reserves of acetylcholine in brain and is prone to dementia and circadian mental status changes.

Naloxone is an opioid receptor antagonist with a relatively short half-life, competitively binding to opioid receptors. Naloxone is not indicated in this setting because the low-dose morphine that could produce sedation, somnolence, and hypoventilation in an elderly patient is unlikely to be the cause of hallucination and restlessness in this scenario.

Physostigmine is a lipophilic cholinesterase inhibitor that, unlike neostigmine and glycopyrrolate, can reach the brain and increase the concentration of acetylcholine.

When the cause of abnormal mental status of a patient is evaluated, hydration status, common electrolytes concentration (sodium, calcium), blood sugar, blood urea nitrogen

(BUN), and creatinine should be taken into consideration. However, the patient symptoms most likely are related to scopolamine.

Ischemic or hemorrhagic stroke in an elderly patient may be responsible for mental status changes. If the patient had any motor or sensory deficit, the probability of a stroke would be even higher. After ruling out all of the other causes and after application of physostigmine IV (1 mg at a time slowly injected), a head CT would be a reasonable option and should not be delayed unnecessarily.

Furthermore, serum electrolyte abnormalities may cause altered mental status. This is especially true of hyponatremia and hypercalcemia. However, the morphine and scopolamine are not likely to have produced sudden electrolyte changes. Remember this is in the preoperative area and was presumably not present before administration of the medications.

Other systemic manifestations of central anticholinergic syndrome include dry mouth, tachycardia, flushed skin, fever, and impaired vision.


**BIBLIOGRAPHY:**

Barash PG, Cullen BF, Stoelting RK, Cahalan MK, Stock MC. *Clinical Anesthesia.* 3rd ed. Philadelphia, PA: Lippincott Raven Publishers; 1997:272-273

Morgan GE, Mikhail MS, Murray MJ. *Clinical Anesthesiology.* 4th ed. New York, NY: McGraw-Hill; 2006:240-241.

Tune LE. Anticholinergic effects of medication in elderly patients. *J Clin Psychiatry.* 2001;62(suppl 21):11-14.


---

| **BOOK A:** | **QUESTION 122** |
|---|---|

## *Answer E*

Physiology

**QUESTION (Choose single best answer):**

For any given $F_{IO_2}$ and $Pa_{CO_2}$, the $Pa_{O_2}$ is lower in a healthy paralyzed patient anesthetized with isoflurane than in the same patient unanesthetized and breathing spontaneously. The primary cause of this difference is

(A) Controlled ventilation.
(B) Increased airway resistance.
(C) Inhibition of hypoxic pulmonary vasoconstriction.
(D) Intraoperative hypothermia.
(E) Preferential ventilation of nondependent lung.

**CORRECT ANSWER: E**

**SUMMARY:**

*When compared with a unanesthetized patient, the $Pa_{O_2}$ will be lower in anesthetized and paralyzed supine patient for several reasons. General anesthesia with muscle relaxation and positive pressure ventilation causes a 15% to 20% reduction in functional residual capacity (FRC), a worsening of V/Q mismatching, and a 5% to 10% increase in venous admixture. While inhibition of hypoxic pulmonary vasoconstriction by volatile anesthetics does occur, its effect is limited at clinically relevant concentrations.*

**EXPLANATION:**

(A) *Incorrect.* Controlled ventilation tends to recruit alveoli, which helps to prevent hypoxia.

(B) *Incorrect.* Increases in airway resistance are generally not seen with general anesthesia alone because of the bronchodilating properties of volatile anesthetics.

Increases in airway resistance, if they occur, are usually due to pulmonary pathology or equipment-related issues.

(C) *Incorrect.* All anesthetics cause an inhibition of hypoxic pulmonary vasoconstriction. This, however, is usually only clinically significant at high concentrations (ED50 ~2 MAC).

(D) *Incorrect.* Intraoperative hypothermia will decrease oxygen consumption but will not cause a hypoxia.

(E) *Correct.* Under normal negative-pressure spontaneous ventilation, the dependent areas of the lung get both an increased perfusion and increased ventilation secondary to the effects of gravity and a more negative intrapleural pressure. Under positive-pressure ventilation, however, the less dependent areas of the lung will get more ventilation and the dependent areas will get more perfusion, resulting in an increased V/Q mismatch and thus a lower $Pao_2$.

### REASONING:

This question tests knowledge of the changes in pulmonary physiology associated with controlled ventilation and anesthesia with an inhalational anesthetic agent. In reality, there are many reasons that the $Pao_2$ is lower in an anesthetized patient in the supine position. Here, the board asks for the single best answer, which for this question is E.

### BIBLIOGRAPHY:

Barash PG, Cullen BF, Stoelting RK, Calahan M, Stock MC. *Clinical Anesthesia.* 6th ed. Philadelphia, PA; Lippincott Williams & Wilkins; 2009:243-246, 248.

Morgan GE, Mikhail MS, Murray MJ. *Clinical Anesthesiology.* 4th ed. New York, McGraw-Hill; 2006:551, 556-557.

---

| BOOK A: | QUESTION 123 |
| --- | --- |

*Answer D*

Basic Science

### QUESTION (Choose single best answer):

Normal pseudocholinesterase

(A) Is highly concentrated at the motor end plate.
(B) Hydrolyzes succinylcholine by Hofmann elimination.
(C) Is produced primarily at nerve terminals.
(D) Is antagonized by acetylcholinesterase inhibitors.
(E) Resists dibucaine inhibition more than its atypical variant.

### CORRECT ANSWER: D

### SUMMARY:

*Both pseudocholinesterase and acetylcholinesterase are enzymes that catalyze the ester hydrolysis of acetylcholine and succinylcholine. Pseudocholinesterase is a soluble enzyme that circulates in the blood (made primarily in the liver), whereas acetylcholinesterase is a membrane-bound enzyme present at the motor end plate. Both these enzymes are inhibited by acetylcholinesterase (or just cholinesterase) inhibitors because these drugs are nonspecific in mechanism. Dibucaine is an amide local anesthetic that can inhibit normal pseudocholinesterase activity by 80%. It also inhibits variant pseudocholinesterase, but to a lesser degree. Dibucaine inhibition can be used to identify patients with low pseudocholinesterase activity and those with enzyme variants. Clinically significant prolongation of succinylcholine neuromuscular blockade only occurs after pseudocholinesterase activity decreases more than 75% from normal levels.*

**EXPLANATION:**

(A) *Incorrect.* Pseudocholinesterase is a soluble enzyme found in the plasma, not at the motor end plate.

(B) *Incorrect.* Pseudocholinesterase degrades succinylcholine by ester hydrolysis, producing succinic acid and choline. Hoffmann elimination is not involved in succinylcholine metabolism.

(C) *Incorrect.* Pseudocholinesterase is produced in the liver and then circulates in the plasma. Acetylcholinesterase, however, is produced and functions at the motor end plate.

(D) *Correct.* Cholinesterase inhibitors are nonspecific agents that block both acetylcholinesterase and pseudocholinesterase.

(E) *Incorrect.* Normal pseudocholinesterase is more sensitive to dibucaine inhibition than its abnormal variant.


**REASONING:**

This question tests knowledge of cholinesterase enzymes. It is important to understand that pseudocholinesterase and acetylcholinesterase are separate enzymes that catalyze similar reactions and that both are inhibited by cholinesterase inhibitors. The reader also should understand that acetylcholinesterase resides at the motor end plate and that pseudocholinesterase is present in the plasma and produced by the liver. The best answer is D.


**BIBLIOGRAPHY:**

Miller RD, Miller ED, Reves JG, et al. *Anesthesia.* 5th ed. New York, NY: Churchill Livingstone; 2000:546.

Morgan GE, Mikhail MS, Murray MJ. *Clinical Anesthesiology.* 3rd ed. New York, NY: McGraw-Hill; 2002:183, 712.

---

**BOOK A:**

**QUESTION 124**

*Answer E*

Pediatrics

**QUESTION (Choose single best answer):**

Thirty-six hours after primary repair of a meningomyelocele, a term newborn has frequent periods of apnea lasting 25 seconds and associated with oxygen desaturation to 80%. The most likely explanation is

(A) Hyperglycemia.
(B) Loss of cerebrospinal fluid.
(C) Obstructive hydrocephalus.
(D) Residual anesthetic effect.
(E) Normal postoperative events.


**CORRECT ANSWER: E**


**SUMMARY:**

*Neural tube defects occur from failed closure of the neural tube in utero and include spina bifida, myelomeningocele, encephalocele, and tethered cord. Myelomeningocele is a defect of the vertebral column of neural tissue partially covered by epithelial tissue and occurs in the lumbosacral region 75% of the time. Ninety-five percent of patients with myelomeningocele also have Arnold-Chiari malformation type II, which is the abnormal displacement of the cerebellum and brainstem into the foramen magnum and even the lower cervical vertebrae. Associated problems include obstructive hydrocephalus, vocal cord paralysis with stridor, dysphagia, apnea, pulmonary aspiration, and cranial nerve deficits.*

*Most infants with a myelomeningocele present for primary closure within 48 hours of life to minimize the risk of infection. Treatment involves surgical resection of the myelomeningocele, ventriculoperitoneal shunting, and decompression of the cerebellum and brainstem.*

**EXPLANATION:**

(A) *Incorrect.* Hyperglycemia is not associated with meningomyelocele or apnea.

(B) *Incorrect.* There is no evidence of loss of cerebrospinal fluid (CSF) and moderate loss of CSF should not cause apnea or desaturation.

(C) *Incorrect.* Obstructive hydrocephalus occurs in 85% of patients with myelomeningocele and is treated surgically with ventriculoperitoneal shunting. Central respiratory dysfunction occurs in approximately 6% of such patients and is due to abnormal development of the brainstem, not hydrocephalus. Infants who have had repair of meningomyelocele are at risk of central respiratory dysfunction despite cervical decompression for Arnold-Chiari malformation or ventriculoperitoneal shunting for hydrocephalus.

(D) *Incorrect.* Residual anesthetic effects should not last 36 hours.

(E) *Correct.* Neonates (especially ex-preterm infants) are at increased risk of postoperative apnea until they are 50 to 60 weeks postconceptional age. Risk factors for postanesthetic apnea include prematurity, anemia ($< 30\%$), hypothermia, sepsis, and neurological abnormalities.

**REASONING:**

The key concepts tested here are that patients are at risk of central respiratory problems even after repair of myelomeningocele, and even with a working ventriculoperitoneal shunt in place. Choices A and B do not explain apnea. Choice C, while it may cause apnea, is usually treated at time of surgery. Choice D is unlikely at 36 hours postoperatively. Finally, while not normal for a healthy patient, central respiratory dysfunction can continue even after surgical repair and therefore is "normal" in patients with meningomyelocele.

**BIBLIOGRAPHY:**


Cote CJ. *A Practice of Anesthesia for Infants and Children.* 4th ed. Philadelphia, PA; Saunders; 2009:494-496.

Cote CJ, Todres D, Goudsouzian NG. *Practice of Anesthesia for Infants and Children,* 3rd ed. Philadelphia, PA; Saunders; 45-48; 513-514; 531-532.

Morgan GE, Mikhail MS, Murray MJ. *Clinical Anesthesiology.* 4th ed. New York, NY: McGraw-Hill; 2006:940.

Oren J, Kelly DH, Todres ID, Shannon DC. Respiratory complications in patients with myelodysplasia and Arnold-Chiari malformation. *Am J Dis Child.* 1986;140:221-224.

Peterson MC, Wolraich M, Sherbondy A, Wagener J. Abnormalities in control of ventilation in newborn infants with myelomeningocele. *J Pediatr.* 1995;126:1011-1015.


---

**BOOK A:**　　　　　**QUESTION 125**

---

*Answer A*

Pediatrics

**QUESTION (Choose single best answer):**

Inhalation induction of anesthesia is more rapid in a 6-month-old infant than in an adult because infants have

(A) A greater ratio of alveolar ventilation to FRC.

(B) A greater ratio of blood volume to body weight.

(C) A greater solubility of anesthetic in blood.

(D) A lower anesthetic requirement.

(E) A lower distribution of cardiac output to vessel-rich organs.

**CORRECT ANSWER: A**

**SUMMARY:**

*Various factors contribute to a more rapid uptake of inhalational anesthetic agents and therefore the rate of inhalational induction in children. First, there is greater alveolar minute ventilation along with a lower functional residual capacity (FRC) compared to adults. In addition, children have a higher cardiac index that correlates with increased alveolar blood flow compared to adults. Neonates and infants also have lower blood/ gas partition coefficients, which translates into lower solubility and more rapid uptake. Finally, a greater proportion of the cardiac output is delivered to vessel-rich organs that extract a greater amount of anesthetic more quickly. Even though minimum alveolar concentration (MAC) is greater in infants and children, care must be taken with induction because the margin of safety between adequate anesthesia and cardiopulmonary is decreased.*

**EXPLANATION:**

(A) *Correct.* The age-related differences in alveolar ventilation to functional residual capacity (VA/FRC) ratio accounts for most of the differences between FA/FI of anesthetics in neonates and adults. The VA/FRC ratio is approximately 5:1 in neonates compared with only 1.5:1 in adults. This results in more rapid uptake of anesthetic agents.

(B) *Incorrect.* Infants do have a greater ratio of blood volume to body weight, but this does not affect rate of induction. However, cardiac output, the rate at which the blood is pumped throughout the body, does affect rate of induction.

(C) *Incorrect.* Greater solubility in blood would slow induction. The blood/gas coefficients, and thus solubility for isoflurane and halothane are actually 18% lower in children than in adults. Blood solubilities of the less soluble anesthetics such as sevoflurane are similar in children and adults.

(D) *Incorrect.* MAC (halothane, isoflurane, desflurane) (preterm infant < term infant < 3- to 6-month-old infant) >> older child > adult > elderly. The MAC of sevoflurane in neonates and infants younger than 6 months is the same, and then it decreases as age increases.

(E) *Incorrect.* Children have a higher distribution of cardiac output to vessel-rich organs.

**REASONING:**

This question tests understanding of the determinants of the rate of induction with inhaled anesthetic agents and the physiologic differences between children and adults. Choice B is misleading because it is a true statement. However, blood volume to body weight ratio does not affect rate of induction. Choice C can be eliminated because it is false and because greater solubility actually slows induction. The reader should be able to recognize that children have greater anesthetic requirements and greater distribution to vessel-rich organs and rule out choices D and E. That leaves choice A, which is true, and explains why induction is more rapid in children.

**BIBLIOGRAPHY:**

Cote CJ. *A Practice of Anesthesia for Infants and Children.* 4th ed. Philadelphia, PA; Saunders; 2009:101-104, 107.

Morgan GE, Mikhail MS, Murray MJ. *Clinical Anesthesiology.* 4th ed. New York, NY: McGraw-Hill; 2006:929 (Table 44-4).

*Answer B*

Pediatrics

**QUESTION (Choose single best answer):**

Which of the following findings is most hazardous in premature infants?

(A) Hematocrit of 55%.
(B) Rectal temperature of 35°C.
(C) Umbilical arterial blood $P_{O_2}$ of 50 mm Hg.
(D) Umbilical arterial blood $P_{CO_2}$ of 45 mm Hg.
(E) Umbilical arterial systolic pressure of 60 mm Hg.

**CORRECT ANSWER: B**

**SUMMARY:**

*Children born before 37 weeks' gestation are termed* premature infants *and include the low–birth-weight (< 2500 g), very-low-birth-weight (< 1500 g), and the extremely low-birth-weight (< 1000 g) infants. All may have immature physiologic systems, including immature pulmonary (surfactant deficiency, apnea), renal, gastrointestinal (feeding intolerance, inadequate absorption), hematopoietic (anemia), and immune function (increased susceptibility to infection); immature cerebral vasculature (increased risk of hemorrhage); patent ductus arteriosus (left to right shunt); and impaired thermoregulation. These high-risk newborns require meticulous anesthetic technique.*

**EXPLANATION:**

(A) *Incorrect.* A hematocrit of 55% is acceptable for a premature infant. Neonatal polycythemia (hematocrit > 65%) may lead to symptoms of hyperviscosity.
(B) *Correct.* A temperature of 35°C is considered hypothermic and should be corrected as it increases oxygen consumption. Premature infants are susceptible to hypothermia as they have little fat for insulation and a large surface area to mass ratio. Hyperthermia leads to increased risk of hypoglycemia, bradycardia, apnea, and metabolic acidosis.
(C) *Incorrect.* Normal $P_{aO_2}$ in newborns range from 60 to 80 mm Hg. An umbilical artery blood $P_{O_2}$ of 50 mm Hg is acceptable as long as there is no acidosis. Oxygen saturation should be maintained around 92% to 96%, which correlates with a $P_{aO_2}$ of approximately 70 to 80 mm Hg in premature infants intraoperatively to minimize the risk of retinopathy of prematurity.
(D) *Incorrect.* An umbilical artery blood $P_{CO_2}$ of 45 mm Hg is acceptable.
(E) *Incorrect.* Umbilical artery systolic blood pressure of 60 mm Hg is within normal range. Average systolic pressure in premature infants range from 55 to 75 mm Hg.

**REASONING:**

Understanding of the range of normal values for premature infants is important to answer this question. Choices A, D, and E are well within normal ranges, so they can be eliminated. Choice C is acceptable. While a $P_{aO_2}$ of 50 mm Hg is not ideal, we have no evidence that it is inadequate for this patient. In fact for patients with mixing congenital cardiac lesions, this may be normal. This leaves choice B that is concerning as premature infants have decreased ability for thermoregulation.

**BIBLIOGRAPHY:**

Cote CJ. *A Practice of Anesthesia for Infants and Children.* 4th ed. Philadelphia, PA: Saunders; 2009:15 (Table 2-8), 18 (Table 2-10), 22, 738.
Morgan CG, Mikhail MS, Murray MJ. *Clinical Anesthesiology.* 4th ed. New York, NY: McGraw-Hill; 2006:939-940.

*Answer E*

Clinical Anesthesia

**QUESTION (Choose single best answer):**

A 40-year-old patient has pain following injection of 8 mL thiopental 2.5% through a right radial artery catheter. His hand remains pink. Which of the following is the most appropriate next step?

(A)  Injection of lidocaine through the catheter.
(B)  Injection of nitroglycerin though the catheter.
(C)  Injection of papaverine through the catheter.
(D)  Right stellate ganglion block.
(E)  No intervention.

**CORRECT ANSWER: E**

**SUMMARY:**

*With intra-arterial thiopental, vasospasm is induced by the local release of norepinephrine and local tissue destruction can occur. Furthermore, there is potential for ischemia, gangrene, and loss of tissue or a limb. There are no well-controlled studies that clearly demonstrate the effectiveness of any given therapy. Any drug that promotes blood flow, such as vasodilators like papaverine and lidocaine, or any procedure to improve blood flow, such as a brachial plexus or stellate ganglion block, could be helpful. In addition, IV heparin can potentially prevent any thrombosis. Because the hand is still pink, the most appropriate next step is to watch the hand carefully and hold off on any interventions. Then, if the hand becomes cyanotic and pain persists, different therapies can be attempted such as elevation of the hand to improve flow, local anesthetic infiltration, extremity sympatholysis, and other chemical therapies.*

**EXPLANATION:**

(A)  *Incorrect.* Although lidocaine may help to vasodilate an artery exposed to thiopental and prevent reflex vasospasm, there are also risks to its administration such as arterial laceration or tissue damage contributing to thrombosis. Thus, it is best to wait and watch the hand very closely.

(B)  *Incorrect.* Nitroglycerin is generally a venodilator rather than an arterial dilator. In addition, injecting nitroglycerin intra-arterially can cause profound, systemic hypotension and is not the best choice to improve blood flow to the affected limb.

(C)  *Incorrect.* Although papaverine could promote blood flow to the limb after accidental intra-arterial thiopental administration, again there exist risks to its intra-arterial administration and it is best not to intervene yet because the hand is still pink.

(D)  *Incorrect.* An ipsilateral stellate ganglion block can produce a sympathectomy in the affected arm, causing vasodilation for a prolonged period of time and improving blood flow to the right arm. However, because the hand is still pink, it is not worth the risk of a pneumothorax, nerve paralysis, local anesthetic toxicity, or spinal injection.

(E)  *Correct.* Because the hand is still pink in this scenario, it is best not to intervene and just to watch the extremity closely. Only if the hand appears ischemic or continues to be quite painful should something be done because vasospasm of the artery can develop with subsequent gangrene and loss of tissue.

**REASONING:**

Thiopental is a water soluble barbiturate, prepared in an alkaline solution with a pH of 10.5. Because of its alkaline state, thiopental has the potential of forming crystals and subsequently occluding smaller arteries and arterioles from where it is actually administered through an arterial catheter. Extravasation into subcutaneous tissue can cause necrosis and inadvertent intra-arterial injection can cause vasospasm, pain, ischemia, gangrene, and the potential loss of tissue or a limb. Although lidocaine and papaverine can be helpful in causing vasodilation in the affected limb, an ipsilateral stellate ganglion block is probably the most efficacious in promoting an increased blood flow to the arm with a sympathectomy. However, in this situation, the hand is still pink with good perfusion and, thus, it is not worth incurring the risks with such therapies yet.


**BIBLIOGRAPHY:**

Ghouri A, Mading W, and Prabaker K. Accidental intraarterial drug injections via intravascular catheters placed on the dorsum of the hand. *Anesth Analg.* 2002;95:487-491.

Morgan CG, Mikhail MS, Murray MJ. *Clinical Anesthesiology.* 4th ed. New York, NY: McGraw-Hill; 2006:185-187.

Stoelting RK, Miller RD. *Basics of Anesthesia.* 3rd ed. Philadelphia, PA: Churchill Livingstone; 1994:62.


---

**BOOK A:**  **QUESTION 128**

---

*Answer D*

Equipment/Physics

**QUESTION (Choose single best answer):**

During nitrous oxide anesthesia, which of the following expands most rapidly?

(A) Air bubble in the blood.
(B) Air in the intestine.
(C) Endotracheal tube cuff.
(D) Pneumothorax.
(E) Sulfahexafluoride bubble in the vitreal cavity.

**CORRECT ANSWER: D**

**SUMMARY:**

*Nitrous oxide is 35 times more soluble than nitrogen in blood. Thus, it will diffuse into air-containing cavities more rapidly than nitrogen is absorbed by the bloodstream. The magnitude of volume increase is influenced by the alveolar partial pressure of nitrous, blood flow to the air-filled cavity, and the duration of the nitrous anesthetic. Nitrous oxide exposed to those places that are noncompliant, such as a gas space created in the eye by a sulfur hexafluoride injection, will cause a rapid increase in pressure rather than volume. On the contrary, the volume rather than the pressure within more compliant places, such as a pneumothorax, bowel, air embolus, and endotracheal cuff, will expand rapidly. The volume of gas in the bowel expands slowly and rarely can such expansion cause a clinically significant difference in an hour. Likewise, the cuff of an endotracheal tube will increase its volume rather slowly, as the nitrous must penetrate different materials.*

**EXPLANATION:**

(A) *Incorrect.* An air bubble in blood will increase its volume rather quickly with a nitrous oxide anesthetic; however, the bubble must remain intact within the circulation for the nitrous oxide to diffuse into this compliant space from the blood. There is no secondary mechanism for nitrous uptake into the bubble like into a pneumothorax. With the latter, there is direct diffusion of nitrous from the alveoli rather than just vascular delivery of this gas into a closed space.

(B) *Incorrect.* The increase in bowel gas is slow compared to the increase in the size of a pneumothorax. Normally, there is only approximately 100 cc of air in the bowel. Thus, after several hours, the nitrous oxide may be delivered in the blood to the bowel to double its gaseous contents which may not even be appreciated by the surgeons.

(C) *Incorrect.* An endotracheal tube cuff is filled with 5 to 7 cc of air. Only after several hours of a nitrous anesthetic will some of the nitrous oxide diffuse into the cuff and potentially increase the pressure exerted on tracheal mucosa. The nitrous oxide must penetrate the cuff first and slowly increase the volume within this compliant, closed space.

(D) *Correct.* A pneumothorax will expand rather quickly, as the insoluble nitrous oxide gas will rapidly leave the blood and enter the air-filled cavity 34 times faster than nitrogen would exit the pneumothorax. The more rapid change with a pneumothorax probably results from the movement of nitrous oxide across the visceral pleura rather than just from the transport of the nitrous oxide into this space from blood alone.

(E) *Incorrect.* Sulfur hexafluoride is an inert gas that is less soluble in blood than is nitrogen and much less soluble than nitrous oxide. Thus, its longer duration of action compared with an air bubble can be advantageous to the ophthalmologist. If a patient is breathing a nitrous anesthetic, the nitrous oxide will quickly entrain the bubble and increase its size before the sulfur hexafluoride has a chance to diffuse into the blood. A 70% nitrous oxide technique will almost double the pressure in a closed eye within 30 minutes. Because it is a rather noncompliant space, its pressure, rather than its volume, expands quickly.

**REASONING:**

Nitrous oxide will cause an increase in pressure in noncompliant spaces, such as those created by sulfahexafluoride injections, and, on the contrary, will cause an increase in volume in compliant spaces, such as the bowel, a pneumothorax, an air embolus, and an endotracheal tube cuff. Of these, a pneumothorax expands the most rapidly probably due to diffusion of nitrous oxide through the visceral pleura besides the delivery and the diffusion of the nitrous oxide in the circulation. Nitrous oxide is quite insoluble in blood; however, it is 35 times more soluble than nitrogen in blood. Hence, anywhere there is air (the majority of which is nitrogen), it will attempt to fill the space quicker than the nitrogen can escape. Both the bowel and endotracheal cuff fill with nitrous oxide rather slowly. An air bubble has the potential to expand rapidly with nitrous oxide if the nitrous is able to diffuse into the bubble before it is dissipated within the circulation.

**BIBLIOGRAPHY:**

Eger E. *Nitrous Oxide.* New York, NY: Elsevier Science Publishing Company, Inc.; 1985:95-99.

Kaur S, Cortiella J, Vacanti C. Diffusion of nitrous oxide into the pleural cavity. *Br J Anaesth.* 2001;87:894-896.

Morgan CG, Mikhail MS, Murray MJ. *Clinical Anesthesiology.* 4th ed. New York, NY: McGraw-Hill;2006:164-166.

Stoelting RK, Miller RD. *Basics of Anesthesia.* 3rd ed. Philadelphia, PA: Churchill Livingstone; 1994:21.

---

**BOOK A:**  **QUESTION 129**

*Answer C*

Equipment/Physics

**QUESTION (Choose single best answer):**

While an anesthesia machine is being checked, opening the oxygen flow–control valve yields no oxygen flow, although the wall-mounted oxygen pipeline supply gauge reads 50 psi (pounds per square inch gauge). Opening the backup oxygen cylinder results in normal oxygen flow. The most likely cause is

(A) Failure of the oxygen pipeline supply.
(B) Failure of the second-stage oxygen pressure regulator.
(C) A malfunctioning check valve in the oxygen pipeline supply inlet.
(D) A malfunctioning fail-safe valve.
(E) A malfunctioning oxygen flow–control valve.

**CORRECT ANSWER: C**

**SUMMARY:**

*The only valve that lies close to the beginning of the oxygen supply from the pipeline is the check valve from the pipeline supply inlet. A faulty valve could prevent oxygen from getting to the flowmeters, whereas, if the cylinder is opened, oxygen could bypass this faulty valve and enter the flowmeter. Because the gauge reads 50 psi, there is no failure with the pipeline. In addition, the oxygen flow–control valve is working appropriately because opening the backup oxygen cylinder results in normal oxygen flow. The second-stage oxygen pressure regulator and the fail-safe valve lie downstream to the oxygen supply from both the pipeline or cylinder and would not prevent oxygen from flowing entirely if they faulty.*

**EXPLANATION:**

(A) *Incorrect.* The oxygen pipeline supply has not failed as the supply gauge still reads 50 psi which is the normal.

(B) *Incorrect.* The second-stage oxygen pressure regulator maintains oxygen flowmeter output as long as at least 12 psi of oxygen pressure is in the system. It lies downstream from both oxygen sources, immediately prior to the flowmeters.

(C) *Correct.* The check valve in the oxygen pipeline supply inlet prevents transfilling of gas cylinders or flow of gas from cylinders into the central supply and lies directly after the start of the pipeline supply into the anesthesia machine. Such a faulty valve may prevent oxygen from the pipeline supply from reaching the flowmeters.

(D) *Incorrect.* The fail-safe valve lies downstream, from the oxygen supply from both the pipeline and cylinder. This valve automatically closes all other gas lines if oxygen pressure falls below 25 psi or 50% of normal to help prevent the possibility of delivering a hypoxic mixture.

(E) *Incorrect.* The oxygen flow–control valve on the flowmeter is not malfunctioning as there is oxygen flow once the source is changed from the pipeline supply to the cylinder.

**REASONING:**

There are several valves within the anesthesia machine, each positioned in a different place within the "circuit" of the machine. The check valve in the pipeline supply inlet prevents backfilling from the cylinders into the pipeline supply and is the only valve directly downstream from only the pipeline supply. Thus, its malfunction could prevent any oxygen from being delivered from this one source that is functioning appropriately with a pressure of 50 psi. Both the fail-safe valve and the second stage pressure regulator lie farther downstream from both the pipeline supply and the oxygen cylinder and, thus, a malfunction in this valve would probably prevent oxygen flow entirely. However, in this particular situation, the opened oxygen–flow control valve had oxygen flow once the cylinder was opened.

**BIBLIOGRAPHY:**

Morgan CG, Mikhail MS, Murray MJ. *Clinical Anesthesiology*. 4th ed. New York, NY: McGraw-Hill; 2006:48-54.

## *Answer A*

### Physiology

**QUESTION (Choose single best answer):**

Which of the following statements concerning pulmonary function in patients with pulmonary fibrosis is true?

(A) Diffusion capacity is decreased.
(B) Pulmonary artery diastolic-to-occlusion pressure gradients are normal.
(C) Ventilation-perfusion relationships are normal.
(D) Static pulmonary compliance is unchanged.
(E) Mechanical ventilation with a slow rate and a large tidal volume is optimal.

**CORRECT ANSWER: A**

**SUMMARY:**

*Pulmonary fibrosis has significant anesthetic implications. There are many different causes, but the end result is the same—progressive inflammation and fibrosis of the pulmonary connective tissue, principally in the alveolar wall with eventual respiratory failure. The tissue remodeling causes chronic hypoxia, decreased diffusing capacity, and secondary pulmonary hypertension. In addition, the decreased FRC results in V/Q mismatching that also contributes to hypoxemia. Low lung compliance leads to high peak pressures with positive-pressure ventilation, and low tidal volume ventilator strategies reduce the risk of barotrauma in these patients.*

**EXPLANATION:**

(A) **Correct.** Parenchymal fibrosis, principally in the alveolar wall, causes a decrease in diffusing capacity of the alveoli.
(B) **Incorrect.** Patients with pulmonary fibrosis have secondary pulmonary hypertension, but left-sided pressures in the heart are normal. Pulmonary artery diastolic pressures are therefore significantly higher than the pulmonary artery occlusion pressure.
(C) **Incorrect.** The ventilation-perfusion ratio is abnormal in restrictive lung disease owing to decreased lung volumes, including the FRC.
(D) **Incorrect.** Static and dynamic lung compliances are both decreased from the continued fibrosis of the lung parenchyma.
(E) **Incorrect.** Large tidal volumes increase the risk of barotrauma that could result in a lethal pneumothorax. The patient should be ventilated with smaller tidal volumes at a rate that does not cause air trapping.

**REASONING:**

This question tests knowledge of the pathophysiology and clinical implications of pulmonary fibrosis. Patients with pulmonary fibrosis develop restrictive lung physiology, characterized by decreased compliance and decreased lung volumes (including FRC and FVC). $FEV_1$ is also decreased, and thus the $FVE_1$/FVC ratio is usually normal. The decrease in diffusion capacity observed with restrictive lung disease such as pulmonary fibrosis can be due to thickening of the alveolar membrane (gas/blood barrier) in addition to loss of lung volume associated with the restrictive disease state. The single best answer is A.

**BIBLIOGRAPHY:**

Barash PG, Cullen BF, Stoelting RK, Calahan M, Stock MC. *Clinical Anesthesia.* 6th ed. Philadelphia, PA: Lippincott Williams & Wilkins; 2009:251-252.

Kumar V, Abbas AK, Fausto N, Aster JC. The lung, chronic diffuse interstitial (restrictive) lung disease. In: Kumar V, Abbas AK, Fausto N, Aster JC, eds. *Robbins and Cotran*

*Pathologic Basis of Disease.* 8th ed. Philadelphia, PA: Saunders Elsevier; 2010: Chap 15.

Morgan GE, Mikhail MS, Murray MJ. *Clinical Anesthesiology.* 4th ed. New York, NY: McGraw-Hill; 2006:578-580.

| BOOK A: | QUESTION 131 |
| --- | --- |

## *Answer C*

### Physiology

**QUESTION (Choose single best answer):**

In which of the following situations is mismatching of ventilation to perfusion in the lung greatest?

(A) Awake patient, spontaneous ventilation, lateral decubitus position.
(B) Anesthetized patient, controlled ventilation, supine position.
(C) Anesthetized patient, controlled ventilation, lateral decubitus position.
(D) Anesthetized patient, controlled ventilation, sitting position.
(E) Anesthetized patient, spontaneous ventilation, prone position.

**CORRECT ANSWER: C**

**SUMMARY:**

*This is an important question for understanding effects of anesthesia and positioning on ventilation and perfusion mismatch. The first important point is that anesthesia has about the same deleterious effects on V/Q mismatch whether spontaneously ventilating or with mechanical ventilation. The second important concept is the effects of positioning on V/Q mismatch. A direct comparison of these positions is difficult to find in the major textbooks. The textbooks describe greater perfusion in the dependent lung and greater ventilation in the nondependent lung. They consistently state that moving from the upright to supine position decreases FRC and causes greater mismatch. A comparison of supine and lateral decubitus positions had to be found in the literature.*

**EXPLANATION:**

(A) *Incorrect.* The lateral decubitus position in an awake, spontaneously breathing patient preserves ventilation-perfusion matching. The dependent lung receives greater perfusion owing to gravity and greater ventilation owing to compliance. Awake patients have better preservation of their FRC and the dependent diaphragm preserves its ability to contract.

(B) *Incorrect.* FRC is decreased with anesthesia by 0.4 to 0.5 L with anesthesia and another 0.8 to 1 L when changing position from upright to supine. Much of these changes are due to loss of respiratory muscle tone. Patients in a lateral decubitus position experience even greater derangements in V/Q mismatching.

(C) *Correct.* A study looking at relationships of V/Q mismatch and atelectasis formation was conducted in the supine and lateral positions. When the patients were turned from supine to the lateral position, further V/Q mismatch was observed in addition to a fall in $Pao_2$ with increased dead space.

(D) *Incorrect.* FRC is decreased with anesthesia by 0.4 to 0.5 L with anesthesia and another 0.8 to 1 L when changing position from upright to supine. Thus the sitting position preserves up to 1 L of FRC.

(E) *Incorrect.* Studies have shown that the worsening of gas exchange caused by anesthesia is about the same in an anesthetized spontaneously ventilating person as in an anesthetized mechanically ventilated person even with paralysis. An improvement in ventilation perfusion mismatch has been noted in the prone position and is thought to be due to regional differences in vascular configuration. Ventilation was more uniform in the prone position.

**REASONING:**
Ventilation perfusion mismatching is one of the major causes of hypoxemia during anesthesia. Having a good understanding of the effects of anesthesia whether spontaneously ventilation or mechanically ventilated is important and knowing that anesthesia affects both groups about the same. Positioning can also cause significant problems such as V/Q mismatching.


**BIBLIOGRAPHY:**
Barash PG, Cullen BF, Stoelting RK, Cahalan MK, Stock MC. *Clinical Anesthesia.* 6th ed. Philadelphia, PA: Lippincott Williams & Wilkins; 2009:244-245, 1040-1042.
Kingstedt C, Heenstierna G, Baehrendtz S, et al. Ventilation-perfusion relationships and atelectasis formation in the supine and lateral positions during controlled mechanical and differentional ventilation. *Aeta Aneaethesiol Scand.* 1990 Aug;34(6):421-429.
Miller RD, Eriksson LI, Fleisher LA, et al. *Miller: Miller's Anesthesia.* 7th ed. Churchill Livingston; 2009:470.

---

**BOOK A:**

**QUESTION 132**

---

*Answer C*

Cardiovascular

**QUESTION (Choose single best answer):**

The following hemodynamic profile is from a 62-year-old man in the intensive care unit (ICU) after coronary artery bypass grafting.

|  | **Entering ICU** | **+30 Minutes** |
|---|---|---|
| Heart rate (bpm) | 90 | 120 |
| Blood pressure (mm Hg) | 125/75 | 80/30 |
| PADP (mm Hg) | 12 | 25 |
| PAOP (mm Hg) | 10 | 25 |
| CVP (mm Hg) | 6 | 8 |

Which of the following is the most likely cause of the changes occurring after 30 minutes?

(A) Anaphylactic reaction.
(B) Left ventricular ischemia.
(C) Pericardial tamponade.
(D) Pulmonary embolism.
(E) Septic shock.


**CORRECT ANSWER: C**


**SUMMARY:**

*Cardiac tamponade after heart surgery is a common perioperative complication that requires surgical reexploration. Tamponade can occur even if the pericardium is left open after surgery. Loculated bleeding and clot formation can cause obstruction to diastolic filling of the right or left sides of the heart independently. The differential diagnosis includes right or left ventricular dysfunction. Classic signs of tamponade include hypotension, tachycardia, shock, and equalization of pressures in the heart such that CVP = PAD = PCWP = 25 mm Hg (although not all signs are always seen). Echocardiography (TTE or TEE) can be helpful in establishing the diagnosis.*


**EXPLANATION:**
(A) *Incorrect.* Anaphylactic reaction would cause distributive shock with low CVP, PAD, and PCWP. Associated symptoms such as rash and bronchospasm may be seen.

(B) *Incorrect.* Electrocardiographic (ECG) changes of ischemia may be noted. It is unusual for left ventricular dysfunction to cause pressure equalization of PAD and PCWP. Echocardiography will help to differentiate these findings.

(C) *Correct.* Tamponade is consistent with these hemodynamic findings.

(D) *Incorrect.* Pulmonary embolus will give rise to elevated right-sided pressures, right ventricular failure, bronchospasm, and hypoxia. It will not cause equalization of pressures across the heart chambers.

(E) *Incorrect.* Septic shock will have a clinical picture significant for a source of infection, fever, elevated white blood cell count, and distributive shock. Unless there was an ongoing active infection, it would be unusual to see septic shock immediately after surgery.

## REASONING:

It is important to have a thorough differential diagnosis for postoperative hypotension after cardiac surgery. Some causes include hypovolemia, biventricular failure, bleeding, tamponade, or pneumothorax. Clinical signs and symptoms can create a confusing picture. Tamponade is the most likely cause of the observed findings in this patient with acute hypotension in ICU after a short period of stability who has pressure equalization without increased chest tube drainage.

## BIBLIOGRAPHY:


Hensley F, Martin DE, Gravlee FP. *Practical Approach to Cardiac Anesthesia.* 4th ed. Philadelphia, PA: Lippincott Williams & Wilkins; 2002:280.

Morgan GE, Mikhail MS, Murray MJ. *Clinical Anesthesiology.* 4th ed. New York, NY: McGraw-Hill; 2002:526-527.


---

## BOOK A:                    QUESTION 133

*Answer D*

Equipment/Physics

## QUESTION (Choose single best answer):

The odor of isoflurane is noted during isoflurane anesthesia with an endotracheal tube and mechanical ventilation. Mean airway pressure is unchanged. A scavenging system with an open interface and an active disposal system is being used. The most likely cause of the isoflurane odor is

(A) A leak in the inspiratory limb of the anesthesia circuit.

(B) Application of an excessive negative pressure to the scavenging interface.

(C) Malfunction of the pop-off valve of the anesthesia machine.

(D) Obstruction of the gas disposal tubing leading from the scavenging interface.

(E) Obstruction of the transfer tubing to the scavenging interface.

## CORRECT ANSWER: D

## SUMMARY:

*The scavenging system described has an active disposal system whereby the disposal tubing is directly connected to the hospital's vacuum system to get rid a gaseous wastes. Such an open interface has a negative-pressure relief valve and a reservoir bag. A leak in the inspiratory limb would cause a drop in mean airway pressures achieved and could not be the source of the operating room (OR) pollution. Application of excessive negative pressure to the scavenging system would cause patient circuit collapse. With a malfunction of the pop-off valve, this would not cause a leak into the atmosphere and, in addition, obstruction of the transfer tubing to the scavenging interface could cause an increase in pressure with barotrauma. Thus, an obstruction of the gas disposal tubing leading from the scavenging interface would most likely cause the venting of gases into the OR as the interface is open to the atmosphere without any valves.*

**EXPLANATION:**

(A) *Incorrect.* A leak in the inspiratory limb would cause a drop in mean airway pressures, pressure alarms would be activated, and tidal volumes would never be achieved.

(B) *Incorrect.* By applying excessive negative pressure to the scavenging system, all the gases would be sucked into the vacuum system leading to collapse of the patient's circuit. Gaseous wastes would not be vented into the OR in this circumstance.

(C) *Incorrect.* Malfunction of the pop-off valve would result in either excessive buildup of gas in the patient's circuit leading to barotrauma rather than venting of gaseous waster into the environment.

(D) *Correct.* By having an obstruction in the gas disposal tubing leading from the scavenging interface into the hospital's vacuum system, there is nowhere for vented gases to escape except out. There are no valves with an open interface so it is open to the atmosphere.

(E) *Incorrect.* Obstruction in the transfer tubing going to the scavenging interface can cause a buildup of pressure and gases into the patient's circuit with a potential for barotraumas.

**REASONING:**

Within an anesthesia machine's scavenging system, there are various reasons for OR pollution. The most common cause is kinking or obstruction of the tubing leading from the scavenging interface. An obstruction at this point would also cause the venting of gases into the OR through an open interface because there are no valves to protect against this hazard. A leak in the inspiratory limb would lead to a decrease in mean airway pressures and obstruction of the transfer tubing or malfunction of the pop-off valve could lead to barotrauma in the patient.

**BIBLIOGRAPHY:**

Morgan CG, Mikhail MS, Murray MJ. *Clinical Anesthesiology*. 4th ed. New York, NY: McGraw-Hill; 2006:45.

---

**BOOK A:**

*Answer E*

Pharmacology

## QUESTION 134

**QUESTION (Choose single best answer):**

Which of the following statements concerning the volume of distribution of a drug is true?

(A) It is equal to the sum of the volumes of the tissue spaces into which it diffuses.
(B) It is equal to the volume to which it is distributed outside the plasma volume.
(C) It is unaltered by the amount bound to red blood cells and plasma proteins.
(D) It depends on elimination from plasma.
(E) It relates the total amount of the drug in the body to the plasma concentration.

**CORRECT ANSWER: E**

**SUMMARY:**

*The volume of plasma that would be necessary to account for the observed plasma concentration is known as a drug's volume of distribution. It can be calculated by dividing the dose of the drug in the body by its plasma concentration. Causes for a small volume of distribution include anything that increases plasma concentration such as high protein binding or ionization. Conversely, anything that decreases plasma concentration will increase the volume of distribution, such as high solubility or binding of the drug in tissues other than plasma (ie, fentanyl in adipose tissue). The volume of distribution does not depend on elimination from the plasma.*

**EXPLANATION:**

(A) *Incorrect.* The volume of distribution only reflects the volume of plasma necessary to account for the plasma concentration of the drug and has nothing to do with volumes of other tissues into which the drug diffuses.

(B) *Incorrect.* The volume of plasma into which the drug is distributed is key to calculating the volume of distribution and the volume outside the plasma is irrelevant to the calculation.

(C) *Incorrect.* The binding of a drug to plasma proteins increases its distribution within the plasma and, therefore, decreases its volume of distribution.

(D) *Incorrect.* A drug's elimination from the plasma does not affect its volume of distribution and the initial calculation once the drug is injected.

(E) *Correct.* The volume of distribution of a drug can be calculated by the total amount of drug administered and the proportion that resides in the plasma.

**REASONING:**

A drug's volume of distribution is reflective of the total amount of drug administered and the amount in the plasma only. This is dependent on the drug's redistribution into other tissues affected by such things as drug ionization, drug protein binding, and drug lipophilicity. To calculate this number, divide the total amount of drug injected (mg) by the concentration of the drug in the plasma (mg/cc).

**BIBLIOGRAPHY:**

Morgan CG, Mikhail MS, Murray MJ. *Clinical Anesthesiology*. 4th ed. New York, NY: McGraw-Hill; 2006:181.

---

| BOOK A: | QUESTION 135 |
|---|---|

*Answer E*

Pharmacology

**QUESTION (Choose single best answer):**

Which of the following statements concerning propofol is true?

(A) Active metabolites can produce residual postoperative sedation.
(B) It causes less cardiovascular depression than an equivalent induction dose of thiopental.
(C) It causes less respiratory depression than an equivalent induction dose of thiopental.
(D) It has analgesic properties.
(E) The vehicle emulsion is associated with hypersensitivity reactions.

**CORRECT ANSWER: E**

**SUMMARY:**

*Propofol (2,6-diisopropylphenol) is one of the most commonly used modern intravenous induction agents. It is formulated in a soybean oil–egg lecithin–glycerol emulsion (Diprivan) that is capable of causing hypersensitivity reactions. Propofol can cause cardiovascular and respiratory depression, and these effects are more pronounced than with thiopental administration. Propofol is thought to work by facilitation of inhibitory neurotransmission by γ-aminobutyric acid (GABA). Propofol does not have any analgesic properties (but can synergize with fentanyl and alfentanil). Propofol is metabolized by the liver, and its subsequent inactive metabolites are eliminated by the kidneys.*

## EXPLANATION:

(A) ***Incorrect.*** Propofol is metabolized in the liver by conjugation with glucuronide and sulfate into inactive water-soluble compounds that are eliminated by the kidneys. Chronic renal failure does not affect the parent drug.

(B) ***Incorrect.*** Propofol causes more cardiovascular depression than an equivalent dose of thiopental.

(C) ***Incorrect.*** Propofol causes more respiratory depression than an equivalent dose of thiopental.

(D) ***Incorrect.*** Propofol has no analgesic properties.

(E) ***Correct.*** Propofol is packaged as an emulsion containing 10% soybean oil, 2.25% glycerol, and 1.2% egg yolk phospholipid. Allergic hypersensitivity reactions can occur to these additives.

## REASONING:

This question tests knowledge of the pharmacologic properties of propofol. It is important for the reader to review the multisystemic effects of propofol and how they differ compared with other anesthetic agents. Propofol does not have analgesic properties, and its metabolites are not active. Propofol is profoundly insoluble in aqueous solution and requires the use of solubilizing agents. Early clinical formulations of propofol (e.g., propofol EL) contained a Cremophor-EL solubilizer that produced a high incidence of allergic reactions and was withdrawn subsequently from clinical testing. Diprivan uses an egg lecithin and soybean oil emulsion to solubilize propofol. Most egg-allergic people are allergic to the egg protein (egg white) and propofol contains egg yolk so reactions are rare. Allergic reactions to these components can occur and are reported at 1 in 45,000 anesthetics for propofol-related immune reactions.


## BIBLIOGRAPHY:

Barash PG, Cullen BF, Stoelting RK, Cahalan MK, Stock MC. *Clinical Anesthesia.* 6th ed. Philadelphia, PA: Lippincott Williams & Wilkins; 2009:452-453.

Bassett CW, Talusan-Canlas E, Holtzin L, et al. An adverse reaction to propofol in a patient with egg hypersensitivity [abstract 476]. *J Allergy Clin Immunol.* 1994;93(1):242.

Laxenaire MC, Maten-Bermejo E, Moneret-Vautrin DA, Gueant JL. Life-threatening anaphylactoid reactions to propofol (Diprivan). *Anesthesiology.* 1992;77:275-280.

Miller RD, Miller ED, Reves JG, et al. *Anesthesia.* 7th ed. New York, NY: Churchill Livingstone; 2009:720-728.

Morgan GE, Mikhail MS, Murray MJ. *Clinical Anesthesiology.* 4th ed. New York, NY: McGraw-Hill; 2006:200-202.

Murphy A, Campbell DE, Bains D, Mehr S. Allergic reactions to propofol in egg-allergic children. *Anesth Analg.* 2011;113(1):140-144.

## Answer C

Cardiovascular

**QUESTION (Choose single best answer):**

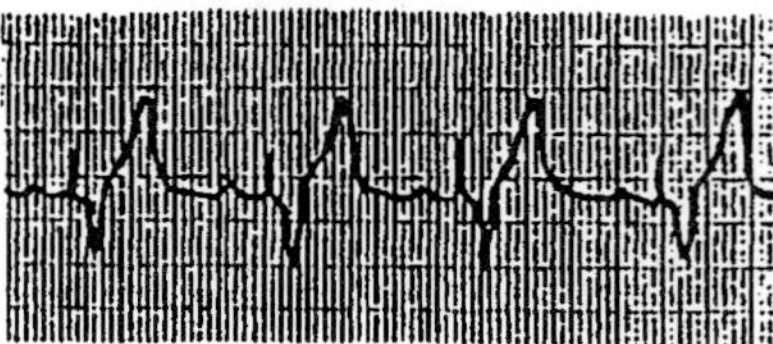

The ECG strip shown here is recorded as a patient with a permanent transvenous DDD pacemaker enters the operating room. These changes indicate that the pacemaker is

(A) Sensing the T waves.
(B) Sensing the retrograde P waves.
(C) Triggering off the intrinsic atrial activity.
(D) Malfunctioning in the atrial pacing mechanism.
(E) Prematurely stimulating the ventricle.

**CORRECT ANSWER: C**

**SUMMARY:**

*Pacemakers are identified by a five-letter coding system. The first letter stands for the chambers being paced, and the second letter indicates the chambers sensed for inherent electrical activity. The third letter indicates the pacemaker response to the sensed P and R waves. The fourth letter denotes the programmability of pacemaker, and the last letter denotes the antitachyarrhythmia therapy. The DDD pacemaker in this patient is dual-chamber paced and dual-chamber sensed and has a dual response to sensing (ie, triggered and inhibited). On ECG, normal intrinsic P waves are visible followed by a pacer spike for QRS stimulation. The pacemaker is triggering off the intrinsic atrial activity.*

**EXPLANATION:**

(A) *Incorrect.* Pacemakers sense atrial and ventricular depolarizing activity as P and R waves, not repolarizing T waves.
(B) *Incorrect.* Retrograde P waves would have different morphology from a sinus node P wave.
(C) *Correct.* A normal P wave is followed by a pacer spike and QRS complex.
(D) *Incorrect.* With atrial pacer malfunction, one may not see P waves or a pacer spike for P waves, and atrial-ventricular synchrony would be lost.
(E) *Incorrect.* The PR interval is normal in this patient and is not consistent with premature simulation of the ventricle.

**REASONING:**

This is a challenging question because it requires interpretation of the ECG to assess pacemaker performance. The reader should review the pacemaker letter coding system to fully understand the function expected of any pacer. Besides clinical history, the ECG is good way to evaluate the pacer activity.

**BIBLIOGRAPHY:**

Barash PG, Cullen BF, Stoelting RK, Cahalan MK, Stock MC. *Clinical Anesthesia.* 6th ed. Philadelphia, PA: Lippincott Williams & Wilkins; 2001:1587-1589
Morgan GE, Mikhail MS, Murray MJ. *Clinical Anesthesiology.* 4th ed. New York, NY: McGraw-Hill; 2006:488.

## *Answer A*

### Pediatrics

**QUESTION (Choose single best answer):**

Acute epiglottitis usually

(A) Requires a lateral radiograph of the neck for diagnosis.
(B) Occurs in children 2 to 4 years of age.
(C) Is treated effectively with racemic epinephrine.
(D) Has a viral etiology.
(E) Requires immediate awake intubation by direct laryngoscopy in the emergency department.

**CORRECT ANSWER: A**

**SUMMARY:**

*Acute epiglottitis is usually caused by a bacterial infection with* Haemophilus influenzae. *It was classically seen in 2- to 6-year-old children but has now become a disease of adults since the introduction of the Hib vaccine in the 1980s. Acute epiglottitis progresses from a sore throat to dysphagia and complete airway obstruction with progressive supraglottic inflammation. A thickened epiglottis is the classic lateral radiographic finding (the classic "thumb print" finding in 73%-86%). At no time should direct laryngoscopy be attempted in an unanesthetized patient as agitation may precipitate the collapse of an already compromised airway.*

**EXPLANATION:**
(A) *Correct.* While fever, drooling, a "hot potato" voice and a preference for sitting and leaning the head forward are characteristic of acute epiglottitis especially in children, a lateral radiograph of a thickened epiglottis is diagnostic.
(B) *Incorrect.* Acute epiglottitis was formerly a disease of children but now occurs mainly in adults at a rate of 2 to 3 per 100,000 per year. The incidence in children is 0.3 to 0.6 per 100,000 per year.
(C) *Incorrect.* Racemic epinephrine is of limited usefulness in acute epiglottitis.
(D) *Incorrect.* The most common etiological agent is *H. influenzae*, although various strep and staph species have also been implicated.
(E) *Incorrect.* Only up to 20% of cases of acute epiglottitis have required an artificial airway. Impending or actual airway obstruction is treated with careful inhalation induction of general anesthesia prior to rigid bronchoscopy or endotracheal intubation. A difficult airway and the possibility of an emergent tracheostomy should be anticipated.

**REASONING:**
Answers B, C, and D are factually incorrect. Answer E is contraindicated in acute epiglottitis. This leaves only answer A.

**BIBLIOGRAPHY:**
Bansal A, Miskoff J, Lis RJ. Otolaryngological critical care. *Crit Care Clin.* 2003;19:55-72.
Miller RD, ed. *Anesthesia.* 7th ed. New York, NY: Churchill Livingstone; 2010:2375.
Morgan CG, Mikhail MS, Murray MJ. *Clinical Anesthesiology.* 4th ed. New York, NY: McGraw-Hill; 2006:943.

## QUESTION 138 (OPTIONAL)

*Answer A*

OB/Regional

**QUESTION (Choose single best answer):**

Characteristics of postdural puncture headache include

(A) Incidence unrelated to the timing of ambulation.
(B) Increased severity with addition of vasoconstrictors to the anesthetic.
(C) Less frequent occurrence if the needle bevel is perpendicular to the direction of dural fibers.
(D) More frequent occurrence in men.
(E) Prevention by prophylactic epidural blood patch.

**CORRECT ANSWER: A**

**SUMMARY:**

*Postdural puncture headache (PDPH) can occur after spinal anesthesia, inadvertent dural puncture while placing an epidural, subarachnoid migration of an epidural catheter, diagnostic lumbar puncture, and myelograms. Characterized as throbbing, the pain typically is frontal, occipital, and retroorbital and extends to the neck. Postural changes are key to the diagnosis of PDPH, with the headache worsened when assuming the upright position and relieved with lying supine. The incidence of PDPH is highest in young women, especially during pregnancy. Technical factors such as needle direction parallel to dural fibers, decreased needle size, and use of pencil point (Whitacre) rather than cutting (Qunicke) needles decrease the incidence of PDPH. Treatment ranges from conservative management with hydration and caffeine to epidural blood patch.*

**EXPLANATION:**

(A) **Correct.** There is no relationship between the timing of ambulation and incidence of PDPH.
(B) **Incorrect.** There is no evidence that the intensity of the headache is increased in patients who have had vasoconstrictors added to the spinal anesthetic.
(C) **Incorrect.** Dural fibers are longitudinal. The incidence of headache is increased if the needle bevel is perpendicular to the direction of the dural fibers. This is likely due to increased leakage of CSF with more traumatic injury to the dura.
(D) **Incorrect.** The incidence of PDPH is higher in women.
(E) **Incorrect.** Epidural blood patch is an effective treatment for PDPH in 90% of patients. In a 2004 study, prophylactic epidural blood patches reduced the duration of symptoms but had no effect on the incidence of PDPH or the need for a therapeutic blood patch.

**REASONING:**

Choices C and D can be eliminated because they are not characteristic of PDPH. There is no evidence that vasoconstrictors alter the quality of the headache, making choice B incorrect. Choice B has not been studied in isolation, but studies examining the efficacy of different local anesthetic combination do not show an increase in intensity in patients who receive epinephrine or other vasoconstrictors in the anesthetic. There is evidence that prophylactic blood patches are not effective, making E incorrect, leaving A as the best answer.

**BIBLIOGRAPHY:**

Bucklin B, Gambling DR, Wlody DJ. *A Practical Approach to Obstetric Anesthesia.* Philadelphia, PA: Lippincott Williams & Wilkins; 2009:297-305.

Chestnut DH, Polley LS, Tsen LC, Wong CA. *Chestnuts Obstetric Anesthesia.* 4th ed. Philadelphia, PA: Mosby Elsevier; 2009:677-700.

Scavone BM, Wong CA, Sullivan JT, Yaghmour E, Sherwani SS, McCarthy RJ. Efficacy of a prophylactic epidural blood patch in preventing post dural puncture headache in parturients after inadvertent dural puncture. *Anesthesiology.* 2004;101(6):1422-1427.

## Answer B

### Physiology

**QUESTION (Choose single best answer):**

Which of the following statements concerning the superior laryngeal nerve is true?

(A) It provides sensory innervation to the subglottic surface of the vocal cord.
(B) It provides sensory innervation to the inferior surface of the epiglottis.
(C) It is a branch of the glossopharyngeal nerve.
(D) It is blocked by injection of anesthetic near the lateral portion of the cricothyroid membrane.
(E) It is the most commonly injured nerve during thyroid surgery.

**CORRECT ANSWER: B**

**SUMMARY:**

*The superior laryngeal nerve (SLN) is a branch of the vagus nerve (X) that in turns arises from the middle of the ganglion nodosum. The SLN has two terminal branches: the internal and external. The internal branch is sensory and innervates the supraglottic area, including the vocal folds, aryepiglottic folds, arytenoids, base of the tongue, and epiglottis. The external branch is motor and innervates the cricothyroid muscle. This nerve is blocked by injection of local anesthetic at the thyrohyoid junction. The recurrent laryngeal nerve is also a branch of the vagus nerve (X). It has sensory innervation below the level of the vocal cords, including the trachea and controls motor function for all muscles of the larynx except the cricothyroid muscle. The recurrent laryngeal nerve is the most commonly injured nerve during thyroid surgery. If the SLN is injured bilaterally, it can cause a hoarse and tiring voice, but unilateral damage has minimal effects.*

**EXPLANATION:**

(A) *Incorrect.* The SLN provides sensory innervation to the supraglottic surface of the vocal cords.
(B) *Correct.* The internal branch of the SLN provides sensory innervation to the epiglottis.
(C) *Incorrect.* The SLN is a branch of the vagus nerve.
(D) *Incorrect.* It is blocked by injection of local anesthetic at the lateral aspect of the thyrohyoid membrane. Complications include intravascular injection of local anesthetic because the carotid sheath lies just posteriorly.
(E) *Incorrect.* The recurrent laryngeal nerve is the most commonly injured nerve during thyroid surgery.

**REASONING:**

This question tests knowledge of the differences in sensory and motor innervation between the superior and recurrent laryngeal nerves. This knowledge would eliminate choice A and make B correct. Also knowing that both these nerves are branches of the vagus would eliminate choice C. Knowledge of the anatomy of the larynx and its associated structures enables elimination of choice D. Choice E is incorrect because the recurrent laryngeal nerve is the most commonly injured. The best answer is B.


**BIBLIOGRAPHY:**

Barash PG, Cullen BF, Stoelting RK, Cahalan MK, Stock MC. *Clinical Anesthesia*. 6th ed. Philadelphia, PA: Lippincott Williams & Wilkins; 2009:775, 1318-1319.
Morgan GE, Mikhail MS, Murray MJ. *Clinical Anesthesiology*. 4th ed. New York, NY: McGraw-Hill; 2006:92-94.

*Answer D*

Pharmacology

**QUESTION (Choose single best answer):**

Which of the following is a complication of glycine used for irrigation during transurethral resection of the prostate?

(A) Epileptiform activity on EEG.
(B) Peripheral neuropathy.
(C) Tachycardia.
(D) Transient blindness.
(E) Transient deafness.

**CORRECT ANSWER: D**

**SUMMARY:**

*The use of 1.5% glycine during a transurethral resection of the prostate (TURP) procedure is common. Glycine is used as an irrigant to distend the bladder and facilitate removal of blood and dissected prostatic tissue. Glycine is inexpensive, nonelectrolytic, and slightly hypo-osmolar. Intravascular absorption may occur if the irrigating fluid pressure exceeds the venous pressure of the prostate. Absorption can be as much as 2 L or more. Absorption of large amounts of glycine can result in visual disturbances and transient blindness. This is thought to occur as a peripheral mechanism because of glycine's inhibitory neurotransmitter properties.* (See also question 35, Book B.)

**EXPLANATION:**

(A) *Incorrect.* Glycine is an inhibitory neurotransmitter.
(B) *Incorrect.* Glycine irrigation during TURP has not been associated with an increased incidence of peripheral neuropathy.
(C) *Incorrect.* This is not a common side effect of glycine irrigation.
(D) *Correct.* Glycine toxicity is a known cause of visual disturbances and transient blindness.
(E) *Incorrect.* Hyperglycinemia can result in visual disturbances but not deafness.

**REASONING:**

This question tests knowledge of the toxicity of glycine used as an irrigant for TURP. In addition to transient blindness, glycine also is associated with ammonia toxicity. Ammonia is a major by-product of the oxidative metabolism of glycine. Elevated ammonia levels can result in nausea and vomiting, negative hemodynamic changes, and decreased mental status to include coma that can last 24 to 48 hours. Absorption of irrigant depends on the duration of resection and the pressure of the irrigation. D is the best answer.

**BIBLIOGRAPHY:**

Barash PG, Cullen BF, Stoelting RK, Cahalan MK, Stock MC. *Clinical Anesthesia.* 6th ed. Philadelphia, PA: Lippincott Williams & Wilkins; 2009:1365.
Morgan GE, Mikhail MS, Murray MJ. *Clinical Anesthesiology.* 4th ed. New York, NY: McGraw-Hill; 2006:760-761.

# QUESTION 141

*Answer C*

Equipment/Physics

**QUESTION (Choose single best answer):**

In the event of a leak in the air flowmeter, which flowmeter arrangement produces the lowest risk for delivering hypoxic gas mixtures?

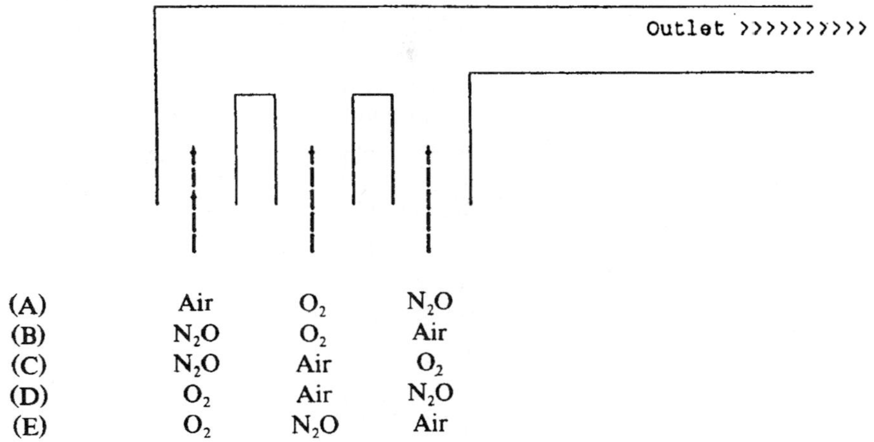


| | | | |
|---|---|---|---|
| (A) | Air | $O_2$ | $N_2O$ |
| (B) | $N_2O$ | $O_2$ | Air |
| (C) | $N_2O$ | Air | $O_2$ |
| (D) | $O_2$ | Air | $N_2O$ |
| (E) | $O_2$ | $N_2O$ | Air |

**CORRECT ANSWER: C**

**SUMMARY:**

*In the presence of a flowmeter leak, especially that involving the air flowmeter, a hypoxic mixture is less likely to occur if the oxygen flowmeter is downstream from all other flowmeters.*

**EXPLANATION:**

(A) *Incorrect.* Nitrous oxide is downstream; oxygen flow passing through the leak results in a greater proportion of nitrous oxide being delivered to the outlet.

(B) *Incorrect.* Oxygen is upstream from the leak, and thus some oxygen flow can pass through the leak, increasing the risk of a hypoxic mixture being delivered to the outlet.

(C) *Correct.* Oxygen is downstream; a portion of nitrous oxide flow passes through air leak, and the remainder advances the entire oxygen flow to the outlet.

(D) *Incorrect.* Nitrous oxide is downstream to all other flowmeters; oxygen flow passing through the leak results in a greater proportion of nitrous oxide being delivered to the outlet.

(E) *Incorrect.* Nitrous oxide is downstream to oxygen, and both are upstream from the leak. Therefore, there is a relatively lower concentration of oxygen in the final gas mixture at the outlet.

**REASONING:**

The key to answering this question correctly is identifying choice C as the only correct option because it places the oxygen flowmeter the farthest downstream and closest to the gas outlet.

**BIBLIOGRAPHY:**

Barash PG, Cullen BF, Stoelting RK, Cahalan MK, Stock MC. *Clinical Anesthesia.* 6th ed. Philadelphia, PA: Lippincott Williams & Wilkins; 2009:657-658.

Eger EI, Hylton RR, Irwin RH, Guadagni N. Anesthetic flowmeter sequence—a cause for hypoxia. *Anesthesiology.* 1963;24:396.

Morgan GE, Mikhail MS, Murray MJ. *Clinical Anesthesiology.* 4th ed. New York, NY: McGraw-Hill; 2006:58-59.

## Answer D

### Neuroanesthesia

**QUESTION (Choose single best answer):**

A 100-kg, 42-year-old woman received enflurane and oxygen for clipping of an intracranial aneurysm lasting 8 hours. In the first 2 postoperative hours, urine output is 2 L. Serum sodium concentration is 152 mEq/L. Urine osmolarity and central venous pressure are low. Which of the following is best used to establish the diagnosis?

(A) Pulmonary artery occlusion pressure.
(B) Serum fluoride concentration.
(C) Serum osmolarity.
(D) Response to antidiuretic hormone.
(E) Response to fluid restriction.

**CORRECT ANSWER: D**

**SUMMARY:**

*Alterations in sodium homeostasis can be seen after neurosurgery, resulting in disturbances such as central diabetes insipidus (DI), syndrome of inappropriate antidiuretic hormone secretion (SIADH), or cerebral salt-wasting syndrome. Central DI is commonly seen as a transient event after neurosurgery or cranial trauma, resulting in hypernatremia, low urine osmolarity, and polyuria. Diagnosis of central DI (as opposed to nephrogenic DI) is made by an increasing urine osmolarity with antidiuretic hormone (ADH) therapy. Enflurane is no longer used clinically but is metabolized by the CYP450 2E1 enzymes to inorganic fluoride, which can impair urine concentrating ability transiently with fluoride levels decreasing rapidly postoperatively, whereas methoxyflurane (also no longer used) was well known to cause dose-dependent polyuric renal failure and nephrogenic DI with fluoride levels above 50 μmol/L.*

**EXPLANATION:**

(A) *Incorrect.* Pulmonary artery occlusion pressure would not be useful in differentiating central versus nephrogenic DI in this case, but it may prove helpful in further evaluation of the patient's volume status if her clinical picture worsened.

(B) *Incorrect.* This was the correct ASA answer in 1993 but is not the best test to establish this patient's diagnosis. Long anesthetics using enflurane in obese patients have been associated with elevated inorganic serum fluoride levels, but no cases of renal dysfunction were noted. Therefore serum fluoride concentration is of little clinical utility because nephrogenic DI from enflurane has not been described, but was historically seen with methoxyflurane.

(C) *Incorrect.* Serum osmolarity can play a role in diagnosing DI (urine osmolarity < serum osmolarity); however, the triad of postoperative polyuria, hypernatremia, and low urine osmolarity in the setting of neurosurgery point to DI and warrant a trial of ADH to differentiate central from nephrogenic causes.

(D) *Correct.* ADH (or an ADH analogue such as DDAVP) is the best test to distinguish central from nephrogenic DI in this patient, as it will improve urine osmolarity in the former and will not change urine osmolarity in the latter.

(E) *Incorrect.* Fluid and water restriction are important in diagnosis and treatment of SIADH, which can been after neurosurgery or hypothalamic lesions and would present with hyponatremia and elevated urine osmolarity, which are not present in this patient.

**REASONING:**

This question is challenging because the noted ASA answer from 1993 was choice B. While transient elevation of serum organic fluoride has been seen with sevoflurane and enflurane anesthetics, it does not necessarily cause renal dysfunction. Therefore, measuring serum fluoride concentration does nothing to distinguish whether this patient's DI is central or renal in etiology. Choices A and E can be easily eliminated. Choice C is challenging because serum osmolarity is part of the DI workup, but not the best test. Therefore, choice D provides both a diagnostic and potentially therapeutic maneuver with ADH to increase urine osmolarity.

**BIBLIOGRAPHY:**

Miller RD, Eriksson LI, Fleisher LA, Wiener-Kronish JP, Young WL. *Miller's Anesthesia.* 7th ed. Philadelphia, PA: Churchill Livingstone; 2010:641, 650, 1707-1709, 2062-2063.

Morgan CG, Mikhail MS, Murray MJ. *Clinical Anesthesiology.* 4th ed. New York, NY: McGraw-Hill; 2006:670, 735.

---

| **BOOK A:** | **QUESTION 143** |
| --- | --- |

## *Answer C*

### Neuroanesthesia

**QUESTION (Choose single best answer):**

The drug that causes does-dependent EEG evidence of both central nervous system excitation and depression is

(A) Lidocaine.
(B) Halothane.
(C) Thiopental.
(D) Nitrous oxide.
(E) Midazolam.

**CORRECT ANSWER: C**

**SUMMARY:**

*EEG monitoring is useful during neurosurgical procedures and can be used in all surgical procedures to assess depth of anesthesia. Anesthetic agents have variable effects on the EEG ranging from activation to depression; most anesthetics initially produce a pattern of activation at subanesthetic doses, followed by a dose-dependent depression of the EEG signal at higher doses (ie, a biphasic pattern). Barbiturates, propofol, and etomidate are the only intravenous agents that induce both burst suppression and electrical silence at high doses. Halothane produces a typical biphasic pattern, while nitrous oxide produces an increase in both frequency and amplitude at escalating doses (high-amplitude activation). Benzodiazepines, such as most anesthetics, produce a typical biphasic pattern; they are unable to produce burst suppression or an isoelectric EEG.*

**EXPLANATION:**

(A) *Incorrect.* Lidocaine toxicity can ultimately manifest as seizures, and thus does not produce both CNS excitation and depression at higher doses.

(B) *Incorrect.* Halothane produces a typical biphasic pattern on the EEG.

(C) *Correct.* Thiopental produces both excitation and depression in a dose-dependent manner, with periods of burst suppression at higher doses, followed by eventual electrical silence at even higher doses.

(D) *Incorrect.* Nitrous oxide produces an increase in both amplitude and frequency at higher doses.

(E) *Incorrect.* Midazolam produces a typical biphasic pattern on the EEG.


### REASONING:

This question tests knowledge of the effects of common anesthetic agents on EEG signals. It is important to understand that the question asks for the drug that causes both activation and depression in a dose-dependent manner (as opposed to a drug that causes activation followed by depression in a dose-dependent manner, ie, the typical biphasic pattern). Both halothane and midazolam are typical, so they can be eliminated. Nitrous oxide only produces high-amplitude activation, so it too can be eliminated. Lidocaine does not induce the pattern of EEG changes that this question refers to. We are left with thiopental, which does cause dose-dependent activation and depression on the EEG. C is the best answer.


### BIBLIOGRAPHY:

Miller RD, Eriksson LI, Fleisher LA, Wiener-Kronish JP, Young WL. *Miller's Anesthesia.* 7th ed. Philadelphia, PA: Churchill Livingstone; 2010:1499-1502.

Morgan GE, Mikhail MS, Murray MJ. *Clinical Anesthesiology.* 4th ed. New York, NY: McGraw-Hill; 2006:624-626.

Stoelting RK, Hillier SC. *Pharmacology & Physiology in Anesthetic Practice.* 4th ed. Philadelphia, PA: Lippincott Williams & Wilkins; 2006:47, 136, 141.

Turcant A, Delhumeau A, Premel-Cabic A, et al. Thiopental pharmacokinetics under conditions of long-term infusion. *Anesthesiology.* 1985;63:50-54.

Yamamura T, Fukuda M, Takeya H, Goto Y, Furukawa K. Fast oscillatory EEG activity induced by analgesic concentrations of nitrous oxide in man. *Anesth Analg.* 1981;60: 283-288.

---

**BOOK A:**　　　　**QUESTION 144**

---

*Answer A*

Physiology

**QUESTION (Choose single best answer):**

Which of the following findings differentiates the pickwickian syndrome from morbid obesity?

(A) Carbon dioxide retention.
(B) Upper airway obstruction.
(C) Decreased forced expiratory volume.
(D) Increased shunt fraction.
(E) Increased FRC.


**CORRECT ANSWER: A**


### SUMMARY:

*Obesity is a growing epidemic in the United States. Approximately 27% of the US population is obese (body mass index [BMI] $\geq$ 30 kg/m$^2$). Obesity is associated with many diseases and has special physiologic consequences and anesthetic implications. Changes in respiratory physiology associated with obesity include increased oxygen demand and consumption, work of breathing, decreased lung volume and capacity, increased $CO_2$ production even at rest, decreased chest wall compliance, decreased FRC, mismatch, and hypoxemia. A special subset of morbidly obese patients have pickwickian syndrome also* *called* obesity-hypoventilation syndrome *(OSH). First described by Charles Dickens as a condition afflicting the character "Fat Boy" in his serial "The Pickwick Papers" published between 1836 and 1837, pickwickian syndrome is characterized by awake chronic hypoxemia with* $Pa_{O_2}$ *less than 65 without a diagnosis of COPD or other primary lung disease. These patients also have BMI of greater than 20 kg/m² and an awake* $P_{CO_2}$ *greater than 45. Chronic hypoventilation from obstructive sleep apnea leads to chronic hypoxemia and hypercarbia. Other associated findings can include impaired central ventilatory drive, cyanosis-induced polycythemia, daytime hypersomnolence, pulmonary hypertension, cor pulmonale, and eventual biventricular failure.*

<table>
<tr><td colspan="3" align="center">Simplified Comparison of Obstructive Sleep Apnea (OSA) and Obesity Hypoventilation Syndrome (OHS) Parameters</td></tr>
<tr><td>Parameter</td><td>OHS</td><td>OSA</td></tr>
<tr><td>Gender distribution</td><td>Males = females</td><td>Males > females</td></tr>
<tr><td>Obesity (BMI ≥ 30 kg/m²)</td><td>Yes</td><td>Maybe (risk increases with obesity)</td></tr>
<tr><td>Ventilation pattern</td><td>Hypoventilation</td><td>Normal (except during apnea)</td></tr>
<tr><td>$Pa_{CO_2}$ (mm Hg)</td><td>Increased (> 45 mm Hg)</td><td>Normal (increased during apnea)</td></tr>
<tr><td>$Pa_{O_2}$ (mm Hg)</td><td>Decreased; most severe during REM sleep</td><td>Normal (decreased during apnea)</td></tr>
<tr><td>$Sa_{O_2}$ (%)</td><td>Decreased</td><td>Normal (decreased during apnea)</td></tr>
<tr><td>Nocturnal upper airway obstruction</td><td>No (except with coexisting OSA)</td><td>Yes; choking or gasping during sleep</td></tr>
<tr><td>Recurrent awakenings from sleep</td><td>No</td><td>Yes</td></tr>
<tr><td>Pulmonary hypertension</td><td>More common and more severe</td><td>Less common</td></tr>
<tr><td>Nocturnal monitoring</td><td>Increased $Pa_{CO_2}$ during sleep to > 10 mm Hg from awake supine values. $O_2$ desaturation during sleep not explained by apnea or hypopnea</td><td>≥ 5 obstructive breathing events per hour of sleep</td></tr>
</table>

BMI, body mass index; REM, rapid eye movement.

## EXPLANATION:

(A) **Correct.** Pickwickian syndrome is uniquely characterized by carbon dioxide retention.

(B) **Incorrect.** Upper airway obstruction can be present with both morbid obesity and pickwickian syndrome.

(C) **Incorrect.** Both can cause decreased forced expiratory volume.

(D) **Incorrect.** Both can cause an increased shunt fraction.

(E) **Incorrect.** Decreased FRC is a characteristic of both morbid obesity and pickwickian syndrome.

## REASONING:

This question tests knowledge of the pathophysiology of morbid obesity and pickwickian syndrome. Morbidly obese patients with pickwickian syndrome develop chronic hypoxemia and hypercarbia owing to alveolar hypoventilation (unlike the classic morbidly obese patient with normocarbia and alveolar hyperventilation). This knowledge leads to choice A as the correct answer. Choices B through D are common to both disorders and can be eliminated. Finally, decreased, not increased, FRC is a feature of both disorders. The best answer is A.


**BIBLIOGRAPHY:**

Barash PG, Cullen BF, Stoelting RK, Cahalan MK, Stock MC. *Clinical Anesthesia.* 6th ed. Philadelphia, PA: Lippincott Williams & Wilkins; 2009:1230-1233, 1234 (Table 47-4).

Dickens C. *The Pickwick Papers.* New York, NY: Penguin Books; 2000. [Originally published in serial form between 1836 and 1837.]

Miller RD, Miller ED, Reves JG, et al. *Anesthesia.* 7th ed. New York, NY: Churchill Livingstone; 2009:1030.

Morgan GE, Mikhail MS, Murray MJ. *Clinical Anesthesiology.* 4th ed. New York, NY: McGraw-Hill; 2006:813-814.

Yanovski SZ, Yanovski JA. Obesity. *N Engl J Med.* 2002;346(8):591-602.


---

**BOOK A:** **QUESTION 145**

---

*Answer B*

OB/Regional

**QUESTION (Choose single best answer):**

Which of the following is the most likely sequela of interscalene brachial plexus block?

(A) Cervical epidural block.
(B) Hemidiaphragmatic paralysis.
(C) Pneumothorax.
(D) Seizure.
(E) Vocal cord paralysis.

**CORRECT ANSWER: B**

**SUMMARY:**

*The interscalene brachial plexus block is most commonly used for shoulder procedures, targeting the plexus at the level of the upper and middle trunks. Because of the proximity of structures such as the stellate ganglion, phrenic nerve, lung pleura, spinal nerve roots, recurrent laryngeal nerve, and vertebral artery, complications can sometimes arise. The most likely sequelae of interscalene block is ipsilateral phrenic nerve blockade with resultant hemidiaphragmatic paresis in 100% of blocks as local anesthetic spreads anteriorly over the anterior scalene muscle. This universally expected outcome can reduce pulmonary function in some patients by 25%, which may not be tolerated in those with poor baseline function. Pneumothorax, direct intra-arterial injection, recurrent laryngeal nerve or epidural block, and neuritis are all rare events. A recent prospective randomized controlled trial using low-volume ropivacaine interscalene brachial plexus block significantly reduced the incidence of diaphragmatic paresis with ultrasound-guided block compared to nerve stimulator-guided block.*

**EXPLANATION:**

(A) *Incorrect.* Cervical epidural, subdural, or subarachnoid blocks are all rare following interscalene brachial plexus block, but they can occur because both the neural foramina and nerve roots are close to the site of local anesthetic injection.

(B) *Correct.* Ipsilateral hemidiaphragmatic paresis occurs in 100% of these blocks. Patients can complain of dyspnea and those with poor baseline lung function are at risk for respiratory failure.

(C) *Incorrect.* Pneumothorax is a rare complication after interscalene block, occurring when the needle is advanced to far laterally and the pleural dome is entered.

(D) *Incorrect.* Seizure, either from direct arterial injection into the vertebral artery or from systemic absorption of local anesthetic is indeed a rare occurrence with interscalene block.

(E) *Incorrect.* Vocal cord paralysis, a rare outcome after interscalene block, is due to local block of the ipsilateral recurrent laryngeal nerve, which may result in hoarseness.

### REASONING:

The key to answering this question correctly is distinguishing the rare complications of interscalene brachial plexus block from the normally expected outcomes. As it is well known that ipsilateral hemidiaphragmatic paresis occurs in all of these blocks, choice B is the clear answer. Epidural block, pneumothorax, seizures, and vocal cord paralysis all occur rarely.

### BIBLIOGRAPHY:


Miller RD, Eriksson LI, Fleisher LA, Wiener-Kronish JP, Young WL. *Miller's Anesthesia.* 7th ed. Philadelphia, PA: Churchill Livingstone; 2010:1640-1643.

Morgan CG, Mikhail MS, Murray MJ. *Clinical Anesthesiology.* 4th ed. New York, NY: McGraw-Hill; 2006:331-332.

Renes SH, Rettig HC, Gielen MJ, Wilder-Smith OH, van Geffen GJ. Ultrasound-guided low-dose interscalene brachial plexus block reduces the incidence of hemidiaphragmatic paresis. *Reg Anesth Pain Med.* 2009;34:498-502.


---

## BOOK A:  QUESTION 146

### *Answer B*

Physiology

### QUESTION (Choose single best answer):

Which of the following is the most reliable indicator of adequate reversal of neuromuscular block?

(A) Inspiratory force equal to $-30$ cmH$_2$O.
(B) Sustained head lift for 5 seconds.
(C) Train-of-four ratio of 0.7.
(D) Twitch height at 100% of control.
(E) Vital capacity of 15 mL/kg.

### CORRECT ANSWER: B

### SUMMARY:

*The correct answer for this question appears to have stemmed from a seminal paper by Pavlin and colleagues in 1989, who exposed a cohort of healthy unanesthetized volunteers to partial neuromuscular blockade with D-tubocurarine. They examined the correlation between a range of maximum inspiratory pressures (MIPs) that gradually diminished with increasing paralysis and various clinical outcome measures such as vital capacity (VC), hand grip strength, and functional assessment of the muscles of airway protection. They found that while an MIP of $-25$ cmH$_2$O was adequate to prevent hypoventilation, but that the MIP50 for return of protective airway muscles was $-42$ cmH$_2$O. They then showed that the MIP50 for a 5-second head lift was $-53$ cmH$_2$O and therefore concluded that the ability to sustain a head lift for 5 seconds was the most sensitive indicator of residual muscle paresis. (Note: Since the initial examination in 1993, the most reliable indicator has been no longer a sustained head lift; see explanation as follows.)*

## EXPLANATION:

(A) *Incorrect.* While an MIP of −30 cmH$_2$O may be sufficient to ensure adequate ventilation, it does not ensure return of adequate protective airway muscle function necessary to prevent aspiration.

(B) *Correct.* Miller originally reported the 5-second head lift as the most sensitive indicator of residual neuromuscular blockade. Pavlin and colleagues went on to show that the MIP50 for a 5-second head lift is −53 cmH$_2$O. This is a more negative inspiratory pressure than the MIP50 of −43 cmH$_2$O associated with return of muscles of airway protection.

(C) *Incorrect.* The train-of-four (TOF) ratio of 0.7 has been associated with decreased grip strength, decreased pharyngeal muscle tone, and inability to sit up without assistance. In addition, decreased upper esophageal pressures and laryngeal aspiration have been detected at TOF ratios of less than 0.9.

(D) *Incorrect.* The twitch height can be at 100% of baseline but could demonstrate significant fade that would indicate residual paralysis.

(E) *Incorrect.* Normal VC is approximately 60 mg/kg and is reduced with ventilatory muscle weakness. This VC is approximately 25% of normal and does not indicate adequate reversal of neuromuscular blockade. Pavlin and colleagues found that an MIP of −38 cmH$_2$O corresponds to a VC that is 77% of control. This observation implies that a patient can have a VC almost 80% of normal and still have inadequate muscle strength to protect the airway.


## REASONING:

This question tests knowledge of clinical indicators of adequate reversal of neuromuscular blockade. The best answer from the choices given stems from the seminal work of Pavlin and colleagues as mentioned above. It is important to note, however, that since the publication of the first edition (1993), Eriksson and colleagues demonstrated that a TOF ratio of greater than 0.9 was required to prevent laryngeal aspiration and for full return of upper airway function. The target for TOF ratio has been thus moved up to more than 0.9. That same year Kopman et al showed that a sustained head lift is associated with an average TOF ratio of 0.6, indicating that the sustained head lift is not the most reliable indicator of residual neuromuscular blockade. Subsequently, fade with 100-Hz tetanic stimulation was shown to be detectable at TOF ratios of 0.8 to 0.9, making 100-Hz tetanic stimulation the current most sensitive test for residual neuromuscular blockade.


## BIBLIOGRAPHY:


Barash PG, Cullen BF, Stoelting RK, Calahan M, Stock MC. *Clinical Anesthesia*. 6th ed. Philadelphia, PA: Lippincott Williams & Wilkins; 2009:522-523.

Capron F, Fortier LP, Racine S, et al. Tactile fade detection with hand or wrist stimulation using train-of-four, double-burst stimulation, 50-hertz tetanus, 100-hertz tetanus, and acceleromyography. *Anesth Analg*. 2006;102:1578.

Eriksson LI, Sundman E, Olsson R, et al. Functional assessment of the pharynx at rest and during swallowing in partially paralyzed humans:simultaneous videomanometry and mechanomyography of awake human volunteers. *Anesthesiology*. 1997;87:1035.

Kopman AF, Yee PS, Neuman GG. Relationship of the train-of-four fade ratio to clinical signs and symptoms of residual paralysis in awake volunteers. *Anesthesiology*. 1997;86(4):765-771.

Miller RD. Antagonism of neuromuscular blockade. *Anesthesiology*. 1976;44:318-329.

Miller RD. How should residual neuromuscular blockade be detected? *Anesthesiology*. 1989;70:379-380.

Morgan GE, Mikhail MS, Murray MJ. *Clinical Anesthesiology*. 4th ed. New York, NY: McGraw-Hill; 2006:230-231.

Pavlin EG, Holle RH, Schoene RB. Recovery of airway protection compared with ventilation in humans after paralysis with curare. *Anesthesiology*. 1989;70:381-385.

*Answer D*

Physiology

**QUESTION (Choose single best answer):**

A 25-year-old man requires exploratory laparotomy following a motor vehicle accident. He is acutely intoxicated with alcohol. Which of the following is the most likely result of the alcohol ingestion?

(A) Hyperdynamic circulation.
(B) Hyperglycemia.
(C) Hyperthermia.
(D) Increased respiratory depression from opioids.
(E) Increased sensitivity to neuromuscular blocking drugs.

**CORRECT ANSWER: D**

**SUMMARY:**

*The anesthetic implications of alcohol depend on the acuity of its use. Chronic use of alcohol often has end-organ effects such as hyperdynamic circulation, hypoglycemia, increased MAC requirements, increased depressant effects of opioids, and a resistance to neuromuscular blockade. Acute intoxication lowers MAC and can synergize with other depressant drugs such as opioids by decreasing hepatic blood flow and affecting clearance of drugs.*

**EXPLANATION:**

(A) *Incorrect.* Chronic not acute alcohol usage results in a hyperdynamic circulation and elevated cardiac output.
(B) *Incorrect.* Hypoglycemia is a consequence of chronic alcohol use.
(C) *Incorrect.* Hyperthermia is not a known consequence of either chronic or acute alcohol ingestion. If anything, hypothermia is a more likely consequence of alcohol intoxication (eg, due to unplanned physical exposure to environmental elements). Nutritional disorders from chronic alcoholism can also lead to hypothermia.
(D) *Correct.* Acute alcohol intoxication can synergize with opioids, resulting in increased respiratory depression.
(E) *Incorrect.* Chronic alcohol use results in resistance to neuromuscular blockers. It can lead also to alcoholic polyneuropathy. It is important to recall that cirrhosis and advanced liver disease can reduce elimination of vecuronium, rocuronium and mivacurium and result in a prolonged duration of neuromuscular blockade.

**REASONING:**

This question tests knowledge of the physiologic differences between acute and chronic alcohol ingestion. Choices B, C, and E can be eliminated because they are not associated with alcohol ingestion. Choice A is a consequence of chronic use, so it also can be eliminated. Choice D remains and is by default the correct answer. Interestingly, acute alcohol intoxication causes respiratory depression by synergizing with opioids, whereas chronic use can cause respiratory depression by impairing the elimination of opioids.

**BIBLIOGRAPHY:**
Barash PG, Cullen BF, Stoelting RK, Cahalan MK, Stock MC. *Clinical Anesthesia.* 6th ed. Philadelphia, PA: Lippincott Williams & Wilkins; 2009:918.
Faust RJ. *Anesthesiology Review.* 3rd ed. New York, NY: Churchill Livingstone; 2002:523-524.

Miller RD, Miller ED, Reves JG, et al. *Anesthesia*. 7th ed. New York, NY: Churchill Livingstone; 2009:1114, 2139-2140.

Morgan GE, Mikhail MS, Murray MJ. *Clinical Anesthesiology*. 4th ed. New York, NY: McGraw-Hill; 2006:659.

| BOOK A: | QUESTION 148 |
|---|---|

*Answer A*

Pharmacology

**QUESTION (Choose single best answer):**

The decreased duration of action of an intravenous dose of fentanyl compared with an intravenous dose of morphine is best explained by

(A) Greater lipid solubility.
(B) Increased hepatic metabolism.
(C) Less protein binding.
(D) Shorter elimination half-life.
(E) Smaller volume of distribution.

**CORRECT ANSWER: A**

**SUMMARY:**

*Both fentanyl and morphine are used commonly for perioperative analgesia. Compared with morphine, fentanyl has a characteristically shorter onset and duration of action. Fentanyl has a much greater lipid solubility. This accounts for both its rapid onset and offset. Fentanyl has a greater fat solubility than morphine which allows to pass the blood-brain barrier quicker. Elimination from these central tissues (brain, heart, and lung) is also rapid because fentanyl distributes to other tissues such as muscle and fat. Compared with morphine, fentanyl has more protein binding and a larger volume of distribution. Both morphine and fentanyl have similar hepatic metabolism.*

**EXPLANATION:**

(A) ***Correct.*** Fentanyl does have a greater lipid solubility than morphine. This explains its rapid onset and decreased duration of action. Redistribution of fentanyl to muscle and fat compartments occurs rapidly and is responsible for its short duration of action.

(B) ***Incorrect.*** Both fentanyl and morphine have an equal degree of hepatic metabolism.

(C) ***Incorrect.*** Fentanyl (84% significantly to red blood cells) has more protein binding compared with morphine (35%).

(D) ***Incorrect.*** Fentanyl actually has a somewhat longer-elimination half-life than morphine (3.1-6.6 vs 1.7-3.3 hours). However, fentanyl has faster initial redistribution to muscle and fat compartments compared with morphine. This explains its shorter duration of action.

(E) ***Incorrect.*** Fentanyl has a larger volume of distribution than morphine (335 vs 224 L).

**REASONING:**

This question tests knowledge of the pharmacokinetic differences between fentanyl and morphine. Realizing that both fentanyl and morphine have equal hepatic metabolism eliminates choice B. Compared with morphine, fentanyl has more protein binding, a longer-elimination half-life, and a larger volume of distribution. This eliminates choices C through E as potential answers. It is important to understand that fentanyl's short duration of action is due to its rapid distribution phase compared with morphine. A is the best answer.

**BIBLIOGRAPHY:**
Barash PG, Cullen BF, Stoelting RK, Cahalan MK, Stock MC. *Clinical Anesthesia.* 6th ed. Philadelphia, PA: Lippincott Williams & Wilkins; 2009:476-479.
Morgan GE, Mikhail MS, Murray MJ. *Clinical Anesthesiology.* 4th ed. New York, NY: McGraw-Hill; 2006:196-197.

**BOOK A:**

*Answer D*

Pediatrics

## QUESTION 149 (OPTIONAL)

**QUESTION (Choose single best answer):**

Which of the following complications of caudal anesthesia with 0.25% bupivacaine is more likely in children than in adults?

(A) Intravascular injection.
(B) Neurotoxicity.
(C) Profound motor block.
(D) Systemic toxicity.
(E) Total spinal block.

**CORRECT ANSWER: D**

**SUMMARY:**

*Caudal anesthesia is a common and valuable regional technique in infants and children. While the potential for inadvertent intrathecal or intravenous injection is always present, the overall rate of complications of pediatric caudal anesthesia is low. Intravascular injection does not occur at a higher rate in children compared with adults, but lower protein binding leading to a greater free fraction of bupivacaine in children younger than 6 months puts these patients at increased risk for systemic toxicity.*

**EXPLANATION:**

(A) *Incorrect.* The risk of intravascular injection should not be increased in pediatric patients. A negative aspiration for blood should precede injection of local anesthetic.

(B) *Incorrect.* Local anesthetics readily cross the blood-brain barrier. Therefore, the risk of CNS toxicity should be the same in adults and children.

(C) *Incorrect.* In a study of 750 caudal anesthetics, the incidence of motor block in children following caudal anesthesia with 0.25% bupivacaine was 54%. There have been no studies demonstrating a greater rate of motor block in children compared with adults using the same concentration and milligram per kilogram dose of local anesthetic. The incidence of motor block is lower using concentrations of less than 0.25%.

(D) *Correct.* After intercostal blocks, caudal blocks result in the highest-peak plasma levels of local anesthetic. All caudal dosing is weight based, and toxicity is a very rare complication in the pediatric complication. However, owing to lower plasma binding secondary to decreased $\alpha_1$ glycoprotein and albumin, children develop a greater free fraction of drug and more potential for systemic toxicity compared with adults at the same milligram per kilogram dose. In short, there is a narrower toxicity window in children than in adults.

(E) *Incorrect.* Although the distance to the intrathecal space is more superficial in children, children have not been shown to have a greater risk of total spinal block. Injection of local anesthetic should take place only after a negative aspiration for CSF. Some clinicians advocate the administration of a test dose, whereas others simply dose the caudal incrementally. The lower end of the dural sac is at S1 in both adults and children (S3 in neonates), therefore making the risk of dural puncture the same in each population.

**REASONING:**
This is a very challenging question and we had a difficult time finding supporting evidence. Few studies have been done to compare the same regional technique in adults and children. Because the overall rate of complications of caudal anesthesia is low, it is difficult to show a significant difference in complication rates. While the dura is more superficial, the sacral hiatus is also easier to identify in children. The only difference between children and adults about a given dose of bupivacaine is a greater free fraction of drug that puts children at higher risk of systemic toxicity.

**BIBLIOGRAPHY:**
Barash PG, Cullen BF, Stoelting RK, Cahalan MK, Stock MC. *Clinical Anesthesia.* 6th ed. Philadelphia, PA: Lippincott Williams & Wilkins; 2010:1218.
Cote CJ, Ryan JF, Todres ID, Goudsouzian NG, eds. *A Practice of Anesthesia for Infants and Children.* 2nd ed. Philadelphia, PA: Saunders; 1993:430-433, 464-466.
Morgan GE, Mikhail MS, Murray MJ. *Clinical Anesthesiology.* 4th ed. New York, NY: McGraw-Hill; 2006:314-316, 937.

---

**BOOK A:**　　　　　**QUESTION 150**

*Answer B*

OB/Regional

**QUESTION (Choose single best answer):**

After an axillary brachial plexus block, the patient feels pain when the surgeon clips the skin over the thenar eminence. The most likely cause is inadequate anesthesia in the distribution of the

(A) Intercostobrachial nerve.
(B) Median nerve.
(C) Musculocutaneous nerve.
(D) Radial nerve.
(E) Ulnar nerve.

**CORRECT ANSWER: B**

**SUMMARY:**

*A complete understanding of brachial plexus anatomy and patterns of innervation is important for the application of this block in clinical practice. Axillary brachial plexus blocks are useful for surgery of the elbow, forearm, and hand with the primary targets of the median, ulnar, and radial nerves. The musculocutaneous nerve needs to be blocked separately. There are various approaches to the axillary block, which include nerve stimulation or ultrasound guidance. The brachial plexus classically arises from the anterior primary rami C5-C8 and T1 spinal nerves. It has five roots, three trunks, six divisions, three cords, and five major terminal nerves. The terminal nerves are median, ulnar, radial, axillary and musculocutaneous. A potential complication of an axillary block is failure to block the median nerve. The median nerve is derived from the lateral and medial cords of the brachial plexus. It runs medial to the brachial artery and the insertion of the biceps tendon at the level of the elbow. The median nerve provides sensory innervation to most of the palmer surface of the hand, including the thenar eminence.*

**EXPLANATION:**
(A) *Incorrect.* The intercostobrachial nerve provides sensory innervation to the medial aspect of the arm, not the hand.
(B) *Correct.* The median nerve typically supplies the palmar surface of the thumb, second, third, and half of the fourth fingers. This includes the thenar eminence of the hand and is a common cause of a failed axillary block.

(C) *Incorrect.* The musculocutaneous nerve supplies the lateral half of the forearm.
(D) *Incorrect.* The radial nerve typically supplies the lateral aspect of the lower arm, a middle strip on the posterior forearm, and most of the posterior aspect of the hand from thumb to third finger.
(E) *Incorrect.* The ulnar nerve typically supplies about half of the fourth finger and the fifth finger on the dorsal and palmer surfaces but not the thenar eminence.

### REASONING:

This question tests knowledge of the sensory innervation of the brachial plexus. A complete knowledge of upper extremity innervation is required to eliminate wrong answers. The reader should review this information carefully because it is commonly tested. Choices A and C can be eliminated because they supply the arm/forearm and not the hand. Choice E can be eliminated because, although it does have palmer innervation, it does not supply the thenar eminence. Choice D can be eliminated because, although it does supply some of the thenar eminence, it does not supply the bulk of it. The median nerve supplies this distribution, and B is the best answer.

### BIBLIOGRAPHY:


Barash PG, Cullen BF, Stoelting RK, Cahalan MK, Stock MC. *Clinical Anesthesia.* 6th ed. Philadelphia, PA: Lippincott Williams & Wilkins; 2009:969-976, 969 (Figure 38-12), 970 (Figure 38-14).

Morgan GE, Mikhail MS, Murray MJ. *Clinical Anesthesiology.* 4th ed. New York, NY: McGraw-Hill; 2006:335-337.


---

**BOOK A:**  **QUESTION 151**

---

*Answer E*

Equipment/Physics

**QUESTION (Choose single best answer):**

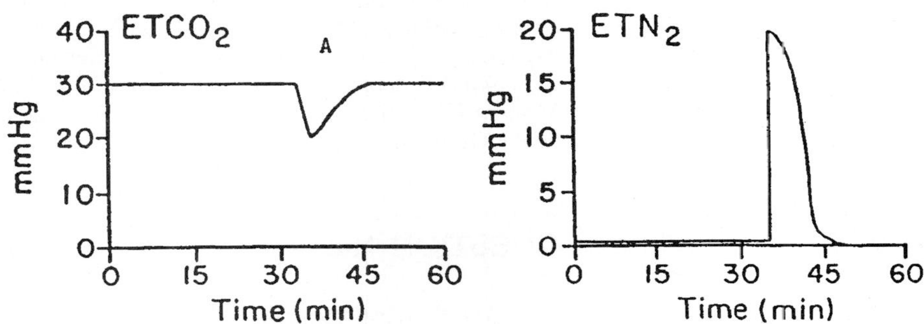


This trend plot above shows end-tidal gases measured during a radical neck dissection. The event occurring at *A* is most likely

(A) Acute hypotension.
(B) Endobronchial intubation.
(C) Kinking of the endotracheal tube.
(D) Rupture of the endotracheal tube cuff.
(E) Venous air embolism.

### CORRECT ANSWER: E

### SUMMARY:

*Analysis of expired gases in an anesthetized patient can provide valuable clinical information. In addition to confirming endotracheal intubation, it also provides information on expired anesthetic concentration and the amount of expired oxygen and carbon dioxide. A sudden increase in expired nitrogen is highly specific for detecting the presence of air embolism, although it is somewhat less sensitive than a decrease in expired carbon dioxide for the detection of subclinical air embolism. Measurement of expired nitrogen also enables the volume of the air embolism to be calculated.*

**EXPLANATION:**

(A) *Incorrect.* Acute hypotension can cause a sudden drop in $ETCO_2$ owing to increased dead space ventilation from decreased perfusion of the lung. However, it would not be associated with an increase in expired nitrogen.

(B) *Incorrect.* Endobronchial intubation would not cause a change in $ETCO_2$, especially an acute drop. It also would not be associated with an increase in expired nitrogen.

(C) *Incorrect.* Kinking of the endotracheal tube might cause a decreased $ETCO_2$, but it would not be associated with an increase in expired nitrogen.

(D) *Incorrect.* Rupture of the endotracheal tube cuff can result in a drop in $ETCO_2$ from the large leak that would develop. This leak also could produce an increase in end-tidal nitrogen, but it would not be transient. A cuff rupture would cause a continued leak with the associated lower $CO_2$ and high nitrogen from the entrainment of air around the leak.

(E) *Correct.* A sudden drop in $ETCO_2$ with an associated rise in end-tidal nitrogen is highly suspicious for a venous air embolism (VAE).

**REASONING:**

This question tests knowledge of the interpretation of expired gas analysis for the detection of air embolism. There are many causes of decreased end-tidal carbon dioxide that the reader should review carefully. However, a sudden rise in end-tidal nitrogen is highly specific for air embolism and is the key to establishing the diagnosis in this patient. The best answer is E.

**BIBLIOGRAPHY:**

Barash PG, Cullen BF, Stoelting RK, Cahalan MK, Stock MC. *Clinical Anesthesia.* 6th ed. Philadelphia, PA: Lippincott Williams & Wilkins; 2009:699-700.

Matjasko J, Petrozza P, Mackenzie CF. Sensitivity of end-tidal nitrogen in venous air embolism detection in dogs. *Anesthesiology.* 1985;63(4):418-423.

Morgan GE, Mikhail MS, Murray MJ. *Clinical Anesthesiology.* 4th ed. New York, NY: McGraw-Hill; 2006:638.

---

**BOOK A:**  **QUESTION 152**

---

*Answer C*

Clinical Anesthesia

**QUESTION (Choose single best answer):**

A 36-year-old woman develops acute airway obstruction 24 hours after total thyroidectomy. The most likely cause is

(A) Bilateral recurrent laryngeal nerve injury.
(B) Unilateral recurrent laryngeal nerve injury.
(C) Hypocalcemia.
(D) Subglottic edema.
(E) Tracheomalacia.

**CORRECT ANSWER: C**

**SUMMARY:**

*Anesthesiologists should be vigilant for signs of airway compromise after thyroid surgery. Airway obstruction after thyroidectomy can occur in the immediate postoperative period, 24 hours after surgery, or even several days postoperatively. Complications such as recurrent laryngeal nerve damage and tracheal compression from a hematoma often can lead to immediate compromise of the airway. Hypocalcemia due to inadvertent removal of parathyroid tissue can lead to airway compromise and usually presents 24 to 96 hours after surgery. Other problems, such as tracheomalacia, can lead to airway issues several days to months postoperatively.*

### EXPLANATION:

(A) *Incorrect.* Bilateral injury to the recurrent laryngeal nerve is extremely rare and can result in stridor and airway problems but usually occurs immediately after extubation or before the first postoperative day.

(B) *Incorrect.* Unilateral injury to the recurrent laryngeal nerve often results in hoarseness or unilateral vocal cord dysfunction but not airway compromise. It is the most common injury and can be transient.

(C) *Correct.* Hypocalcemia due to inadvertent removal of the parathyroid gland can lead to stridor that can progress to laryngospasm and acute airway obstruction.

(D) *Incorrect.* Subglottic edema also can result in airway obstruction. However, the timing and acuity of the airway obstruction in this patient suggest that it is more likely due to hypocalcemia.

(E) *Incorrect.* Tracheomalacia can lead to airway obstruction but usually beyond the 24- to 48-hour period.

### REASONING:

The clinical presentation of acute airway obstruction 24 hours after thyroid surgery helps narrow down the options. Choices A and B can be readily eliminated because they are more likely to manifest immediately after surgery. Choices D and E can be eliminated because they are more likely to occur after 24 hours. This leaves choice C, a classic complication that is the most likely cause of airway obstruction 24 hours after surgery.

### BIBLIOGRAPHY:


Barash PG, Cullen BF, Stoelting RK, Cahalan MK, Stock MC. *Clinical Anesthesia.* 6th ed. Philadelphia, PA: Lippincott Williams & Wilkins; 2009:1282.

Morgan GE, Mikhail MS, Murray MJ. *Clinical Anesthesiology.* 4th ed. New York, NY: McGraw-Hill; 2006:808.


---

| **BOOK A:** | **QUESTION 153** |
|---|---|

*Answer D*

Cardiovascular

### QUESTION (Choose single best answer):

Arterial pressure in the radial artery is 155/70 mm Hg measured by a correctly calibrated catheter-transducer system. At the same time, aortic pressure is 140/75 mm Hg using a high-fidelity catheter tip transducer. The most likely cause of this discrepancy is

(A) A large amount of air in the dome of the radial artery transducer.
(B) Coarctation of the aorta.
(C) Peripheral vascular constriction produced by sympathetic stimulation.
(D) Physiologic amplification of the waveform from the aorta to the radial artery.
(E) Too high a frequency response in the catheter-transducer system.

### CORRECT ANSWER: D

### SUMMARY:

*Arterial blood pressure measurement is affected by the site at which this measurement is done. This phenomenon is called distal pulse amplification or pulse wave amplification (PWA). There are two main contributors to the differences in arterial waveform shape and measurements between different sites. One is the wave reflection, a phenomenon resulting from the bouncing back and forth of the pressure wave inside the systemic arterial tree. The second is the increasing stiffness of the peripheral arteries, which becomes maximum at the arteriolar level. The result is an increasing systolic pressure, decreasing diastolic pressure, and wider pulse pressure as the measure is taken distal. The mean arterial pressure (MAP), however, is only slightly decreased.*

### EXPLANATION:

(A) ***Incorrect.*** A large air bubble will overdampen the system, resulting in a lower radial than aortic pressure measurement.

(B) ***Incorrect.*** Depending of the level, coarctation of the aorta will cause a blood pressure disparity between left and right upper extremities or between upper and lower extremities.

(C) ***Incorrect.*** It is not clear from the question that this patient has a reason for sympathetic stimulation. Regardless, the effect of sympathetic stimulation (ie, strenuous exercise) on PWA has been studied. Roswell and colleagues examined changes in radial artery and aortic arch pressure waveforms at rest and during upright exercise requiring up to 100% maximal oxygen uptake in a cohort of young healthy men. They found that MAPs were essentially the same when measured at both sites, ranging from 87 to 104 mm Hg from mild to maximal exercise. However, systolic pressures were higher and diastolic pressures were lower at the radial artery site. In addition, while pulse pressures at the central aortic arch site increased 1.95-fold with maximal exercise, the measured radial pulse pressure increased 2.60-fold. The authors postulate that the increased PWA observed at the peripheral site is due to local vasoconstriction. They corroborate their theory with the finding that reactive hyperemia and peripheral vasodilatation from increased heat load during exercise significantly decrease peripheral amplification. Thus, while local vasoconstriction may be responsible for increased peripheral PWA observed with sympathetic stimulation, we have no reason to suspect that PWA in this patient should be increased above baseline. It is certainly not the most likely cause of the observed discrepancy. This answer is correct. Because of the decreasing compliance of the vascular tree with age, the radial artery pressure will be higher and the diastolic pressure will be lower than the aortic root pressure.

(D) ***Correct.*** Physiologic amplification of the waveform from the aorta to the radial arteries occurs which results in an increasing systolic pressure, decreasing diastolic pressure, and wider pulse pressure as the measure is taken distally. However, MAP decreases only slightly.

(E) ***Incorrect.*** This would result in underdamping of the system and an artificially elevated systolic and diastolic pressure when comparing the radial to aortic pressure waveforms.

### REASONING:

The key to this question is remembering the shape of the arterial waveform from the radial artery and comparing it to the shape of the aortic root waveform. The aortic waveform is rounder and slightly smaller than the radial thus a lower systolic pressure and the drops off less at diastole thus a higher diastolic at the root.

### BIBLIOGRAPHY:


Miller RD, Eriksson LI, Fleisher LA, et al. *Miller: Miller's Anesthesia.* 7th ed. New York, NY: Churchill Livingstone; 2009. Retrieved January 25, 2012 from http://www. mdconsult.com/books/linkTo?type=bookPage&isbn=978-0-443-06959-8&eid=4-u1.0-B978-0-443-06959-8..00040-6-s0050.

Morgan GE, Mikhail MS, Murray MJ. *Clinical Anesthesiology.* 4th ed. New York, NY: McGraw-Hill; 2006:119, 429.

O'Rourke MF, Blazek JV, Morreels CL Jr, Krovetz LJ. Pressure wave transmission along the human aorta. *Circ Res.* 1968;23:567-579.

Roswell LB, Brengelmann GL, Blackmon JR, et al. Disparities between aortic and peripheral pulse pressures induced by upright exercise and vasomotor changes in man. *Circulation.* 1968;37:954-964.

## Answer A

### Neuroanesthesia

**QUESTION (Choose single best answer):**

During insertion of a Harrington rod with deliberate hypotension for correction of spinal scoliosis, accurate interpretation of somatosensory evoked potentials requires

(A) Core temperature greater than 35°C.
(B) Hematocrit of at least 25%.
(C) Mean arterial pressure greater than 70 mm Hg.
(D) $Po_2$ of at least 80 mm Hg.
(E) Reversal of neuromuscular block.

**CORRECT ANSWER: A**

**SUMMARY:**

*Accurate interpretation of somatosensory evoked potentials (SSEPs) requires minimal changes to the anesthetic technique with a limited amount of inhalational agent, stable hemodynamics and oxygenation, and normothermia. Hypothermia can increase latency and decrease amplitude so a core temperature of greater than 35°C is required. As long as the hematocrit is reasonable and stable and, in addition, the MAP and saturation do not fluctuate dramatically, SSEPs are reliable. Neuromuscular blockade will not affect SSEPs because motor potentials from the ventral spinal cord are not being monitored.*

**EXPLANATION:**

(A) *Correct.* Below 35°C, the amplitude is reduced and latency of SSEPs is increased. In addition, marked hyperthermia can also alter SSEPs.
(B) *Incorrect.* A hematocrit of 25% would not interfere with SSEPs interpretation as long as this blood level has been relatively stable throughout the operation. If the patient has suffered an acute loss of blood from a hematocrit of 45 to 25 within minutes, this change would alter SSEPs.
(C) *Incorrect.* Hemodynamic stability is key to interpreting SSEPs. If an MAP of 70 remains somewhat stable throughout the surgery, SSEPs are reliable. Frequently, deliberate hypotension is mandated by the surgeon and an MAP of 70 is common in this type of surgery. However, again, if the patient had an MAP of 110 throughout the surgery and it suddenly drops to 70, there may be a change in the SSEPs.
(D) *Incorrect.* A $Po_2$ of 80 mm Hg corresponds to saturation greater than 90%. Hypoxia will alter SSEPs; however, with this oxygen tension and a corresponding saturation greater than 90%, evoked potentials should be accurate.
(E) *Incorrect.* Neuromuscular blockade will not interfere with SSEPs. The majority of the blood supply to the motor tracts derives from the anterior spinal artery, while the spinal tracts are supplied by posterior spinal arteries. Thus, SSEPs do not monitor change in motor tracts and neuromuscular blockade can be present.

**REASONING:**

SSEPs are produced by application of small electric currents that stimulate a peripheral nerve. The evoked potential reflects the integrity of neurological pathways from the periphery, to the spinal cord, and then to the somatocortex. Besides the influence from anesthetic agents, a patient must be normothermic for the accurate interpretation of SSEPs. In particular, nitrous oxide does not affect latency, etomidate increases both latency and amplitude, and ketamine only increases amplitude. In addition, large swings in hemodynamics, oxygenation, and blood levels must be avoided for SSEPs to be reliable. Extreme hypotension (MAP < 50-60), severe anemia, and oxygen saturations below 90% will interfere with SSEPs. As soon as one realizes that there has been a change in SSEPs, change the simple things to ensure that the alteration is due to surgical manipulation. Place the patient on 100% oxygen, get the blood pressure up, and check an ABG.

**BIBLIOGRAPHY:**

Morgan CG, Mikhail MS, Murray MJ. *Clinical Anesthesiology*. 4th ed. New York, NY: McGraw-Hill; 2006:146, 147, 626.

---

| **BOOK A:** | **QUESTION 155** |
|---|---|

*Answer E*

Clinical Anesthesia

**QUESTION (Choose single best answer):**

During insufflation of the peritoneal cavity with carbon dioxide at the start of laparoscopy, heart rate increases to 140 bpm, blood pressure decreases to 70/40 mm Hg, and a loud murmur is heard through the esophageal stethoscope. The most appropriate immediate step is to

(A) Administer a vasoconstrictor.
(B) Infuse crystalloid solution rapidly.
(C) Discontinue the inhaled anesthetic.
(D) Insert a central venous catheter.
(E) Deflate the abdomen.

**CORRECT ANSWER: E**

**SUMMARY:**

*Laparoscopy is common surgical procedure. It relies on the creation of a pneumoperitoneum using $CO_2$ that is insufflated through the trocars into the abdomen. This cause increased intra-abdominal pressure with subsequent atelectasis, decreased cardiac output, and hypercarbia. Surgical complications include hollow viscus or major blood vessel injury, hemorrhage, subcutaneous emphysema, pneumomediastinum, pneumothorax, and VAE.*

**EXPLANATION:**

(A) *Incorrect.* The patient experiencing a VAE may undergo circulatory depression and collapse. It is appropriate to support the pressure with a vasopressor, but this is not the first step in the management of VAE in this case.

(B) *Incorrect.* Infusing crystalloid solution will increase the preload but in this case will not help with prevention of further air entrainment. This is because the pressure in the abdomen is driving the VAE through open veins in the abdomen and one would be unable to generate enough central venous pressure to counteract the abdominal pressure.

(C) *Incorrect.* This could help with the hemodynamics in this case, but it is not the first treatment. One should quickly discontinue any nitrous oxide because it will increase the size of the VAE.

(D) *Incorrect.* Once again, this is a valid treatment option to attempt to remove the air from the right-sided heart, but this is not the first step in the treatment.

(E) *Correct.* This should be the first step. The air is entering the venous system through an open vein in the abdomen and is being driven through the pressure created by the insufflated abdomen. Release of the pneumoperitoneum will stop further air entrainment into the venous system.

The key to this question is the statement in the question "the most appropriate immediate step." Several of the answers are correct for the treatment of VAE, but the first step should be to deflate the abdomen to prevent further air entrainment.

**BIBLIOGRAPHY:**

Miller RD, Eriksson LI, Fleisher LA, et al. *Miller: Miller's Anesthesia.* 7th ed. New York, NY: Churchill Livingstone; 2009. Retrieved January 25, 2012 from http://www.mdconsult.com/books/linkTo?type=bookPage&isbn=978-0-443-06959-8&eid=4-u1.0-B978-0-443-06959-8..00068-6.

Morgan GE, Mikhail MS, Murray MJ. *Clinical Anesthesiology.* 4th ed. New York, NY: McGraw-Hill; 2006:583-584.

---

**BOOK A:**

*Answer E*

Pain

## QUESTION 156

**QUESTION (Choose single best answer):**

A 35-year-old man has acute onset of low back pain, lower extremity weakness, and bladder dysfunction. He had a lumbar laminectomy 2 years ago. A myelogram shows disk herniation at L4-5. The most appropriate management is

(A) Bed rest.
(B) Administration of a nonsteroidal anti-inflammatory agent.
(C) Epidural administration of a corticosteroid.
(D) Epidural administration of a local anesthetic.
(E) Surgical decompression.

**CORRECT ANSWER: E**

**SUMMARY:**

*A patient with acute low back pain and signs of neurologic compromise (both new lower extremity weakness and bladder dysfunction) requires emergent surgical decompression. Failure to decompress expeditiously may lead to permanent neurologic injury. Short-term bed rest is appropriate for low back sprain marked by low back pain. Nonsteroidal anti-inflammatory drug (NSAID) use may relieve some pain associated with low back sprain, but it is not the primary intervention in a patient with neurologic compromise. Epidural corticosteroid appears to be effective in reducing the time to resolution of lumbar radiculopathy (pain radiating from the back below the knee). Epidural local anesthetic has an unclear role in back pain and in this case might only mask further neurologic deterioration.*

**EXPLANATION:**

(A) *Incorrect.* Bed rest, NSAIDs, and epidural corticosteroids are reasonable approaches to acute low back pain without severe or rapidly progressive neurologic signs but are inadequate in the face of acute onset of low back pain, lower extremity weakness, and bladder dysfunction.

(B) *Incorrect.* See above.

(C) *Incorrect.* See above.

(D) *Incorrect.* Epidural local anesthetics are contraindicated in this case because they do not address the emergent nature of the injury and could mask further neurologic compromise.

(E) *Correct.* Spinal cord compression from disk herniation with acute neurologic changes requires immediate surgical decompression to prevent further neurologic compromise.

Indications for emergent surgical decompression of a herniated lumbar disk are severe or rapidly progressive radicular neurologic deficit or the cauda equina syndrome (ie, bladder, bowel, and sexual dysfunction). In properly selected patients, lumbar diskectomy has an 80% to 90% success rate. In the absence of these symptoms, conservative treatment can be pursued. Conservative treatment includes bed rest (2-3 days) and NSAIDs. The sooner patients resume normal activity, the more likely they are to recover fully. They should be encouraged to pursue aerobic exercise and avoid heavy lifting. Most patients will experience resolution of symptoms within 4 to 6 weeks if there is no distinct underlying pathology. While most patients (90%) will experience relief with these measures, the use of epidural steroids reduces the amount of time until resolution of symptoms.

BIBLIOGRAPHY:

Gordon D. Diagnosis and management of lumbar disk disease. *Mayo Clin Proc.* 1996;71(3):283-287.

Morgan GE, Mikhail MS, Murray MJ. *Clinical Anesthesiology.* 4th ed. New York, NY: McGraw-Hill; 2006:403-404.

---

**BOOK A:**  **QUESTION 157**

---

*Answer B*

OB/Regional

**QUESTION (Choose single best answer):**

A patient with chronic obstructive pulmonary disease is undergoing spinal anesthesia to a T6 sensory level. The most pronounced effect on pulmonary function will be a decrease in

(A)  Minute ventilation.
(B)  Peak expiratory flow.
(C)  Physiologic dead space.
(D)  Tidal volume.
(E)  Vital capacity.


**CORRECT ANSWER: B**


**SUMMARY:**

*The respiratory effects of neuraxial blockade are relatively minimal. Tidal volume, minute ventilation, dead space, arterial blood gas tensions, and shunt fraction are minimally affected. Sensory levels affecting abdominal and intercostal musculature can have an effect on respiratory function by decreasing active exhalation and therefore decreasing expiratory reserve volume (ERV). Patients with impaired respiratory function due to obstructive or restrictive pulmonary disease may depend on active exhalation and have compromised oxygenation with neuraxial anesthesia extending to a high thoracic sensory level.*


**EXPLANATION:**

(A)  *Incorrect.* Minute ventilation is not changed with spinal anesthesia to a T6 sensory level.
(B)  *Correct.* Peak expiratory flow is accomplished by active exhalation, which requires mainly abdominal muscle function. Blockade of these muscles due to a T6 sensory level will cause paralysis of the abdominal musculature and significantly impair active exhalation.
(C)  *Incorrect.* Anatomic dead space is the gas in nonrespiratory airways, and alveolar dead space is the gas in alveoli that are not perfused. The sum of the two is the physiologic dead space, and it is not changed with neuraxial anesthesia to thoracic sensory levels.

(D) *Incorrect.* Tidal volume is the volume of air in each normal breath. It is unchanged
     with thoracic neuraxial anesthesia.
(E) *Incorrect.* Vital capacity (VC) is the maximum volume of gas that can be exhaled
     following maximal inspiration. While this maneuver depends on intercostal and
     abdominal muscular function, VC changes less than 10% with neuraxial blockade.


### REASONING:

This question tests changes in respiratory function associated with neuraxial anesthesia.
Choices A, C, and D could be eliminated early because these parameters do not change
with neuraxial anesthesia. Choices B and E both decrease with high sensory levels, but
this question asks what would have the *most pronounced effect*. VC will be decreased in
this situation. However, the effect is minimal compared with the decrease in peak expiratory flow, a maneuver that requires abdominal muscular strength. The best answer is B.


### BIBLIOGRAPHY:


Barash PG, Cullen BF, Stoelting RK, Cahalan M, Stock M. *Clinical Anesthesia*. 6th ed.
     Philadelphia, PA: Lippincott Williams & Wilkins; 2010:947.
Miller RD, Eriksson LI, Fleisher LA, Wiener-Kronish JP, William YL. *Miller's Anesthesia*.
     7th ed. Philadelphia, PA: Churchill Livingstone; 2010:1618.
Morgan GE, Mikhail MS, Murray MJ. *Clinical Anesthesiology*. 4th ed. New York, NY:
     McGraw-Hill; 2006:297, 545 (Figure 22-4).



## BOOK A:  QUESTION 158

### Answer D

### Cardiovascular

### QUESTION (Choose single best answer):

A 70-year-old patient is shivering and has chest pain in the PACU following a cholecystectomy. Heart rate is 120 bpm, and blood pressure is 220/120 mm Hg. $Spo_2$ is 97% at
an $Fio_2$ of 0.4. An ECG shows ST–T-wave changes that are not affected by intravenous
administration of nitroglycerin. Which of the following is the most appropriate next step?

(A) Administration of esmolol.
(B) Administration of hydralazine.
(C) Administration of nitroprusside.
(D) Application of a warming blanket.
(E) Increasing $Fio_2$.


### CORRECT ANSWER: D


### SUMMARY:

*Postoperative shivering causes an enormous rise in oxygen consumption (up to 800%),
$CO_2$ production, and myocardial oxygen demand. These physiologic responses are not
well tolerated in patients with limited cardiopulmonary reserve. The patient in this clinical scenario is likely developing myocardial ischemia owing to increased demand placed
on the compromised heart. Treatment should be directed at correcting the inciting event,
in this case shivering.*


### EXPLANATION:

(A) *Incorrect.* Esmolol would decrease myocardial oxygen demand by lowering the heart
     rate but would not treat the underlying cause of the event.
(B) *Incorrect.* Hydralazine would decrease myocardial oxygen demand by lowering the
     blood pressure but again would not treat the underlying cause of the ischemia.

(C) *Incorrect.* See above.

(D) *Correct.* Application of a warming blanket would treat the hypothermia causing the shivering that is thought to be the root cause of the increased myocardial oxygen demand responsible for the ischemia.

(E) *Incorrect.* Increasing the $F_{IO_2}$ would improve oxygenation but would not treat the underlying cause of the ischemia.


**REASONING:**

This question tests knowledge of the physiologic response to hypothermia and the consequence of such a response in patients with a compromised cardiopulmonary system. It is important to direct efforts initially at correcting hypothermia with forced-air warming and small doses of meperidine. Intubation with paralysis and mechanical ventilation while actively rewarming should be considered if the hypothermia and myocardial oxygen supply-demand imbalance are profound or hemodynamic instability ensues. D is the best answer.


**BIBLIOGRAPHY:**

Barash PG, Cullen BF, Stoelting RK, Cahalan MK, Stock MC. *Clinical Anesthesia.* 6th ed. Philadelphia, PA: Lippincott Williams & Wilkins; 2001:1074.

Morgan GE, Mikhail MS, Murray MJ. *Clinical Anesthesiology.* 4th ed. New York, NY: McGraw-Hill; 2006:1008.

---

**BOOK A:**  **QUESTION 159**

---

*Answer E*

Clinical Anesthesia

**QUESTION (Choose single best answer):**

A 24-year-old man who sustained multiple rib fractures in a motor vehicle accident has air leaks through bilateral chest tubes. Which of the following is most likely following initiation of high-frequency jet ventilation?

(A) Airway pressure will be measured most reliably at the proximal (external) end of the endotracheal tube.

(B) Atelectatic areas of the lungs will reexpand.

(C) Changes in end-tidal carbon dioxide tension measured at the tip of the endotracheal tube will match changes in $Pa_{CO_2}$.

(D) Hypercarbia will develop.

(E) The air leaks will be proportional to peak airway pressure.


**CORRECT ANSWER: E**


**SUMMARY:**

*This patient has bilateral pneumothoraces that can present significant ventilation challenges owing to poor lung compliance resulting from the injury and the need to keep airway pressures low. High-frequency jet ventilation (HFJV) uses a small catheter to send a jet of gas from a high-pressure source into the airway. The small gas jet entrains additional gas via the Venturi effect to provide ventilation. The lower airway pressures and smaller tidal volumes produced by HFJV would be beneficial in this patient and help reduce the amount of air leakage from the pneumothoraces.*


**EXPLANATION:**

(A) *Incorrect.* The small high-pressure jet at the proximal end of the endotracheal tube generates a subatmospheric pressure gradient via the Venturi principle that entrains additional gas to achieve ventilation. Airway pressures at the proximal (external) end would not accurately reflect tracheal airway pressures at the tip of the endotracheal tube.

(B) *Incorrect.* HFJV provides high-frequency (100-400 breaths/min) low-tidal-volume breaths to achieve lower peak airway pressures. These small tidal volumes would not likely significantly reexpand areas of the atelectatic lung. Gas transport in HFJV may depend more on molecular diffusion, high-velocity flow, and coaxial gas flow in the airways.

(C) *Incorrect.* Gottschalk and colleagues demonstrated that a significant gradient between arterial and end-tidal $CO_2$ tension exists during supraglottic jet ventilation ($13.4 \pm 6.8$ mm Hg) compared with conventional ventilation through an endotracheal tube ($5.7 \pm 5.2$ mm Hg).

(D) *Incorrect.* HFJV can be an effective method of ventilation in this situation, and hypercarbia would not be likely with adequate ventilation.

(E) *Correct.* The air leaks from the chest tube represent air moving through the bronchial airways out the pneumothorax and into the chest tube. Higher peak airway pressures would generate larger air leaks. This is why HFJV is beneficial for this patient.


### REASONING:

This is a challenging question that tests knowledge of the management of HFJV in a patient who cannot tolerate high peak airway pressures. Many of the finer points of this question involve detailed knowledge of the principles of HFJV, and thus HFJV should be reviewed carefully. However, most readers would be able to reason that air leakage from the pneumothoraces would be proportional to peak airway pressures, even without detailed knowledge of HFJV. E is the single best answer.


### BIBLIOGRAPHY:

Baer G. Complications and technical aspects of jet ventilation for endolaryngeal procedures. *Acta Anaesthesiol Scand.* 2000;44(10):1273.

Barash PG, Cullen BF, Stoelting RK, Cahalan MK, Stock MC. *Clinical Anesthesia.* 6th ed. Philadelphia, PA: Lippincott Williams & Wilkins; 2009:1312, 1315.

Gottschalk A, Mirza N, Weinstein GS, Edwards MW. Capnography during jet ventilation for laryngoscopy. *Anesth Analg.* 1997;85(1):155-159.

Morgan GE, Mikhail MS, Murray MJ. *Clinical Anesthesiology.* 4th ed. New York, NY: McGraw-Hill; 2006:1034-1035.

Patel C, Diba A. Measuring tracheal airway pressures during transtracheal jet ventilation: an observational study. *Anaesthesia.* 2004;59(3):248-251.


## BOOK A:　QUESTION 160

*Answer D*

Clinical Anesthesia

### QUESTION (Choose single best answer):

Which of the following statements concerning the risk of acquiring hepatitis from a blood transfusion is true?

(A) Most patients with posttransfusion hepatitis become clinically jaundiced.
(B) Most cases of posttransfusion hepatitis are caused by the hepatitis B virus.
(C) The risk for hepatitis is less than that for AIDS.
(D) The risk for posttransfusion hepatitis is less than 1% per unit transfused.
(E) The incidence of posttransfusion hepatitis has remained unchanged over the past decade.


### CORRECT ANSWER: D


### SUMMARY:

*Within the last 10 years, the incidence of posttransfusion hepatitis has decreased from 7% to 10% to less than 1% per unit of blood transfused. Because of improvement in virus nucleic acid testing for hepatitis C, most posttransfusion hepatitis now results from hepatitis B virus. Although rare, patients who present with posttransfusion hepatitis usually are not jaundiced. The transmission of human immunodeficiency virus (HIV) following blood transfusions has an estimated incidence of 1 in 1,215,000 transfusions.*

## EXPLANATION:

(A) *Incorrect.* Most patients with posttransfusion hepatitis do not become clinically jaundiced. About 75% of patients are anicteric, 50% develop chronic liver disease, and of the latter, 10% to 20% develop cirrhosis. Fewer than one-third of these patients develop jaundice.

(B) *Incorrect.* Ninety percent of *posttransfusion hepatitis* is caused by the hepatitis C virus.

(C) *Incorrect.* According to the 2003 statistics from the American Red Cross, after a blood transfusion the risk for HIV (1/2,135,000) is much less than that for hepatitis B virus (HBV 1/205,000).

(D) *Correct.* The risk for posttransfusion hepatitis is significantly less than 1% per unit transfused.

(E) *Incorrect.* Since 1985, the incidence of *posttransfusion hepatitis* has decreased, probably for three reasons. The first is improved donor screening. In 1984, donors who were in a high-risk category for AIDS were requested not to donate blood on a volunteer basis. Second, in 1985 all donor blood was tested for antibodies to HIV (see Acquired Immunodeficiency Syndrome). Third, a specific test for hepatitis C was developed.

## REASONING:

Over the last decade, testing the blood supply has decreased the potential risk of transfusion-transmitted infections dramatically. With virus nucleic acid testing, hepatitis C transmission has decreased to 1 in 1,935,000 transfusions according to the American Red Cross in 2003, making its transmission even rarer than hepatitis B (1/205,000 transfusions). HIV testing also has improved drastically, with a transfusion-related incidence of infection that is 1 in 1,315,000. Overall, the risk of posttransfusion hepatitis is much less than 1%, and most of those who get infected do not become jaundiced. One needs to remember that this examination was written in 1993. Current statistics make D correct.

## BIBLIOGRAPHY:


Morgan GE, Mikhail MS, Murray MJ. *Clinical Anesthesiology*. 3rd ed. New York, NY: McGraw-Hill; 2002:553.

Miller RD, et al. *Anesthesia*. 7th ed. Philadelphia, PA: Churchill Livingstone; 2010: 1755-1756.

Pomper GJ, Wu Y, Snyder EL. Risks of transfusion-transmitted infections. *Curr Opin Hematol*. 2003;10:412-418.


---

**BOOK A:**       **QUESTION 161**

---

*Answer D*

Pharmacology

### QUESTION (Choose single best answer):

Which of the following is more likely to occur with use of trimethaphan to induce hypotension than with use of nitroprusside?

(A) A predictable decrease in mean arterial pressure.

(B) Increased mixed venous $P_{O_2}$.

(C) Increased serum lactate concentration.

(D) Mydriasis.

(E) Reflex tachycardia.

**SUMMARY:**

*Trimethaphan is a short-acting nicotinic ganglion blocker formerly used as intravenous antihypertensive agent. Trimethaphan works by blocking acetylcholine receptors in autonomic ganglia and relaxing vascular smooth muscle producing peripheral vasodilatation. It is no longer used due to its rapid onset of tachyphylaxis, associated with a wide range of side effects, including fixed pupillary dilation, diminished cardiac contractility with moderate tachycardia, profound inhibition of gastrointestinal and genitourinary motility, and exaggerated or paradoxical response to autonomic agents. Nitroprusside relaxes both arteriolar and venous smooth muscle through the production of nitric oxide. It is metabolized to thiocyanate and cyanide, and high doses may cause impaired utilization of oxygen by the cells. Because nitroprusside is not selective, it may cause pulmonary vasodilation with V/Q mismatch and decreased $Pao_2$.*

**EXPLANATION:**

(A) *Incorrect.* Both nitroprusside and trimethaphan produce a reliable and predictable decrease in blood pressure.

(B) *Incorrect.* Unlike nitroprusside, trimethaphan does not inhibit hypoxic pulmonary vasoconstriction; thus it will not affect mixed venous $Po_2$.

(C) *Incorrect.* Trimethaphan's metabolism does not result in cyanide production; it thus would not be associated with increased serum lactate levels.

(D) *Correct.* Trimethaphan blocks parasympathetic ganglia and can cause mydriasis.

(E) *Incorrect.* Trimethaphan is associated with an increased heart rate, but it is caused by parasympathetic ganglionic blockade rather than reflex tachycardia.

**REASONING:**

Unlike nitroprusside, trimethaphan is not a common drug in the OR, and the key to this question is what you know about nitroprusside, to eliminate the answers associated with nitroprusside. This only leaves mydriasis, which is the correct answer.

**BIBLIOGRAPHY:**

Barash PG, Cullen BF, Stoelting RK, Cahalan MK, Stock MC. *Clinical Anesthesia.* 6th ed. Philadelphia, PA: Lippincott Williams & Wilkins; 2009:344, 365.

Michel T, Hoffman BB. Treatment of myocardial ischemia and hypertension. In: Brunton LL, Chabner BA, Knollmann BC, eds. *Goodman & Gilman's The Pharmacological Basis of Therapeutics.* 12th ed. 2011:chap 27. Retrieved January 25, 2012 from http://www.accessmedicine.com/content.aspx?aID=16667490.

Morgan GE, Mikhail MS, Murray MJ. *Clinical Anesthesiology.* 4th ed. New York, NY: McGraw-Hill; 2006:256-258.

Pappano AJ. Cholinoceptor-blocking drugs. In: Katzung BG, Masters SB, Trevor AJ, eds. *Basic & Clinical Pharmacology.* 11th ed. 2009:chap 8. Retrieved January 25, 2012 from http://www.accessmedicine.com/content.aspx?aID=4511453.


---

**BOOK A:** **QUESTION 162**

*Answer E*

Basic Science

**QUESTION (Choose single best answer):**

Local anesthetics block nerve conduction by

(A) Closing calcium channels.
(B) Decreasing intracellular calcium concentration.
(C) Decreasing potassium conductance.
(D) Causing extrusion of intracellular potassium.
(E) Inhibiting cellular influx of sodium.

## CORRECT ANSWER: E

### SUMMARY:

*Local anesthetics slow the rate of depolarization of nerve membranes by reversibly binding to specific receptors inside of sodium channels in their inactivated state. This prevents the sodium channel from opening, and the nerve impulse in the form of an action potential from propagating because the membrane does not reach the threshold potential of −55 mV. Local anesthetics do not block nerve conduction by closing calcium channels, decreasing intracellular calcium, decreasing potassium conductance, or causing the extrusion of intracellular potassium. The resting membrane potential of the nerve is also unaffected.*

### EXPLANATION:

(A) *Incorrect.* Calcium channel blockers, but not local anesthetics, close intracellular calcium channels by plugging them (nifedipine) or binding them in their depolarized inactivated state (verapamil).

(B) *Incorrect.* Local anesthetics do not decrease intracellular calcium concentrations.

(C) *Incorrect.* The nerve cell membrane is much more permeable to potassium than sodium, accounting for a negative resting membrane potential of −70 mV. With decreased intracellular sodium, there will be a decrease in potassium conductance outside of the cell and a slowing of the rate of depolarization. However, a slow outflow of potassium is not the mechanism of action of local anesthetics.

(D) *Incorrect.* Local anesthetics do not cause an extrusion of intracellular potassium.

(E) *Correct.* Local anesthetics inhibit sodium channel activation. Without the influx of sodium, the membrane potential does not increase enough to reach threshold and there is no action potential propagation.

### REASONING:

This question tests basic knowledge of the mechanism of the site of action of local anesthetics, which is the sodium channel or choice E.

### BIBLIOGRAPHY:

Barash PG, Cullen BF, Stoelting RK, Cahalan M, Stock M. *Clinical Anesthesia.* 6th ed. Philadelphia, PA: Lippincott Williams & Wilkins; 2010:531-536.

Morgan GE, Mikhail MS, Murray MJ. *Clinical Anesthesiology.* 4th ed. New York, NY: McGraw-Hill; 2006:263-265, 417.



---

**BOOK A:**      **QUESTION 163**

---

## *Answer B*

## Pharmacology

### QUESTION (Choose single best answer):

Which of the following drugs decreases lower esophageal sphincter tone?

(A) Edrophonium.
(B) Glycopyrrolate.
(C) Metoclopramide.
(D) Prochlorperazine.
(E) Succinylcholine.

### CORRECT ANSWER: B

SUMMARY:

*The lower esophageal sphincter (LES) is a 2- to 3-cm band of circular muscle fibers located above and below the diaphragm that is under increased pressure (resting tone of 10-15 cmH$_2$O). The likelihood for reflux is related to the barrier pressure or the difference between the LES pressure and gastric pressure. The LES is innervated by vagal and sympathetic nerves. Certain drugs with anticholinergic effects, including atropine, glycopyrrolate, and tricyclic antidepressants, have been shown to relax the LES. Lower LES tone is associated with pregnancy, obesity, hiatal hernia, and gastroesophageal reflux disease (GERD). A number of medications that increase acetylcholine activity, including succinylcholine, prochlorperazine, metoclopramide, edrophonium, and neostigmine, will also increase LES tone.*

EXPLANATION:

(A) *Incorrect.* Edrophonium, an acetylcholinesterase inhibitor, stimulates gastrointestinal ACh receptors, leading to increased LES tone.

(B) *Correct.* Glycopyrrolate, an anticholinergic, has been shown to lower LES tone.

(C) *Incorrect.* Metoclopramide is a benzamide that acts centrally as a dopamine antagonist and peripherally as a cholinomimetic, increasing Ach transmission in receptors on intestinal smooth muscle as well as increasing LES tone.

(D) *Incorrect.* Prochlorperazine (Compazine) is a phenothiazine that antagonizes dopaminergic receptors in the chemoreceptor trigger zone in the medulla. Like metoclopramide, it also increases LES tone peripherally.

(E) *Incorrect.* Succinylcholine is a depolarizing muscle relaxant that mimics ACh. It causes abdominal wall fasciculations and increases intragastric pressure and LES tone.

REASONING:

This question tests knowledge of drug mechanisms of action on LES tone. A good guess can be made on the basis that one of the drugs listed, namely glycopyrrolate, antagonizes acetylcholine activity while all of the others have a cholinomimetic effect.

BIBLIOGRAPHY:

Barash PG, Cullen BF, Stoetling RK, Cahalan MK, Stock MC. *Clinical Anesthesia.* 6th ed. Philadelphia, PA: Lippincott-Raven Publishers; 2009:1139, 1221-1222.

Brock-Utne JG, Rubin J, Welman S, Dimopoulos GE, Moshal MG, Downing JW. The action of commonly used anti-emetic drugs on the lower oesophageal sphincter. *Br J Anaesth.* 1978;50(3):295-298.

Morgan GE, Mikhail MS, Murray MJ. *Clinical Anesthesiology.* 4th ed. New York, NY: McGraw-Hill; 2006:210-215, 228-229, 238-240, 279-281.

---

**BOOK A:**     **QUESTION 164**

---

*Answer A*

Basic Science

QUESTION (Choose single best answer):

In patients homozygous for atypical pseudocholinesterase, which of the following best explains the prolonged action of succinylcholine?

(A) An increased proportion of the dose reaches the neuromuscular junction.

(B) Diffusion away from the neuromuscular junction is slowed.

(C) Hepatic clearance of succinylcholine is decreased.

(D) Prejunctional activity is unopposed.

(E) Succinylmonocholine induces neuromuscular block.

**CORRECT ANSWER: A**

**SUMMARY:**

*Most of the succinylcholine administered to a patient is metabolized by pseudocholinesterase in the bloodstream to succinylmonocholine, a metabolite with minimal neuromuscular blocking properties. Only 5% of the injected drug ever reaches the neuromuscular junction. The block ends when succinylcholine diffuses into the extracellular space. Prolonged block occurs in individuals homozygous for one of more than 20 identified mutations for atypical pseudocholinesterase. In these individuals, the enzyme is absent or has a markedly decreased affinity for succinylcholine. As a consequence, more succinylcholine reaches the neuromuscular junction. After the usual 1 to 1.5 mg/kg dose of succinylcholine, NMB may be prolonged to 3 to 6 hours until urinary excretion and protein binding effectively clear the drug.*

**EXPLANATION:**

(A) *Correct.* In patients homozygous for atypical pseudocholinesterase, less succinylcholine is metabolized in the plasma and a large percentage of the drug reaches the neuromuscular junction, resulting in prolonged block.

(B) *Incorrect.* In patients homozygous for atypical pseudocholinesterase, there is more succinylcholine in the end plate area and its diffusion into the extracellular fluid will probably be increased. In any case, it is the higher drug concentration in the neuromuscular junction and not a slower diffusion away that accounts for its prolonged effects.

(C) *Incorrect.* While pseudocholinesterase is produced by the liver, succinylcholine does not undergo hepatic metabolism.

(D) *Incorrect.* Prejunctional activity is opposed by the inhibition of motor end plate repolarization by succinylcholine.

(E) *Incorrect.* Succinylmonocholine, the metabolite of succinylcholine by pseudocholinesterase, is a very weak neuromuscular blocker with 1/20 to 1/80th the potency of succinylcholine. It is quickly hydrolyzed to succinic acid in the plasma. Patients homozygous for atypical pseudocholinesterase would have reduced levels of succinylmonocholine in the plasma.

**REASONING:**

Answers B, C, D, and E are clearly incorrect. Prolonged block is due mainly to the increased proportion of the dose of drug reaching the neuromuscular junction.

**BIBLIOGRAPHY:**

Barash PG, Cullen BF, Stoetling RK, Cahalan MK, Stock MC. *Clinical Anesthesia.* 6th ed. Philadelphia, PA: Lippincott-Raven Publishers; 2009:127, 504-506.

Morgan GE, Mikhail MS, Murray MJ. *Clinical Anesthesiology.* 4th ed. New York, NY: McGraw-Hill; 2006:201-215.

Stoelting RK. *Pharmacology and Physiology in Anesthetic Practice.* 2nd ed. Philadelphia, PA: Lippincott Williams & Wilkins; 1991:178.

## Answer E

### OB/Regional

**QUESTION (Choose single best answer):**

Recognized side effects of magnesium sulfate used for the treatment of preeclampsia that would be of anesthetic concern include each of the following *except*

(A)  Maternal pulmonary edema.
(B)  Neonatal hypotonia.
(C)  Increased maternal sensitivity to succinylcholine.
(D)  Increased maternal sensitivity to vecuronium.
(E)  Maternal hypokalemia.

**CORRECT ANSWER: E**

**SUMMARY:**

*Magnesium sulfate is a commonly used medication for the treatment of preeclamptic patients. Normal levels range from 1.7 to 2.4 mg/dL; therapeutic effects are reached at levels between 4.8 and 8.4 mg/dL. Patellar reflex testing is used to screen for toxicity. Loss of patellar reflexes are found at levels of approximately 12 mg/dL. Higher levels will cause respiratory arrest (15-20 mg/dL), and asystole (> 25 mg/dL). Other side effects include chest pain, palpitations, nausea, blurred vision, lethargy, hypotension, increased sensitivity to neuromuscular blockers, and rarely pulmonary edema. Management of acute toxicity includes discontinuation of the infusion and administration of calcium gluconate (1 g IV) over 10 minutes.*

*Magnesium sulfate crosses the placenta and may cause neonatal hypotonia if severe hypermagnesemia is present at delivery.*

**EXPLANATION:**

(A)  *Incorrect.* The combination of preeclampsia and magnesium increases the risk for maternal pulmonary edema.
(B)  *Incorrect.* Magnesium crosses the placenta increasing the risk of fetal hypotonia.
(C)  *Incorrect.* There is an increased sensitivity to both depolarizing and nondepolarizing neuromuscular agents in patients receiving magnesium.
(D)  *Incorrect.* There is an increased sensitivity to both depolarizing and nondepolarizing neuromuscular agents in patients receiving magnesium.
(E)  *Correct.* Hypokalemia is not associated with hypermagnesemia, but with the administration of tocolytics such as ritodrine and terbutaline.

**REASONING:**

Because magnesium sulfate has shown to be the most effective agent in prevention and recurrence of eclamptic seizures, it is important for the anesthesiologist to be familiar with the side effects and toxicity of the agent both in mother and neonate.

**BIBLIOGRAPHY:**

Chestnut DH, Polley LS, Tsen LC, Wong CA. *Chestnut's Obstetric Anesthesia: Principles and Practice: E-Book.* 4th ed. Philadelphia, PA: Mosby; 2009.

Cunningham FG, Leveno KJ, Bloom SL, Hauth JC, Rouse DJ, Spong CY. Pregnancy hypertension. In: Cunningham FG, Leveno KJ, Bloom SL, Hauth JC, Rouse DJ, Spong CY, eds. *Williams Obstetrics.* 23rd ed. 2010:chap 34. Retrieved January 25, 2012 from http://www.accessmedicine.com/content.aspx?aID=6032899.

Morgan GE, Mikhail MS, Murray MJ. *Clinical Anesthesiology.* 4th ed. New York, NY: McGraw-Hill; 2006:911, 919.

## Answer B

### Neuroanesthesia

**QUESTION (Choose single best answer):**

A comatose 40-year-old man is to undergo evacuation of an acute subdural hematoma. His left pupil is dilated, and blood is present behind the left tympanic membrane. Each of the following is an acceptable intervention *except*

(A) Application of 5 cmH$_2$O positive end-expiratory pressure.
(B) Blind nasotracheal intubation.
(C) Use of isoflurane.
(D) Use of nitrous oxide.
(E) Use of succinylcholine.

**CORRECT ANSWER: B**

**SUMMARY:**

*Patients with neurologic injury often have competing indications and contraindications for the use of medications and anesthetic techniques. Management of increased intracranial pressure (ICP) must be considered when assessing clinical techniques for managing and securing the airway. "The most important therapeutic maneuvers in these patients are aimed at normalizing ICP, CPP, and oxygen delivery." 1 CPP = MAP − ICP (or CVP, whichever is greater). These maneuvers include moderate hyperventilation, elevating the head of the bed, administration of mannitol and Lasix, and placement of interventricular drains. The dilated pupil of this patient suggests an elevated ICP, whereas hemotympanum is associated with a basilar skull fracture.*

**EXPLANATION:**

(A) ***Incorrect.*** Positive end-expiratory pressure (PEEP) increases central venous pressure, as well as ICP in those with decreased ventricular compliance, which can decrease CPP. Despite this, PEEP is not contraindicated and its benefit on oxygenation must be carefully balanced with its potentially deleterious effects on cerebral perfusion.
(B) ***Correct.*** Blind nasotracheal intubation (BNTI) in this patient may result in inadvertent placement of an endotracheal tube into the cranial vault. One case report in the anesthesia literature has described inadvertent intracranial placement during BNTI in a patient with fracture of the nasal fossa and a complex skull fracture. There have been numerous reports of inadvertent placement of nasogastric tubes into the cranial vault after basilar skull fractures. Therefore, BNTI is relatively contraindicated in the setting of severe facial trauma or basilar skull fracture.
(C) ***Incorrect.*** Isoflurane is perfectly acceptable for patients with increased ICP.
(D) ***Incorrect.*** The effects of nitrous oxide on ICP are mild, but they should be avoided when there is air entrapped within the cranium or during periods of hypotension.
(E) ***Incorrect.*** Succinylcholine can cause a transient increase in ICP and its use is controversial, especially in closed head injuries. In a trauma situation this risk may be outweighed by the importance of quickly and safely securing the airway. In any case, BNTI (answer choice B) is definitely contraindicated, making E an incorrect selection.

**REASONING:**

This question tests knowledge of the anesthetic management of a patient with signs of increased ICP and possible skull fracture. The choices for this question vary from perfectly acceptable (isoflurane), to acceptable (nitrous), to less than ideal but acceptable (succinylcholine), to not necessarily harmful (PEEP), to an unacceptable intervention (BNTI).

One must use clinical judgment when weighing several alternatives in anesthetic management. B is the best answer.


**BIBLIOGRAPHY:**

Barash PG, Cullen BF, Stoelting RK, Cahalan MK, Stock MC. *Clinical Anesthesia.* 6th ed. Philadelphia, PA: Lippincott Williams & Wilkins; 2009:898-901.

Bouzarth WF. Intracranial nasogastric tube intubation. *J Trauma.* 1978;18:818-819.

Fremstad JD, Martin SH. Lethal complication from insertion of nasogastric tube after severe basilar skull fracture. *J Trauma.* 1978;18:820-822.

Gregory A, Turner P, Reynolds A. A complication of nasogastric intubation: Intracranial penetration. *J Trauma.* 1978;18:823-824.

Horellou MF, Mathe D, Feiss P. A hazard of nasotracheal intubation. *Anaesthesia.* 1978;33:73-74.

Morgan GE, Mikhail MS, Murray MJ. *Clinical Anesthesiology.* 4th ed. New York, McGraw-Hill; 2006:639-640, 867, 1039.

Pointer JE. Nasotracheal intubation. In: Dailey RH, Simon B, Young CP, Stewart RD, eds. *The Airway Emergency Management.* St Louis, MO: Mosby; 1992:101-110.


---

| **BOOK A:** | **QUESTION 167** |
| --- | --- |

*Answer C*

Clinical Anesthesia

**QUESTION (Choose single best answer):**

A jaundiced patient requires general anesthesia for portocaval shunt. He has a long history of alcohol abuse and is cirrhotic with ascites. Special considerations relevant to induction of anesthesia for this patient include each of the following *except* that

(A) Denitrogenation by mask may be more rapid than expected.
(B) The risk of aspiration is increased.
(C) The dose of thiopental necessary for induction will be predictably reduced.
(D) The duration of succinylcholine action may be prolonged.
(E) Alfentanil would be an appropriate supplement.

**CORRECT ANSWER: C**

**SUMMARY:**

*Cirrhosis is a multisystem disease. There are many special considerations relevant to the induction of anesthesia for patients with chronic alcoholism, cirrhosis and ascites. There is an increased risk of aspiration, and a slower clearance of drugs that are hepatically metabolized (eg, alfentanil) or that are degraded by pseudocholinesterase, an enzyme manufactured in the liver (eg, succinylcholine). These patients often have a primary respiratory alkalosis from hyperventilation and hypoxemia secondary to intrapulmonary shunting, a decreased FRC, and a restrictive ventilatory defect from large amounts of ascites. Additionally, there is often an unpredictable CNS response to anesthetic agents such as thiopental and the dose cannot be predictably reduced.*

**EXPLANATION:**

(A) *Incorrect.* Denitrogenation by mask ventilation may be more rapid with an increased baseline respiratory rate in cirrhotic patients who often present with respiratory alkalosis secondary to hyperventilation.

(B) *Incorrect.* The risk of aspiration is increased in alcoholic patients as alcohol delays gastric emptying and decreases LES tone. Aspiration risk is also increased by ascites, which mechanically increases gastric pressure.

(C) *Correct.* While the hypoalbuminemia seen in cirrhosis results in a predictable increase in the unbound or active fraction of thiopental, the total plasma clearance, volume of distribution, and elimination half-life are unchanged and the average dose of thiopental may not be different from nonalcoholic patients. The CNS response to thiopental can be unpredictable in patients with alcoholic cirrhosis. Patients with a history of chronic alcohol abuse may exhibit tolerance or an increased sensitivity.

(D) *Incorrect.* Levels of pseudocholinesterase, the enzyme that metabolizes ester drugs such as succinylcholine and mivacurium, may be reduced by severe liver disease and there may be a mild but clinically insignificant prolongation of succinylcholine action.

(E) *Incorrect.* Alfentanil would be an appropriate supplement, but the dose should be reduced as the free fraction and the elimination half-time of this hepatically cleared drug will be prolonged in a patient with cirrhosis.

## REASONING:

Answers A and D can be excluded as they suggest outcomes that "may" or may not occur with an alcoholic cirrhotic patient. There is no absolute contraindication to using alfentanil in a patient with liver disease, ruling out answer E, and answer B is correct because ascites and alcohol use clearly increase aspiration risk. Answer C is the best choice.

## BIBLIOGRAPHY:

Barash PG, Cullen BF, Stoelting RK, Cahalan MK, Stock MC. *Clinical Anesthesia.* 6th ed. 2009:506, 1262-1267, 1272.

Morgan GE, Mikhail MS, Murray MJ. *Clinical Anesthesiology.* 4th ed. New York, McGraw-Hill; 2006:792-796.

---

| **BOOK A:** | **QUESTION 168** |
| --- | --- |

*Answer B*

Clinical Anesthesia

### QUESTION (Choose single best answer):

A patient being ventilated mechanically in the ICU requires wound debridement twice daily. Each of the following agents would be appropriate for induction of brief general anesthesia *except*

(A) Nitrous oxide.
(B) Etomidate.
(C) Ketamine.
(D) Methohexital.
(E) Midazolam.

### CORRECT ANSWER: B

### SUMMARY:

*Anesthesiologists generally administer medications to induce hypnosis and amnesia, analgesia, and muscle relaxation for surgical cases. Many different anesthetic techniques can be used for the proposed procedure. The patient is being ventilated mechanically, and airway management is not a concern. We presume that the patient has reasonable hemodynamic stability. The MAC of nitrous oxide is 106%. This limits its effectiveness as a single agent, but it may be sufficient to induce anesthesia with supplemental narcotic administration during the brief maintenance period of anesthesia. Ketamine, methohexital, and midazolam all can provide adequate hypnosis and amnesia during the wound debridement. However, etomidate can cause adrenal suppression after even one dose, making it a poor choice for frequent induction of anesthesia in a critically ill ICU patient.*

### EXPLANATION:

(A) *Incorrect.* Nitrous oxide typically is not used as a sole anesthetic agent because its MAC is 106%. However, administration of 70% nitrous oxide with supplemental narcotic as needed is a reasonable technique in this patient who requires brief periods of anesthesia for wound debridement.

(B) *Correct.* Etomidate can cause adrenal suppression after even one dose, and its adrenal suppression has been implicated in the increased mortality of critically ill patients sedated with etomidate infusions. For this reason alone, frequent induction with etomidate is a poor choice in a critically ill ICU patient.

(C) *Incorrect.* Ketamine is used often for dressing changes because it provides both good analgesia and hypnosis with a rapid return to normal function.

(D) *Incorrect.* Methohexital is a short-acting barbiturate with rapid redistribution and awakening.

(E) *Incorrect.* Midazolam can be used for induction of anesthesia in this patient.

### REASONING:

The key to this question is identifying the side-effect profile of etomidate and the impact of adrenal suppression in a critically ill ICU patient. Many readers may have considered nitrous oxide as the initial answer because it is used rarely as a sole anesthetic agent for induction. In this patient, however, it is a more reasonable technique than administration of etomidate. B is the best answer.

### BIBLIOGRAPHY:


Barash PG, Cullen BF, Stoelting RK, Cahalan MK, Stock MC. *Clinical Anesthesia.* 6th ed. Philadelphia, PA: Lippincott Williams & Wilkins; 2009:454-455.

Miller RD, Eriksson LI, Fleisher LA, et al. *Anesthesia*, 7th ed. New York, NY: Churchill Livingstone; 2010:732-733, 738-739, 746-747, 749-750.

Morgan GE, Mikhail MS, Murray MJ. *Clinical Anesthesiology.* 4th ed. New York, NY: McGraw-Hill; 2006:199-200.

Wagner RL, White PF, Kan PB. Inhibition of adrenal steroidogenesis by the anesthetic etomidate. *N Engl J Med.* 1984;310:1415.


---

**BOOK A:**  **QUESTION 169**

---

*Answer C*

Cardiovascular

### QUESTION (Choose single best answer):

A computer program for hemodynamic calculations has the following input values: body surface area, arterial blood pressure, heart rate, pulmonary artery occlusion pressure, pulmonary artery pressure, and cardiac output. Each of the following values can be derived with this program *except*

(A) Cardiac index.
(B) Stroke volume index.
(C) Systemic vascular resistance.
(D) Pulmonary vascular resistance.
(E) Left ventricular stroke work index.

### CORRECT ANSWER: C

### SUMMARY:

*It is important to be able to calculate and interpret various hemodynamic variables to help guide the anesthetic care of critically ill or unstable patients. Certain parameters can be measured directly, such as heart rate, cardiac output, and blood pressure. Other variables, such as stroke volume, can be computed from these measures. SVR cannot be calculated from the available data because it requires a measure of central venous pressures.*

**EXPLANATION:**
(A) *Incorrect.* Cardiac index = cardiac output (CO)/body surface area (BSA) (normally 2.2-4.2 L/min/m$^2$).
(B) *Incorrect.* Stroke volume = index stroke volume (SV)/BSA = (CO/heart rate)/BSA (normally 20-65 mL/beat/m$^2$).
(C) *Correct.* Systemic vascular resistance (SVR) = 80 × ([mean arterial pressure] MAP – [central venous pressure] CVP)/CO (normally 1200-1500 dyn · s · cm$^{-5}$). We are not given the CVP, so this value cannot be computed.
(D) *Incorrect.* Pulmonary vascular resistance (PVR) = 80 × ([pulmonary artery pressure] PAP – [pulmonary artery occlusion pressure] PAOP)/CO (normally 100-300 dyn · s · cm$^{-5}$).
(E) *Incorrect.* Left ventricular stroke work index – work index = 0.0136(MAP – PAOP) × stroke index (SI) (normally 45-60 g · m/beat/m$^2$).

**REASONING:**
This question tests knowledge of the computation of various hemodynamic variables. The reader is encouraged to review the equations for calculating these parameters.

**BIBLIOGRAPHY:**
Barash PG, Cullen BF, Stoelting RK, Cahalan MK, Stock MC. *Clinical Anesthesia.* 6th ed. Philadelphia, PA: Lippincott Williams & Wilkins; 2009:706 (Table 27-4).
Morgan GE, Mikhail MS, Murray MJ. *Clinical Anesthesiology.* 4th ed. New York, NY: McGraw-Hill; 2006:138.

---

**BOOK A:**

## QUESTION 170

*Answer D*

OB/Regional

**QUESTION (Choose single best answer):**

A successful ankle block for transmetatarsal amputation of the first and second toes should include each of the following nerves *except* the

(A) Saphenous.
(B) Deep peroneal.
(C) Superficial peroneal.
(D) Sural.
(E) Tibial.

**CORRECT ANSWER: D**

**SUMMARY:**

*The ankle block is a simple and safe regional anesthetic technique for surgeries involving the foot. It involves blocking five nerves at the level of the ankle. The saphenous nerve is a branch of the femoral nerve. The remaining nerves—deep and superficial peroneal, sural, and tibial—all derive from the sciatic nerve.*

**EXPLANATION:**
(A) *Incorrect.* The saphenous nerve is anesthetized by infiltrating 5 mL local anesthetic around the saphenous vein as it passes anterior to the medial malleolus. It supplies sensory input for the superficial component of the anteromedial foot.

(B) *Incorrect.* The deep peroneal nerve is blocked by injecting 5 mL local anesthetic lateral to the pulsation of the anterior tibial artery at the level of the skin crease on the anterior midline surface of the ankle. It provides sensation to the medial half of the dorsal foot.

(C) *Incorrect.* The superficial peroneal nerve is blocked by infiltrating a ridge of local anesthetic along the skin crease between the anterior tibial artery and the lateral malleolus. It provides sensation to the cutaneous portion of the dorsal foot and all the toes.

(D) *Correct.* The sural nerve provides sensation to the lateral foot, which would not be needed for surgery involving the first and second toes. It is blocked with a ridge of local anesthetic behind the lateral malleolus.

(E) *Incorrect.* The tibial nerve provides sensation for the heal, the medial sole, and part of the lateral sole of the foot. It can be blocked with a fan-shaped injection of local anesthetic in a triangle bounded by the posterior tibial artery, Achilles tendon, and the tibia.

### REASONING:

This question tests knowledge of the anatomy and distribution of nerves anesthetized by an ankle block. This question relies on knowing the sensory component to each nerve of the foot. A thorough understanding of the anatomy is essential to derive the correct answer.

### BIBLIOGRAPHY:

Barash PG, Cullen BF, Stoelting RK, Cahalan M, Stock M. *Clinical Anesthesia.* 6th ed. Philadelphia, PA: Lippincott Williams & Wilkins; 2010:998-999.

Morgan GE, Mikhail MS, Murray MJ. *Clinical Anesthesiology.* 4th ed. New York, NY: McGraw-Hill; 2006:352-353.

---

## BOOK A:     QUESTION 171 (OPTIONAL)

*Answer A*

Pharmacology

### QUESTION (Choose single best answer):

Each of the following contributes to hypotension following induction of anesthesia with propofol *except*

(A) Central vagal stimulation.
(B) Decreased central sympathetic tone.
(C) Direct myocardial depression.
(D) Resetting of arterial baroreceptors.
(E) Systemic vasodilation.

### CORRECT ANSWER: A

### SUMMARY:

*Propofol induces systemic hypotension via multiple mechanisms. Myocardial depression may result from inhibition of transsarcolemmal calcium influx, which decreases the available intracellular calcium and thus decreases inotropy. Propofol induces both arterial vasodilation and venodilation; this is due to both a decrease in sympathetic tone, as well as a direct effect on vascular smooth muscle via changes in either intracellular calcium or local nitric oxide production. Propofol's alteration of the baroreflex mechanism results in a lesser increase in heart rate for a given degree of arterial hypotension; this may account for the greater magnitude of hypotension induced by propofol as compared to thiopental.*

**EXPLANATION:**

(A) ***Correct.*** There is some controversial evidence in the literature to suggest that propofol possesses vagotonic properties and may increase central vagal stimulation. These studies mainly cite observations of bradycardia or even asystole with propofol anesthesia. However, this evidence does not demonstrate conclusively that the etiology of these observations is a propofol-induced increase in central vagal stimulation. It has been shown recently in animal models that propofol-induced bradycardia cannot be prevented by pretreatment with atropine. The decrease in heart rate that is sometimes observed with propofol may be due to decreased sympathetic cardioaccelerator tone rather than vagomimetic activity. There is also some evidence to suggest that propofol, in a dose-dependent manner, decreases cardiac parasympathetic tone. Standard anesthesia texts state that heart rate does not change significantly with an induction dose of propofol. In summary, current evidence does not support the notion that hypotension after induction of anesthesia with propofol is due to central vagal stimulation.

(B) ***Incorrect.*** Propofol decreases central sympathetic tone.

(C) ***Incorrect.*** Propofol causes direct myocardial depression. Myocardial depression may result from inhibition of transsarcolemmal calcium influx, which decreases the available intracellular calcium and thus decreases inotropy.

(D) ***Incorrect.*** Propofol does reset or inhibit the arterial baroreceptor response. The alteration of the baroreflex mechanism results in a lesser increase in heart rate for a given degree of arterial hypotension.

(E) ***Incorrect.*** Propofol causes systemic vasodilation. It induces both arterial vasodilation and venodilation; this is due to both a decrease in sympathetic tone, as well as a direct effect on vascular smooth muscle via changes in either intracellular calcium or local nitric oxide production.

**REASONING:**

This question tests detailed knowledge of the physiologic effects responsible for propofol-induced hypotension. The examiners are asking for the incorrect statement, which in this case is choice A. Choices B, C, and E can be eliminated easily because induction with propofol causes a drop in blood pressure by decreasing sympathetic tone and inducing systemic vasodilation and myocardial depression. This leaves only choices A and D as possibilities. Choice D is a correct statement because propofol can impair or reset the arterial baroreceptor response. Thus A is the best answer.

**BIBLIOGRAPHY:**

Baraka A. Severe bradycardia following propofol-suxamethonium sequence. *Br J Anaesth*. 1988;61:482-483.

Barash PG, Cullen BF, Stoelting RK, Cahalan MK, Stock MC. *Clinical Anesthesia*. 6th ed. Philadelphia, PA: Lippincott Williams & Wilkins; 2009:452.

Egan TD, Brock-Utne JG. Asystole after anesthesia induction with a fentanyl, propofol, and succinylcholine sequence. *Anesth Analg*. 1991;73:818-820.

Hashiba E, Hirota K, Suzuki K, Matsuki A. Effects of propofol on bronchoconstriction and bradycardia induced by vagal nerve stimulation. *Acta Anaesthesiol Scand*. 2003;47:1059-1063.

Kanaya N, Hirata N, Kurosawa S, Nakayama M, Namiki A. Differential effects of propofol and sevoflurane on heart rate variability. *Anesthesiology*. 2003;98:34-40.

Krassioukov AV, Gelb AW, Weaver LC. Action of propofol on central sympathetic mechanisms controlling blood pressure. *Can J Anaesth*. 1993;40:761-769.

Miller RD, Eriksson LI, Fleisher LA, Wiener-Kronish JP, Young WL. *Miller's Anesthesia*. 7th ed. Philadelphia, PA: Churchill Livingstone; 2010:724-726.

Morgan GE, Mikhail MS, Murray MJ. *Clinical Anesthesiology*. 4th ed. New York, NY: McGraw-Hill; 2006:201.

Sellgren J, Ejnell H, Elam M, Ponten J, Gunnar WB. Sympathetic muscle nerve activity, peripheral blood flows, and baroreceptor reflexes in humans during propofol anesthesia and surgery. *Anesthesiology*. 1994;80:534-454.

*Answer A*

OB/Regional

**QUESTION (Choose single best answer):**

Inhibition of labor by terbutaline causes each of the following maternal side effects *except*

(A) Hyperkalemia.
(B) Hypotension.
(C) Ventricular dysrhythmias.
(D) Hyperglycemia.
(E) Pulmonary edema.

**CORRECT ANSWER: A**

**SUMMARY:**

*Terbutaline and ritodrine are β-adrenergic agonists used to treat preterm labor. They exert their tocolytic effects by binding to uterine $\beta_2$ receptors, causing cyclic adenosine monophosphate (cAMP)–mediated relaxation of uterine smooth muscle. Increased cardiac output, stroke volume, heart rate, and left ventricular ejection fraction are a result of $\beta_1$-receptor activation and may result in arrhythmias, myocardial ischemia, and congestive heart failure. Other side effects include hyperglycemia, pulmonary edema, hypokalemia, anxiety, nervousness, and hypotension.*

**EXPLANATION:**

(A) **Correct.** *Hypokalemia* is a side effect of β-agonist therapy. This is due to insulin-mediated intracellular movement of glucose and potassium and activation of sodium/potassium ATPase in skeletal muscle cells.

(B) **Incorrect.** Hypotension can occur due to β-receptor–mediated vasodilation.

(C) **Incorrect.** $\beta_1$-Receptor activation leads to increased heart rate, stroke volume, left ventricular ejection fraction, and cardiac output. This can result in dysrhythmias, including premature ventricular contractions, nodal contractions, atrial fibrillation, and myocardial ischemia.

(D) **Incorrect.** Hyperglycemia occurs with β-agonist therapy as a result of activation of hepatic phosphorylase, resulting in increased glycogen breakdown and glucose production.

(E) **Incorrect.** Pulmonary edema is the most frequent serious complication of β-agonist therapy. Although the mechanism is not clearly understood, increased fluid retention due to β-receptor therapy is a key component. Additionally, patients at risk of cardiogenic pulmonary edema will be more likely to develop this complication when exposed to the cardiac effects of β-adrenergic receptor stimulation.

**REASONING:**

This question tests knowledge of the pharmacology and side effects of terbutaline. To answer this question correctly, one must know that terbutaline is a β-adrenergic receptor agonist and recall the physiologic effects of these drugs. Choices B, C, and D are all effects of β-agonists. Choice E occurs more commonly in pregnant patients treated with these medications. Choice A is clearly incorrect because hypokalemia is associated with β-receptor agonists.

**BIBLIOGRAPHY:**

Chestnut DH, Polley LS, Lawrence CT, Wong CA. *Chestnut's Obstetrical Anesthesia: Principles and Practice: E-Book.* 4th ed. Philadelphia, PA: Mosby; 2009:766-767.

Morgan GE, Mikhail MS, Murray MJ. *Clinical Anesthesiology.* 4th ed. New York, NY: McGraw-Hill; 2006:245-246.

## *Answer A*

### Pharmacology

**QUESTION (Choose single best answer):**

A 66-year-old man with chronic obstructive pulmonary disease who underwent colectomy 12 hours ago has been receiving an epidural infusion of fentanyl at a rate of 100 µg/h. Which of the following is *least* likely to develop?

(A) Hypotension.
(B) Nausea.
(C) Pruritus.
(D) Respiratory depression.
(E) Urinary retention.

**CORRECT ANSWER: A**

**SUMMARY:**

*Epidural opiates cause many side effects. These include early respiratory depression, delayed respiratory depression, pruritus, nausea, urinary retention, sedation, and ileus. The most worrisome side effect is delayed respiratory depression, which occurs because of cephalad diffusion of opiates in CSF affecting the medullary respiratory center. This is dose dependent. Epidural opioids can also cause early respiratory depression seen within 1 to 2 hours of administration. This is thought to be systemic uptake of opioids via spinal blood vessels. Hypotension is a common side effect of local anesthetics in the epidural space, not opiates.*

**EXPLANATION:**

(A) *Correct.* Hypotension is not a common side effect of epidural opiates.
(B) *Incorrect.* Nausea, pruritus, respiratory depression, and urinary retention are all likely side effects from epidural opiates.
(C) *Incorrect.* See above.
(D) *Incorrect.* See above.
(E) *Incorrect.* See above.

**REASONING:**

This question test knowledge of the side effects commonly associated with epidural opioid administration. Common side effects are nausea, pruritus, respiratory depression, and urinary retention (choices B through E). Hypotension is a common side effect associated with epidural administration of local anesthetics, not opiates. A is the least likely and is the best answer.

**BIBLIOGRAPHY:**

Barash PG, Cullen BF, Stoelting RK, Cahalan MK, Stock MC. *Clinical Anesthesia.* 6th ed. Philadelphia, PA: Lippincott Williams & Wilkins; 2009:1482-1490.
Morgan GE, Mikhail MS, Murray MJ. *Clinical Anesthesiology.* 4th ed. New York, NY: McGraw-Hill; 2006:397-398.

*Answer B*

Clinical Anesthesia

**QUESTION (Choose single best answer):**

A 65-year-old man is disoriented and has a headache and nausea in the recovery room 30 minutes after transurethral resection of the prostate with glycine irrigation performed under spinal anesthesia. Heart rate is 50 bpm, and blood pressure is 180/110 mm Hg. Which of the following is *least* likely?

(A) Decreased serum osmolality.
(B) Serum sodium concentration of 132 mEq/L.
(C) Increased serum ammonia concentration.
(D) Bibasilar rales.
(E) Jugular venous distension.

**CORRECT ANSWER: B**

**SUMMARY:**

*Transurethral resection of the prostate (TURP) syndrome is caused by the absorption of hypotonic irrigation solution from prostatic venous sinuses during TURP. The signs and symptoms relate to three issues: hypervolemia, hypo-osmolar hyponatremia, and chemical effects of the solute in the irrigation. Irrigation fluid dilutes blood, causing decreased serum osmolality and hyponatremia. Hypervolemia can lead to bibasilar rales and jugular venous distension. Metabolism of absorbed glycine causes hyperammonemia and hyperglycinemia. However, the neurologic symptoms described do not develop until serum sodium concentration drops closer to 120 mEq/L.*

**EXPLANATION:**

(A) *Incorrect.* Decreased serum osmolarity is found in virtually all patients with TURP syndrome.
(B) *Correct.* It would be unlikely to observe the patient's symptoms with the mild hyponatremia of 132 mEq/L.
(C) *Incorrect.* Glycine absorption likely will result in some increase in ammonia concentration.
(D) *Incorrect.* Bibasilar rales are likely to occur with the significant volume overload associated with TURP syndrome.
(E) *Incorrect.* Jugular venous distension is likely to occur owing to the significant volume overload associated with TURP syndrome.

**REASONING:**

This question tests knowledge of the symptoms associated with TURP syndrome. All the choices could be found following a TURP. The patient's elevated blood pressure following spinal anesthesia suggests fluid overload, and bibasilar rales with an elevated jugular venous pressure would be quite possible. However, fluid overload alone will not result in the nausea and disorientation described. These are most likely due to hyponatremia, which typically would be asymptomatic with a sodium of 132 mEq/L. The patient's sodium is likely much lower. Increased serum ammonia results from metabolism of the absorbed glycine. Thus, while all the choices might be found following a TURP, the symptoms described would likely be seen only in a patient with a more serious hyponatremia. B is the best answer.

**BIBLIOGRAPHY:**

Barash PG, Cullen BF, Stoelting RK, Cahalan MK, Stock MC. *Clinical Anesthesia.* 6th ed. Philadelphia, PA: Lippincott Williams & Wilkins; 2009:1365-1367.
Morgan GE, Mikhail MS, Murray MJ. *Clinical Anesthesiology.* 4th ed  New York, NY: McGraw-Hill; 2006:760-761.

*Answer E*

Physiology

**QUESTION (Choose single best answer):**

A 70-year-old man sustains injuries to both carotid bodies during bilateral carotid endarterectomies performed 4 days apart. Two hours after the second procedure, the patient is breathing room air in the PACU. Which of the following sets of arterial blood gas values is *least* likely?

|     | pH  | $Pco_2$ (mm Hg) | $Po_2$ (mm Hg) |
| --- | --- | --- | --- |
| (A) | 7.3 | 50 | 58 |
| (B) | 7.3 | 50 | 86 |
| (C) | 7.4 | 40 | 86 |
| (D) | 7.4 | 42 | 58 |
| (E) | 7.5 | 32 | 58 |

**CORRECT ANSWER: E**

**SUMMARY:**

*Both carotid body stretch receptors and chemoreceptors can be damaged by surgical manipulation during carotid endarterectomy (CEA). The baroreceptor reflex functions as a negative feedback loop, stimulating the cardiovascular center of the medulla when systolic blood pressure rises to decrease sympathetic outflow, while carotid chemoreceptors normally respond to acidosis (pH) and hypoxemia ($Pao_2$) by stimulating medullary respiratory centers to increase ventilation. Surgical injury to bilateral carotid bodies can abolish the normal ventilatory response to acute hypoxia and the normal cardiovascular response to hypertension postoperatively. When this occurs, the central chemoreceptors become the primary ventilation control mechanism.*

**EXPLANATION:**

(A) *Incorrect.* Postoperative respiratory acidosis in the setting of hypoxemia could occur in this patient as the medullary ventilatory response has been abolished due to peripheral carotid chemoreceptor damage.

(B) *Incorrect.* This was the original ABA answer in 1993. According to the alveolar gas equation ($Pao_2 = Fio_2 \times [Patm - pH20] - [Paco_2/0.8]$), the alveolar $Pao_2$ on room air would be 87.5 mm Hg when the $Pco_2$ is 50, resulting in an A-a gradient of 1.5 mm Hg, an unlikely value in a patient who just underwent an anesthetic, but still possible.

(C) *Incorrect.* A normal blood gas and $Pao_2$ on room air is entirely possible in the recovery room despite damage to the carotid bodies.

(D) *Incorrect.* This blood gas is also possible as a normal acid-base status, and hypoxemia could be expected in the recovery room due to atelectasis and V/Q mismatch from the anesthetic.

(E) *Correct.* With a $Pao_2$ of 58 mm Hg on room air, the patient's impaired ventilatory drive would not be expected to mount a response to acute hypoxia. Also, as pain is not typically great after CEA, hyperventilation from pain is also not likely. Therefore, blood gas evidence of respiratory alkalosis and hyperventilation is the least likely of all blood gases listed.

**REASONING:**

The key to answering this question correctly requires an understanding of how bilateral damage to the carotid bodies blunts the ventilatory response to acidosis and hypoxia. The original ABA examination answer, choice B, is not correct because an acute respiratory acidosis can occur in the recovery room with a normal $Pao_2$. Choices A, C, and D are also possible because none show evidence of hyperventilation with respiratory alkalosis. Choice E is correct because the patient would not be expected to mount a significant respiratory response to hypoxemia.


**BIBLIOGRAPHY:**
Miller RD, Eriksson LI, Fleisher LA, Wiener-Kronish JP, Young WL. *Miller's Anesthesia.* 7th ed. Philadelphia, PA: Churchill Livingstone; 2010:707-709, 2033.
Morgan GE, Mikhail MS, Murray MJ. *Clinical Anesthesiology.* 4th ed. New York, NY: McGraw-Hill; 2006:533.

# ANSWERS TO
# BOOK B EXAMINATION

## *Answer A*

### Equipment/Physics

**QUESTION (Choose single best answer):**

The need for increased doses of nondepolarizing muscle relaxants in patients with extensive burns is best explained by

(A) Increased protein binding.
(B) Hypermetabolism.
(C) Increased glomerular filtration rate.
(D) Proliferation of receptors on burned muscle.
(E) Decreased volume of distribution.

**CORRECT ANSWER: A**

*Miller's Anesthesia* **states clearly that burn injury cases upregulation of both fetal and mature acetylcholine receptors, which is associated with resistance to nondepolarizing neuromuscular blockers and increased sensitivity to succinylcholine. This occurs by 72 hours after injury and in patients with burns over 25% of the total body surface area. Reference: Miller's Anesthesia, 7th ed. Page 900.**

**SUMMARY:**

*Burn patients have a relative resistance to nondepolarizing muscle relaxants (NDMRs) because of altered protein binding and the proliferation of neuromuscular junctional and extrajunctional acetylcholine receptors. The proliferation of acetylcholine receptors occurs not on burned muscle but on viable tissue. Altered protein binding in burn patients is a consequence of decreased serum albumin immediately after injury (for up to 60 days) and increases in $a_1$-acid glycoprotein (AAG). The free fraction of NDMRs is reduced owing to binding with AAG. The net effect is thought to be a relative resistance to NDMRs and the requirement of a higher dose to reach clinical effect.*

**EXPLANATION:**

(A) ***Correct.*** Highly protein-bound drugs circulate longer in plasma and are not available to the site of action (eg, the neuromuscular junction [NMJ]) as quickly as non–protein-bound drugs. In burn patients there is upregulation of AAG leading to higher dose requirements of drug to achieve the same clinical effect.

(B) ***Incorrect.*** Although burn patients exhibit hypermetabolic states, the primary effect of this change is on increased oxygen consumption and $CO_2$ production, leading to increased alveolar ventilation. Although there may be some effect on the rate of metabolism of drugs, the initial potency of NDMRs used in the clinical burn setting (usually as single-dose administration for intubation) is more affected by protein binding, volume of distribution, and receptor expression.

(C) ***Incorrect.*** While it is true that glomerular filtration rate (GFR) has been shown to rise in burn patients, its effect on an initial bolus dose of NDMRs likely would be small. This statement assumes that the drug effect is terminated during the distribution phase because then the GFR would not contribute to an increased need for drug (at least not in a single-dose setting). However, if drug plasma levels are still effective during the elimination phase of the drug, an increased GFR may shorten drug action.

(D) ***Incorrect.*** The proliferation of acetylcholine receptors in burn patients occurs not on burned muscle but in extrajunctional and junctional nondamaged tissue.

(E) ***Incorrect.*** The volume of distribution of drug reflects the volume of plasma that would account for the plasma concentration observed after administering a dose of drug, that is,

$$V_d = \frac{dose}{plasma\ concentration}$$

Burn patients have an increased vascular permeability owing to decreased capillary integrity (especially in the first 24-48 hours). However, the volume of distribution ($V_d$) of NDMR is unchanged or decreased. A decreased $V_d$ would require a smaller amount of drug to achieve the desired plasma concentration.

## REASONING:

This question tests knowledge of the pathophysiology associated with burn injury and its effects on the pharmacokinetics of muscle relaxants. It is challenging because the wording used in choice D attempts to lead you down a path that is clearly wrong once the choice is examined carefully. Burned muscle tissue does not regenerate acetylcholine receptors. Rather, the sites of healthy tissue (both intra- and extrajunctional) have been correlated with increased expression of acetylcholine receptors. Choices B and C can be eliminated because they do not significantly affect the pharmacokinetics of muscle relaxants. Choice A is the best answer because the direction of association is correct (increased protein binding leading to decreased drug potency), and the pharmacokinetics involved relate directly to drug potency. It is important to note that depolarizing muscle relaxants should not be administered to burn patients after the first 24 hours (owing to proliferation of acetylcholine receptors) because they can cause severe hyperkalemia leading to cardiac arrest. This effect is thought to peak 20 to 90 days after the injury but has been reported to persist for up to 2 years.

## BIBLIOGRAPHY:

Bonate PL. Clinical pharmacology of muscle relaxants in patients with burns. *Clin Pharmacokinet*. 1980;5(6):548-556.

Gronert GA. A possible mechanism of succinylcholine-induced hyperkalemia. *Anesthesiology*. 1980;53(4):356.

Gronert GA, Dotin LN, Ritchey CR, Mason AD, Jr. Succinylcholine-induced hyperkalemia in burned patients, part II. *Anesth Analg*. 1969;48(6):958-962.

Gronert GA, Theye RA. Pathophysiology of hyperkalemia induced by succinylcholine. *Anesthesiology*. 1975;43(1):89-99.

Jaede U, Sorgel F. Clinical pharmacokinetics in patients with burns. *Clin Pharmacokinet*. 1995;29(1):15-28.

Leibel WS, Martyn JA, Szyfelbein SK, Miller KW. Elevated plasma binding cannot account for the burn-related D-tubocurarine hyposensitivity. *Anesthesiology*. 1981; 54(5):378-382.

Loirat P, Rohan J, Baillet A, et al. Increased glomerular filtration rate in patients with major burns and its effect on the pharmacokinetics of tobramycin. *N Engl J Med*. 1978;299(17):915-919.

Marathe PH, Dwersteg JF, Pavlin EG, et al. Effect of thermal injury on the pharmacokinetics and pharmacodynamics of atracurium in humans. *Anesthesiology*. 1989;70(5): 752-755.

Martyn J, Goldhill DR, Gousouzian NG. Clinical pharmacology of muscle relaxants in patients with burns. *Clin Pharmacol*. 1986;26(8):680-685.

Martyn JA, Matteo RS, Greenblatt DJ, et al. Pharmacokinetics of D-tubocurarine in patients with thermal injury. *Anesth Analg*. 1982;61(3):241-246.

Martyn JA, Matteo RS, Szyfelbein SK, Kaplan RF. Unprecedented resistance to neuromuscular blocking effects of metocurine with persistence after complete recovery in a burned patient. *Anesth Analg*. 1982;61(7):614-617.

Morgan GE, Mikhail MS, Murray MJ. *Clinical Anesthesiology*. 3rd ed. New York, NY: McGraw-Hill; 2002:803, 190 (Table 9-7 Diseases With Altered Responses to Muscle Relaxants).

Schaner PJ, Brown RL, Kirksey TD, et al. Succinylcholine-induced hyperkalemia in burned patients, part I. *Anesth Analg*. 1969;48(5):764-770.

Viby-Mogensen J, Hanel HK, Hansen E, et al. Serum cholinesterase activity in burned patients. *Acta Anaesthesiol Scand*. 1975;9(3):159-179.

*Answer D*

Pediatrics

**QUESTION (Choose single best answer):**

Which of the following parts of the infant's airway determines the appropriate diameter of a nasotracheal tube?

(A)  Nares.
(B)  Glottis.
(C)  Vocal cords.
(D)  Cricoid cartilage.
(E)  Third tracheal ring.

**CORRECT ANSWER: D**

**SUMMARY:**

*The infant larynx has a funnel shape and is narrowest at the level of the cricoid cartilage. The cricoid cartilage size determines the diameter of both oral and nasal endotracheal tubes with a leak pressure of 20 to 30 cmH$_2$O being adequate. Too small a tube size with excessive leak can impede ventilation, while too large a tube can cause mucosal trauma and airway edema. New evidence shows that the adult airway is not narrowest at the level of the glottic opening, but actually at the level of the cricoid cartilage in most adults. Ultrasound imaging of the pediatric cricoid cartilage can aid in determining proper endotracheal tube size.*

**EXPLANATION:**

(A)  *Incorrect.* The diameter of the nares must accommodate the outer diameter of a nasal endotracheal tube, but it is not, in fact, a determinant of tube diameter.

(B)  *Incorrect.* The glottic opening is larger than the subglottic area in infants due to the funnel shape of the infant airway. Previously, the glottic opening was thought to be the narrowest portion of the adult airway, but adult cadaveric data have shown that the cricoid cartilage is the narrowest portion of the airway in about 70% of adults.

(C)  *Incorrect.* The distance between the vocal cords is larger than the cricoid cartilage diameter in both infants and in most adults.

(D)  *Correct.* The infant larynx is funnel shaped and is narrowest at the level of the cricoid cartilage. Multiple formulae exist for estimating proper pediatric endotracheal tube diameter and length, including height, weight, and age. Recently, the use of preinduction ultrasound-guided imaging of the pediatric cricoid cartilage in determining proper endotracheal tube size has been validated.

(E)  *Incorrect.* This part of the trachea is below the cricoid cartilage and is not involved in endotracheal tube selection.

**REASONING:**

Choice A is tempting, but the cricoid cartilage, ultimately, is the determinant of any endotracheal tube diameter, whether oral or nasal. Choices B and C can be eliminated because both the cords and glottic opening are larger than the cricoid cartilage diameter due to the funnel shape of the infant larynx. Choice D plays no role in tube selection. An excessively small endotracheal tube can contaminate the operating room with volatile anesthetic and decrease ventilation of the infants lungs, while an excessively large-tube diameter can damage airway mucosa and lead to postextubation croup or stridor.

**BIBLIOGRAPHY:**

Miller RD, Eriksson LI, Fleisher LA, Wiener-Kronish JP, William YL. *Miller's Anesthesia.* 7th ed. Philadelphia, PA: Churchill Livingstone; 2010:2562, 2578 (Table 82-6 Recommended Sizes and Distance of Insertion of Endotracheal Tubes and Laryngoscope Blades for Use in Pediatric Patients).

Morgan GE, Mikhail MS, Murray MJ. *Clinical Anesthesiology.* 4th ed. New York, NY: McGraw-Hill; 2006:936.

Shibasaki M, Nakajima Y, Ishii S, et al. Prediction of pediatric endotracheal tube size by ultrasonography. *Anesthesiology.* 2010;113(4):819-824.


---

## BOOK B:                    QUESTION 3

---

*Answer C*

Pharmacology

**QUESTION (Choose single best answer):**

Administration of 200 mEq of sodium bicarbonate during cardiopulmonary resuscitation is associated with

(A)  Cerebrospinal fluid (CSF) alkalosis.
(B)  Hypercalcemia.
(C)  Hypercarbia.
(D)  Hyperkalemia.
(E)  Shift of the oxyhemoglobin dissociation curve to the right.

**CORRECT ANSWER: C**

**SUMMARY:**

*Administration of sodium bicarbonate is associated with $CO_2$ production owing to neutralization of $H^+$ ion, which initially produces carbonic acid. It is immediately broken down to $CO_2$ and water. Other effects include metabolic alkalosis, hypernatremia, hyperosmolarity, and leftward shift of the oxyhemoglobin dissociation curve.*

**EXPLANATION:**

(A)  *Incorrect.* $CO_2$ produced from bicarbonate administration causes CSF acidosis from rapid passage of $CO_2$ across cell membranes.
(B)  *Incorrect.* Alkalosis produces hypocalcemia by altering the equilibrium of ionized and bound calcium.
(C)  *Correct.* The neutralization of hydrogen ion produces carbonic acid that immediately dissociates to $CO_2$ and water. $CO_2$ is eliminated in the lungs through expiration. Inadequate alveolar ventilation can result in hypercarbia and worsening acidosis.
(D)  *Incorrect.* Alkalosis produces hypokalemia.
(E)  *Incorrect.* Sodium bicarbonate administration produces alkalosis, resulting in a leftward shift of oxyhemoglobin curve.

**REASONING:**

This question is challenging because two choices, A and C, seem like plausibly correct choices. Most readers recognize that sodium bicarbonate administration causes an elevation in serum bicarbonate, leading to alkalosis. Most readers also recognize that sodium bicarbonate administration is associated with a transient hypercarbia. The key to this question is that choice A refers to CSF, and not serum alkalosis, which makes it incorrect. C is the best answer.

**BIBLIOGRAPHY:**

Barash PG, Cullen BF, Stoelting RK, Cahalan M, Stock M. *Clinical Anesthesia*. 6th ed. Philadelphia, PA: Lippincott Williams & Wilkins; 2009:293, 1544.

Morgan GE, Mikhail MS, Murray MJ. *Clinical Anesthesiology*. 4th ed. New York, NY: McGraw-Hill; 2006:562-563, 682, 719.


---

**BOOK B:**

## QUESTION 4

*Answer C*

Pharmacology

**QUESTION (Choose single best answer):**

When compared with diazepam, midazolam

(A)  Metabolites contribute more significantly to the sedative effect.
(B)  Elimination is less dependent on hepatic metabolism.
(C)  Has more predictable action after intramuscular administration.
(D)  Produces less respiratory depression.
(E)  Produces less hypotension during induction of anesthesia with opioids.

**CORRECT ANSWER: C**

**SUMMARY:**

*The differences between midazolam and diazepam are tested frequently on board examinations. These drugs differ primarily in onset and duration of action, route of administration, extent of biotransformation to active metabolites, and suitability for use in the intraoperative setting. Midazolam is a highly protein-bound benzodiazepine that is suitable for intravenous, oral, and intramuscular administration. It is associated with rapid onset of action and elimination, lack of active metabolites, and significant respiratory depression at higher dosages, especially in elderly patients. Diazepam is suitable for oral and intravenous administration but not for intramuscular usage owing to pain at the site of injection and unreliability of action when given via the intramuscular route. Diazepam has active metabolites that prolong its duration of action. The duration of action of both diazepam and midazolam is dependent on hepatic clearance.*

**EXPLANATION:**

(A)  *Incorrect.* Diazepam metabolites contribute more significantly to the sedative effect. Midazolam has virtually no active metabolites.

(B)  *Incorrect.* Both midazolam and diazepam are dependent on hepatic metabolism for clearance. They both undergo oxidation and conjugation reactions in the liver prior to clearance. These reactions are affected most commonly by age, cirrhosis, and coadministration of other drugs (especially those metabolized by the cytochrome P-450 enzyme system).

(C)  *Correct.* Midazolam has a much more reliable onset and action when given intramuscularly than diazepam. Diazepam is also painful on injection.

(D)  *Incorrect.* Midazolam is associated with greater respiratory depression because of increased potency of the drug compared with diazepam. After initial Food and Drug Administration (FDA) approval of midazolam, there were deaths related to inadvertent overdosing that led to fatal respiratory depression. A decrease in the dosing recommendations as well as unit repackaging ensued.

(E)  *Incorrect.* Benzodiazepines and high-dose narcotics have been reported to produce hypotension during induction for coronary bypass surgery. A study by Liang and colleagues found no significant differences in hemodynamic changes associated with induction of anesthesia with fentanyl (5 μg/kg) and midazolam (0.3 mg/kg) versus fentanyl (5 μg/kg) and diazepam (0.3 mg/kg).

**REASONING:**

This is a somewhat challenging question that reflects the often-tested pharmacodynamic and pharmacokinetic comparisons between midazolam and diazepam. The reader should ensure that these differences are understood clearly. Choice D can be eliminated with knowledge of midazolam's sixfold increased intrinsic potency compared with diazepam. One might also have used this knowledge to exclude choice E. Knowledge of the Liang study similarly would have excluded choice E. Similarly, choice A can be eliminated if the reader recalls that diazepam has two active metabolites, whereas midazolam does not have any. Choice B is incorrect because all benzodiazepines are dependent on hepatic clearance for elimination. This leaves choice C, which makes empirical sense because diazepam is not given intramuscularly in the clinical setting.


**BIBLIOGRAPHY:**

Buhrer M, Maitre PO, Crevoisier C, Stanski DR. Electroencephalographic effects of benzodiazepines: II. Pharmacodynamic modeling of the electroencephalographic effects of midazolam and diazepam. *Clin Pharmacol Ther.* 1990;48(5):555-567.

Liang SW. Studies of midazolam, diazepam and thiopentone on respiratory and cardiovascular function during induction anesthesia. *Zhonghua Wai Ke Za Zhi.* 1991;29(3): 161-164, 205.

Miller RD, Miller ED, Reves JG, et al. *Anesthesia.* 7th ed. New York, NY: Churchill Livingstone; 2009.

Morgan GE, Mikhail MS, Murray MJ. *Clinical Anesthesiology.* 4th ed. New York, NY: McGraw-Hill; 2006.

Mould DR, DeFeo TM, Reele S, et al. Simultaneous modeling of the pharmacokinetics and pharmacodynamics of midazolam and diazepam. *Clin Pharmacol Ther.* 1995;58(1):35-43.

Tuman KJ, McCarthy RJ, el-Ganzouri AR, et al. Sufentanil-midazolam anesthesia for coronary artery surgery. *J Cardiothorac Anesth.* 1990;4(3):308-313.


---

## BOOK B:      QUESTION 5

*Answer A*

Pharmacology

**QUESTION (Choose single best answer):**

Which of the following statements concerning a patient who has been receiving nitroprusside for several days is true?

(A) Biotransformation of cyanide requires a sulfur donor.
(B) Formation of methemoglobin increases cyanide toxicity.
(C) Increased serum thiocyanate concentrations are innocuous.
(D) Mixed venous $P_{O_2}$ decreases as cyanide toxicity develops.
(E) Serum thiocyanate concentrations reflect the degree of cyanide toxicity.

**CORRECT ANSWER: A**

**SUMMARY:**

*Sodium nitroprusside (SNP) is metabolized to cyanide ions, which can combine with methemoglobin, thiosulfate, or cytochrome oxidase. It is the interaction with cytochrome oxidase that interrupts cellular respiration. This leads to anaerobic respiration and accumulation of lactic acid, acidosis, and increased mixed venous oxygen owing to a cellular inability to use oxygen. Untreated, this process eventually causes cell death. Toxic blood cyanide levels (> 100 mg/dL) are associated with greater than 1 mg/kg SNP infused over 2 hours or more than 0.5 mg/kg/h administered within 24 hours.*

**EXPLANATION:**

(A) **Correct.** Cyanide ions are metabolized by rhodanase enzyme present in the liver and kidney to produce thiocyanate. Rhodanase requires thiosulfate ions as sulfur donors to catalyze this reaction.

(B) **Incorrect.** The nitroprusside moiety breaks down to yield five cyanide radicals and one NO molecule. These cyanide radicals can be cleared by one of the three mechanisms. CN can combine with methemoglobin to give cyanomethemoglobin. Therefore, formation of methemoglobin does not increase cyanide toxicity. On the contrary, it leads to safe elimination of cyanide.

(C) **Incorrect.** Elevated thiocyanate levels (5-10 mg/dL) can cause central nervous system (CNS) abnormalities.

(D) **Incorrect.** Mixed venous $Po_2$ increases because $CN^-$ prevents use of oxygen as the final electron acceptor in the electron transport pathway involved with cellular respiration.

(E) **Incorrect.** Thiocyanate is cleared by the kidney. Its accumulation in renal failure produces toxicity characterized by nausea, muscle weakness, altered mental state, and thyroid dysfunction. Kidney or liver disease does not increase the likelihood of cyanide toxicity.

**REASONING:**

A commonly tested complication to chronic SNP infusion is the potential for toxicity related to cyanide and thiocyanate. It should be noted that toxicity is unlikely if a constant rate infusion is kept below 0.5 µg/kg/min (for chronic infusion, ie, > 3 hours). For infusions of short duration, the dose can go up to 8 to 10 µg/kg/min. Cyanide toxicity occurs by interfering with mitochondrial respiration. This produces acidosis, increased mixed venous oxygen saturation, and ultimately death. Increasing dose requirements to achieve pharmacologic effect (tachyphalaxis) may be the first clue to the onset of cyanide toxicity. Treatment consists of termination of the SNP infusion, ventilation with 100% oxygen, and infusion of thiosulfate (as a sulfur donor) and sodium nitrate (to produce methemoglobin). Administration of hydroxocobalamine instead of thiosulfate is recommended in patients with coexisting renal failure.

**BIBLIOGRAPHY:**

Barash PG, Cullen BF, Stoelting RK Cahalan M, Stock M. *Clinical Anesthesia.* 4th ed. Philadelphia, PA: Lippincott Williams & Wilkins; 2001:773-775 (Figure 28-13).

Morgan GE, Mikhail MS, Murray MJ. *Clinical Anesthesiology.* 4th ed. New York, NY: McGraw-Hill; 2006.

Stoelting RK. Pharmacology and Physiology in Anesthetic Practice, 3d ed. Philadelphia, Lippincott Williams & Wilkins, 1999, p. 316.

---

**BOOK B:**  **QUESTION 6**

*Answer C*

OB/Regional

**QUESTION (Choose single best answer):**

Which of the following increases the cephalad spread of hyperbaric intrathecal local anesthetics?

(A) Cephalad-directed needle bevel.
(B) Coughing.
(C) Lithotomy position.
(D) Obesity.
(E) Rapid injection.

**CORRECT ANSWER: C**

**SUMMARY:**

*Hyperbaric local anesthetic solutions are by definition denser than CSF, and their distribution therefore is governed largely by gravity. Patient position is one of the most important factors in the spread of these agents, especially the Trendelenburg, lateral, and jackknife positions. Factors that affect the spread of local anesthetics include age, height, direction of the needle opening during injection (dependent on needle type, ie, Whitacre), anatomic configuration of the spinal column, site of injection, volume and density of CSF, dosage of anesthetic, and volume of anesthetic solution. Factors that have been shown to have limited clinical importance include gender, direction of the needle bevel, turbulence, composition of CSF, CSF pressure, CSF circulation, addition of vasoconstrictors, and weight of the patient.*

**EXPLANATION:**

(A) *Incorrect.* When studied, the direction of the needle bevel had no effect on the distribution of local anesthetic in the CSF. When a solution is injected through a standard beveled lumbar puncture needle, the solution exits in a straight line regardless of the needle bevel direction. Exceptions to this may be the Whitacre and Tuohy needles, which have different bevel openings, but the question does not specifically ask about these types of needles.

(B) *Incorrect.* Although CSF pressure increases with coughing, studies demonstrate that it does not have an effect on the spread of local anesthetic.

(C) *Correct.* Although other patient positions have a significant effect on spread of hyperbaric local anesthetics, lithotomy position does not. Lithotomy position may remove the pooling effect of the lumbar lordosis on local anesthetic distribution, but the thoracic kyphosis decreases cephalad spread.

(D) *Incorrect.* Weight does not have an effect on local anesthetic spread. This question was written prior to information generated by a 2011 paper by Carvalho et al, which showed that weight had no dependence on block height for cesarean delivery using modest doses of bupivacaine. This is no longer a valid answer.

(E) *Incorrect.* When studied, the level of sensory anesthesia was the same with varying injection rates up to 0.5 mL/s.

**REASONING:**

This question had many possible choices, including some that are intuitively correct but have been refuted when studied. Because hyperbaric solutions will follow gravity, choice A could be eliminated. Choices B and E are controversial at best and refuted in many studies. D has also been refuted in a recent study. C is the correct answer due to gravity-dependent distribution of local anesthetic.

**BIBLIOGRAPHY:**

Barash PG, Cullen BF, Stoelting RK, Cahalan M, Stock M. Clinical Anesthesia. 6th ed. Philadelphia, PA: Lippincott Williams & Wilkins; 2010:937-941.

Carvalho B, Collins J, Drover DR, et al. ED(50) and ED(95) of intrathecal bupivacaine in morbidly obese patients undergoing cesarean delivery. *Anesthesiology.* 2011;114(3): 529-535.

Morgan GE, Mikhail MS, Murray MJ. *Clinical Anesthesiology.* 4th ed. New York, NY: McGraw-Hill; 2006:305-308, 305, (Table 16-2 Factors Affecting the Level of Spinal Anesthesia).

Singh SI, Morley-Forster PK, Shamsah M, et al. Influence of injection rate of hyperbaric bupivacaine on spinal block in parturients: a randomized trial. *Can J Anaesth.* 2007;54(4):290-295.

## Answer B

### Pharmacology

**QUESTION (Choose single best answer):**

Compared with a patient without liver disease, a patient with cirrhosis will have

(A) Greater accumulation of vecuronium with infusion.
(B) Increased unbound plasma vecuronium concentration.
(C) More frequent occurrence of phase II block after succinylcholine administration.
(D) Prolonged elimination half-life of atracurium.
(E) Unchanged volume of distribution for pancuronium.

**CORRECT ANSWER: B**

**SUMMARY:**

*Vecuronium is metabolized by the liver to a limited extent. It is cleared largely by biliary excretion and to a small extent by renal excretion (25%). Muscle relaxants are water-soluble drugs with increased volume of distribution in disease states such as liver or renal failure. Multiple factors affect dose and duration of action of neuromuscular blocking agents.*

**EXPLANATION:**

(A) *Incorrect.* Vecuronium is metabolized by the liver to a limited extent, but, according to *Miller's Anesthesia*, "has been shown to have decreased clearance, a prolonged elimination half-life, and a prolonged neuromuscular blockade in patients with cirrhosis." The increased volume of distribution can also contribute to a longer-elimination half-life. According to *Clinical Anesthesiology*, "the duration of action of vecuronium is usually not significantly prolonged in patients with cirrhosis unless doses greater than 0.15 mg/kg are given." It seems that at usual clinical doses, accumulation of vecuronium is not clinically significant, making answer choice B a better selection.

(B) *Correct.* Vecuronium exhibits a moderate to high protein-binding capacity of 60% to 80%. Cirrhosis usually is accompanied by hypoalbuminemia, leading to increased plasma concentration of the unbound drug.

(C) *Incorrect.* Decreased levels of pseudocholinesterase that occur in liver disorders produce prolonged phase I block.

(D) *Incorrect.* Atracurium is degraded primarily by the Hofmann reaction and nonspecific ester hydrolysis, with less than 10% being excreted unchanged by renal and biliary routes. Thus its elimination is independent of renal or hepatic function.

(E) *Incorrect.* Liver failure produces increased volume of distribution for water-soluble drugs such as pancuronium. Thus there is a need for larger initial dose and less frequent maintenance doses in these patients.

**REASONING:**

This question is challenging because two choices, A and B, are plausibly correct. Greater drug accumulation plausibly can occur in patients with impaired hepatic elimination. However, the high protein-binding capacity of vecuronium, coupled with the knowledge that the duration of action is usually not significantly prolonged in cirrhotic patients, makes B the best answer.

**BIBLIOGRAPHY:**
Barash PG, Cullen BF, Stoelting RK, Cahalan M, Stock M. *Clinical Anesthesia*. 6th ed. Philadelphia, PA: Lippincott Williams & Wilkins; 2009:509, 1272.

Miller RD, Eriksson LI, Fleisher LA, et al. *Anesthesia*. 7th ed. New York, NY: Churchill Livingstone; 2010:2139-2140.

Morgan GE, Mikhail MS, Murray MJ. *Clinical Anesthesiology*. 4th ed. New York, NY: McGraw-Hill; 2006:220, 223-224, 795.

---

| **BOOK B:** | **QUESTION 8** |

## *Answer E*

### Pharmacology

**QUESTION (Choose single best answer):**

Intrathecally administered opioids exert their analgesic effects primarily in the

(A) Brain stem.
(B) Fourth ventricle.
(C) Spinal nerve roots.
(D) Spinothalamic tracts.
(E) Substantia gelatinosa.

**CORRECT ANSWER: E**

**SUMMARY:**

*Opioids are administered in the intrathecal or epidural space to manage acute or chronic pain. Intrathecal opioids produce analgesia by binding to opioid receptors, mostly μ-receptors, in the substantia gelatinosa (Rexed's lamina II) located in the dorsal horn of the spinal cord. In contrast to intravenous administration of opioids, intrathecal opioids are not associated with sympathetic nervous system denervation, skeletal muscle weakness, or loss of proprioception.*

**EXPLANATION:**

(A) *Incorrect.* See above.
(B) *Incorrect.* See above.
(C) *Incorrect.* See above.
(D) *Incorrect.* See above.
(E) *Correct.* Opioid receptors are nonuniformly distributed throughout the CNS. However, the primary site of action of intrathecal opioids is the substantia gelatinosa because of its high density of opioid receptors and the role of these receptors in modulating neuronal pain pathways.

**REASONING:**

This question tests knowledge of how intrathecal opioids produce analgesia. Opioid receptors are located throughout the CNS, including all of the above answer choices. However, the question focuses on intrathecal opioids primary site of action which is the substantia gelatinosa. Understanding the pain pathways in the CNS would help determine that receptors in the substantia gelatinosa would be the most effective in modulating the pathways and producing analgesia, making E the best answer.

**BIBLIOGRAPHY:**

Barash PG, Cullen BF, Stoelting RK, Cahalan MK, Stock MC. *Clinical Anesthesia*. 6th ed. Philadelphia, PA: Lippincott Williams & Wilkins; 2009:466-468.

Chestnut DH, Polley LS, Lawrence CT, Wong CA. *Chestnut's Obstetric Anesthesia Principles and Practice*. 4th ed. Philadelphia, PA: Mosby Elsevier; 2009:263-266.

Stoelting RK, Miller RD. *Basics of Anesthesia*. 5th ed. Philadelphia, PA: Churchill Livingstone; 2007:113-114.

## *Answer D*

## Clinical Anesthesia

**QUESTION (Choose single best answer):**

During laser excision of vocal cord polyps in a 5-year-old boy, dark smoke suddenly appears in the surgical field. The trachea is intubated, and anesthesia is being maintained with halothane, nitrous oxide, and oxygen. The most appropriate initial step is to

(A) Change from oxygen and nitrous oxide to air.
(B) Fill the oropharnyx with water.
(C) Instill water into the endotracheal tube.
(D) Remove the endotracheal tube.
(E) Ventilate with carbon dioxide.

**CORRECT ANSWER: D**

**SUMMARY:**

*Airway fire due to laser is the number one complication (and most disastrous) of laser surgery of the airway, with a cited incidence of 0.14%. The first step is to extubate the trachea. Prevention involves avoiding the use of a tracheal tube if possible (jet ventilation or a mask/apnea technique), avoiding combustible $N_2O$, using the lowest $F_{IO_2}$ possible (21% if tolerated), limiting laser time by the surgeon, insufflating the cuff with methylene blue and saline, or substituting a metal-wrapped tracheal tube. Tubes made of polyvinyl chloride (PVC) are highly susceptible to fire from $CO_2$ lasers, while Nd:YAG lasers are less prone to cause fire with PVC but can still ignite if blood or secretions coat the tube. After mask ventilation and reintubation, bronchoscopy can be used to diagnose further airway damage.*

**EXPLANATION:**

(A) *Incorrect.* Changing to room air is not part of the airway-fire protocol. This would actually be a strategy to prevent airway fire. Also, changing to air does not immediately remove the combustible gases, $O_2$ and $N_2O$, already present in the airway.

(B) *Incorrect.* This maneuver is also not part of the airway-fire protocol. If the source of the fire is coming from the blow-torch phenomenon at the distal end of the tracheal tube, water into the oropharynx would not address this issue.

(C) *Incorrect.* Loose or charred pieces of the tracheal tube or damaged tissue could potentially be pushed into distal airways if water is instilled into the tube. After extubation and mask ventilation, the entire tube should be placed in water.

(D) *Correct.* Extubation and discontinuation of ventilation is the first step. This removes all three of the fire sources from the patient's airway: the fuel (tracheal tube), combustion gases ($O_2$ and $N_2O$), and the ignition source (laser). Currently used volatile anesthetics are not flammable and not explosive.

(E) *Incorrect.* This maneuver plays no role in treating airway fire.

**REASONING:**

This question requires familiarity with the algorithm for airway fire. Extubating the trachea is of primary importance because the combustion gases ($N_2O$ and $O_2$) and the flammable source (tracheal tube) are still in the surgical field where the ignition source (laser) is being used. Choice E can be eliminated easily in this case. Choice A is challenging because it does substitute the combustion agents for air, but is actually a preventive technique and not a treatment. Choice C is tempting, but false because the tube, once removed, should be entirely submerged in water. Choice B does not address the fire if the portion of the burned tube is below the level of the cords and not in direct contact with the oropharynx.

**BIBLIOGRAPHY:**

Miller RD, Eriksson LI, Fleisher LA, Wiener-Kronish JP, William YL. *Miller's Anesthesia.* 7th ed. Philadelphia, PA: Churchill Livingstone; 2010:2412-2413.

Morgan GE, Mikhail MS, Murray MJ. *Clinical Anesthesiology.* 4th ed. New York, NY: McGraw-Hill; 2006:26, 28, 839-840 (Table 39-3 Airway-Fire Protocol).

---

**BOOK B:**  **QUESTION 10**

---

*Answer E*

Neuroanesthesia

**QUESTION (Choose single best answer):**

During craniotomy in the sitting position, end-tidal carbon dioxide tension suddenly decreases. Ventilatory excursion of the chest is normal. Further evaluation is most likely to show a decrease in

(A) Alveolar-to-arterial oxygen tension difference.
(B) Alveolar-to-arterial carbon dioxide tension difference.
(C) Dead space ventilation.
(D) Pulmonary artery pressure.
(E) Pulmonary artery occlusion pressure (POAP).

**CORRECT ANSWER: E**

**SUMMARY:**

*The incidence of air embolism is highest during sitting craniotomies (20%-40%). Because of the 10% to 25% population incidence of patent foramen ovale, there is a significant risk of paradoxical air embolus. Clinical signs of air embolism include a decrease in end-tidal carbon dioxide tension ($ETco_2$) and a decrease in $Spo_2$ owing to increased dead space ventilation (increased A–a gradient for $O_2$ and $CO_2$), as well as hypotension. A large volume of air in the right ventricle can lead to right ventricular outflow tract (RVOT) obstruction and increased pulmonary artery pressures. RVOT obstruction will lead to decreased left ventricular preload and decreased PAOP.*

**EXPLANATION:**

(A) *Incorrect.* There is an increase in the A–a $O_2$ gradient.
(B) *Incorrect.* There is an increase in the A–a $CO_2$ gradient.
(C) *Incorrect.* Dead space ventilation increases.
(D) *Incorrect.* The pulmonary artery pressure is increased with air embolism.
(E) *Correct.* RVOT obstruction will lead to decreased left ventricular preload, resulting in a decreased PAOP.

**REASONING:**

This question tests knowledge of the signs of venous air embolism (VAE) in a patient undergoing craniotomy in the sitting position. VAE can occur anytime the surgical area is above the level of the heart and there are large venous sinuses or plexuses that can entrain air. Clinical signs of VAE under anesthesia depend on the amount and rate of entrainment and the preexisting cardiopulmonary derangement. Signs can range from subtle to catastrophic cardiorespiratory collapse. It is common to see a decrease in $ETco_2$ and $Spo_2$ in VAE. Rapid sudden rise in the end-tidal nitrogen concentration is also seen. Hypotension often can present as the first sign. Right ventricular outflow tract and pulmonary arterial obstruction leads to increased pulmonary artery pressure, right ventricular strain and failure, and cardiovascular collapse. The key is to understand that RVOT obstruction leads to decreased forward flow through the pulmonary circulation and subsequent decrease in left ventricular preload, reflected by a decreased PAOP. E is the single best answer.

**BIBLIOGRAPHY:**

Barash PG, Cullen BF, Stoelting RK, Cahalan M, Stock M. *Clinical Anesthesia.* 6th ed. Philadelphia, PA: Lippincott Williams & Wilkins; 2009:1019, 1380-1381.

Miller RD, Eriksson LI, Fleisher LA, et al. *Anesthesia.* 7th ed. New York, NY: Churchill Livingstone; 2010:2055-2058, 2057f.

Morgan GE, Mikhail MS, Murray MJ. *Clinical Anesthesiology.* 4th ed. New York, NY: McGraw-Hill; 2006:638-639.

---

| **BOOK B:** | **QUESTION 11** |
|---|---|

*Answer A*

OB/Regional

**QUESTION (Choose single best answer):**

Which of the following is a cardiorespiratory effect of epidural block to a T4 sensory level?

(A) Decreased expiratory reserve volume.
(B) Decreased tidal volume.
(C) Increased circulating catecholamine concentrations.
(D) Increased heart rate.
(E) Unchanged vital capacity.

**CORRECT ANSWER: A**

**SUMMARY:**

*Epidural anesthesia results in blockade of sympathetic fibers two to six levels above the sensory level, resulting in decreased heart rate, cardiac output, and blood pressure. In healthy individuals, respiratory effects of neuraxial blockade are relatively minimal. Tidal volume, minute ventilation (MV), dead space, arterial blood gas tensions, and shunt fraction are minimally affected. Sensory levels affecting abdominal and intercostal musculature can have an effect on respiratory function by decreasing active exhalation and therefore decreasing expiratory reserve volume (ERV). Of note is the fact that apnea associated with neuraxial block is due to hypoperfusion of the brain stem respiratory centers rather than diaphragmatic or phrenic nerve paralysis.*

**EXPLANATION:**

(A) *Correct.* Epidural blockade with a $T_4$ sensory level is associated with abdominal and intercostal muscle relaxation, which can impair active exhalation and therefore decrease ERV.

(B) *Incorrect.* Tidal volume remains unchanged.

(C) *Incorrect.* Epidural anesthesia is associated with blockade of sensory afferent fibers associated with the stress response to surgery, and therefore levels of catecholamines are reduced.

(D) *Incorrect.* Because of the differential blockade of nerve fibers associated with neuraxial anesthesia, the sympathetic fibers two to six levels above the sensory level will be affected. A $T_4$ sensory level will be associated with blockade of the cardioaccelerator fibers at $T_{1-4}$ and will result in decreased heart rate.

(E) *Incorrect.* Vital capacity includes ERV. Because the ERV is decreased, vital capacity must decrease.

## REASONING:
The key concepts for answering this question involve understanding differential blockade, the components of pulmonary volumes and capacities, and the physiologic effects of neuraxial blockade. Because ERV is a component of vital capacity, choice E can be eliminated. Knowledge of the effects of sympathetic blockade eliminates choices C and D, and understanding that unless the brain stem is hypoperfused with an unusually high block, the MV should remain unchanged eliminates choice B.


## BIBLIOGRAPHY:
Barash PG, Cullen BF, Stoelting RK, Cahalan M, Stock M. *Clinical Anesthesia.* 6th ed. Philadelphia, PA; Lippincott Williams & Wilkins; 2010:947.

Miller RD, Eriksson LI, Fleisher LA, Wiener-Kronish JP, William YL. *Miller's Anesthesia.* 7th ed. Philadelphia, PA: Churchill Livingstone; 2010:1616-1618.

Morgan GE, Mikhail MS, Murray MJ. *Clinical Anesthesiology.* 4th ed. New York, NY: McGraw-Hill; 2006;297, 545 (Figure 22-4).


---

**BOOK B:**      **QUESTION 12**

---

*Answer E*

Physiology

**QUESTION (Choose single best answer)**

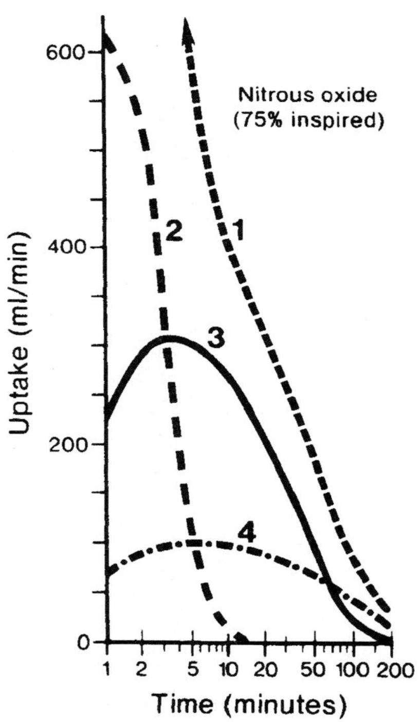


This figure describes the uptake of nitrous oxide 75% by individual tissue groups (vessel-rich group [VRG], muscle group [MG], fat group [FG]) and their sum (total uptake [TU]). Which set of labels accurately describes the curves?

|     | **1** | **2** | **3** | **4** |
|-----|-----|-----|-----|-----|
| (A) | MG  | FG  | VRG | TU  |
| (B) | VRG | MG  | FG  | TU  |
| (C) | FG  | MG  | TU  | VRG |
| (D) | TU  | FG  | MG  | VRG |
| (E) | TU  | VRG | MG  | FG  |

**CORRECT ANSWER: E**

**SUMMARY:**

*The uptake of inhaled anesthetics by tissues is influenced by blood gas solubility, blood flow, and the partial pressure difference (arterial and venous blood). The vessel-rich group (VRG) has a rapid uptake and limited capacity, so it gets saturated quickly (curve 2). The muscle group has less blood supply but greater capacity, so it can have continued uptake for hours (curve 3). The fat group has poor blood supply but enormous capacity for gases with increased lipid solubility. Because fat can have prolonged uptake (days), total uptake by the body will continue, albeit at a lower rate.*

**EXPLANATION:**

(A) *Incorrect.* For all inhaled anesthetics, greatest uptake in the initial period occurs in the VRG group. The VRG organs, such as the brain, heart, kidney, liver, and endocrine system, have limited capacity and are saturated rapidly, and uptake decreases.

(B) *Incorrect.* The muscle group has smaller blood supply and huge capacity and continues to take up anesthetic for hours.

(C) *Incorrect.* The fat group has poor blood supply and the greatest capacity. It will have continued uptake for days (except for $N_2O$).

(D) *Incorrect.* See above.

(E) *Correct.* See above.

**REASONING:**

This is a challenging question that tests knowledge of uptake and distribution of inhaled anesthetics. Curve 2 fits the description of the VRG, and only answer E has curve 2 in the correct order. By this reasoning, the reader can disregard all other answers. E is the best answer.

**BIBLIOGRAPHY:**

Barash PG, Cullen BF, Stoelting RK, Cahalan M, Stock M. *Clinical Anesthesia*. 6th ed. Philadelphia, PA: Lippincott Williams & Wilkins; 2009:416-417.

Morgan GE, Mikhail MS, Murray MJ. *Clinical Anesthesiology*. 4th ed. New York, NY: McGraw-Hill; 2006;157-159.

---

**BOOK B:**

**QUESTION 13**

---

*Answer B*

OB/Regional

**QUESTION (Choose single best answer):**

A 67-year-old man undergoes spinal anesthesia with hyperbaric tetracaine 10 mg for transurethral resection of the prostate (TURP). At the end of the 50-minute procedure, the level of anesthesia is T6, and blood pressure is 120/70 mm Hg. Within 2 minutes of transfer to a stretcher, the patient has nausea, and his blood pressure decreases to 76/42 mm Hg. Which of the following is the most likely cause of the acute hypotension?

(A) Acute congestive heart failure.
(B) Decreased venous return.
(C) Dilutional hyponatremia.
(D) Progression of sympathetic block.
(E) Unrecognized bladder perforation.

**CORRECT ANSWER: B**

**SUMMARY:**

*TURP can be associated with excessive fluid absorption and subsequent fluid overload. The resulting clinical signs and symptoms are due to hyponatremia and increased intravascular volume and are collectively termed TURP syndrome. This syndrome is characterized clinically by restlessness, confusion, nausea, vomiting, lethargy, hypertension, bradycardia, tachypnea, and seizures. This constellation of symptoms is difficult to assess in a patient under general anesthesia. For this reason, regional techniques, especially spinal anesthesia, are popular for this procedure. While spinal block is considered preferable to general anesthesia for TURP, the patient is still vulnerable to its cardiovascular effects. These include decreased arterial vascular sympathetic tone, decreased venous return, and decreased cardiac output, and they can be exacerbated by changes in position during the procedure. When complications occur, the astute clinician must be able to differentiate between complications attributable to the procedure and those attributable to the anesthetic technique.*

**EXPLANATION:**

(A) *Incorrect.* Acute congestive heart failure (CHF), presumably due to fluid overload, is unlikely in this case because the patient did not exhibit any of the symptoms of TURP syndrome prior to his hemodynamic instability.

(B) *Correct.* Spinal anesthesia results in decreased venous return. The position commonly used for TURP is lithotomy with Trendelenburg position, which facilitates venous return. When the patient was transferred out of this position and his legs were placed in a dependent position, venous return was decreased. Combined with the sympathectomy from the spinal block, this change in position resulted in severe hypotension secondary to the inability to compensate by increasing vascular tone.

(C) *Incorrect.* Dilutional hyponatremia occurs following TURP owing to excessive fluid absorption. It causes many of the clinical symptoms associated with TURP syndrome, including lethargy, confusion, and seizures. TURP syndrome is also associated with hypertension, which is not seen in this situation, so it is unlikely.

(D) *Incorrect.* Progression of sympathetic block is unlikely in this situation because the patient was hemodynamically stable until movement to the stretcher. While tetracaine is a local anesthetic with a long duration of action, it is likely that the block is stable after 50 minutes.

(E) *Incorrect.* Bladder perforation is a complication of TURP. It manifests as abdominal pain, commonly referred to the shoulder, even in patients with adequate neuraxial blockade. This pain tends to have a temporal relationship to the perforation and typically occurs during the procedure.

**REASONING:**

The key to this question is the timing of this patient's hypotension. It occurs after the procedure and is associated with moving to the stretcher. It is important to know the signs and symptoms of TURP syndrome to recognize that this patient does not appear to have this condition. Therefore, choices A and C can be eliminated. The timing of the hypotension eliminates choices C and D. Lack of abdominal pain makes choice E unlikely. The best answer is B.

**BIBLIOGRAPHY:**

Barash PG, Cullen BF, Stoelting RK, Cahalan M, Stock M. *Clinical Anesthesia.* 6th ed. Philadelphia, PA: Lippincott Williams & Wilkins; 2010:945-946.

Miller RD, Eriksson LI, Fleisher LA, Wiener-Kronish JP, William YL. *Miller's Anesthesia.* 7th ed. Philadelphia, PA: Churchill Livingstone; 2010:1616-1618.

Morgan GE, Mikhail MS, Murray MJ. *Clinical Anesthesiology.* 4th ed. New York, NY: McGraw-Hill; 2006:759-761, 760 (Figure 33-2 Manifestations of the TURP syndrome).

*Answer A*

OB/Regional

**QUESTION (Choose single best answer):**

A 26-year-old woman has persistent uterine bleeding following a normal spontaneous delivery without anesthesia. The uterus is firm on manual examination. Which of the following anesthetics is most appropriate for manual extraction of the placenta?

(A) Sevolfurane.
(B) Pudendal block with lidocaine.
(C) Subarachnoid tetracaine.
(D) Thiopental.
(E) Vecuronium.

**CORRECT ANSWER: A**

**SUMMARY:**

*Retained products of conception that require manual extraction are a common cause of postpartum hemorrhage and occur in up to 3.3% of deliveries. An important distinction is whether the patient requires analgesia and/or uterine relaxation. If the patient has a functioning epidural or spinal block, this may be adequate for manual extraction if the uterus is not contracted. If the uterus has contracted, it will be virtually impossible for the obstetrician to extract the placenta without relaxation. Classically, this has been done with volatile anesthetic agents (equipotent doses of halothane, sevoflurane, and desflurane cause equivalent uterine relaxation), frequently requiring induction of general anesthesia and endotracheal intubation for airway protection. More recently, nitroglycerin (intravenous or sublingual) or terbutaline has been used with great success. Hypotension with nitroglycerin has not been a clinically significant problem, and the risk of hypotension is outweighed by the advantages of not requiring an anesthetic machine, protection of airway reflexes, avoidance of general anesthesia, and the short duration of action.*

**EXPLANATION:**

(A) ***Correct.*** The question mentions that the uterus is firm and that manual extraction of the placenta is required. This cannot be accomplished without uterine relaxation, and halothane is the only agent among the choices that will provide uterine relaxation.

(B) ***Incorrect.*** Pudendal block will anesthetize the S2-4 nerves associated with the pain of the second stage of labor but will not relax the uterus.

(C) ***Incorrect.*** Subarachnoid tetracaine will provide spinal anesthesia, which does not relax the uterus. Of note, tetracaine will have a prolonged onset and long duration of action in this patient who is bleeding and has the potential for hemodynamic instability. Thus it would not be a preferable agent for spinal anesthesia.

(D) ***Incorrect.*** Thiopental will induce general anesthesia but will not provide uterine relaxation.

(E) ***Incorrect.*** Vecuronium is an NDMR. It will not relax the uterus, and its administration to this patient would result in a paralyzed, awake patient with an unprotected airway.

**REASONING:**

This question is straightforward, provided that one knows that the patient and obstetrician require uterine relaxation for manual extraction of the placenta. The only agent among the list of choices that provides uterine relaxation is sevoflurane. Current practice is to use nitroglycerin for this procedure, but at the time the test question was written, it may not have been in widespread use.

**BIBLIOGRAPHY:**

Bucklin B, Gambling DR, Wlody DJ. *A Practical Approach to Obstetric Anesthesia.* Philadelphia, PA: Lippincott Williams & Wilkins; 2009:253-254.

Chestnut DH, Polley LS, Lawrence CT, Wong CA. *Chestnut's Obstetric Anesthesia Principles and Practice.* 4th ed. St. Louis, MO: Mosby Elsevier; 2009:368, 823.

---

| **BOOK B:** | **QUESTION 15 (OPTIONAL)** |
|---|---|

## *Answer B*

### Physiology

**QUESTION (Choose single best answer):**

Compared with intermittent positive-pressure ventilation (IPPV), intermittent mandatory ventilation (IMV)

(A) Better maintains cardiac output.
(B) Provides less than full mechanical ventilatory support.
(C) Requires a greater level of sedation.
(D) Requires a higher $F_{IO_2}$.
(E) Requires a lower inspiratory flow rate.

**CORRECT ANSWER: B**

**SUMMARY:**

*Controlled mechanical ventilation (CMV), that is, using positive pressure to ventilate the lungs, is commonly used in the operating rooms and on intensive care units (ICUs). Intermittent positive-pressure ventilation (IPPV), continuous positive-pressure ventilation (CPPV) (IPPV + PEEP), and intermittent mandatory ventilation (IMV) are among the common modes of mechanical ventilation. IPPV is best suited for paralyzed patients without spontaneous breathing. Respiratory rate (RR) is set and minute ventilation (MV) is depending on the tidal volume, which is constant if ventilation is volume controlled. Patient is unable to breathe between the mechanical breaths. In contrast, IMV allows the patient to breathe between the breaths if needed. The RR in IMV guarantees a minimum of backup ventilation. Hence, the MV can be variable depending on the patient's own RR.*

**EXPLANATION:**

(A) ***Uncertain.*** The effects of positive-pressure ventilation on the cardiovascular system are too complex and depend on the specific situation of the patient such as hypovolemia, compromised myocardial function, pulmonary disease, etc. In general, an increase in the intrathoracic pressure caused by positive-pressure ventilation may reduce the venous return to the right atrium and cause a decrease in cardiac output. This effect is more prominent when the patient is hypovolemic. To compare the effects of the two ventilation modes, the exact settings must be known. IMV in a heavily sedated patient does not differ from IPPV when the settings are comparable. In patients with compromised cardiac pump function, positive-pressure ventilation may improve the cardiac output.

(B) ***Correct.*** This answer is correct if the patient has some amount of spontaneous ventilation, because in that case the patient can breathe between the mandatory mechanical breaths. In a paralyzed or heavily sedated patient, IMV can be similar to IPPV and provide full ventilatory support.

(C) ***Incorrect.*** Because IPPV does not allow the patient to breathe spontaneously between the mechanical breaths, it is suitable for a paralyzed or heavily sedated patient. In contrast, IMV does not require heavy sedation. IMV is advantageous when weaning the patient from the ventilator is the goal.

(D) ***Incorrect.*** Any level of $F_{IO_2}$ can be used with either ventilation modes.

(E) *Incorrect.* The flow rate can be set according to the ventilatory parameters. Lower flow rate is not a specification of IMV.

**REASONING:**

A basic knowledge of mechanical ventilation is key to answering this question. The simplest mode of mechanical ventilation is IPPV that is broadly used in the operating room. With this mode the ventilator delivers the preset breaths regardless of what the patient is doing. The patient would encounter a closed valve if he/she attempted a spontaneous breath. As an improvement and as a step forward toward weaning a patient from the ventilator, the IMV was created. For this type of ventilation, patients can attempt spontaneous breathing between the mechanical breaths, even though some breaths may collide with the mandatory mechanical breaths. By varying the rate and tidal volume of the mandatory breaths in IMV, the ventilatory support can be tailored to the patient's needs.

**BIBLIOGRAPHY:**

Hall JB, Schmidt GA, Wood LDH. *Principles of Critical Care.* 3rd ed. 2005, Chapter 44, pp 625-637.
Morgan GE, Mikhail MS, Murray MJ. *Clinical Anesthesiology.* 4th ed. New York, NY: McGraw-Hill; 2006:77-79.
Shekerdemian L, Bohn D. Cardiovascular effects of mechanical ventilation. *Arch Dis Child.* 1999;80:475-480.

---

| **BOOK B:** | **QUESTION 16** |
|---|---|

## *Answer D*

### Neuroanesthesia

**QUESTION (Choose single best answer):**

Which of the following findings would be considered normal in the electroencephalogram (EEG) of an adult?

(A) Decreased frequency during induction with halogenated anesthetics.
(B) Decreased frequency in frontal areas with administration of nitrous oxide 50%.
(C) Dominance of beta rhythm at 20 to 30 Hz during the awake relaxed state.
(D) Electrical silence with administration of isoflurane 2.5 minimum alveolar concentration (MAC).
(E) The presence of burst suppression during natural sleep.

**CORRECT ANSWER: D**

**SUMMARY:**

*EEG is a commonly used monitor during anesthetics in which cerebral perfusion is of concern. Isoflurane is unique in that it produces an isoelectric EEG pattern at clinically used doses of 1 to 2 MAC, which would persist at levels of 2.5 MAC. However, desflurane and sevoflurane will not produce an isoelectric EEG pattern at clinically used doses but can produce burst suppression. Nitrous oxide is unique in producing a high-frequency high-amplitude activation pattern on the EEG.*

**EXPLANATION:**

(A) *Incorrect.* The biphasic EEG pattern seen with many anesthetics begins with EEG activation during induction (high-frequency, low-voltage waves) and progresses to depression (low-frequency, high-voltage) as the dose escalates.

(B) **_Incorrect._** Nitrous oxide is unique in that it produces a high-amplitude activation of the EEG (high-frequency, high-amplitude) and at levels of 50% produces this pattern predominantly in the anterior EEG leads.

(C) **_Incorrect._** Beta rhythms (> 12 Hz) are high-frequency low-amplitude waves and are the most common pattern during the awake arousal state, while alpha rhythms (8-12 Hz) are the dominant pattern of the awake relaxed state.

(D) **_Correct._** Isoflurane is unique among the volatile anesthetics in that it produces an isoelectric EEG pattern (ie, it is abolished) at clinically used doses of 1 to 2 MAC, with adequate preservation of hemodynamic parameters. The isoelectric EEG would be expected to persist at isoflurane levels as high as 2.5 MAC.

(E) **_Incorrect._** Burst suppression does not occur during sleep but can occur with many intravenous and inhalational anesthetics.

## REASONING:

This question requires familiarity with both basic EEG wave types and those produced by inhalational anesthetics. Because burst suppression does not occur during sleep and beta patterns are the primary wave during arousal, choices E and C can be eliminated, respectively. Knowing that nitrous oxide increases EEG frequencies eliminates choice B, while remembering that the biphasic EEG pattern results first in activation during induction leaves choice D as the only possible correct answer.

## BIBLIOGRAPHY:

Barash PG, Cullen BF, Stoelting RK, Cahalan M, Stock M. *Clinical Anesthesia.* 6th ed. Philadelphia, PA: Lippincott Williams & Wilkins; 2010:424-426, 1009-1010.

Morgan GE, Mikhail MS, Murray MJ. *Clinical Anesthesiology.* 4th ed. New York, NY: McGraw-Hill; 2006:chap 25, 624-625 (Table 25-2 Electroencephalographic Changes During Anesthesia).

---

## BOOK B:     QUESTION 17

*Answer B*

Equipment/Physics

### QUESTION (Choose single best answer):

Proper zeroing of an arterial pressure transducer attached to a supine anesthetized patient is best accomplished by

(A) Continuous flow of fluid through the intravascular catheter.
(B) Opening the system to air at heart level.
(C) Placement of the transducer diaphragm at heart level.
(D) Proper damping of the transducer system.
(E) Zeroing the transducer during the expiration phase of mechanical ventilation.

### CORRECT ANSWER: B

### SUMMARY:

*Accuracy of invasive arterial blood pressure monitoring depends on correct zeroing and leveling procedures. Zeroing is accomplished by exposing the transducer to atmospheric pressure by opening the stopcock to air and pressing the zero-pressure button on the monitor. Leveling assigns the zero reference point to a specific position on the patient's body, which is the level of the heart found at the midchest midaxillary line in the supine position.*

**EXPLANATION:**

(A) *Incorrect.* Zero reference point is defined as atmospheric pressure, not a continuous flow of fluid through the catheter.

(B) *Correct.* Opening the system to air at heart level will accomplish both zeroing and level of the transducer to allow for accurate measurements.

(C) *Incorrect.* Placement of the transducer diaphragm at heart level levels the transducer but fails to set a zero reference point.

(D) *Incorrect.* The damping coefficient is a measure of how long it takes an oscillating system to come to rest, which is important for accurate measurements but is not involved in the zeroing procedure.

(E) *Incorrect.* Zeroing is used to measure atmospheric pressure and thus ventilation has no effect on zeroing.

**REASONING:**

This question tests knowledge of proper zeroing and leveling of a catheter-fluid arterial pressure transducer system. Answers A and D can be eliminated because they are not involved in the zeroing process. Ventilation has no effect on zeroing; thus answer E can be eliminated. Answer C is tempting, but it describes only leveling and not zeroing the system. Answer B describes proper zeroing and is the correct answer.

**BIBLIOGRAPHY:**

Miller RD, Eriksson LI, Fleisher LA, Weiner-Kronish JP, Young WL. *Miller's Anesthesia.* 7th ed. Philadelphia, PA: Churchill Livingstone; 2010:1277-1281.

Morgan GE, Mikhail MS, Murray MJ. *Clinical Anesthesiology.* 4th ed. New York, NY: McGraw-Hill; 2006:126-130.

---

## BOOK B:      QUESTION 18

*Answer B*

Pediatrics

**QUESTION (Choose single best answer):**

A 1-month-old infant becomes hypoxemic faster during apnea than an adult. Which of the following is the primary cause of this difference?

(A) Functional residual capacity in an infant is half that of an adult.
(B) Metabolic rate in an infant is twice that of an adult.
(C) Resting $Pao_2$ in an infant is lower than that in an adult.
(D) The number of alveoli in an infant is 12% the number in an adult.
(E) The hemoglobin dissociation curve in an infant is shifted to the right.

**CORRECT ANSWER: B**

**SUMMARY:**

*Infant hemoglobin desaturates faster than that of an adult during periods of apnea primarily due to an elevated metabolic rate and rate of oxygen consumption (7-9 mL/kg/min infant, 3 mL/kg/min adult). Although tidal volumes are similar between infants and adults (6-7 mL/kg), RR and MV are both higher in infants. Infant functional residual capacity (FRC) is slightly less than that of an adult, but a higher MV/FRC ratio leaves less oxygen available in the FRC during apnea. Also, infants have a higher work of breathing due to their compliant chest wall and less fatigue-resistant type I muscle fibers in the diaphragm.*

**EXPLANATION:**

(A) *Incorrect.* Infant FRC (27-30 mL/kg) is slightly less than that of an adult, but not half. This can contribute to faster desaturation during apnea, but it is not the primary reason.

(B) *Correct.* Infants have a higher rate of oxygen consumption (two to three times higher) compared to adults, which is the primary reason for faster hypoxemia during apnea. The higher MV/FRC ratio leaves less available oxygen in the FRC component during apnea.

(C) *Incorrect.* Normal resting $Pao_2$ is 85 to 90 mm Hg between the ages of 1 and 10 months, with adult values slightly higher at 100 mm Hg. This small difference does not contribute to rapid desaturation.

(D) *Incorrect.* Infant alveoli are fewer in number and smaller in size than those of an adult, approaching adult values by age 8. While this can contribute to a reduced surface area for oxygen exchange, it is not the primary reason for hemoglobin desaturation during infant apnea.

(E) *Incorrect.* Hemoglobin F (HbF) constitutes 70% to 80% of total hemoglobin at birth and decreases markedly by the age of 3 to 6 months. HbF causes a left shift, not a right shift, in the oxyhemoglobin dissociation curve and does not contribute to the faster desaturation during infant apnea.

### REASONING:

This question is challenging because choices B and C are both true statements regarding infant respiratory physiology, but only choice B is the primary reason for desaturation during apnea. Choice A significantly overestimates the FRC difference and choice D overestimates the alveolar anatomical difference. Choice E is clearly wrong because HbF causes a left shift in the curve.

### BIBLIOGRAPHY:


Barash PG, Cullen BF, Stoelting RK, Cahalan M, Stock M. *Clinical Anesthesia*. 6th ed. Philadelphia, PA: Lippincott Williams & Wilkins; 2010:1174.

Morgan GE, Mikhail MS, Murray MJ. *Clinical Anesthesiology*. 4th ed. New York, NY: McGraw-Hill; 2006:chap 44, 923-924 (Table 44-1 Characteristics of Neonates and Infants That Differentiate Them From Adult Patients).

Stoelting RK, Miller RD. *Basics of Anesthesia*. 5th ed. Philadelphia, PA: Churchill Livingstone; 2007:507-509.


## BOOK B:     QUESTION 19

*Answer B*

Clinical Anesthesia

### QUESTION (Choose single best answer):

During extracorporeal shock wave lithotripsy, the shock wave should be synchronized with

(A) The P wave of the ECG (electrocardiogram).
(B) The R wave of the ECG.
(C) The T wave of the ECG.
(D) Peak inspiration.
(E) End expiration.

### CORRECT ANSWER: B

### SUMMARY:

*Extracorporeal shock wave lithotripsy (ESWL) is used to treat kidney stones in the upper two-thirds of ureters or kidneys. Repetitive high-energy shock waves are generated and focused on the stone, which cause it to fragment by shear and tear forces. Dissipation of shock wave energy can cause tissue injury, including mechanical stress on the cardiac conduction system leading to arrhythmias. Synchronization of shock waves to the R wave of the ECG decreases the incidence of arrhythmias.*

**EXPLANATION:**
(A) *Incorrect.* The shock waves are timed to be 20 milliseconds after the R wave of the ECG to correspond with the ventricular refractory period. Synchronizing with the P or T wave will induce arrhythmias.
(B) *Correct.* The shock waves are timed to be 20 milliseconds after the R wave of the ECG to correspond with the ventricular refractory period.
(C) *Incorrect.* See answer A.
(D) *Incorrect.* Lung tissue is susceptible to injury by the shock waves because its air-tissue interface can cause dissipation of energy. However, the lungs are typically not in the path of the shock wave in ESWL, and shocks do not need to be synchronized with the ventilatory cycle. This procedure is often performed in patients under regional anesthesia where they are maintaining spontaneous ventilation.
(E) *Incorrect.* See answer D.


**REASONING:**

This question tests knowledge of ESWL and its complication of causing cardiac arrhythmias. Answers D and E can be eliminated as ESWL can be performed under regional anesthesia with the patient spontaneously breathing. To decrease the incidence of arrhythmias, the shock wave during ESWL should coincide with the refractory period of the ventricle, making answer B the best choice.


**BIBLIOGRAPHY:**

Miller RD, Eriksson LI, Fleisher LA, Weiner-Kronish JP, Young WL. *Miller's Anesthesia.* 7th ed. Philadelphia, PA: Churchill Livingstone;2010:2124-2126.
Morgan GE, Mikhail MS, Murray MJ. *Clinical Anesthesiology.* 4th ed. New York, NY: McGraw-Hill; 2006:762-764.

---

<table>
<tr><td>BOOK B:</td><td>QUESTION 20</td></tr>
</table>

*Answer E*

Cardiovascular

**QUESTION (Choose single best answer)**

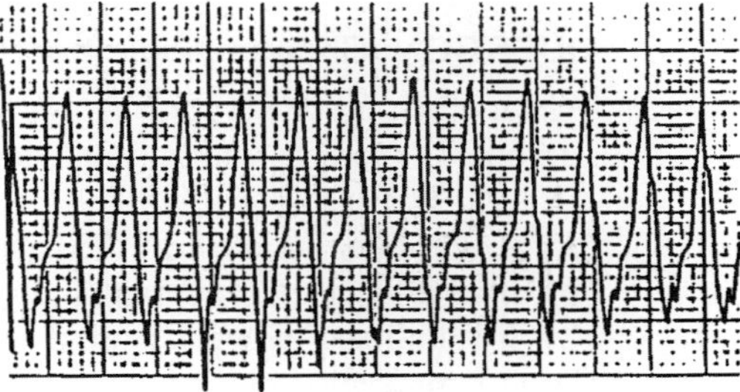

The cardiac rhythm shown here appeared suddenly in an anesthetized patient. The most appropriate management is

(A) Administration of adenosine.
(B) Administration of digoxin.
(C) Administration of epinephrine.
(D) Overdrive pacing.
(E) Synchronous cardioversion.


**CORRECT ANSWER: E**

SUMMARY:

*Stable monomorphic VT is treated with synchronized cardioversion (E) or antiarrhythmic drugs such as amiodarone, sotalol, procainamide, or lidocaine. PEA or VT/VF should be treated with immediate defibrillation and CPR.*

EXPLANATION:

(A) *Incorrect.* Adenosine is incorrect. Adenosine is used in the treatment of SVT and narrow and wide complex tachycardia of supraventricular origin. Adenosine also helps differentiate between wide complex tachycardia of supraventricular and nonsupraventricular origin.

(B) *Incorrect.* Digoxin is incorrect. It is not used in the acute management of ventricular tachycardia.

(C) *Incorrect.* Epinephrine is incorrect. Epinephrine is first-line therapy in the current ACLS (advanced cardiovascular life support) guidelines for PEA and VT/VF.

(D) *Incorrect.* Overdrive pacing is incorrect. Overdrive pacing may be useful in polymorphic ventricular tachycardia with a prolonged QT.

(E) *Correct.* The correct treatment is synchronized cardioversion (initial recommended dose monophasic 100-200 J; biphasic 50-100 J).

REASONING:

Synchronous cardioversion is correct. Given the information in the question stem, assume monomorphic VT with a pulse and unknown cardiac function. The treatment is synchronized cardioversion (initial recommended dose monophasic 100-200 J; biphasic 50-100 J). In stable patients with wide-QRS tachycardia and preserved LV function, you may consider an antiarrhythmic infusion of procainamide, amiodarone, or sotalol.

BIBLIOGRAPHY:

American Heart Association. 2010. Guidelines for CPR and Emergency Cardiovascular Care. Miller RD, Eriksson LI, Fleisher LA, Wiener-Kronish JP, William YL. *Miller's Anesthesia.* 7th ed. Philadelphia, PA: Churchill Livingstone; 2009:Chap 97.

---

## BOOK B:     QUESTION 21

*Answer B*

Clinical Anesthesia

QUESTION (Choose single best answer):

Which of the following statements concerning hyperkalemia after succinylcholine administration to a patient with a spinal cord injury is true?

(A) It is unlikely to occur if the lesion is located below T6.
(B) It is unlikely to occur within 24 hours of the injury.
(C) It is unlikely to occur more than 60 days after the initial injury.
(D) It is prevented by pretreatment with small doses of a nondepolarizing agent.
(E) It is decreased in magnitude by pretreatment with calcium chloride.

CORRECT ANSWER: B

SUMMARY:

*Succinylcholine normally raises serum potassium levels by 0.5 mEq/L. In skeletal muscle injuries or atrophy caused by spinal cord injury, there is upregulation of acetylcholine receptors outside the NMJ. Widespread depolarization of these receptors can result in life-threatening potassium levels (up to 14 mEq/L), causing irreversible cardiac arrest and dysrhythmias, a process that peaks between 7 days and 5 months after injury. Administration of succinylcholine is unlikely to cause hyperkalemia during the first 24 hours after an injury, but it should be avoided after that time. Although the risk of hyperkalemia probably decreases 6 months after the injury, the use of NDMRs is preferred.*

**EXPLANATION:**

(A) *Incorrect.* Injuries below T1 and above L4 result in paraplegia, which places patients at risk for succinylcholine-induced hyperkalemia.

(B) *Correct.* Succinylcholine-induced hyperkalemia is unlikely to occur within 24 hours of a spinal cord injury.

(C) *Incorrect.* While most sources report that the risk of hyperkalemia after a spinal cord injury probably decreases after 6 months, the true duration is unknown. An NDMR must be used 60 days after a spinal cord injury when there is still significant risk of hyperkalemia.

(D) *Incorrect.* Life-threatening hyperkalemia after succinylcholine administration is not reliably prevented by pretreatment with an NDMR.

(E) *Incorrect.* Hyperkalemia is not decreased in magnitude by pretreatment with calcium chloride. The cardiac arrest that can occur with succinylcholine-induced hyperkalemia after a spinal cord injury may be refractory to normal cardiopulmonary resuscitation including treatment with calcium chloride.

**REASONING:**

Choice B is clearly correct. The risk of a hyperkalemic response peaks at 7 to 10 days after an injury, yet it is considered safe to administer succinylcholine to a normokalemic patient within 24 hours after a spinal cord injury. Choices A, D, and E are clearly incorrect. Choice C is likely, but because succinylcholine administration is not recommended 24 hours after a spinal cord injury. Choice A is the best answer.

**BIBLIOGRAPHY:**

Barash, PG, Cullen BF, Stoetling RK, Cahalan M, Stock M. *Clinical Anesthesia*. 6th ed. Philadelphia, PA: Lippincott-Raven Publishers; 2009;1377.

Morgan GE, Mikhail MS, Murray MJ. *Clinical Anesthesiology*. 4th ed. New York, NY: McGraw-Hill; 2006:210,1654-1655.

---

## BOOK B: QUESTION 22

*Answer E*

Physiology

**QUESTION (Choose single best answer):**

The severity of chronic bronchitis is best assessed by measuring

(A) Tidal volume.
(B) Carbon dioxide diffusing capacity.
(C) Sputum production over 24 hours.
(D) Forced vital capacity.
(E) Arterial blood gases.

**CORRECT ANSWER: E**

**SUMMARY:**

*Chronic bronchitis is characterized clinically by a productive cough present for 3 consecutive months for at least 2 consecutive years. Hypertrophy of the bronchial mucus glands results in increased airway secretions. Patients with chronic bronchitis develop hypercarbia and hypoxemia earlier than those with emphysema and are predisposed to early cor pulmonale. Therefore, preoperative assessment of patients with chronic bronchitis should include an arterial blood gas sample if the severity of the disease is in question.*

EXPLANATION:
(A) *Incorrect.* Residual volume may be increased, but tidal volume remains near normal in patients with chronic bronchitis.
(B) *Incorrect.* Restrictive lung disease such as pulmonary fibrosis can result in decreased carbon dioxide diffusion capacity. DLco tends to be normal in obstructive lung disease.
(C) *Incorrect.* Patients with chronic bronchitis produce copious amounts of sputum owing to hypertrophy of mucus glands. However, measuring 24-hour sputum production is not an accurate assessment of disease severity.
(D) *Incorrect.* While patients with chronic obstructive pulmonary disease (COPD) can have a decreased $FEV_1/FVC$ ratio on pulmonary function tests (PFTs), measuring FVC alone is not the best assessment of severity.
(E) *Correct.* Arterial blood gas sampling is the best assessment of disease severity. Patients with chronic bronchitis are at risk for hypoxemia and hypercarbia earlier than those with emphysema. Chronic hypoxemia eventually can lead to right ventricular failure or cor pulmonale.


REASONING:

The key to this question is to remember the progression of chronic bronchitis. Think of the "blue bloater." The most severe result of chronic bronchitis is the development of corpulmonale that carries a high mortality rate. The greatest risk factors for the development of this condition, hypoxemia and hypercarbia, can be detected by arterial blood gases.


BIBLIOGRAPHY:
Morgan GE, Mikhail MS, Murray MJ. *Clinical Anesthesiology*. 3rd ed. New York, NY: McGraw-Hill; 2002:516-519, 516 (Table 23-3 Signs and Symptoms of CCPD).
Stoelting RK, Miller RD. *Basics of Anesthesia*. 4th ed. New York, NY: Churchill Livingstone; 2000:279 (Table 19-2 Comparative Features of COPD).

---

| BOOK B: | QUESTION 23 |
| --- | --- |

*Answer B*

Pediatrics

QUESTION (Choose single best answer):

An 8-kg, 1-year-old boy is scheduled for a bilateral inguinal hernia repair. If regional anesthesia is to be used for postoperative analgesia, which of the following statements is true?

(A) Caudal administration of 0.25% bupivacaine will provide analgesia without evidence of motor block.
(B) Caudal administration of 0.125% bupivacaine is as effective as caudal administration of 0.25% bupivacaine.
(C) Caudal analgesia is more difficult to achieve in young children than in adults.
(D) The recommended volume of local anesthetic used for caudal analgesia in children is 3 mL per year of age.
(E) The volume of 0.25% bupivacaine required for bilateral ilioinguinal and iliohypogastric nerve blocks would be too large.


CORRECT ANSWER: B


SUMMARY:
*Caudal anesthesia can provide effective postoperative analgesia for pediatric patients undergoing inguinal hernia repair. Bupivacaine 0.125% is as effective as 0.25% in providing postoperative analgesia and produces less motor block. The caudal space is accessed via the sacral hiatus and is typically easier to identify in children than adults. Potential complications include spinal, intravenous, or interosseous injection, but the overall rate is low. Other side effects include residual motor block and urinary retention in the early postoperative period.*

**EXPLANATION:**

(A) *Incorrect.* Bupivacaine caudal anesthesia is associated with motor blockade. A retrospective study of 750 consecutive patients reported the incidence to be 54%. Another study demonstrated that motor block with bupivacaine increases with higher concentration.

(B) *Correct.* A study of 105 infants and children who received caudal anesthesia for postoperative pain control found that 0.125% bupivacaine was as effective as 0.25% with significantly less motor blockade. In a recent study comparing pain scores and oral analgesic administration postoperatively, there was no significant difference between patients who received caudal analgesia using 0.125% versus 0.25% bupivacaine in combination with fentanyl.

(C) *Incorrect.* Caudal analgesia is easier to achieve in young children than in adults. Calcification of the sacrococcygeal ligament in adults can make identification of the caudal space more difficult.

(D) *Incorrect.* Recommended volumes of local anesthetic used for caudal analgesia are based on weight (0.5-1 mL/kg), not age.

(E) *Incorrect.* Bilateral ilioinguinal and iliohypogastric nerve blocks also can provide postoperative analgesia following hernia repair. These blocks can be performed safely with a volume of local anesthetic under the toxic bupivacaine dose.

**REASONING:**

This question tests knowledge of regional anesthesia for postoperative analgesia in children. This question is challenging because there is some conflict in the literature regarding the optimal bupivacaine dose for intraoperative caudal anesthesia. However, because the question concerns postoperative analgesia, B is the best answer.

**BIBLIOGRAPHY:**

Dalens B, Hasnaoui A. Caudal anesthesia in pediatric surgery: success rate and adverse effects in 750 consecutive patients. *Anesth Analg*. 1989;68(2):83-89.

Gunter JB, Dunn CM, Bennie JB, et al. Optimum concentration of bupivacaine for combined caudal-general anesthesia in children. *Anesthesiology*. 1991;75(1):57-61.

Joshi W, Connelly NR, Dwyer M, et al. A comparison of two concentrations of bupivacaine and adrenaline with and without fentanyl in paediatric inguinal herniorrhaphy. *Paediatr Anaesth*. 1999;9(4):317-320.

Morgan GE, Mikhail MS, Murray MJ. *Clinical Anesthesiology*. 3rd ed. New York, NY: McGraw-Hill; 2002:273-274.

Wolf AR, Valley RD, Fear DW, et al. Bupivacaine for caudal analgesia in infants and children: the optimal effective concentration. *Anesthesiology*. 1988;69(1):102-106.

---

| **BOOK B:** | **QUESTION 24** |
| --- | --- |

*Answer A*

Clinical Anesthesia

**QUESTION (Choose single best answer):**

After a left-sided double-lumen endotracheal tube is inserted, both cuffs are inflated. When the right (tracheal) lumen is clamped, breath sounds are heard only in the lower right lung field. When the left (bronchial) lumen is clamped, breath sounds are heard over the entire left lung field. Where is the tube positioned?

(A) Tracheal orifice above the carina and bronchial limb in the right bronchus.

(B) Tracheal orifice above the carina and bronchial limb in the left bronchus.

(C) Tracheal orifice and bronchial limb both above the carina.

(D) Tracheal cuff and bronchial limb both in the right bronchus.

(E) Tracheal orifice and bronchial limb both in the left bronchus.

**CORRECT ANSWER: A**

**SUMMARY:**

*Double-lumen endotracheal tubes (DLTs) are used for single-lung ventilation or separation of the two lungs. DLTs are designed for either the right lung or the left lung because there are differences between the anatomy of the two sides, including that (1) the right mainstem takes off at a smaller angle than the left mainstem; (2) there are three branches of the right mainstem bronchus and two branches of the left mainstem bronchus—the takeoff of the right upper lobe bronchus is closer to the carina than the first branch of the left mainstem. Right-sided DLTs have an orifice in the bronchial cuff that allows for ventilation of the right upper lobe when positioned in the right main bronchus. Left-sided DLTs do not have such an orifice. (Also see question 33 in Book B for indications of single-lung ventilation.)*

**EXPLANATION:**

(A) *Correct.* This is the wrong way to position a left-sided double-lumen tube, but it satisfies the clinical description: Clamping the left (bronchial) lumen will insufflate air into the right lung while clamping the right (tracheal) lumen will insufflate air into the right lower field because the right upper lobe bronchus is occluded by the bronchial cuff.

(B) *Incorrect.* This is how a left-sided double-lumen tube *should* be positioned: bronchial lumen and cuff in the left main bronchus and tracheal orifice and cuff in the trachea above the carina. However, this configuration does not satisfy the clinical description.

(C) *Incorrect.* Positioning both the tracheal orifice and the bronchial limb above the carina is no different than having a single-lumen endotracheal tube. You should not hear any difference in breath sounds by clamping either lumen.

(D) *Incorrect.* Positioning both the tracheal cuff and the bronchial limb in the right bronchus would be similar to inserting a single-lumen endotracheal tube into the right mainstem bronchus. No air should be entering the left lung.

(E) *Incorrect.* Positioning both the tracheal orifice and the bronchial limb in the left bronchus is similar to inserting a single-lumen endotracheal tube into the left mainstem bronchus. The only difference would be that the tracheal cuff might not be deep enough in the left bronchus to prevent air from escaping to the right lung.

**REASONING:**

This is a straightforward question that only requires an understanding the differences between right and left lung anatomy and the design of right and left-sided endotracheal tubes. With that knowledge, the reader should be able to figure out that choice A, albeit malpositioned, is the only configuration that would satisfy the clinical description.

**BIBLIOGRAPHY:**

Morgan GE, Mikhail MS, Murray MJ. *Clinical Anesthesiology*. 4th ed. New York, NY: McGraw-Hill; 2006:589-594 (Figure 24-6-8).

*Answer A*

Clinical Anesthesia

**QUESTION (Choose single best answer):**

A 27-year-old man with type 1 von Willebrand disease requires internal fixation of an open fracture of the femur. Prothrombin time, partial thromboplastin time, and platelet count are normal. During surgery, there is significant oozing from the wound, and the surgeon notes poor clot quality. The most appropriate therapy at this time is administration of

(A) Cryoprecipitate.
(B) Desmopressin.
(C) Fresh frozen plasma.
(D) Lyophilized factor VII concentrate.
(E) Platelets.

**CORRECT ANSWER: A**

**SUMMARY:**

*In von Willebrand disease (vWD), occurring in approximately 0.1% of the general population, there is a defective or low level of von Willebrand factor (vWF), a carrier for factor VIII and promoter of platelet aggregation and adherence. In type 1 disease (70%-80% of vWD), levels of normal vWF are decreased. Patients have a prolonged bleeding time, low vWF levels, decreased factor VIII activity, but normal prothrombin time (PT), partial thromboplastin time (PTT), and platelet counts. Cryoprecipitate, which contains vWF and factor VIII, can be given for urgent correction of this disorder. Currently, virus-inactivated factor VIII concentrate, containing VIII and vWF, is preferred over cryoprecipitate, which is pooled from many donors and poses an infectious risk.*

**EXPLANATION:**

(A) **Correct.** The patient in the question is oozing from his wound and requires immediate replacement of vWF and factor VIII. Cryoprecipitate, which is prepared by the slow thawing of fresh frozen plasma (FFP), contains both proteins as well as a high concentration of fibrinogen. Cryoprecipitate is now less commonly used because of its potential for transmission of viral disease. Virus-inactivated plasma-derived concentrates of factor VIII and vWF complex (Humate-P) are the mainstay of treatment of serious bleeding in patients with type 1 vWD.

(B) **Incorrect.** Desmopressin promotes the release of vWF but does not reach peak effect until after 30 minutes when the hemostatic levels of vWF and factor VIII are maintained for 6 to 8 hours. While this may have been an effective therapy given prior to surgery, this patient requires hemostasis immediately and DDAVP would not be the optimal choice.

(C) **Incorrect.** FFP contains all of the plasma proteins, including clotting factors and vWF. It is indicated for the immediate reversal of warfarin therapy, treatment of specific factor deficiencies for which factor concentrates are not available, or for coagulopathies due to liver failure. FFP is not used to treat vWD due to the large volume required to be clinically effective.

(D) **Incorrect.** Factor VII is not deficient in vWD.

(E) **Incorrect.** Platelets counts are normal in vWD.

**REASONING:**

Choices C, D, and E are clearly incorrect because they are not therapies used to treat vWD. Choice B is a first-line therapy for type 1 vWD, but it should be given 30 minutes prior to incision. As this patient has an open femur fracture and requires immediate inadequate hemostasis, choice B is the most appropriate therapy.

BIBLIOGRAPHY:

Barash PG, Cullen BF, Stoelting RK, Cahalan M, Stock M. *Clinical Anesthesia*. 6th ed. Philadelphia, PA: Lippincott Williams & Wilkins; 2010:396-397, 404.

Morgan GE, Mikhail MS, Murray MJ. *Clinical Anesthesiology*. 4th ed. New York, NY: McGraw-Hill; 2006:786-787.

---

## BOOK B:                    QUESTION 26

---

*Answer E*

Clinical Anesthesia

**QUESTION (Choose single best answer):**

A 30-year-old man is brought to the emergency department after being rescued from a house fire. With the trachea intubated and $F_{IO_2}$ at 1.0, arterial blood gas values are $Pa_{O_2}$ 495 mm Hg, $Pa_{CO_2}$ 28 mm Hg, and pH 7.28. Hemoglobin saturation measured by co-oximeter is 50%. The most appropriate next step is to

(A)  Add positive end-expiratory pressure.
(B)  Add *n*-acetylcysteine to the inhaled gases.
(C)  Administer sodium bicarbonate intravenously.
(D)  Transfuse 2 units of packed red blood cells.
(E)  Transfer to a hyperbaric chamber.

**CORRECT ANSWER: E**

**SUMMARY:**

*Carbon monoxide poisoning is an early and major cause of mortality in smoke inhalation. CO causes tissue hypoxia because it has 200 times the affinity of oxygen for hemoglobin and shifts the oxygen dissociation curve to the left, decreasing the release of oxygen to tissues. CO also interferes with mitochondrial functioning, directly causing metabolic acidosis and acting as a myocardial toxin. CO poisoning should be suspected when pulse oximetry readings are normal and a co-oximeter reads a low oxygen saturation. Arterial blood gas will reveal a normal $Po_2$, a $Pco_2$ that is reduced by hyperventilation, and acidosis secondary to tissue anoxia. A hyperbaric chamber is useful for severe cases.*

**EXPLANATION:**

(A)  *Incorrect.* Adding positive end-expiratory pressure (PEEP) will not increase the displacement of carbon monoxide from hemoglobin.
(B)  *Incorrect.* N-acetylcysteine (Mucomyst) is a mucolytic used in patients with viscous secretions. It also replenishes glutathione and is used to treat acetaminophen toxicity but is not a recommended therapy for carbon monoxide poisoning.
(C)  *Incorrect.* Sodium bicarbonate may ameliorate the metabolic acidosis caused by tissue anoxia but would not treat tissue hypoxia secondary to severe CO poisoning.
(D)  *Incorrect.* This patient is not anemic and packed red cells are not indicated.
(E)  *Correct.* The treatment for CO poisoning is 100% oxygen, which displaces the carbon monoxide molecule, shortening its half-life from 4 hours to approximately 40 minutes. Even greater levels of oxygen may be delivered to the blood in a hyperbaric chamber and facilitate the displacement of CO from hemoglobin. Hyperbaric oxygen treatment is recommended for patients with carboxyhemoglobin saturations greater than 30%.

**REASONING:**

The key to answering this question is realizing that the patient is suffering from severe carbon monoxide poisoning secondary to smoke inhalation. The patient is already intubated and on an $F_{IO_2}$ of 1.0, the best immediate treatment for carbon monoxide poisoning. Choice E, the only listed therapy for carbon monoxide toxicity, is the best answer.

**BIBLIOGRAPHY:**
Barash PG, Cullen BF, Stoetling RK. *Clinical Anesthesia*. 4th ed. Philadelphia, PA: Lippincott-Raven Publishers; 2009:909-910.
Morgan GE, Mikhail MS, Murray MJ. *Clinical Anesthesiology*. 4th ed. New York, NY: McGraw-Hill; 2006:1044, 1063.

---

**BOOK B:**

## QUESTION 27

*Answer A*

Physiology

**QUESTION (Choose single best answer):**

A 60-kg, 45-year-old woman who takes digoxin for atrial fibrillation receives furosemide 40 mg and mannitol 60 g during resection of a supratentorial meningioma. After initiation of hyperventilation to decrease $Paco_2$ from 35 to 20 mm Hg, multifocal premature ventricular contractions are noted on the ECG. The most likely cause is

(A)  Acute hypokalemia.
(B)  Cerebral ischemia.
(C)  Impending herniation of the brain stem.
(D)  Paradoxical air embolism.
(E)  Surgical manipulation of the meningioma.

**CORRECT ANSWER: A**

**SUMMARY:**
*Acute hypokalemia can result from (1) loss of total body potassium stores or from (2) shifts into intracellular spaces. Most people are asymptomatic until the serum potassium level falls below 3 mEq/L. Cardiovascular signs are common and include ECG changes, arrhythmias, labile blood pressures due to autonomic dysfunction, and decreased myocardial contractility. Hypokalemia in patients on digoxin can predispose to it cardiac toxicity. Other signs and symptoms of hypokalemia include muscle weakness, renal abnormalities, and glucose intolerance.*

**EXPLANATION:**
(A)  *Correct.* Diuretics increase the renal loss of potassium. Hyperventilation causes respiratory alkalosis and results in the intracellular shift of potassium. Hypokalemia and hypercalcemia can interact with digoxin to produce toxicity.
(B)  *Incorrect.* Arrhythmias are unlikely to be the initial and only signs in focal or global cerebral ischemia. Brain death in later stages can produce arrhythmia secondary to massive sympathetic outflow.
(C)  *Incorrect.* Raised intracranial pressure (ICP) and impending herniation are unlikely in the patient with open dura. Bradycardia and hypertension are the classic signs of impending herniation.
(D)  *Incorrect.* Paradoxical air embolus can produce stroke, myocardial or other visceral ischemia. It is associated with other signs of air embolus. Coronary air will manifest as ST-T changes in inferior leads (right coronary territory), and there can be various arrhythmias.
(E)  *Incorrect.* Surgical manipulation in the brain stem area (not the meningioma) is more prone to cardiovascular changes.

**REASONING:**
The objective of this question is to be aware of the causes and effects of hypokalemia and its drug interaction with digoxin. Considering all the changes occurring in the

patient—diuresis, acute respiratory alkalosis, preexisting digoxin therapy—acute hypokalemia is highest on the differential for premature ventricular contractions (PVCs). Though choices B and D can produce arrhythmias, they are unlikely in the absence of other signs.

**BIBLIOGRAPHY:**

Morgan GE, Mikhail MS, Murray MJ. *Clinical Anesthesiology.* 4th ed. New York, NY: McGraw-Hill; 2006:677-680, 720.

---

| **BOOK B:** | **QUESTION 28** |

## *Answer D*

### Neuroanesthesia

**QUESTION (Choose single best answer):**

A 50-year-old woman with subarachnoid hemorrhage and left hemiparesis undergoes clipping of a right cerebral aneurysm. On the second postoperative day, mental status deteriorates. Blood pressure is 110/70 mm Hg. A cerebral angiogram shows vasospasm. The most appropriate management is to

(A) Administer dexamethasone.
(B) Administer mannitol.
(C) Administer phentolamine.
(D) Expand intravascular volume.
(E) Intubate and hyperventilate to a $Paco_2$ of 28 mm Hg.

**CORRECT ANSWER: D**

**SUMMARY:**

*Cerebral vasospasm is a complication of subarachnoid hemorrhage (SAH) that can be detected on angiogram in up to 70% of patients, with half of these patients having delayed ischemic neurologic deficits (DINDS). Rarely occurring within the first 3 days after aneurysm rupture, the peak incidence of vasospasm after SAH is between 7 and 10 days. Despite the lack of adequate evidence, the cornerstone of treatment continues to be "triple H" therapy: hypervolemia, hypertension, and hemodilution. The goal is to increase cerebral blood flow (CBF). Patients with SAH receive the calcium channel nimodipine to prevent vasospasm, as it is the only pharmacologic therapy, with the exception of statins, proven to improve neurologic outcomes.*

**EXPLANATION:**

(A) *Incorrect.* Corticosteroids are used to reduce cerebral edema, not to increase blood flow.
(B) *Incorrect.* Mannitol can transiently increase CBF as an osmotic agent, but it promotes diuresis, with the end result being hypovolemia.
(C) *Incorrect.* Phentolamine is an $\alpha$-blocker that can dilate blood vessels but leads to an overall reduction in blood pressure, which decreases cerebral perfusion.
(D) *Correct.* Expanding intravascular volume, hypervolemia, continues to be one of the mainstays (remember: "triple H") of treatment of cerebral vasospasm.
(E) *Incorrect.* Hyperventilation to decrease $Paco_2$ is an intervention that results in decreased CBF.

**REASONING:**

This question tests knowledge of the treatment of cerebral vasospasm after SAH. Most of the available answer choices are more appropriate for treatment of increased ICP. "Triple H" therapy is designed to overcome the resistance from vasospasm and increase perfusion to the brain. Expanding the intravascular volume can produce hypervolemia and can also provide beneficial hemodilution (improved microcirculation) of the circulating blood.

**BIBLIOGRAPHY:**

Barash PG, Cullen BF, Stoelting RK, Cahalan M, Stock M. *Clinical Anesthesia*. 6th ed. Philadelphia, PA: Lippincott Williams & Wilkins; 2009:1449-1450.

Morgan GE, Mikhail MS, Murray MJ. *Clinical Anesthesiology*. 4th ed. New York, NY: McGraw-Hill; 2006:632-633, 642-643.

Velat GJ, Kimball MM, Mocco JD, et al. Vasospasm after aneurysmal subarachnoid hemorrhage: review of randomized controlled trials and meta-analyses in the literature. *World Neurosurg*. 2011;76(5):446-454.

---

## BOOK B:      QUESTION 29

*Answer B*

Neuroanesthesia

**QUESTION (Choose single best answer):**

Which of the following statements concerning cerebral blood flow (CBF) during anesthesia is true?

(A) CBF changes minimally when $Paco_2$ increases from 30 to 40 mm Hg.
(B) CBF changes minimally when $Po_2$ decreases from 160 to 100 mm Hg.
(C) CBF is autoregulated when mean arterial pressure (MAP) is 40 mm Hg.
(D) CBF is coupled to cerebral metabolism during isoflurane anesthesia.
(E) CBF is unaffected by 1.2% isoflurane at a $Paco_2$ of 40 mm Hg.

**CORRECT ANSWER: B**

**SUMMARY:**

*Coupling of CBF and cerebral metabolic rate (CMR) describes the parallel adjustment of CBF to meet the needs of CMR. In a normotensive adult, CBF is kept nearly constant between mean arterial blood pressures (MAP) of 60 to 160 mm Hg. This autoregulation curve can be shifted to the right in patients with chronic hypertension. Outside the limits, CBF becomes pressure dependent. Whereas CBF increases significantly only when $Pao_2$ drops below 50 mm Hg, CBF changes proportionately with $Paco_2$ between 20 and 80 mm Hg.*

**EXPLANATION:**

(A) *Incorrect.* A 33% increase in $Paco_2$ from 30 to 40 mm Hg results in a more than minimal proportionate increase in CBF. Blood flow changes approximately 1 to 2 mL/100 g/min per mm Hg change in $Paco_2$.

(B) *Correct.* CBF does not change in the range of $Pao_2$ 160 to 100 mm Hg. Hypoxemia with $Pao_2$ less than 50 mm Hg will increase CBF. Hyperoxemia may minimally decrease CBF. However, $Pao_2$ from 50 to 175 CBF remains relatively constant.

(C) *Incorrect.* At 40 mm Hg $Pao_2$, CBF is not autoregulated, that is, the brain depends on MAP to maintain perfusion.

(D) *Incorrect.* CBF remains coupled to CMR during low-dose isoflurane. Isoflurane causes heterogeneous changes throughout the brain, which explains the conflicting conclusions about whether CBF is coupled to CMR. The net effect is an increase in the CBF/CMR ratio. High doses of isoflurane result in dominance of the vasodilatory effect and an increase in CBF.

(E) *Incorrect.* CBF is increased by 1.2% isoflurane at a $Paco_2$ of 40 mm Hg. As with sevoflurane and desflurane, increase in CBF may be prevented by simultaneous hyperventilation. This is in contrast to hyperventilation with halothane or enflurane, for which hyperventilation must be initiated prior to use.

**REASONING:**
Important concepts for answering this question include an understanding of factors that affect cerebral blood flow. The reader should be able to rule out choice A because 33% is more than a minimal change. Choice B can be ruled out because there is no change in CBF in that range of $Pao_2$. Because 40 mm Hg $Pao_2$ is out of the range of normal autoregulation, choice C can also be eliminated. Knowledge that $Paco_2$ of 40 mm Hg is not enough to abolish the increase of CBF to isoflurane helps rule out choice E. That leaves choice D that is controversial depending on how "coupling" is interpreted. Even if one uses the strict interpretation that CBF should increase with CMR, by eliminating the other choices, the reader is left with the correct answer. In fact, isoflurane increases the CBF/CMR ratio such that there is more perfusion than is required by CMR (luxury perfusion).

**BIBLIOGRAPHY:**
Miller, 7th Edition, pg 316-320.
Morgan GE, Mikhail MS, Murray MJ. Clinical Anesthesiology. 4th ed. New York, NY: McGraw-Hill; 2006:616-630.

---

## BOOK B:

## QUESTION 30

---

*Answer C*

Pharmacology

**QUESTION (Choose single best answer):**
Which of the following drugs is contraindicated in patients with Parkinson disease?

(A) Atropine.
(B) Dopamine.
(C) Droperidol.
(D) Fentanyl.
(E) Isoflurane.

**CORRECT ANSWER: C**

**SUMMARY:**
*Parkinson disease is a neurologic disorder characterized by dyskinetic movements, gait disorders, and abnormal facial expression. The disease process is largely due to progressive depletion of dopamine in the substantia nigra of the midbrain. Medications that worsen the clinical effect of dopamine depletion or worsen the symptoms associated with Parkinson disease would be relatively contraindicated. Droperidol may worsen dyskinetic movements in Parkinson disease patients by blocking dopamine receptors. Other medications that should be avoided in Parkinson disease patients include phenothiazines (eg, thorazine, compazine, and promethazine) and metoclopramide.*

**EXPLANATION:**
(A) *Incorrect.* Atropine is an antimuscarinic that counteracts the effect of vagus nerve stimulation. Effects of atropine include increased heart rate, decreased mucus production and secretion, increased blood pressure, pupilary dilation, decreased intestinal motility, and urinary retention. None of these effects would be particularly problematic in Parkinson disease patients.

(B) *Incorrect.* Dopamine is the neurotransmitter that is depleted in Parkinson disease patients. Levodopa is the most common drug used to treat Parkinson disease. It is converted to dopamine in vivo and exerts its clinical effect in that form. Therefore, dopamine would not be contraindicated in Parkinson patients.

(C) *Correct.* Droperidol is a butyrophenone (of the same class as the antipsychotic drug haloperidol) that acts by blocking dopamine receptors. Because Parkinson disease patients already have depleted dopamine, administration of droperidol is relatively contraindicated in Parkinson disease patients and can worsen the symptoms associated with the disease.

(D) *Incorrect.* Fentanyl is a rapidly acting opioid that blocks μ opioid receptors and interferes with substance P in the spinal cord. μ Receptors are not involved in the Parkinson disease process.

(E) *Incorrect.* Isoflurane is a halogenated hydrocarbon that is not known to have an effect on dopamine transmission in the CNS.

### REASONING:

This question tests knowledge of basic pharmacology and pathophysiology of Parkinson disease. Choices A, D, and E are incorrect because these drugs do not exert their effects on dopaminergic neurons. Choice B is incorrect because drugs that are converted to dopamine are used to treat Parkinson disease, and dopamine is known to improve symptoms in Parkinson patients. Choice C is the only agent that interferes directly with dopaminergic neurons in a manner that would worsen rather than improve symptoms.

### BIBLIOGRAPHY:

Barash PG, Cullen BF, Stoelting RK. *Clinical Anesthesia.* 6th ed. Philadelphia, PA: Lippincott Williams & Wilkins; 2009:630-631.

Morgan GE, Mikhail MS, Murray MJ. *Clinical Anesthesiology.* 3rd ed. New York, NY: McGraw-Hill; 2002:586-587.

---

| **BOOK B:** | **QUESTION 31** |
| --- | --- |

## *Answer C and D*

Clinical Anesthesia

### QUESTION (Choose single best answer):

A 70-kg patient with no acute bleeding has a preoperative platelet count of 40,000/mm$^3$. Following preoperative transfusion of platelets 10 units, the predicted platelet count would be

(A) 50,000/mm$^3$.
(B) 80,000/mm$^3$.
(C) 90,000/mm$^3$.
(D) 140,000/mm$^3$.
(E) 190,000/mm$^3$.

### CORRECT ANSWER: C and D

### SUMMARY:

*Platelets are an essential part of the hemostasis mechanism that includes the various coagulation factors. In general, platelet transfusions are not necessary for patients without bleeding until the platelet count reaches 10,000 to 20,000/mm$^3$ below which there is an increased risk of spontaneous hemorrhage. For patients undergoing surgery, platelet counts less than 50,000/mm$^3$ are associated with increased blood loss. However, the threshold for transfusion should take into consideration the type of surgery, chance of blood loss, number and function of platelets, and the etiology of the thrombocytopenia and/or platelet dysfunction. Platelet concentrates are prepared from a single unit of whole blood whereas an apheresis unit is* *equivalent to 6 to 8 standard units in a concentrated lower volume unit. The majority of platelets now are obtained by apharesis. A common practice is to administer either 1 unit of apharesis per adult patient or 1 unit of platelet concentrate per 10 kg bodyweight.*

## EXPLANATION:

For a 70-kg adult, one unit of platelet concentrate will increase the platelet count by 7000 to 10,000/mm³ under ideal circumstances. Barash et al state that the count will increase 5000 to 10,000/mm³. Therefore, with a starting platelet count of 40,000/mm³, a transfusion of 10 units would raise the count by 50,000 to 100,000/mm³ to 90,000 to 140,000/mm³.

(A) *Incorrect.* 50,000/mm³ is much lower than would be expected.
(B) *Incorrect.* 80,000/mm³ is lower than expected, but not impossible.
(C) *Correct.* Possibly true: 90,000/mm³ is the lower limit of what would be expected.
(D) *Correct.* Possibly true: 140,000/mm³ is the upper limit of what would be expected.
(E) *Incorrect.* 190,000/mm³ is much greater than would be expected.

## REASONING:

The key concept for answering this question is understanding how much the platelet count would rise with a transfusion of a given number of units of platelets. This would be a straightforward question if it was not for the fact that different texts give different estimates for the expected results. For adults, Barash et al give a range of 5000 to 10,000/mm³/unit increase whereas Miller gives a range of 7000 to 10,000/mm³/unit increase. For children, 0.1 to 0.3 U/kg body weight should raise platelet count by 20,000 to 70,000/mm³. Alternatively, 10 cc/kg of platelet concentrate will raise count by 50,000/mm³. In practice, each patient will respond differently depending on what caused the thrombocytopenia: for example splenomegaly, autoimmune destruction, bleeding, and whether there is ongoing bleeding. Thus, the correct answer is either choice C or D depending on the lower or upper limit. In practice one should assume the worst outcome and correlate with clinical signs (ongoing coagulopathy or bleeding) and/or laboratory tests (coags, bleeding time, or platelet count). For purposes of this examination, choice D should be correct under optimal circumstances.

## BIBLIOGRAPHY:

Barash PG, Cullen BF, Stoelting RK, Cahalan M, Stock M. *Clinical Anesthesia*. 6th ed. Philadelphia, PA: Lippincott Williams & Wilkins; 2010:379-380.
Miller, 5th Edition, pg 1636-1637.
Cote CJ. *A Practice of Anesthesia for Infants and Children*. 4th ed. Philadelphia, PA: Saunders; 2009:198-199.
Johns Hopkins Hospital; Jason RJ, Shilkofski N. *Harriet Lane Handbook*. 18th ed. St. Louis, MO: Mosby; 2008:384.
Morgan GE, Mikhail MS, Murray MJ. *Clinical Anesthesiology*. 4th ed. New York, NY: McGraw-Hill; 2006:699-700.

---

**BOOK B:**      **QUESTION 32**

---

## *Answer D*

## Cardiovascular

### QUESTION (Choose single best answer):

Two hours after coronary artery bypass grafting, a 60-year-old man has a heart rate of 140 bpm and a blood pressure of 80/60 mm Hg. Cardiac index is 1.5 L/min/m². Central venous pressure is 23 mm Hg, with large *a* waves in the right atrial pressure tracing. A pulsus paradoxus of 6 mm Hg is noted. Which of the following is the most likely diagnosis?

(A) Atrial flutter.
(B) Cardiac tamponade.
(C) Hypovolemia.
(D) Junctional tachycardia.
(E) Tension pneumothorax.

**CORRECT ANSWER: D**

**SUMMARY:**

*The differential diagnosis for postoperative hypotension and tachycardia in cardiac surgery patient includes bleeding, hypovolemia, tamponade, and ventricular dysfunction. Junctional tachycardia may result in hypotension, shock, and increased central venous pressure (CVP). Cannon waves are seen in junctional rhythms.*

**EXPLANATION:**

(A) *Incorrect.* Arrhythmias are common after cardiac surgery; however, atrial flutter presents with a loss of the *a* wave. Flutter waves are seen on ECG.

(B) *Incorrect.* Cardiac tamponade may occur in the postoperative period from a loculated clot within the open pericardium. However, pulsus paradoxus of greater than 10 to 12 mm Hg is universal (not 6 mm Hg as in the question stem). The CVP tracing would show a dominant *x* descent and an attenuated *y* descent.

(C) *Incorrect.* Hypovolemia could cause hypotension and tachycardia, but the CVP should be low.

(D) *Correct.* Junctional tachycardia produces large *a* waves from AV dissociation because the normal sequence of atrial and ventricular contraction is altered. Atrial contraction occurs when the tricuspid valve is already closed and a tall cannon *a* wave is seen on the CVP tracing.

(E) *Incorrect.* Tension pneumothorax can cause hypotension, tachycardia, and elevated CVP. This would be an unusual presentation 2 hours postoperatively, and other symptoms would include elevated airway pressure, hypoxia, and mediastinal shifts.

**REASONING:**

This question focuses on the ability to be able to interpret the physiologic values obtained from anesthetic monitoring. Cardiac index = CO/BSA and is a measure of cardiac function. Normal values are usually 2.5 to 4.2. If less than 1.8 L/min/m$^2$, the patient may be in cardiogenic shock. CVP is traditionally used for monitoring volume status and gives a crude estimate of left atrial pressure. Normal CVP values are 2 to 8 mm Hg. The sequence of events seen in a typical CVP trace corresponds to specific events in the cardiac cycle, and *a* waves result from atrial contraction. They are absent in atrial fibrillation and atrial flutter and are exaggerated (cannon waves) in junctional rhythms, including junctional tachycardia. Pulsus paradoxus is an exaggerated decreased in systolic blood pressure during inspiration of greater than 10 to 12 mm Hg. It is universal in cardiac tamponade.

There are numerous confounding events that can cause postoperative hypotension in cardiac surgical patient. It is important to differentiate between the surgical and medical causes. Few diagnoses cause large *a* waves in the right atrial pressure tracing so junctional tachycardia is the most correct answer to this question

**BIBLIOGRAPHY:**

Miller RD, Eriksson LI, Fleisher LA, Wiener-Kronish JP, William YL. *Miller's Anesthesia.* 7th ed. Philadelphia, PA: Churchill Livingstone; 2009:Chap 40.

Morgan GE, Mikhail MS, Murray MJ. *Clinical Anesthesiology.* 4th ed. New York, NY: McGraw-Hill; 2006:132, 420.

www.csaol.cn/img/2007asa/RCL_src/102_Mark.pdf.

*Answer C*

Clinical Anesthesia

**QUESTION (Choose single best answer):**

Which of the following is the strongest indication for one-lung ventilation?

(A)  Descending thoracic aortic aneurysm.
(B)  Esophageal resection.
(C)  Lobectomy for lung abscess.
(D)  Lobectomy for tumor.
(E)  Pneumonectomy for tumor.

**CORRECT ANSWER: C**

**SUMMARY:**

*Separation of the two-lung and/or one-lung ventilation involves placing DLTs or bronchial blockers both of which require skill and special equipment to perform successfully. Absolute indications include isolation of the one lung to prevent infection or blood from spilling into the other lung as in cases of abscess or hemorrhage, control of the distribution of ventilation as in cases of bronchopleural fistula or unilateral lung disease, and for unilateral bronchial lavage. Another absolute indication is video-assisted thoracotomy (VAT) surgery. Relative indications mainly encompass optimization of surgical exposure for open thoracic procedures such as thoracic aortic aneurysm, pneumonectomy, thoracic spine surgery, or esophageal surgery.*

**EXPLANATION:**
(A)  *Incorrect.* Surgical exposure for repair of descending thoracic aortic aneurysm is a relative indication for one-lung ventilation.
(B)  *Incorrect.* Surgical exposure for esophageal resection is a relative indication for one-lung ventilation.
(C)  *Correct.* Isolation of the lungs to prevent contamination of lung abscess into the contralateral lung is an absolute indication for one-lung ventilation.
(D)  *Incorrect.* Surgical exposure for lobectomy for tumor resection is a relative indication for one-lung ventilation.
(E)  *Incorrect.* Surgical exposure for pneumonectomy for tumor is a relative indication for one-lung ventilation.

**REASONING:**

The key concept for answering this question is understanding the relative and absolute indications for one-lung ventilation. Choices A, B, D, and E are all relative indications because the main purpose for one-lung ventilation is to optimize surgical exposure. Choice C is the only situation where isolation of the one lung may protect the other, presumably healthier, lung from being infected if the abscess should rupture.

**BIBLIOGRAPHY:**
Barash PG, Cullen BF, Stoelting RK, Cahalan M, Stock M. *Clinical Anesthesia.* 6th ed. Philadelphia, PA: Lippincott Williams & Wilkins; 2010:1042-1053.
Miller, 7th Edition, pg 1833-1838.
Morgan GE, Mikhail MS, Murray MJ. *Clinical Anesthesiology.* 4th ed. New York, NY: McGraw-Hill; 2006:529.

*Answer C*

Clinical Anesthesia

**QUESTION (Choose single best answer):**

In a 65-year-old man, which of the following findings on preoperative pulmonary function testing is associated with the highest risk for respiratory insufficiency following pneumonectomy?

(A) Maximum voluntary ventilation at 65% of predicted.
(B) Mean pulmonary artery pressure of 28 mm Hg.
(C) Predicted postoperative forced expiratory volume in 1 second ($FEV_1$) of 800 mL.
(D) Residual volume to total lung capacity (RV/TLC) ratio of 0.35.
(E) Vital capacity of 3 L.

**CORRECT ANSWER: C**

**SUMMARY:**

*Candidates for pneumonectomy are selected based on anatomic staging and postoperative risk of the pulmonary tumor resection. The extent of lung impairment preoperatively correlates with postoperative mortality and morbidity. Spirometry is one of many PFTs, and it can assess a patient's vital capacity, forced vital capacity, and forced expiratory volume over a time interval. The most common method to determine resectability is by calculating the predicted postoperative $FEV_1$ (PPO $FEV_1$). This is calculated by multiplying the percentage of the total pulmonary blood flow (determined by radionuclide scan) of the remaining lung and the preoperative $FEV_1$. This therefore assumes that the percentage of blood flow to each lung is proportionate to the lung's total contribution of $FEV_1$. Traditionally, a PPO $FEV_1$ of less than 800 mL has been used as a cutoff. To account for patient age and height, current guidelines now recommend using the percentage predicted postoperative FEV (%PPO $FEV_1$), which is the percentage of blood flood multiplied with the %$FEV_1$. A %PPO $FEV_1$ of less than 40% reports a postoperative mortality as high as 50%. However, with the increasing popularity of VATS for lung resection, these rates may be improving. Other predictors of poor postoperative respiratory function include a maximum voluntary ventilation (MVV) of less than 50%, RV/TLC ratio of greater than 0.5, and vital capacity of less than 2 L.*

**EXPLANATION:**

(A) *Incorrect.* MVV is effort dependent and is the largest volume of gas that can be inspired in 1 minute. MVV reflects the endurance of the muscles of respiration. A typical MVV of a healthy adult is 170 L/min. An MVV of less than 50% predicted, not 65%, generally is considered high risk.

(B) *Incorrect.* Postoperative stress on the remaining pulmonary vasculature and right ventricle may occur after pneumonectomy owing to increased pulmonary vascular resistance (PVR) from the reduced pulmonary vascular bed. This postresection pulmonary physiology can be simulated by using a special pulmonary artery catheter to occlude the pulmonary artery of the lung that will be resected. The patient may not be able to tolerate pneumonectomy if the mean pulmonary artery pressure (PAP) rises greater than 40 mm Hg, $Pao_2$ is less than 60 mm Hg, or $Paco_2$ is greater than 45 mm Hg with this maneuver. Although not specifically mentioned, we assume that the reported PAP was measured during a unilateral pulmonary artery occlusion test.

(C) *Correct.* A postoperative predicted $FEV_1$ (PPO $FEV_1$) of less than 800 mL is associated with a 20% to 50% mortality. More commonly, the %PPO $FEV_1$, which accounts for age and height, is calculated as % perfusion of the remaining lung multiplied with %$FEV_1$, with a value less than 40% having mortality as high as 50%.

(D) **Incorrect.** A normal RV/TLC ratio is 0.20 to 0.25. An RV/TLC ratio of 0.4 or less is associated with only 7% mortality. An RV/TLC ratio of 0.5 is generally considered high risk.

(E) **Incorrect.** A vital capacity of three times the tidal volume is required for an effective cough. Normal vital capacity is about 60 mL/kg or about 4200 mL for the average adult. A vital capacity of less than 2 L is predictive of increased postoperative mortality and morbidity following pneumonectomy.

### REASONING:

This question tests knowledge of the role of preoperative pulmonary function testing in assessing postoperative function after lung resection. These tests and the associated clinical assessment algorithm should be reviewed carefully by the reader. The general approach is to begin with studies of whole-lung function (FVC, $FEV_1$, VC, etc) and progress to split-lung function testing and even pulmonary artery occlusion testing if indicated. Pulmonary function testing can help answer three questions: (1) Which patients will benefit from bronchodilators, (2) which patients have increased need for postoperative mechanical ventilation, and (3) which patients have increased risk of mortality following lung resection surgery? Of the available choices in this answer, choice C is associated with the highest postoperative mortality.

### BIBLIOGRAPHY:

Barash PG, Cullen BF, Stoelting RK. *Clinical Anesthesia.* 4th ed. Philadelphia, PA: Lippincott Williams & Wilkins; 2001:814-816 (Figure 30-3).

Collice G, Shafazand S, Griffen J, Keenan R, Bolliger C. Physiologic evaluation of the patient with lung cancer being considered for resectional surgery: ACCP evidence-based clinical practice guidelines (2nd ed). *Chest.* 2007;132;161S-177S.

Morgan GE, Mikhail MS, Murray MJ. *Clinical Anesthesiology.* 3rd ed. New York, NY: McGraw-Hill; 2002:535-536.

---

| **BOOK B:** | **QUESTION 35** |
|---|---|

*Answer C*

Clinical Anesthesia

### QUESTION (Choose single best answer):

During transurethral resection of the prostate (TURP), intravascular absorption of glycine irrigant most commonly produces

(A) Alkalosis.
(B) Hemolysis.
(C) Hypertension.
(D) Tachycardia.
(E) Wheezing.

### CORRECT ANSWER: C

### SUMMARY:

*Continuous irrigation is used during a TURP to facilitate visualization and removal of excised tissue. Ideal irrigants are nonhemolytic, nonionized, and isotonic. Excessive absorption of irrigant fluid (at least 2 L) may lead to intravascular fluid overload, water intoxication, and solute toxicity. Although the average absorption of irrigant during resection of the prostate is 20 mL/min and at times as high as 200 mL/min, poor correlation is seen between the duration of surgery and amount of irrigant absorbed except when lasting longer than 150 minutes. Systemic absorption of this irrigant occurs through venous sinuses that are exposed during resection of the prostate tissue. Hence, TURP syndrome is more likely to occur if the prostate capsule is violated during surgery or if the hydrostatic pressure of the irrigant solution is high (the latter depending on the height of the irrigation pole that should not be more than 60 cm and ideally should be 30 cm above the table initially and less than 15 cm near conclusion of the procedure). The typical progression of TURP syndrome begins with acute volume overload, resulting in initial hypertension and bradycardia. Continued absorption eventually will lead to left-sided heart failure, pulmonary edema, and cardiovascular collapse. Dilutional hyponatremia can ensue, resulting in cerebral and neuronal edema, restlessness, and confusion that eventually progress to loss of consciousness and seizures. Glycine is one of the more commonly used irrigation solutions, and although not specifically illustrated in the answer choices, it has unique side effects. It is a direct cardiac output depressant (average CO decrease of 17.5%) and can cause transient visual blindness secondary to retina toxicity that can last 8 to 48 hours postoperatively and seizures through its ability to potentiate NMDA receptors. Additionally, glycine metabolites are ammonia and oxalic acid that can cause encephalopathy from hyperammonemia and can worsen renal function in patients with coexisting renal disease secondary to hyperoxaluria respectively. (See also question 140 in Book A.)*

## EXPLANATION:

(A) *Incorrect.* Alkalosis is not commonly associated with glycine absorption during TURP.

(B) *Incorrect.* Glycine can be used as an irrigant because it is only mildly hypotonic compared with normal plasma osmolality. Hemolysis therefore is less likely to occur.

(C) *Correct.* Volume overload from TURP syndrome initially causes hypertension.

(D) *Incorrect.* Volume overload causes a reflex bradycardia, not tachycardia. Increased volume sensed by baroreceptors in the carotid sinus and aortic arch cause an increase in vagal tone. Increased vagal tone produces a relative vasodilation and slower heart rate in an attempt to decrease blood pressure.

(E) *Incorrect.* Excessive irrigant absorption can result in CHF and pulmonary edema. Although rales or crackles are more commonly observed with pulmonary edema, wheezing in conjunction with CHF, termed *cardiac asthma*, can also occur. However, hypertension is most likely to precede the development of pulmonary edema, and of those with hypertension who develop CHF/pulmonary edema at most, only one-third present with wheezing, and those patients are more likely to have concomitant baseline lung disease. Hypertension is therefore the best answer.

## REASONING:

This question tests knowledge of TURP syndrome and the side effects that can develop from excessive absorption of irrigant solutions. It is important to remember that the main pathophysiology of TURP syndrome is fluid overload. Acute volume overload, first and foremost, results in hypertension and bradycardia. Other side effects can occur later and are less common.

## BIBLIOGRAPHY:

Barash PG, Cullen BF, Stoelting RK. *Clinical Anesthesia*. 4th ed. Philadelphia, PA: Lippincott Williams & Wilkins; 2001:1019-1021.

Jorge S, Becquemin MH, Delerme S, et al. Cardiac asthma in elderly patients: incidence, clinical presentation and outcome. *BMC Cardiovasc Disord*. 2007 May 14;7:16

Morgan GE, Mikhail MS, Murray MJ. *Clinical Anesthesiology*. 3rd ed. New York, NY: McGraw-Hill; 2002:695-697.

Yao FS, Fontes ML, Malhotra V, eds. *Yao and Artusio's Anesthesiology Problem-Oriented Patient Management*. 6th ed. Philadelphia, PA: Lippincott Williams & Wilkins; 2008:797-821.

*Answer D*

Pediatrics

**QUESTION (Choose single best answer):**

A 2.2-kg, 6-hour-old neonate is to undergo gastrostomy followed by repair of a tracheo-esophageal fistula. During induction with halothane, air, and oxygen, the abdomen becomes distended. Appropriate management is to

(A) Intubate and assist spontaneous ventilation.
(B) Intubate and control ventilation.
(C) Insert an orogastric tube.
(D) Allow the patient to breathe spontaneously by mask until gastrostomy.
(E) Control ventilation by mask until gastrostomy.

**CORRECT ANSWER: D**

**SUMMARY:**

*Congenital tracheoesophageal fistula is present in 1/3000 live births, with the gross C/Vost IIIb types being the most common (90%), in which the upper esophagus is a blind pouch and the distal esophagus forms a posterior tracheal fistula. Today, primary closure is the standard of care, with preoperative gastrostomy tubes reserved for higher-risk patients with large fistulas or concomitant airway anomalies. Prior to placement of the gastrostomy under local anesthesia, it is prudent to avoid positive-pressure ventilation that could worsen gastric distention and impair ventilation of the lungs. Once the gastrostomy is placed and vented, intubation can proceed, with careful placement of the endotracheal tube tip between the fistula and carina.*

**EXPLANATION:**

(A) *Incorrect.* This was the official ABA answer in 1993 when gastrostomy placement prior to TE fistula repair was much more common. Today, however, primary repair is the standard of care. Intubation should be performed after placement of a gastrostomy to allow direct venting or suctioning of the gastrostomy to decrease gastric distention.

(B) *Incorrect.* The combination of intubation and positive-pressure ventilation could worsen gastric distention, decrease lung expansion, and impair ventilation.

(C) *Incorrect.* In most cases, type C/IIIB, an orogastric tube would not pass into the stomach but would end in the upper esophageal blind pouch, not playing any role in stomach decompression.

(D) *Correct.* Avoiding positive-pressure ventilation is key prior to gastrostomy. Major concerns prior to elective repair must address fluid and electrolyte deficits, any underlying aspiration pneumonia as well as other congenital anomalies (29% will have coexisting cardiac anomalies). Although 67% of the tracheoesophageal fistulas occur more than 1 cm above the carina, 11% will occur at the carina itself.

(E) *Incorrect.* Again, positive-pressure ventilation should be avoided, even if by facemask alone. There is no indication that this patient cannot maintain spontaneous ventilation.

**REASONING:**

The key to answering this question is understanding the anatomy of the most common tracheoesophageal fistula type (type C/IIIB) and how positive-pressure ventilation would cause further gastric distention and impair ventilation. Choices A and B both involve intubation, which is not recommended prior to the gastrostomy tube. Although choice C could be useful to suction upper blind pouch secretions, it would not affect gastric distention.

Choice E provides positive-pressure ventilation, which should be avoided. Choice D is correct as spontaneous ventilation is maintained.

**BIBLIOGRAPHY:**
Barash PG, Cullen BF, Stoelting RK, Cahalan M, Stock M. *Clinical Anesthesia.* 6th ed. Philadelphia, PA: Lippincott Williams & Wilkins; 2010:1196-1197.
Broemling N, Campbell F. Anesthetic management of congenital tracheoesophageal fistula. *Pediatr Anesth.* 2010;3:1-8.
Morgan GE, Mikhail MS, Murray MJ. *Clinical Anesthesiology.* 4th ed. New York, NY: McGraw-Hill; 2006:941-942.

---

## BOOK B:             QUESTION 37

*Answer A*

Equipment/Physics

**QUESTION (Choose single best answer):**

Which of the following is an advantage of a circle system over a Mapleson D system?

(A)  Better anesthetic conservation.
(B)  Lower dead space.
(C)  Lower circuit resistance.
(D)  More efficient scavenging.
(E)  More rapid changes in inspired gas concentration.

**CORRECT ANSWER: A**

**SUMMARY:**

*The circle system used in anesthesia has several advantages over Mapleson D circuits. Because of the unidirectional intake and outflow valves, the dead space in a circle system includes only the tubing distal to the Y-piece where inspiratory and expiratory gases mix. Therefore, the length of the breathing tube proximal to the Y-piece in a circle system does not add to the circuit dead space. This is not true for Mapleson D circuits, where tubing length adds to dead space. Other advantages of the circle system over the Maple-son D circuit include (1) greater preservation of anesthetic gases, (2) conservation of airway heat and humidity, and (3) more reliable scavenging. The Mapleson D circuit is efficient during controlled (vs spontaneous) ventilation, is lightweight, and allows more rapid adjustments of inspired gas concentrations. However, it is associated with variable control of anesthetic depth, inability to conserve heat and humidity, and variable scavenging of anesthetic gases.*

**EXPLANATION:**
(A)  ***Correct.*** Anesthetic gases are conserved in a circle system because they are rebreathed after being exhaled (eg, closed-circuit anesthesia). This is not true with Mapleson D circuits, where expired gases are primarily wasted.
(B)  ***Incorrect.*** Although tubing length contributes to dead space in Mapleson D circuits (unlike circle systems), this is a poor choice because tubing length is not specified in the question.
(C)  ***Incorrect.*** Resistance is higher in circle systems than in Mapleson D circuits.
(D)  ***Incorrect.*** Mapleson D circuits have variable scavenging capabilities and are not as effective as circle systems in scavenging waste gases.
(E)  ***Incorrect.*** Mapleson D circuits have the advantage here—they are better at making rapid changes in inspired gas concentrations because there is little to no mixing of inspired and expired gases.

This question tests fairly specific knowledge of the circle system (the circuits on most modern anesthesia machines) and the Mapleson D circuit. Choices C and E can be eliminated immediately with knowledge that these options actually are advantages of the Mapleson D circuit compared with the circle system. Choice B is very tempting and is correct if a Mapleson D circuit with significant tubing length is used for the comparison. However, tubing length is not specified, and this makes B a poor choice. The same is true of choice D because scavenging is variable with Mapleson D circuits. This leaves choice A, which is true for all Mapleson D circuits—there is little conservation of anesthetic because exhaled gases go out into the environment.

**BIBLIOGRAPHY:**

Barash PG, Cullen BF, Stoelting RK, Cahalan M, Stock M. *Clinical Anesthesia*. 6th ed. Philadelphia, PA: Lippincott Williams & Wilkins; 2009:671-673.

Morgan GE, Mikhail MS, Murray MJ. *Clinical Anesthesiology*. 4th ed. New York, NY: McGraw-Hill; 2006:33-41, 35 (Table 3-2).

---

## BOOK B:    QUESTION 38

### *Answer C*

Neuroanesthesia

**QUESTION (Choose single best answer):**

A 27-year-old man with a 1-month history of quadriplegia at a C6 level is given general anesthesia for cystoscopy. During the cystoscopy, blood pressure suddenly increases to 220/120 mm Hg. Further evaluation is most likely to show

(A)  Atrial fibrillation (ventricular rate 100 bpm).
(B)  Paroxysmal atrial tachycardia (160 bpm).
(C)  Sinus bradycardia.
(D)  Piloerection above the level of C6.
(E)  Sweating above the level of C6.

**CORRECT ANSWER: C**

**SUMMARY:**

*Patients with spinal cord transection at T6 and above are at risk for autonomic hyperreflexia. Stimulation below the level of the transection, such as surgical stimulation or distension of viscera, can cause unopposed reflex sympathetic discharge below the level of the lesion. The patient develops hypertension and vasoconstriction below the injury level. Vasodilation (flushing) occurs above the injury level. Baroreceptor-mediated bradycardia occurs via vagal reflexes in response to systemic hypertension. Autonomic hyperreflexia can be prevented by regional and deep general anesthesia. Though once it occurs, the initial step is to remove the offending stimulus, such as emptying the distended bladder during cystoscopy, then to deepen the anesthetic and administer direct acting vasodilators and a-adrenergic blocking agents as needed.*

**EXPLANATION:**

(A)  *Incorrect.* Arrhythmias may occur, but the patient is most likely to have sinus bradycardia via vagal baroreceptor stimulation.
(B)  *Incorrect.* See above.
(C)  *Correct.* Baroreceptors in the aortic arch and carotid sinus sense the increased pressure, producing an increase in vagal tone. This causes bradycardia.
(D)  *Incorrect.* Piloerection is sympathetically mediated; thus it will not occur above the level of cord transection. Piloerection may be present below the transection.

(E) *Incorrect.* Sweating is sympathetically mediated. The patient will be flushed above the level of transection but will not be sweating.


**REASONING:**

This question tests knowledge of the signs and symptoms of autonomic hyperreflexia and understanding which physiologic responses are sympathetically versus parasympathetically mediated. Below the level of the transection, sympathetic tone predominates because there is no opposing tone coming from higher centers (the pathway is transected). Above the transection, there is opposing tone, leading to a predominance of parasympathetic control. Piloerection and sweating are both sympathetic responses, and they will not predominate above the cord injury. The first three choices are all possibilities. However, the most likely is a straightforward sinus bradycardia. C is the single best answer.


**BIBLIOGRAPHY:**

Barash PG, Cullen BF, Stoelting RK, Cahalan M, Stock M. *Clinical Anesthesia.* 6th ed. Philadelphia, Lippincott Williams & Wilkins, 2009, p. 1028, 1377.
Morgan GE, Mikhail MS, Murray MJ. *Clinical Anesthesiology.* 4th ed. New York, NY: McGraw-Hill; 2006:655, 867.

---

| **BOOK B:** | **QUESTION 39** |
| --- | --- |

*Answer D*

Cardiovascular

**QUESTION (Choose single best answer):**

Which of the following is the primary factor regulating normal coronary blood flow?

(A)  Aortic diastolic pressure.
(B)  Coronary perfusion pressure.
(C)  Heart rate.
(D)  Myocardial oxygen consumption.
(E)  Systolic wall tension.


**CORRECT ANSWER: D**


**SUMMARY:**

*Within the ranges of normal coronary perfusion pressure (50-120 mm Hg), coronary blood flow is a function of coronary arterial tone and is regulated primarily by myocardial metabolic needs (ie, myocardial oxygen consumption). This is in contrast to the primary determinant of coronary blood flow at elevated perfusion pressures (> 120 mm Hg). At higher pressures, coronary blood flow depends primarily on coronary perfusion pressure (equal to aortic diastolic pressure minus left ventricular end-diastolic pressure [LVEDP]). This question asks you to distinguish these two scenarios and presents you with options for both.*


**EXPLANATION:**

(A) *Incorrect.* Although aortic diastolic pressure is the primary determinant of perfusion pressure (coronary perfusion pressure = aortic diastolic pressure − LVEDP), perfusion pressure does not dictate blood flow under normal conditions.
(B) *Incorrect.* Perfusion pressure is not the primary determinant of coronary blood flow under normal conditions.
(C) *Incorrect.* Although heart rate is a component of myocardial oxygen demand, it does not directly cause changes in arteriolar tone.

(D) **Correct.** Myocardial oxygen consumption determines myocardial metabolic needs, which, in turn, regulate coronary arteriolar tone at normal perfusion pressures. Thus the demand of the heart itself plays a large part in determining vascular tone and coronary blood flow.

(E) **Incorrect.** Systolic wall tension is not the primary determinant, although it may contribute to smaller changes in coronary blood flow.

**REASONING:**

This question tests knowledge of coronary autoregulation and the determinants of coronary arterial blood flow at normal and high systemic arterial pressures. Under normal conditions, myocardial oxygen demand (and thus metabolism) dictates coronary arteriolar tone, whereas at high pressures it is perfusion pressure that determines coronary artery tone. Choice A, aortic diastolic pressure, is the primary determinant of coronary perfusion pressure (choice B) and contributes largely to coronary blood flow, but only at very high pressures. You can eliminate choices C and E because they do not play a major role in determining coronary blood flow or perfusion pressure. This leaves choice D, which is the primary determinant of coronary blood flow under normal physiologic conditions.

**BIBLIOGRAPHY:**

Barash PG, Cullen BF, Stoelting RK, Cahalan M, Stock M. *Clinical Anesthesia.* 6th ed. Philadelphia, PA: Lippincott Williams & Wilkins; 2009;225.
Morgan GE, Mikhail MS, Murray MJ. *Clinical Anesthesiology.* 4th ed. New York, NY: McGraw-Hill; 2006;432.

---

**BOOK B:**  **QUESTION 40**

---

*Answer D*

Equipment/Physics

**QUESTION (Choose single best answer):**

Which of the following statements concerning pressure support ventilation is true?

(A) Continuous positive airway pressure is provided during inspiration and expiration.
(B) Delivered tidal volume remains the same with decreasing lung compliance.
(C) Inspiratory effort of less than −2 cmH$_2$O is not assisted.
(D) The overall work of breathing decreases when weaning from mechanical ventilation.
(E) The patient will need more sedation than during IMV.

**CORRECT ANSWER: D**

**SUMMARY:**

*Pressure support ventilation (PSV) was designed to support spontaneously breathing, intubated (can also be used with laryngeal mask airway [LMA]) patient with decreased lung/thorax compliance and increased airway resistance. Every inspiratory effort by the patient is supported by a preset positive pressure to reduce the work of breathing. When the inspiratory flow decreases, the ventilator allows the patient to exhale.*

**EXPLANATION:**

(A) **Incorrect.** During the breath cycle in PSV mode, the airway pressure is not necessarily continuously positive. Positive pressure is seen during inspiration and expiration if PEEP is used. The initial portion of inhalation can show negative pressure due to the patient's active inhalation efforts.

(B) *Incorrect.* Because inhalation is pressure controlled, tidal volume will vary with changes in lung/thorax compliance. With decreasing compliance, the preset pressure is reached earlier, resulting in lower tidal volume.

(C) *Incorrect.* The sensitivity of the ventilator can be changed to accommodate the patient's respiratory needs. If the negative-pressure sensitivity is set low enough, the ventilator may even sense the low negative pressure of $-2$ cmH$_2$O.

(D) *Correct.* PSV helps reduce the work of breathing by assisting the patient to overcome the airway resistant and elastic recoil of the lung and thorax.

(E) *Incorrect.* It is actually the opposite. PSV can be used as a weaning mode and requires a spontaneously breathing patient who is not heavily sedated.

### REASONING:

PSV is a mode of assisting and augmenting the breath in a spontaneously breathing patient and thus not appropriate for full ventilatory support. During PSV the ventilator detects the patient's inspiratory effort, which produces a negative deviation of proximal airway pressure from baseline. The ventilator sensitivity can be adjusted to detect larger or smaller patient efforts. The patient, therefore, determines the breaths per minute. Once activated by the patient's effort, the ventilator augments the patient's breath by providing a constant amount of positive airway pressure until the inspiratory flow rate drops to 25% of the maximal inspiratory flow rate. The ventilator then allows the pressure to return to baseline. The baseline pressure may either be zero or an independently preselected PEEP value.

PSV is a mode of assisting each breath of a spontaneously breathing patient with a preset amount of positive pressure sufficient to create adequate tidal volume in the individual patient. This mode activates the ventilatory support only if it detects active respiratory efforts; therefore, the MV depends on the patient's RR and lung/thorax compliance and can be variable during the course of breathing. The ventilatory support of a breath cycle will stop when, after an initial peak, the inspiratory flow decreases about 25% of the peak flow.

### BIBLIOGRAPHY:


Banner MJ, Kirby RR, MacIntyre NR. Patient and ventilator work of breathing and ventilatory muscle loads at different levels of pressure support ventilation. *Chest.* 1991; 100(2):531-533.

Barash PG, Cullen BF, Stoelting RK. *Clinical Anesthesia.* 3rd ed. Philadelphia, PA: Lippincott-Raven Publishers; 1997:1374.

Marino P. *The ICU Book.* 3rd ed. Baltimore, MD: Lippincott Williams & Wilkins; 2007:512-516.

Morgan GE, Mikhail MS, Murray MJ. *Clinical Anesthesiology.* 4th ed. New York, NY: McGraw-Hill; 2006:1030-1033


---

**BOOK B:**  **QUESTION 41**

*Answer D*

Pharmacology

### QUESTION (Choose single best answer):

If administered epidurally in equipotent doses, which of the following opioids will produce analgesia over the greatest number of dermatomes?

(A) Fentanyl.
(B) Hydromorphone.
(C) Meperidine.
(D) Morphine.
(E) Sufentanil.

**CORRECT ANSWER: D**

**SUMMARY:**

*The onset and migration of epidurally administered opioids depend on the density, $pK_a$, molecular weight, protein binding, and lipid solubility of the drug. Of these, lipid solubility is the most influential factor controlling drug onset and degree of dermatomal spread. Highly lipid-soluble (thus hydrophobic) drugs such as sufentanil and fentanyl have relatively low dermatomal spread rostrally because of binding to lipophilic structures within the spinal cord that prevent spread. They will, therefore, not induce analgesia across as many dermatomes as lipid-insoluble or hydrophobic drugs such as morphine and hydromorphone. Morphine is slightly more hydrophilic than hydromorphone and is associated with the highest degree of rostral spread. Unfortunately, this also can lead to undesirable respiratory depression.*

**EXPLANATION:**

(A) *Incorrect.* Fentanyl is highly lipophilic and associated with a low degree of rostral dermatomal spread.
(B) *Incorrect.* Hydromorphone, although relatively hydrophilic, is not as hydrophilic as morphine.
(C) *Incorrect.* Meperidine is not as hydrophilic as morphine.
(D) *Correct.* Morphine is the most hydrophilic and lipid-insoluble drug listed and is associated with the greatest degree of dermatomal spread.
(E) *Incorrect.* Sufentanil is the most lipophilic drug listed and will lead to the least dermatomal spread.

**REASONING:**

This question tests knowledge of opioids and their spread in the epidural space. Knowing that lipid-soluble drugs are associated with a small amount of rostral spread can assist the reader in eliminating fentanyl and sufentanil because these are highly lipophilic drugs. Although meperidine is not particularly lipid-soluble, it is less hydrophilic than morphine and Dilaudid and can be eliminated. This leaves morphine and hydromorphone (which makes sense because these are the two most commonly administered epidural opioids in clinical practice). Morphine is just slightly more hydrophilic than hydromorphone (relative lipid solubility is 1 for morphine and 1.5 for hydromorphone). This makes morphine, choice D, the best answer.

**BIBLIOGRAPHY:**

Barash PG, Cullen BF, Stoelting RK. *Clinical Anesthesia.* 5th ed. Philadelphia, PA: Lippincott Williams & Wilkins; 2006:1426.

Morgan GE, Mikhail MS, Murray MJ. *Clinical Anesthesiology.* 4th ed. New York, NY: McGraw-Hill; 2006:397 (Table 18-15).

Wagemans MFM, Zuurmond WWA, de Lange JJ. Long-term spinal opioid therapy in terminally ill cancer pain patients. *Oncologist.* 1997;2:70-75.

---

**BOOK B:**  **QUESTION 42**

---

*Answer E*

Pharmacology

**QUESTION (Choose single best answer):**

Which of the following is decreased by alkalinization of a 1.5% lidocaine solution?

(A) Concentration of free base.
(B) Dose required for anesthesia.
(C) Duration of anesthesia.
(D) Intracellular concentration of ionized lidocaine.
(E) Time to onset of anesthesia.

**CORRECT ANSWER: E**

## SUMMARY:

*Alkalinization of local anesthetic solutions has been used to hasten the onset of anesthesia for more than a century. There are many likely reasons why alkalinization affects local anesthetic activity. Prepackaged local anesthetic solutions typically are acidotic, especially when they contain additional epinephrine. Alkalinizing these solutions increases the lipid-soluble neutral form of local anesthetic in solution that can cross into the neuronal cytoplasm to achieve effect. Alkalinization also may potentiate the vasoconstrictive effects of epinephrine in situ. Alkalinization of the local neuronal environment also can inhibit neuronal impulse conduction.*

## EXPLANATION:

(A) *Incorrect.* The concentration of free base would increase with alkalinization of lidocaine.

(B) *Incorrect.* Addition of alkalinizing agents such as bicarbonate does not affect the dose of anesthetic required for adequate analgesia because it does not alter the drug potency or duration of action.

(C) *Incorrect.* The duration of action of local anesthetics depends primarily on protein binding, tissue vascularity, use of vasoconstricting agents such as epinephrine, and the rate of drug elimination. None of these is altered by alkalinization.

(D) *Incorrect.* Alkalinization of lidocaine increases the intracellular concentration of its lipid-soluble neutral form (un-ionized). Once inside the cell, the neutral form will reach an equilibrium with the ionized form, which is the form that binds to the receptor within the sodium channel.

(E) *Correct.* Time to onset of lidocaine (and other local anesthetics) is reduced with the addition of bicarbonate. See above.

## REASONING:

This question tests knowledge of the effects of alkalinization on the pharmacology of local anesthetic agents. Choice A can be eliminated easily because the base concentration would increase with alkalinization. Choices B and C can be eliminated because alkalinization does not affect potency or duration of action. Choice D is challenging and requires an understanding of the relationship between the degree of un-ionized fraction of drug and ease of movement across the cell membrane. Because it is primarily un-ionized drug that crosses the cell membrane, choice D does not make sense. E is the best choice because bicarbonate is the agent of choice for speeding onset of local anesthetics.

## BIBLIOGRAPHY:

Barash PG, Cullen BF, Stoelting RK. *Clinical Anesthesia.* 5th ed. Philadelphia, PA: Lippincott Williams & Wilkins; 2006:459-460.

Curatolo M, Petersen-Felix S, Arendt-Nielsen L, et al. Adding sodium bicarbonate to lidocaine enhances the depth of epidural blockade. *Anesth Analg.* 1998;86(2):341-347.

Morgan GE, Mikhail MS, Murray MJ. *Clinical Anesthesiology.* 4th ed. New York, NY: McGraw-Hill; 2006:268.

Wong K, Strichartz GR, Raymond SA. On the mechanisms of potentiation of local anesthetics by bicarbonate buffer: drug structure-activity studies on isolated peripheral nerve. *Anesth Analg.* 1993;76(1):131-143.

## Answer A

### Pharmacology

**QUESTION (Choose single best answer):**

Cyanide toxicity from nitroprusside is unlikely in patients with renal dysfunction because

(A)  Renal excretion of thiosulfate is decreased.
(B)  Metabolic acidosis inactivates cyanide.
(C)  Anemia inhibits breakdown of nitroprusside by oxyhemoglobin.
(D)  Thiocyanate is formed in the liver.
(E)  The dose of nitroprusside necessary to lower blood pressure is greatly decreased.

**CORRECT ANSWER: A**

**SUMMARY:**

*Sodium nitroprusside (SNP) is a potent arteriolar and venous smooth muscle dilator that is used commonly as a hypotensive agent. Its mechanism of action involves the formation of nitric oxide. In patients with renal failure, elimination of SNP is reduced, increasing the risk of accumulating nitroprusside's toxic metabolites, including methemoglobin, cyanide, and thiocyanate. Patients with renal dysfunction accumulate thiocyanate, but they are not at increased risk of cyanide toxicity.*

**EXPLANATION:**

(A)  *Correct.* Renal excretion of thiocyanate is decreased in renal failure, resulting in a milder reaction from thiocyanate toxicity. However, there is no evidence that renal failure increases the risk of cyanide toxicity.
(B)  *Incorrect.* Cyanide toxicity produces metabolic acidosis from its interaction with cytochrome oxidase enzymes.
(C)  *Incorrect.* SNP receives an electron from oxyhemoglobin inside red blood cells to produce methemoglobin and cyanide ions. Anemia is characterized by fewer red blood cells, but it does not inhibit the breakdown of SNP.
(D)  *Incorrect.* Thiocyanate is formed in the liver by thiosulfate and cyanide ion in a reaction catalyzed by the enzyme rhodanese and vitamin $B_{12}$. Thiocyanate accumulates in patients with renal dysfunction because it is cleared primarily by the kidney.
(E)  *Incorrect.* The dose of SNP necessary to lower blood pressure is not decreased. In fact, patients with renal failure and hypertension may require higher doses of SNP if they develop tolerance to the hypotensive effect. Tachyphylaxis or acute tolerance to SNP may be an early sign of cyanide toxicity.

**REASONING:**

SNP can generally be used for days without problems, although cyanide and thiocyanate poisoning may develop in renal failure. The major difference with renal failure patients exposed to SNP is that they do not clear thiocyanate as well as patients with normal renal function. Thiocyanate toxicity is more likely to develop in patients with renal failure.

**BIBLIOGRAPHY:**

Morgan GE, Mikhail MS, Murray MJ. *Clinical Anesthesiology*. 4th ed. New York, NY: McGraw-Hill; 2006:256-258 (Figure 13-2 The metabolism of sodium nitroprusside).

## *Answer D*

## OB/Regional

**QUESTION (Choose single best answer):**

Twelve hours after an uneventful hysterectomy with lidocaine epidural anesthesia, a 70-year-old woman has partial paralysis of the lower extremities. She is receiving morphine 0.5 mg/h through an epidural catheter and is pain-free. On examination, definite motor loss is noted in the lower extremities, but no other deficits are apparent. The most appropriate action at this time is to

(A) Administer naloxone.
(B) Substitute fentanyl for morphine infusion.
(C) Remove the epidural catheter.
(D) Obtain a magnetic resonance imaging (MRI) of the lumbar spine.
(E) Reassure the patient.

**CORRECT ANSWER: D**

**SUMMARY:**

*Rare but potentially devastating neurologic complications associated with epidural anesthesia include epidural abscess or hematoma. Epidural hematomas can be associated with placement or removal of an epidural catheter and are seen most commonly in patients with a known coagulopathy, either drug-induced or owing to a disease process. The symptoms of abscess or hematoma can include sharp back or leg pain with progression to numbness, motor weakness, or urinary and/or anal sphincter dysfunction. It is important to note that local anesthetics or narcotics being infused through the catheter may mask these symptoms. When this complication is suspected, immediate action must be taken. Neurologic imaging, preferably MRI, should be done to obtain a diagnosis with the catheter left in place. The treatment is surgical decompression.*

**EXPLANATION:**

(A) *Incorrect.* The neurologic symptoms are not a result of morphine and would not be reversed by naloxone, as opioids do not usually cause motor blockade.

(B) *Incorrect.* Epidural narcotics do not cause motor blockade and are not likely to be responsible for the symptoms in this patient. Changing from morphine to fentanyl will not correct the problem.

(C) *Incorrect.* Removal of the catheter has been associated with epidural hematoma in patients with coagulopathy. The question states that the procedure was uneventful and does not mention any reason for the patient to be coagulopathic. However, it would be best to do further testing such as MRI and coagulation studies prior to removing the catheter. The faster the diagnosis and treatment, the less chance of permanent neurologic sequelae.

(D) *Correct.* The patient has an unexplained neurologic deficit after epidural blockade. She should have an MRI to rule out the worst-case scenario, which would be epidural hematoma (incidence of 1:150,000) or abscess (incidence varies widely from 1:6500 to 1:500,000). It is important to note that the patient likely does not have pain associated with her symptoms because of the epidural morphine she is receiving.

(E) *Incorrect.* While every effort should be made to communicate with this patient and provide reassurance, this should be done *in addition* to determining the diagnosis. Reassurance and no action in this case could have devastating consequences, including permanent paralysis.

**REASONING:**

This patient has motor blockade after a seemingly uneventful epidural anesthetic and surgical procedure. She is only receiving epidural morphine and no local anesthetic. This should provide analgesia without motor blockade. Twelve hours have passed since she received epidural lidocaine, which normally lasts 2 to 3 hours; therefore, the likelihood of residual block is minimal. Given the clinical situation, one must rule out a neurologic complication and obtain a spine MRI, which makes D the best answer. In many cases, good neurologic recovery has been seen with decompression within 8 to 12 hours.

**BIBLIOGRAPHY:**

Miller RD, Eriksson LI, Fleisher LA, Wiener-Kronish JP, William YL. *Miller's Anesthesia.* 7th ed. Philadelphia, PA: Churchill Livingstone; 2010:1633-1634.

Morgan GE, Mikhail MS, Murray MJ. *Clinical Anesthesiology.* 4th ed. New York, NY: McGraw-Hill; 2006:320.

---

| **BOOK B:** | **QUESTION 45** |
|---|---|

*Answer A*

Equipment/Physics

**QUESTION (Choose single best answer):**

Equipment that is attached to a patient should have leakage current no greater than

(A) 10 μA.
(B) 100 μA.
(C) 1 mA.
(D) 10 mA.
(E) 100 mA.

**CORRECT ANSWER: A**

**SUMMARY:**

Leakage current *is the current that leaks out of electric equipment because of contact between internal electric equipment and capacitance coupling or insulation that is defective. The threshold for causing ventricular fibrillation in a patient owing to transcutaneous electric shock is approximately 100 mA. The maximum leakage current allowed in the operating room equipment is 10 μA. It should be noted that current that is delivered directly to the heart through low-impedance tissues (ie, directly to the myocardium or through blood) can cause cardiac arrest with much smaller current (100 μA).*

**EXPLANATION:**

(A) *Correct.* 10 μA is the maximum allowable leakage current because it is well below the level that can induce ventricular fibrillation if delivered in the form of microshock.
(B) *Incorrect.* 100 μA is the level at which microshock can induce ventricular fibrillation.
(C) *Incorrect.* 1 mA is 10 times the current that can induce ventricular fibrillation in the setting of microshock.
(D) *Incorrect.* 10 mA is 100 times the current that can induce ventricular fibrillation in the setting of microshock.
(E) *Incorrect.* 100 mA is 1000 times the current that can induce ventricular fibrillation in the setting of microshock.

**REASONING:**

This question tests knowledge of microshock and macroshock. In general terms, 100 μA is the minimum level of electric shock associated with potentially fatal arrhythmias. Even if the reader did not know that the current standard leakage limit is less than 10 μA, one might reason that a safe cutoff for electric equipment would provide a margin of safety of either 1/10 or 1/100 that value. Given that 1 μA is not an option, your best choice is 10 μA. A is the single best answer.

**BIBLIOGRAPHY:**
Barash PG, Cullen BF, Stoelting RK. *Clinical Anesthesia*. 6th ed. Philadelphia, PA: Lippincott Williams & Wilkins; 2009:175-180.
Morgan GE, Mikhail MS, Murray MJ. Clinical Anesthesiology. 4th ed. New York, NY: McGraw-Hill; 2006:23.

---

**BOOK B:**

*Answer C*

Basic Science

**QUESTION 46**

**QUESTION (Choose single best answer):**

When the inspired gas is changed from air to 20% oxygen and 80% nitrous oxide, $Pao_2$ increases because

(A) Increased pulmonary artery pressure perfuses alveoli that previously enhanced dead space.
(B) Nitrous oxide stimulates the respiratory center.
(C) Rapid absorption of nitrous oxide increases alveolar oxygen concentration.
(D) Replacement of nitrogen by nitrous oxide expands atelectatic alveoli.
(E) Respiratory depression from nitrous oxide shifts the oxyhemoglobin dissociation curve.

**CORRECT ANSWER: C**

**SUMMARY:**

*The addition of inspired nitrous oxide can increase the alveolar partial pressure of other gases. This observation is explained by the concentrating effect—one of two components that describe the concentration effect. The initial alveolar gas (ie, air) consists of 21% oxygen. The new gas mixture consists of 20% oxygen and 80% nitrous oxide. Because nitrous oxide is more diffusible than oxygen, it will be absorbed more quickly from the alveolus. Theoretically, if half the nitrous oxide were absorbed rapidly, this would leave 20 parts oxygen and 40 parts nitrous oxide, approximately 20/60, or 33%, oxygen. A higher $F_{IO_2}$ will lead to increased $Pao_2$.*

**EXPLANATION:**
(A) *Incorrect.* Pulmonary artery resistance is increased slightly by administration of $N_2O$. This results in constriction of the pulmonary vasculature that would have the opposite effect on dead space (leading to decreased perfusion of ventilated lung).
(B) *Incorrect.* $N_2O$ may cause an increase in RR, but it also decreases tidal volume, resulting in MV that is essentially unchanged.
(C) *Correct.* This describes the concentrating effect of $N_2O$ on $Pao_2$ (alveolar partial pressure of oxygen). When alveolar oxygen concentration rises, the $Pao_2$ also increases. Please note that the second-gas effect is a special instance of the concentrating effect that describes administration of nitrous oxide in conjunction with a potent inhalational anesthetic. Technically, this question does not describe the second-gas effect.
(D) *Incorrect.* Nitrous oxide does not expand atelectatic alveoli.
(E) *Incorrect.* Administration of $N_2O$ does not shift the oxyhemoglobin dissociation curve.

**BIBLIOGRAPHY:**
Barash PG, Cullen BF, Stoelting RK, Cahalan M, Stock M. *Clinical Anesthesia*. 6th ed. Philadelphia, PA: Lippincott Williams & Wilkins; 2009:418-420.
Morgan GE, Mikhail MS, Murray MJ. *Clinical Anesthesiology*. 4th ed. New York, NY: McGraw-Hill; 2006:160-161.


| BOOK B: | QUESTION 47 |
| --- | --- |

*Answer B*

Pharmacology

**QUESTION (Choose single best answer):**

Which of the following characteristics of local anesthetics is associated with long duration of action?

(A)  High degree of lipid solubility.
(B)  High degree of protein binding.
(C)  High molecular weight.
(D)  High $pK_a$.
(E)  Presence of ester linkage.


**CORRECT ANSWER: B**


**SUMMARY:**
*The duration of action of local anesthetics is predominantly affected by the degree of protein binding of drug (the higher the proportion of protein-bound drug, the longer is the duration of action). Protein binding is a key factor determining duration of action because more prominent binding to membrane proteins near the sodium channel of nerves is thought to result in a longer mean residence time of the drug at the site of action. The most protein-bound local anesthetics include bupivacaine (95%), ropivacaine (94%), and etidocaine (95%). Other factors influencing the duration of action of local anesthetics include dose (directly related), degree of tissue vascularity (inversely related), use of epinephrine (directly related), and rate of elimination (inversely related).*


**EXPLANATION:**
(A)  *Incorrect.* The degree of lipid solubility determines potency of local anesthetics because lipid-soluble drugs insert more easily into nerve cell membranes
(B)  *Correct.* Duration of action of local anesthetics is determined primarily by the degree of protein binding of the drug.
(C)  *Incorrect.* Molecular weight does not affect duration of action.
(D)  *Incorrect.* The $pK_a$ of the drug relates to its speed of onset, not its duration of action.
(E)  *Incorrect.* Ester linkages are found in ester-type local anesthetics (eg, procaine, tetracaine, and chloroprocaine). These drugs are metabolized by plasma pseudocholinesterases and, as a group, have a shorter duration of action than amides. However, protein binding is the stronger determinant of duration of action.

**REASONING:**

This question tests knowledge of local anesthetic pharmacokinetics. Choices A and D can be eliminated by understanding that these properties determine onset, not duration of action, of local anesthetics. Choice D is incorrect because molecular weight is not a pharmacokinetic property of these drugs. Choice E is tempting because it refers to a category of local anesthetics that are associated with a shorter duration of action. However, the degree of protein binding is the most influential factor even within these two categories of drugs (both esters and amides), and thus B is the best answer.

**BIBLIOGRAPHY:**

Morgan GE, Mikhail MS, Murray MJ. *Clinical Anesthesiology.* 3rd ed. New York, NY: McGraw-Hill; 2002:235.

Stoelting RK. *Pharmacology and Physiology in Anesthetic Practice.* 3rd ed. Philadelphia, PA: Lippincott Williams & Wilkins; 1999:160 (Table 7-1).

---

| **BOOK B:** | **QUESTION 48** |
|---|---|

## *Answer B*

Pharmacology

**QUESTION (Choose single best answer):**

Which of the following drugs used to produce or reverse muscle relaxation has the greatest prolongation of action in a patient with end-stage renal disease?

(A) Atracurium.
(B) Neostigmine.
(C) Pancuronium.
(D) Succinylcholine.
(E) Vecuronium.

**CORRECT ANSWER: B**

**SUMMARY:**

*Most neuromuscular blocking drugs are associated with some degree of renal elimination. Among the NDMRs, pancuronium is associated with the highest degree of renal excretion (up to 60%) and should be avoided in patients with renal failure. Atracurium and cisatracurium are metabolized by nonspecific plasma esterases and degradation via Hoffmann elimination. These elimination pathways are independent of renal function. Succinylcholine is metabolized by pseudocholinesterases that can be decreased (but not profoundly) in the setting of renal failure. They have a minimal effect on duration of action. Neostigmine is associated with a 50% to 55% renal clearance, and the duration of action is increased two- to threefold in the setting of renal failure. Vecuronium is eliminated predominately by the liver, but it has about 30% renal excretion. An intubating dose of vecuronium has approximately 50% prolonged duration of action in the setting of end-stage renal disease.*

**EXPLANATION:**

(A) *Incorrect.* Atracurium is metabolized by nonspecific plasma esterases and by Hoffmann degradation. Both are not influenced by renal function.

(B) *Correct.* The duration of action of neostigmine may be increased two- to threefold in the setting of renal failure because renal elimination accounts for approximately 50% to 55% of its clearance. In comparing the duration of action of neostigmine with that of nondepolarizing agents (NDMRs), Stoelting states that the duration of action is as long as, if not longer than, that of NDMRs, making the occurrence of recurarization unlikely. The dosage of anticholinesterases does not have to be altered in patients with reduced renal.

(C) *Incorrect.* Although the duration of action of pancuronium is increased in the setting of renal failure, the extent of this change is less than with the anticholinesterase drugs (eg, neostigmine, edrophonium, and pyridostigmine).

(D) *Incorrect.* There is minimally significant prolongation of action with succinylcholine in the setting of renal failure.

(E) *Incorrect.* Vecuronium is metabolized primarily by the liver and has only about 30% renal excretion. Its duration of action is prolonged in end-stage renal disease, but not to the extent of neostigmine.

## REASONING:

This question tests knowledge of the elimination pathways of common anesthetic agents. Choices A, D, and E can be eliminated immediately because these drugs are not eliminated primarily by the kidney. The duration of action for both pancuronium and neostigmine is prolonged in renal failure, and therefore both could be appropriate choices. However, the extent of the increase in duration of action is higher with anticholinesterase drugs than with neuromuscular blocking drugs, including pancuronium. The single best answer is B.

## BIBLIOGRAPHY:


Barash PG, Cullen BF, Stoelting RK. *Clinical Anesthesia.* 4th ed. Philadelphia, PA: Lippincott Williams & Wilkins; 2001:1012-1014.

Cronnelly R, Stanski DR, Miller RD, et al. Renal function and the pharmacokinetics of neostigmine in anesthetized man. *Anesthesiology.* 1979;51(3):222-226.

Cronnelly R, Stanski DR, Miller RD, Sheiner LB. Pyridostigmine kinetics with and without renal function. *Clin Pharmacol Ther.* 1980;28(1):78-81.

Morgan GE, Mikhail MS, Murray MJ. *Clinical Anesthesiology.* 3rd ed. New York, NY: McGraw-Hill; 2002;194-195.

Morris RB, Cronnelly R, Miller RD, et al. Pharmacokinetics of edrophonium in anephric and renal transplant patients. *Br J Anaesth.* 1981;53(12):1311-1314.

Stoelting RK. *Pharmacology and Physiology in Anesthetic Practice.* 3rd ed. Philadelphia, PA: Lippincott Williams & Wilkins; 1999;203, 226-228 (Table 9-1).


---

**BOOK B:**　　　　　　　　　**QUESTION 49**

---

*Answer B*

Neuroanesthesia

### QUESTION (Choose single best answer):

In a patient with chronic congestive heart failure, the safest pharmacologic approach to nonvasogenic brain swelling during a craniotomy is

(A) Dexamethasone.
(B) Furosemide.
(C) Mannitol.
(D) Thiopental.
(E) Urea.

### CORRECT ANSWER: A or B, unanswerable

### SUMMARY:

*Treatment of intracranial hypertension is directed at decreasing the volume of one of three components of the cranial compartment: brain, blood, or cerebral spinal fluid. Agents that are effective include osmotic diuretics such as mannitol and urea, diuretics such as furosemide, and corticosteroids such as dexamethasone. Barbiturates can be used to achieve burst suppression on EEG, but they can cause adverse cardiac outcomes in those with congestive heart failure (CHF). Nonpharmacologic treatment includes proper positioning, hypothermia, sedation, hyperventilation, and surgical decompression and/or drainage of CSF.*

**EXPLANATION:**

(A) *Incorrect.* Dexamethasone, a glucocorticoid, is effective in treating intracranial hypertension from vasogenic edema due to tumor or abscess and promotes repair of the blood-brain barrier. It has not been shown to have any benefit in cerebral edema due to head trauma. It has little effect on the cardiovascular system. However, dexamethasone can cause hyperglycemia that might worsen clinical outcome in the setting of ischemic brain injury if left untreated.

(B) *Correct.* Furosemide, a loop diuretic, lowers intracranial water and decreases CSF formation. It may benefit the patient in CHF by lowering preload through diuresis, but may also result in profound electrolyte abnormalities.

(C) *Incorrect.* Mannitol, an osmotic diuretic, effectively lowers ICP by extracting water from the intracranial compartment into the intravascular space. This may result in acute fluid overload and pulmonary edema in a patient with CHF.

(D) *Incorrect.* Thiopental, a barbiturate, can decrease cerebral blood flow and facilitate absorption of CSF, and therefore reduce ICP. It can also be used to achieve burst suppression coma as a last resort for treatment of intracranial hypertension. However, it may cause direct myocardial depression through profound hypotension and should not be used in a patient with CHF.

(E) *Incorrect.* Urea is an osmotic diuretic with the same mechanism and contraindications for use as mannitol.


**REASONING:**

It is important to understand the pathophysiology of intracranial hypertension and CHF. Choices C and E can be easily ruled out because the mechanism of osmotic diuresis can result in fluid overload. Choice D can also be eliminated because thiopental is not a first-line agent to treat intracranial hypertension, and can cause hypotension and decreased cardiac output. The decision between choices A and B is difficult. Both furosemide and dexamethasone are commonly used, safe medications with potentially dangerous side effects in this setting—electrolyte abnormalities and hyperglycemia, respectively. However, dexamethasone is only effective for vasogenic brain edema. These side effects can be easily monitored and treated in the OR and ICU settings.


**BIBLIOGRAPHY:**


Cottrell JE, Smith JS. *Anesthesia and Neurosurgery.* 4th ed. St. Louis, MO: Mosby; 2001:210-211.

Hardman, JG, Limbird, LE, Goodman, AG. *Goodman and Gilman's The Pharmacologic Basis of Therapeutics.* 10th ed. New York, NY: McGraw-Hill; 2001:767-769.

Morgan GE, Mikhail MS, Murray MJ. *Clinical Anesthesiology.* 4th ed. New York, NY: McGraw-Hill; 2006:185-186, 618, 621, 632.

Pasternak JJ, McGregor DG, Lanier WL. Effect of single-dose dexamethasone on blood glucose concentration in patients undergoing craniotomy. *Neurosurg Anesthesiol.* 2004;16(2):122-125.


---

**BOOK B:**  **QUESTION 50**

*Answer A*

Clinical Anesthesia

**QUESTION (Choose single best answer):**

In clinical anesthesia practice, the term "informed consent" is best described as a legal concept in which patients

(A) Agree to anesthesia care based on full disclosure of facts needed to make the decision intelligently.

(B) Are told of all possible risks of anesthesia and anesthetic procedures.

(C) Delegate all decisions regarding anesthesia care to the anesthesiologist.

(D) Release the physicians from liability.

(E) Sign global consent forms for surgical procedures that cover the administration of anesthesia care.

**CORRECT ANSWER: A**

**SUMMARY:**

*On establishing a doctor-patient relationship, an anesthesiologist assumes the general responsibilities that all physicians have in the care of patients. Among these are obtaining informed consent and adherence to a standard of care while providing treatment to the patient. Informed consent may be written, verbal, or implied, with the main objective that the patient is provided a fair and reasonable account of the proposed procedure. Disclosure of all possible risks is unrealistic, and the guideline requires discussion within the scope of reasonable risk for the individual patient. Anesthetic procedures are distinct from surgical procedures and therefore cannot be covered under surgical consent. With the exception of individuals who are unconscious or unable to consent, where the concept of a "reasonable patient" is used to assume implied consent, treatment of patients without informed consent places the anesthesiologist at risk for criminal battery charges. An anesthesiologist still can be held liable in a malpractice suit if breach of duty, reasonable causation, or damage occurs during anesthetic care.*

**EXPLANATION:**

(A) *Correct.* See above.
(B) *Incorrect.* Discussion of *all* possible risks of anesthesia to a layperson is often not feasible, and in certain instances, some risks are not foreseeable.
(C) *Incorrect.* Part of informed consent is to assist patients in making intelligent decisions when given the pertinent information. The patient still makes decision regarding his or her anesthetic care. Once the patient is sedated or unconscious, it is the anesthesiologist's responsibility to act within the reasonable scope of the patient wishes.
(D) *Incorrect.* See above.
(E) *Incorrect.* See above.

**REASONING:**

This question tests knowledge of informed consent. The reader should be able to identify the correct answer even without detailed knowledge of the legal definition. Phrases such as *all possible risks, global consent,* and *all decisions* should be viewed with the suspicion usually placed on all such absolute and inclusionary phrasing. A is the best answer.

**BIBLIOGRAPHY:**
Barash PG, Cullen BF, Stoelting RK, Cahalan M, Stock M. *Clinical Anesthesia.* 6th ed. Philadelphia, PA: Lippincott Williams & Wilkins; 2009:88-89.
Morgan GE, Mikhail MS, Murray MJ. *Clinical Anesthesiology.* 4th ed. New York, NY: McGraw-Hill; 2006:10-11.

---

| **BOOK B:** | **QUESTION 51** |
|---|---|

*Answer C*

OB/Regional

**QUESTION (Choose single best answer):**

The low fetal/maternal plasma ratio of bupivacaine compared with lidocaine is due to

(A) Fetal tissue binding.
(B) Fetal plasma protein binding.
(C) Maternal plasma protein binding.
(D) Ionization in maternal blood.
(E) Ionization in fetal blood.

**CORRECT ANSWER: C**

**SUMMARY:**
*Fetal plasma drug concentration depends on delivery of drug to the placenta via the uterine artery, transfer of drug across the placenta (compounds < 500 Da can cross the placenta and local anesthetics are < 300 Da), and fetal uptake. Assuming constant uterine artery blood flow, transfer of free drug (ie, not protein-bound) from the maternal to fetal circulation can be described by the Fick equation, that is,*

$$\frac{\Delta q}{\Delta t} = \frac{KA(C_m - C_f)}{X}$$

*where $\Delta q/\Delta t$ represents rate of transfer of the drug, A is the surface area of the membrane, $C_m$ is the maternal drug concentration, $C_f$ is the fetal drug concentration, X is the thickness of the membrane, and K is a diffusion constant determined by drug properties such as molecular weight, lipid solubility, degree of ionization, and spatial configuration. Simply put, the surface area and membrane thickness will remain constant, so nonionized, lipid-soluble, non–protein-bound drugs will cross the placenta more readily. Bupivacaine is highly protein bound and therefore does not cross the placenta as easily as lidocaine.*

**EXPLANATION:**
(A) *Incorrect.* Local anesthetics have limited fetal tissue binding.
(B) *Incorrect.* Fetal plasma protein binding is less than maternal for both lidocaine and bupivacaine and therefore would facilitate transfer from the fetal circulation to maternal circulation.
(C) *Correct.* Bupivacaine is approximately 95% protein bound compared with lidocaine, which is approximately 50% protein bound.
(D) *Incorrect.* Both lidocaine and bupivacaine are weak bases. The $pK_a$ of lidocaine is 7.8, and the $pK_a$ of bupivacaine is 8.1. However, only the non–protein-bound free drug is available for ionization, which is significantly less with bupivacaine than with lidocaine. The difference in $pK_a$ is not enough to compensate for the high protein binding of bupivacaine.
(E) *Incorrect.* Ionization in fetal blood occurs when fetal acidosis is present. The difference in pH between the maternal and fetal circulations causes increased concentration of the ionized form of the local anesthetic and impedes transfer. This question does not refer to the acidotic fetus.

**REASONING:**
To answer this question, one must know that placental transfer of local anesthetic occurs when the drug is small, nonionized, and non–protein-bound. Bupivacaine is the most protein bound of the local anesthetics in common obstetrical practice. Choice A refers to fetal tissue binding, which is not a significant property of local anesthetics. Choice B can be eliminated because fetal protein binding would cause a high fetal-to-maternal plasma concentration ratio. Choice E can be eliminated because the question does not refer to the acidotic fetus. Differentiating between choices C and D is difficult because the difference in $pK_a$ between lidocaine and bupivacaine actually would result in more un-ionized form of bupivacaine, which intuitively would lead to more placental transfer. However, the important concept is that bupivacaine is so highly protein bound that the amount of free, nonionized drug available for transfer across the placenta is less than lidocaine. C is the best answer.

**BIBLIOGRAPHY:**

Bucklin B, Gambling DR, Wlody DJ. *A Practical Approach to Obstetric Anesthesia.* Philadelphia, PA: Lippincott Williams & Wilkins; 2009:32-33.

Miller RD, Eriksson LI, Fleisher LA, Wiener-Kronish JP, William YL. *Miller's Anesthesia.* 7th ed. Philadelphia, PA: Churchill Livingstone; 2010:1618.

---

**BOOK B:** | **QUESTION 52**

*Answer B*

Clinical Anesthesia

**QUESTION (Choose single best answer):**

A previously healthy 28-year-old man is admitted to the emergency department with a probable opioid overdose. Arterial blood gas values are $Pao_2$ 49 mm Hg, $Paco_2$ 76 mm Hg, and pH 7.12 while breathing room air. Which of the following statements is true?

(A) Aspiration of gastric contents must have occurred.
(B) Hypoventilation alone can explain the acidosis and hypoxemia.
(C) The hypoxemia probably is due to noncardiogenic pulmonary edema.
(D) Naloxone should be administered only if the patient is normothermic.
(E) Pure oxygen is contraindicated.

**CORRECT ANSWER: B**

**SUMMARY:**

*Acute respiratory acidosis may take time to correct because of delayed renal compensation. These arterial blood gas values demonstrate a pure respiratory acidosis, as approximated by the decrease in pH of 0.08 unit for every 10 mm Hg increase in $Paco_2$ above 40 mm Hg. It is important to ensure adequate oxygenation in this patient with impaired ventilation. If an opioid overdose is suspected, naloxone should be administered to antagonize its effect and possibly circumvent tracheal intubation and mechanical ventilation.*

**EXPLANATION:**

(A) *Incorrect.* Significant gastric aspiration can result in hypoxia secondary to pulmonary shunting, along with pulmonary edema, pulmonary hypertension, and hypercapnia. Physical findings such as wheezing, tachycardia, and tachypnea also would be expected to occur with such a significant acidosis. Although this choice is possible, the absence of these findings makes it less likely to be correct.

(B) *Correct.* Acute respiratory acidosis due to hypoventilation may be extreme owing to the limited buffering capacity of hemoglobin and exchange of extracellular H+ ion for intracellular cations. Renal compensatory response is slow, requiring days to achieve an effect. In general, every 10 mm Hg increase in $Paco_2$ yields a corresponding decrease in pH of 0.08 in the setting of acute respiratory acidosis.

(C) *Incorrect.* Noncardiogenic pulmonary edema reflects disruption of the alveolar/capillary membrane in the setting of nonelevated (< 18 mm Hg) PAOP and results in shunting and hypoxemia. Noncardiogenic pulmonary edema can be seen after neurologic injury (neurogenic pulmonary edema), in transfusion-related acute lung injury (TRALI), or even after vigorous inspiration against a closed glottis (negative-pressure pulmonary edema). This patient was previously healthy, and there is no indication that these injuries have occurred.

(D) *Incorrect.* Hypothermia is not a contraindication to naloxone administration. There is no indication in this scenario that the respiratory acidosis is due to hypothermia.

(E) *Incorrect.* Tissue hypoxia can be significant in severe acidosis. Cardiovascular function and response to catecholamines are already compromised. Adequate oxygenation is essential for a hypoxic patient, and delivery of 100% oxygen is important for the patient's treatment.

This question tests knowledge of interpretation of arterial blood gas analyses. One always should be wary of obligatory statements such as "must have occurred" or inclusionary statements such as "hypoventilation alone can explain. . . ." In this case, choice A can be excluded easily because aspiration of gastric contents cannot be diagnosed definitively solely from blood gas analysis. Choices C, D, and E reasonably can be excluded with a basic understanding of the principles of blood gas interpretation. The reader should take a moment to ensure a thorough understanding of acid-base interpretation and treatment. The best answer is B.

**BIBLIOGRAPHY:**

Barash PG, Cullen BF, Stoelting RK. Clinical Anesthesia, 4th ed. Philadelphia, Lippincott Williams & Wilkins, 2001, pp. 165–170.

Morgan GE, Mikhail MS, Murray MJ. Clinical Anesthesiology, 3d ed. New York, McGraw-Hill, 2002, pp. 252, 652.

| **BOOK B:** | **QUESTION 53** |
| --- | --- |

## *Answer A*

## Cardiovascular

**QUESTION (Choose single best answer):**

In which of following clinical circumstances does downregulation of β-adrenergic receptors occur?

(A) Chronic congestive heart failure.
(B) Hypothyroidism.
(C) Long-term clonidine administration.
(D) Long-term metoprolol administration.
(E) Stable angina.

**CORRECT ANSWER: A**

**SUMMARY:**

*β-Receptor downregulation is associated with any condition with chronically elevated circulating catecholamines. It is seen in chronic congestive heart failure (CHF). Changes in the density of the receptors are also seen in thyroid disease states. The receptors are increased in hyperthyroidism and reduced in hypothyroidism.*

**EXPLANATION:**

(A) **Correct.** $\beta_1$ Receptors are downregulated during chronic catecholamine stimulation and in CHF. $\beta_2$ Receptors are unaffected in CHF.

(B) **Correct.** According to *Miller's Anesthesia*, this is also a correct answer. Thyroid hormone increases β-adrenergic receptors in hyperthyroidism and decreases it in hypothyroidism. However, CHF is the more commonly known answer.

(C), (D), and (E) **Incorrect.** These conditions are not associated with elevated levels of catecholamines. On the contrary, long-term therapy with clonidine and metoprolol are associated with upregulation of β receptors.

**REASONING:**

This question tests the knowledge of β-receptor physiology and its clinical implication. There is an inverse relationship between the receptor density and the level of catecholamines. Although, there are two correct answers, for the sake of boards, I would choose the one that is better known.

**BIBLIOGRAPHY:**
*Braunwald's Heart Disease.* 9th ed. 2011:1835.
Miller RD, Eriksson LI, Fleisher LA, Wiener-Kronish JP, William YL. *Miller's Anesthesia.* 7th ed. Philadelphia, PA: Churchill Livingstone; 2009:275-278.

---

| **BOOK B:** | **QUESTION 54** |
| --- | --- |

---

*Answer E*

Clinical Anesthesia

**QUESTION (Choose single best answer):**

Which of the following is the most likely cause of apnea occurring after a retrobulbar block?

(A) Epidural injection.
(B) Increased intracranial pressure.
(C) Oculopontine reflex.
(D) Ophthalmic artery injection.
(E) Subarachnoid injection.

**CORRECT ANSWER: E**

**SUMMARY:**

*Retrobulbar block, for eye surgery, involves the injection of local anesthetic into the muscle cone behind the eye. Within the cone lie the optic nerve, ophthalmic artery and vein, and ciliary ganglion. The most common complication is retrobulbar hemorrhage secondary to vessel puncture. The "postretrobulbar apnea syndrome" is due to infiltration of local anesthetic into the CSF, probably from penetration of meningeal sheaths that encase the optic nerve. Besides apnea, signs of CSF infiltration may include unconsciousness, shivering, paraplegia (hemi, para or quad), hyperreflexia, and cranial nerve blockade.*

**EXPLANATION:**
(A) *Incorrect.* There is no "epidural" space as surrounds the spinal cord.
(B) *Incorrect.* The block is not performed intracranially so is not likely to cause increased ICP. Increased ICP may cause respiratory derangements (Cushing triad), but it is a late sign.
(C) *Incorrect.* This is a distractor to make you think of the oculocardiac reflex that causes bradycardia.
(D) *Incorrect.* Intra-arterial injection causes seizures.
(E) *Correct.* High levels of local anesthetic into the CSF cause unconsciousness and apnea.

**REASONING:**

Retrobulbar blocks are done "blindly"; that is, the needle is advanced into the orbit, without seeing what structures are encountered along the way or where, exactly, the needle is placed. Thus the local anesthetic may be injected into any structure: vein, artery, nerve, or eye itself. Complications follow the inadvertent injections.

**BIBLIOGRAPHY:**
Barash PG, Cullen BF, Stoelting RK, Cahalan M, Stock M. *Clinical Anesthesia.* 6th ed. Philadelphia, PA: Lippincott Williams & Wilkins; 2010:1333-1334.
Morgan GE, Mikhail MS, Murray MJ. *Clinical Anesthesiology.* 4th ed. New York, NY: McGraw-Hill; 2006:831-832.

*Answer E*

Cardiovascular

**QUESTION (Choose single best answer):**

A 40-year-old man is undergoing open reduction and internal fixation of a fractured femur. During anesthesia with fentanyl, enflurane, and oxygen, his heart rate decreases to 20 bpm, and 6 premature ventricular contractions per minute are noted. No pulse is detected. The most appropriate next step is to

(A)  Administer atropine.
(B)  Administer epinephrine.
(C)  Administer lidocaine.
(D)  Apply a transthoracic pacemaker.
(E)  Start cardiopulmonary resuscitation.


**CORRECT ANSWER: E**


**SUMMARY:**

*Enflurane, as well as isoflurane and halothane, depresses the sinoatrial (SA) node rate and prolongs conduction through the atrioventricular (AV) node, which can result in junctional rhythms or slow sinus rates with escape beats. Regardless of the type of anesthetic used, a patient without a detectable pulse has insufficient tissue perfusion, and cardiopulmonary resuscitation (CPR) should be initiated immediately. This patient shows electrical activity on the monitor but no detectable pulse. This clinical presentation is described as* pulseless electrical activity (PEA). *The most common causes of PEA are known as the "five H's and five T's"—hypovolemia,* hypoxia, hydrogen ion acidosis, hyper/hypokalemia, and hypothermia; and tablets (overdose), tamponade, tension pneumothorax, coronary thrombosis, and pulmonary thrombosis. After initiating supportive measures for the patient with PEA, the root cause should be identified and treated.*


**EXPLANATION:**

(A)  *Incorrect.* Atropine may increase the electrical rate but not pressure. Without a pulse, there will not be any mechanism to circulate the drug.
(B)  *Incorrect.* Epinephrine has both chronotropic and vasopressor properties. Without a pulse, there will not be any mechanism to circulate the drug.
(C)  *Incorrect.* Lidocaine has some antiarrhythmic properties, but like all local anesthetics, it decreases depolarization rates and has negative inotropic properties. Lidocaine typically is used for premature ventricular beats, stable ventricular tachycardia, and refractory ventricular fibrillation/pulseless ventricular tachycardia. However, without a pulse, there will not be any mechanism to circulate the drug.
(D)  *Incorrect.* A transthoracic pacemaker will take precious time to institute and will only increase rate, not provide for a blood pressure. The American Heart Association describes transthoracic pacing as a "disappointing" treatment for PEA.
(E)  *Correct.* CPR is the most appropriate next step in a patient without a pulse.


**REASONING:**

The patient with PEA may need all the interventions listed in the choices to survive. However, without a discernible pulse pressure, medication administered may not be distributed to the sites of action. The primary survey for a patient with PEA involves chest compressions; the secondary survey has the rescuer administering drugs and assessing for pseudo-PEA (blood flow present but too low to be felt by palpation), and finally treating for reversible causes.

**BIBLIOGRAPHY:**

*Advanced Cardiac Life Support.* Dallas, TX: American Heart Association; 2010:38, 85, 99.

Miller RD, Miller ED, Reves JG, et al. *Anesthesia.* 7th ed. Philadelphia, PA: Churchill Livingstone; 2010:2988-2989.

Morgan GE, Mikhail MS, Murray MJ. *Clinical Anesthesiology.* 4th ed. New York, NY: McGraw-Hill; 2006:996.

---

**BOOK B:**  **QUESTION 56**

---

*Answer D*

Cardiovascular

**QUESTION (Choose single best answer):**

A 35-year-old woman with systemic lupus erythematosus is admitted to the critical care unit following sudden onset of severe chest pain. Examination shows tachycardia, hypotension, pulmonary edema, and a blowing systolic murmur in the left parasternal region. The most appropriate management is

(A)  Aerosol administration of terbutaline.
(B)  Intravenous infusion of phenylephrine and nitroglycerin.
(C)  Intravenous infusion of esmolol.
(D)  Intravenous infusion of epinephrine and nitroprusside.
(E)  Volume loading with lactated Ringer solution.

**CORRECT ANSWER: D**

**SUMMARY:**

*Systemic lupus erythematosus (SLE) can have various cardiac manifestations, including pericarditis, myocarditis, coronary artery disease, dysrhythmias, and valvular disease. Over 50% of patients with SLE have been shown to have valvular abnormalities on transesophageal studies. These are commonly noninfectious vegetations affecting the mitral and aortic valves. Valvular disease includes thickening and fibrosis that may eventually cause retraction of the valves, resulting in insufficiency or stenosis. The clinical constellation described is one of acute mitral insufficiencies. Mitral regurgitation causes volume overload of the left ventricle, resulting in decreased cardiac output and elevated left atrial pressure. This is manifested clinically by tachycardia, hypotension, and pulmonary edema.*

**EXPLANATION:**

(A)  *Incorrect.* Aerosolized terbutaline, a $\beta_2$-adrenergic agonist, is used to treat asthma. The patient's presentation is inconsistent with an asthma exacerbation.

(B)  *Incorrect.* Intravenous infusion of phenylephrine will raise blood pressure, but also increase systemic vascular resistance (SVR) and therefore worsen regurgitation. Nitroglycerin might help vasodilate the coronary arteries, but may also dilate venous capacitance vessels, resulting in undesirable decreased preload.

(C)  *Incorrect.* Intravenous infusion of esmolol is contraindicated because a goal of management is to maintain a normal to slightly elevated heart rate (80-100 bpm). This serves to decrease time for regurgitation in the cardiac cycle and improve cardiac output.

(D)  *Correct.* Intravenous infusion of epinephrine may positively assist contractility and chronotropy. Nitroprusside may decrease SVR promoting forward flow and decreasing the regurgitant flow.

(E)  *Incorrect.* Volume loading with lactated Ringer solution is contraindicated because the problem is not inadequate preload, but inability of the left ventricle to maintain forward flow. Volume loading will increase SVR and further volume overload the left ventricle, increasing the amount regurgitated.

**REASONING:**

Answering this question requires identifying acute mitral regurgitation in a high-risk patient and knowing the appropriate treatment. Choice A can be immediately eliminated by knowing that the problem is cardiac in origin. The next step is to figure out that the pathology is valvular regurgitation from the signs and symptoms. This is especially tricky because the symptoms could be consistent with aortic insufficiency (AI) as well. Knowing that the murmur of AI is primarily diastolic would help differentiate between the two. Fortunately, goals in management are similar for both mitral and aortic regurgitation: maintaining normal to elevated heart rate, gentle vasodilation, maintaining cardiac output, and avoiding fluid overloading. Thus choices B, C, and E may also be ruled out.

**BIBLIOGRAPHY:**

Braunwald D, Zipes P. *Heart Disease*. 6th ed. Philadelphia, PA; W.B Saunders; 2001; 2204-2206.
Miller, 7th Edition, pg 1929-1931.
Morgan GE, Mikhail MS, Murray MJ. *Clinical Anesthesiology*. 4th ed. New York, NY: McGraw-Hill; 2006:464, 469-472.

---

**BOOK B:**

## QUESTION 57

*Answer A*

Pharmacology

**QUESTION (Choose single best answer):**

The following table shows the pharmacokinetic effects of a new neuromuscular blocker.

| | Normal | Renal Failure |
|---|---|---|
| Volume of distribution | 15 L | 21 L |
| Clearance | 200 mL/min | 100 mL/min |

In a patient with renal failure, which of the following will result in a response to this drug most similar to that of a normal individual?

(A) Increased loading dose.
(B) The same maintenance dose.
(C) Decreased maintenance dose interval.
(D) Avoidance of continuous infusion.
(E) Increased dose of anticholinesterase for reversal.

**CORRECT ANSWER: A**

**SUMMARY:**

*The volume of distribution ($V_d$) is the apparent volume in which a drug is distributed. It is determined by a drug's lipid solubility, amount of protein binding, and organ perfusion. A large $V_d$ implies extensive spread and tissue uptake of a drug so that a smaller fraction is available at the effector site. In a patient with a large $V_d$, as in renal failure, a larger dose may be required initially to achieve the same therapeutic level. The clearance is the rate of a drug's elimination either by metabolism or excretion, and along with redistribution it helps terminate the drug effect. Administering the same maintenance dose given to a normal patient or using continuous infusion when a drug's clearance is compromised by renal failure can result in undesirable prolonged drug effects. Decreasing the maintenance dose interval is a possible option, but it may result in periods of subtherapeutic drug levels. The volume of distribution of the anticholinesterase drug neostigmine is not affected significantly by renal failure, and the loading dose would not need to be increased.*

**EXPLANATION:**

(A) *Correct.* A larger $V_d$ means that a larger loading dose is necessary to achieve the same drug plasma concentration. We assume that the response in the question is the time to onset of neuromuscular blockade.

(B) *Incorrect.* This will result in drug accumulation.

(C) *Incorrect.* This will result in drug accumulation.

(D) *Incorrect.* This is a somewhat vaguely worded choice. If the continuous infusion were adjusted to clearance (half the rate), this would not be a problem. We are not given this information and assume that the constant infusion is at the same rate as for a healthy patient. This would result in drug accumulation.

(E) *Incorrect.* The pharmacokinetics of neostigmine has been studied in patients with renal failure using a two-compartment model. The volume of distribution is not affected significantly, and the loading dose of neostigmine would not need to be increased.

## REASONING:

This question tests knowledge of pharmacokinetics and the concept of volume of distribution. A decreased renal clearance does not preclude use of a continuous infusion as long as the maintenance dose or dosing interval or both are decreased. There is considerable ambiguity regarding what "response" is being measured and the proposed dose of the continuous infusion. An increased loading dose and an increased dosing interval or a reduced infusion rate would be the most complete answer to this question. Considering these limitations, A seems like the best answer.

## BIBLIOGRAPHY:


Barash PG, Cullen BF, Stoelting RK. *Clinical Anesthesia.* 4th ed. Philadelphia, PA: Lippincott Williams & Wilkins; 2001:249-254.

Cronnelly R, Stanski DR, Miller RD, et al. Renal function and the pharmacokinetics of neostigmine in anesthetized man. *Anesthesiology.* 1979;51(3):222-226.

Morgan GE, Mikhail MS, Murray MJ. *Clinical Anesthesiology.* 3rd ed. New York, NY: McGraw-Hill; 2002;153.


---

## BOOK B:

## QUESTION 58

*Answer A*

Physiology

QUESTION (Choose single best answer)

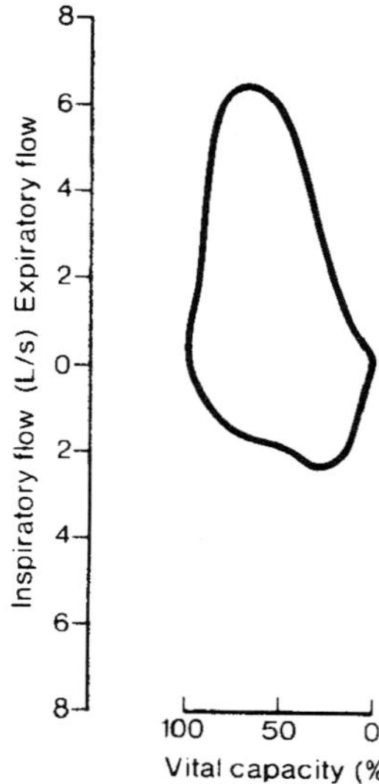


The flow-volume loop shown here is most likely from a patient with which of the following?

(A) Bilateral vocal cord paralysis.

(B) Chronic bronchitis.

(C) Tracheal stenosis 6 months after a previous tracheostomy.

(D) Tumor of the lower trachea.

(E) Normal respiratory status.

**CORRECT ANSWER: A**

## SUMMARY:

*Flow-volume loops can be used to differentiate between different types of obstructive and restrictive pulmonary diseases. The subject is asked to inhale fully to total lung capacity, then to exhale completely, and finally to inhale maximally back to total lung capacity. The flow generated is plotted against the volume inspired/expired forming the flow-volume loop. Obstructive pulmonary diseases result in decreased flows whereas restrictive diseases result in decreased volumes. The loop can also distinguish between variable intrathoracic and extrathoracic obstruction because of decreases in expiratory and inspiratory flows respectively. Finally, fixed large airway obstruction will result in decreases in both inspiratory and expiratory flows. Imaging techniques such as MRI give more precise and useful information on airway obstruction and have superseded the use of flow-volume loops, which are now considered outdated.*

## EXPLANATION:

(A) *Correct.* Bilateral vocal cord paralysis is an example of variable extrathoracic obstruction. The inspiratory loop is flattened because negative pressure during inspiration causes airway collapse resulting in reduced flow. Expiratory flow is unchanged as positive intrathoracic pressure pushes the paralyzed cords into an abducted state.

(B) *Incorrect.* Chronic bronchitis is an example of diffuse airway obstruction. The flow-volume loop would show abnormally decreased flow ("scooped out") on end expiration.

(C) *Incorrect.* Tracheal stenosis from tracheostomy is an example of fixed obstruction. The flow-volume loop shows a plateau during both the inspiratory and expiratory effort-dependent portions of the curve because the airway diameter does not change due to the obstruction.

(D) *Incorrect.* Tumor of the lower trachea is an example of variable intrathoracic obstruction. The flow-volume loop shows a plateau during the expiratory phase because negative inspiratory pressure is no longer maintaining airway patency.

(E) *Incorrect.* This is not an example of normal respiratory status because the expiratory flow is much greater than the inspiratory flow.

## REASONING:

The key concept for answering this question is understanding the flow-volume loop and how different pathologic states generate different loops. The reader should be able to recognize that the flow volume loop shown demonstrates decreased inspiratory flow with relatively normal expiratory flow. This is consistent with variable extrathoracic obstruction (choice A). The other choices are examples of other pathologic states that would have flow-volume loops different from that shown. Flow-volume loops have fallen out of favor with the advent of modern imaging technologies.

## BIBLIOGRAPHY:

Barash PG, Cullen BF, Stoelting RK, Cahalan M, Stock M. Clinical Anesthesia. 6th ed. Philadelphia, PA: Lippincott Williams & Wilkins; 2009:249.

Morgan GE, Mikhail MS, Murray MJ. *Clinical Anesthesiology*. 4th ed. New York, NY: McGraw-Hill; 2006:601-602, 604f.

*Answer C*

Cardiovascular

**QUESTION (Choose single best answer):**

A 66-year-old patient with aortic stenosis is scheduled for aortic valve replacement. Examination shows blood pressure of 110/60 mm Hg and sinus rhythm at a rate of 75 bpm. POAP is 20 mm Hg with a prominent *a* wave on the tracing. Which of the following is the most appropriate management?

(A) Increasing myocardial contractility.
(B) Maintaining PAOP below 20 mm Hg.
(C) Maintaining sinus rhythm.
(D) Promoting mild tachycardia.
(E) Decreasing peripheral resistance.

**CORRECT ANSWER: C**

**SUMMARY:**
*The pathophysiology of aortic stenosis involves the gradual development of obstruction to flow through the aortic valve. This leads to left ventricular hypertrophy (LVH), impaired diastolic function, and eventually compromises the systolic function of the left ventricle. The stiff ventricle is dependent on normal atrial function for filling  The classic presentation of the symptomatic patient with AS is dyspnea on exertion, angina, and syncope.*

**EXPLANATION:**
(A) *Incorrect.* The LV is already operating maximally or has lost the ability to increase contractility. Increased contractility will increase oxygen demand, further stressing the heart.
(B) *Incorrect.* The high wedge pressure is a reflection of the stiff ventricle. The PAOP should be maintained at a high level to ensure adequate LV filling and cardiac output.
(C) *Correct.* Sinus rhythm ensures that the atrial volume will fill the ventricle and the atrial kick helps distend the LV to get in this volume.
(D) *Incorrect.* Tachycardia leaves less time in diastole for LV filling and increases oxygen demand.
(E) *Incorrect.* Afterload reduction, in general, increases forward flow. However, in the patient with AS, there is a fixed obstruction, the valve, which will not be reduced. Decreasing afterload may lead to a drop in preload and a decrease in filling and cardiac output. In addition, low pressure beyond the valve may lead to decreased coronary artery perfusion.

**REASONING:**
The patient with symptomatic aortic valve stenosis has a dismal prognosis without valve replacement. The patient with AS managed inappropriately under anesthesia also has a dismal prognosis. The key to a successful anesthetic is maintaining homeostasis. Preload must be kept high enough to fill a noncomplaint LV. Afterload is relatively fixed. Rate is neither too high (as explained in the answer) nor too low that decreases cardiac output. The left atrium can contribute as much as 40% of LV filling. Loss of this volume, as in atrial fibrillation, will dramatically decrease CO; hypotension develops with decreased coronary perfusion, and decreased preload follows along with ischemia and further decreased filling, decreased CO, etc. This quickly degenerates into a vicious cycle that is difficult to correct.

**BIBLIOGRAPHY:**

Morgan GE, Mikhail MS, Murray MJ. *Clinical Anesthesiology*. 4th ed. New York, NY: McGraw-Hill; 2006:473-475.

| | |
|---|---|
| **BOOK B:** | **QUESTION 60** |

*Answer D*

Clinical Anesthesia

**QUESTION (Choose single best answer):**

During rapid-sequence induction prior to an emergency surgical procedure, a 20-year-old patient vomits gastric contents containing particulate matter. An endotracheal tube is easily inserted, and ventilation with pure oxygen is initiated. Despite the presence of bilateral breath sounds, $SpO_2$ is 90%. Which of the following is the most appropriate next step?

(A) Administration of broad-spectrum antibiotics.
(B) Intravenous administration of high-dose methylprednisolone.
(C) Bronchial lavage with normal saline solution.
(D) Bronchoscopy to remove particulate matter.
(E) Cancellation of the surgical procedure.

**CORRECT ANSWER: D**

**SUMMARY:**

*The treatment of aspiration of gastric contents is controversial. Intubation with supportive management is the mainstay of therapy in the symptomatic patient. Pharmacologic treatment is not indicated during the initial approach to aspiration. Large particles may be amenable to removal by bronchoscopy, especially if they are of a size to obstruct airways. Otherwise, leave it alone. Any attempt at lavage or removal may push the gastric contents further down the respiratory tree.*

**EXPLANATION:**

(A) *Incorrect.* Indiscriminate use of antibiotics may select for a more virulent strain, and many patients never develop an infection if left untreated. Targeted antibiotic therapy may benefit a patient with documented cultures or the patient with bowel obstruction.
(B) *Incorrect.* Steroids have not been shown to conclusively benefit patients with aspiration.
(C) *Incorrect.* Lavage may disperse gastric contents further throughout the lungs enlarging the area of injury.
(D) *Correct.* Large particles may be suctioned out via bronchoscopy, particularly if they are obstructing the airways.
(E) *Incorrect.* This is an emergency procedure. Presumably, you would not have begun an elective case without fasting the patient an appropriate amount of time. An elective case complicated by an aspiration of this magnitude should be cancelled.

**REASONING:**

Aspiration of gastric contents can lead to aspiration pneumonitis that is a chemical injury (also known as *Mendelson syndrome*) and aspiration pneumonia that is an infection. Aspiration may have dramatic effects: wheezing, coughing, shortness of breath, pulmonary edema, hypotension, hypoxemia, adult respiratory distress syndrome (ARDS), and death. Thankfully, in a study of patients undergoing anesthesia who had witnessed aspiration 63% had no symptoms. Unfortunately, several patients died. The treatment in the short term is supportive—mainly oxygenation and ventilation. Later, as other symptoms present, the treatment is targeted.

**BIBLIOGRAPHY:**

Marik PE. Aspiration pneumonitis and aspiration pneumonia. *N Engl J Med.* 2001; 344(9):665-671.

Morgan GE, Mikhail MS, Murray MJ. *Clinical Anesthesiology.* 4th ed. New York, NY: McGraw-Hill; 2006:288.

---

**BOOK B:**

**QUESTION 61 (OPTIONAL)**

---

*Answer B*

Equipment/Physics

**QUESTION (Choose single best answer):**

A radial artery catheter is to be used for blood pressure measurement during a sitting craniotomy. When zeroing the transducer, which of the following describes the best levels for placement of the transducer and opening of the system to air?

|     | **Transducer** | **Opening to Air** |
| --- | --- | --- |
| (A) | Head | Wrist |
| (B) | Head | Head |
| (C) | Head | Heart |
| (D) | Heart | Heart |
| (E) | Heart | Wrist |

**CORRECT ANSWER: B**

**SUMMARY:**

*Pressure transducer accuracy depends on proper zeroing and leveling of the transducer. These two distinct and separate steps often are performed simultaneously by the anesthesiologist. Zeroing the transducer involves turning the stopcock most proximal to the transducer toward the arterial line tubing connected to the patient. This effectively eliminates any contact between the pressure transducer and the patient. The pressure transducer is now exposed solely to atmospheric pressure, and the "zero" button on the anesthesia monitor is selected. This maneuver establishes the current atmospheric pressure as a zero reference point. When the stopcock is returned to its original position, connection with the patient is reestablished and the arterial waveform measures pressure relative to the zero reference point. Leveling the transducer involves moving the transducer to the top of the fluid column of the chamber or vessel you wish to monitor. In the supine position, the midchest midaxillary plane estimates the level of the heart and is used to measure systemic arterial pressures. During a sitting craniotomy, the clinician is most concerned with the cerebral perfusion pressure, for which the level of the ear is used to approximate the pressure in the circle of Willis. Leveling of the transducer does not significantly affect the zero reference point initially established by opening the transducer to air. For instance, atmospheric pressure does not change significantly between the wrist and the head in the sitting position. Using the relationship*

$$log_{10} \, P \approx 5 - \frac{height}{15,500}$$

*where P is pressure, we can calculate that atmospheric pressure decreases 0.00129% with a 1-m increase from sea level. This change is not clinically significant. Therefore, the transducer can be opened to air at any point and does not need to be rezeroed when the transducer is releveled. (See also question 17, Book B.)*

**EXPLANATION:**

(A) *Incorrect.* The transducer is at the correct level. Atmospheric pressure does not change appreciably from the wrist to the head (< 0.00129%). Opening the transducer to air at the wrist still would provide an accurate zero reference point. This choice is only incorrect because it is not the "theoretically" best location. This difference is clinically insignificant.

(B) **Correct.** The transducer is at the correct level. Theoretically, the zero reference point (opening the transducer to air) is most accurately measured here, but the difference is not clinically significant.

(C) **Incorrect.** The transducer is at the correct level. Atmospheric pressure does not change appreciably from the heart to the head.

(D) **Incorrect.** The transducer should be leveled at the head during a sitting craniotomy so that it provides a better estimate of cerebral perfusion pressure to the brain.

(E) **Incorrect.** See above.

### REASONING:

This is a challenging question because it implies that rezeroing (opening the transducer to air) is necessary when a transducer is releveled. This is not the case. Atmospheric pressure does not vary significantly between the wrist, heart, and head. Zeroing (opening the transducer to air) at any of these locations would provide an accurate atmospheric zero reference point. Leveling of the transducer to the top of the fluid column of a specific chamber or vessel simply establishes the arterial pressure at that location. The pressure difference between the head and the wrist is simply the hydrostatic pressure of the fluid column between the two sites (7.46-mm Hg decrease in pressure for every 10-cm increase in height, assuming 1.34 cmH$_2$O = 1 mm Hg). Choices A, B, and C all will provide clinically accurate zero reference points. On an actual examination, we would select choice B only because it is theoretically the "best" location for zeroing and leveling. This difference, however, is not clinically significant.

### BIBLIOGRAPHY:


*Environmental Test Methods and Engineering Guidelines.* US Department of Defense Military Standard 810E. Washington, DC, US Government Printing Office; 1989.

Miller RD, Miller ED, Reves JG, et al. *Anesthesia.* 7th ed. Philadelphia, PA: Churchill Livingstone; 2010:1277-1279.

Morgan GE, Mikhail MS, Murray MJ. *Clinical Anesthesiology.* 4th ed. New York, NY: McGraw-Hill; 2006;103-105.


---

| **BOOK B:** | **QUESTION 62** |
|---|---|

*Answer B*

Equipment/Physics

**QUESTION (Choose single best answer):**

The gauge pressure on a cylinder of nitrous oxide

(A) Varies with the size of the cylinder.
(B) Is the same for full and half-full cylinders.
(C) Is the same as that of a full cylinder of oxygen if both are full.
(D) Is independent of the temperature of the cylinder.
(E) Reliably indicates the amount of nitrous oxide in the cylinder.

**CORRECT ANSWER: B**

### SUMMARY:

*Nitrous oxide is an inorganic, colorless, compressible, and odorless inhaled anesthetic agent that is a gas at room temperature but can be stored as a liquid while under pressure. These unique properties account for the characteristic of the gas in compressed tanks. Oxygen cylinder pressure readings reflect the quantity of gas left in the tank. In contrast, nitrous oxide will have the same cylinder pressure (745 psi [pounds per square inch])* *until the liquid $N_2O$ is exhausted. As $N_2O$ is depleted, the liquid vaporizes at the same rate as it is being consumed from the tank until there is no liquid left. The only accurate method to estimate the amount of $N_2O$ in a cylinder is to weigh the tank and subtract the tare weight (weight of the empty tank).*

**EXPLANATION:**

(A) *Incorrect.* The pressure of a tank of $N_2O$ will read 745 psi regardless of the tank size because liquid $N_2O$ is vaporized at the same rate at which it is consumed (at normal ambient temperature and assuming that the cylinder is not completely devoid of liquid $N_2O$).

(B) *Correct.* The pressure in a cylinder of $N_2O$ will be the same until the tank is nearly empty (about 400 L of $N_2O$) and no more liquid is available to vaporize as the gas is being consumed. This is so because the rate at which the liquid converts to the gaseous phase is the same as the rate of gas consumption from the cylinder until there is no liquid left to convert.

(C) *Incorrect.* A full cylinder of oxygen has a pressure of 1800 to 2200 psi at 20°C. The pressure of a cylinder of $N_2O$ at the same temperature is 745 psi.

(D) *Incorrect.* $N_2O$ is a compressible gas. Increases in temperature cause transformation of some liquid to the gaseous phase, but this is not usually accompanied by a significant increase in pressure. Large increases in temperature may overcome the compressibility of the gas and result in increased cylinder pressures.

(E) *Incorrect.* Only the weight of the tank can reliably indicate the amount of $N_2O$ remaining because the pressure will be constant until only 400 L of $N_2O$ is left in the tank and liquid $N_2O$ is depleted (the point where the tank pressure will begin to fall).

**REASONING:**

This question tests knowledge of the properties of compressed anesthetic gases in cylinders. Choice A can be eliminated because the size of a cylinder has nothing to do with the vapor pressure of a gas. Choice C is clearly incorrect based on the standard tank pressures for $N_2O$ and $O_2$. Choice D is incorrect regarding large increases in temperature (although small temperature changes do not result in significant increases in pressure). The magnitude of temperature change is not a specified, making choice D a poor one. The best answer is B.

**BIBLIOGRAPHY:**


Barash PG, Cullen BF, Stoelting RK, Cahalan M, Stock M. *Clinical Anesthesia*. 6th ed. Philadelphia, PA: Lippincott Williams & Wilkins; 2009:653-655.

Morgan GE, Mikhail MS, Murray MJ. *Clinical Anesthesiology*. 4th ed. New York, NY: McGraw-Hill; 2006:19-20.


---

**BOOK B:**　　　　　**QUESTION 63**

---

*Answer A*

Neuroanesthesia

**QUESTION (Choose single best answer):**

Immediately after sustaining severe head injury, a 20-year-old man has a blood pressure of 150/90 mm Hg and an intracranial pressure (ICP) of 35 mm Hg. After 1 hour of thiopental infusion, blood pressure is 105/60 mm Hg, ICP is 20 mm Hg, central venous pressure (CVP) is 5 mm Hg, and temperature is 36°C. The EEG shows slow-wave activity. The most appropriate next step is administration of

(A) Additional thiopental.
(B) A corticosteroid.
(C) Furosemide.
(D) Nimodipine.
(E) Phenylephrine.

**CORRECT ANSWER: A**

**SUMMARY:**

*In severe head injury neurologic insult may be followed from elevations in ICP, preventing arterial inflow and reducing CPP leading to tissue hypoxia and cell death. The Brain Trauma Foundation recommends that the goal in the management of these patients involve reduction of less than 20 mm Hg in ICP and the maintenance of cerebral perfusion. Recall that CPP = MAP − ICP. They recommend a target $P_{CO_2}$ of between 30 and 35 mm Hg with a CPP of more than 60 mm Hg. While an elevated CPP is clearly harmful, there is controversy regarding the optimal goal. One recent study that aimed at lowering edema in head injury proposes a CPP as low as 50 mm Hg using β-blockers as required and the reduction in cerebral metabolic demand with barbiturates.*

**EXPLANATION:**

(A) *Correct.* Thiopental may be continued with a goal of an ICP of less than 20 mm Hg in the setting of severe head injury.

(B) *Incorrect.* Corticosteroids are contraindicated. Numerous studies have failed to show benefit from the use of corticosteroids in head trauma.

(C) *Incorrect.* Volume reduction with furosemide use in a patient with a lowered central venous pressure (CVP) may lower ICP at the expense of lowered CPP and should be avoided.

(D) *Incorrect.* Nimodipine is a useful drug in preventing and treating vasospasm that can occur after SAH. It does not decrease ICP.

(E) *Incorrect.* Hypotension from barbiturate therapy may offset the ICP lowering effects on cerebral perfusion pressure. This should be taken into account in patients that may not tolerate hypotension. However, mild hypotension is usually well tolerated in healthy 20-year-old men.

**REASONING:**

Choice A is the best answer. The key to this question is identifying the goals of preventing secondary physiologic insult following severe head injury. CPP should be maintained while ICP is lowered. ICP of greater than 20 mm Hg is associated with worse outcome and should be managed aggressively.

**BIBLIOGRAPHY:**

Morgan GE, Mikhail MS, Murray MJ. *Clinical Anesthesiology.* 4th ed. New York, NY: McGraw-Hill; 2006:640.

---

| **BOOK B:** | **QUESTION 64** |
|---|---|

*Answer E*

Cardiovascular

**QUESTION (Choose single best answer):**

Following induction of anesthesia with sufentanil and pancuronium, a patient with left main coronary artery disease has a decrease in blood pressure from 110/70 to 60/40 mm Hg. There is no change in heart rate or ECG. The most appropriate management of the hypotension is administration of

(A) Calcium chloride.
(B) Ephedrine.
(C) Epinephrine.
(D) Isoproterenol.
(E) Phenylephrine.

**CORRECT ANSWER: E**

**SUMMARY:**

*The learning objective in this question is to understand the clinical significance of left main disease, myocardial oxygen supply, and demand. Patients with left main disease or severe three-vessel disease are at greatest risk for cardiac complications. It is vital to restore any myocardial supply demand imbalance immediately by treating any hypotension, tachycardia, or hypertension. Treatment with phenylephrine increases diastolic BP without concomitant tachycardia.*

**EXPLANATION:**

(A) ***Incorrect.*** Although calcium increases blood pressure, it also increases contractility, thus increasing myocardial oxygen demand.

(B) ***Incorrect.*** Ephedrine increases blood pressure, but because it also has $\beta_1$ and $\beta_2$ effects, it has positive inotropic and chronotropic effects, increasing myocardial oxygen demand.

(C) ***Incorrect.*** Epinephrine activates all adrenergic receptors and causes tachycardia and increased contractility, increasing myocardial oxygen demand.

(D) ***Incorrect.*** Isoproterenol is a pure $\beta$-agonist and can cause tachycardia and arrhythmias, making it a poor choice in this clinical scenario.

(E) ***Correct.*** It is important to have a clear understanding of all the factors that affect myocardial supply and demand. In this patient with left main coronary artery disease, hypotension affects the entire left ventricle. If not treated immediately, this can lead to death spiral, by the way of hypotension producing global LV ischemia, contributing to hypotension, hypoperfusion, acidosis, etc. One should choose a pharmacologic agent that will improve myocardial perfusion pressure without increasing the oxygen demand. Phenylephrine, with its $\alpha_1$ effect, increases perfusion pressure by increasing diastolic BP without tachycardia.

**REASONING:**

Key concept in this question is optimizing myocardial oxygen supply and demand while understanding the significance of left main coronary artery disease. The treatment is to elevate the diastolic blood pressure, thus improving the oxygen delivery while keeping the oxygen demand low by avoiding tachycardia, hypertension, and increased wall tension or chamber size.

**BIBLIOGRAPHY:**

Hensley AF, Martin ED, Gravlee PG. *Practical Approach to Cardiac Anesthesia*. 3rd ed. Philadelphia, PA: Lippincott Williams & Wilkins; 280-282 (Chapter 11 Anesthetic Management of Myocardial Revascularization).

Miller RD, Eriksson LI, Fleisher LA, Wiener-Kronish JP, William YL. *Miller's Anesthesia*. 7th ed. Philadelphia, PA: Churchill Livingstone; 2009:282-286 (Chapter 12).

Morgan GE, Mikhail MS, Murray MJ. *Clinical Anesthesiology*. 4th ed. New York, NY: McGraw-Hill; 2006:456-457, 462.

## Answer D

### Pharmacology

**QUESTION (Choose single best answer):**

In a 35-year-old patient, which of the following is associated with an increased duration of clinical narcosis following infusion of a total dose of 10 mg/kg thiopental over 3 hours?

(A) Alcoholism in remission.
(B) Asthma.
(C) Fever.
(D) Obesity.
(E) Use of appetite suppressants.

**CORRECT ANSWER: D**

**SUMMARY:**

*Thiopental is a barbiturate used for induction of anesthesia. Its sedative-hypnotic effects result from activation of γ-aminobutyric acid (GABA) inhibitory neurotransmitters. The quick onset of an induction dose is due to rapid equilibration of blood levels with the highly perfused brain, and the quick offset is due to redistribution to the intermediately perfused lean tissue such as muscle. Poorly perfused organs such as adipose tissue take up thiopental much more slowly accounting for the prolonged duration of effect if a large induction dose is given, or a continuous infusion is administered. The induction dose of thiopental should be based on lean body mass rather than actual body weight.*

**EXPLANATION:**

(A) *Incorrect.* Chronic alcohol intake does not change thiopental anesthetic requirement, pharmacokinetics, or pharmacodynamics. The study by Swerdlow et al also examined the pharmacokinetics and pharmacodynamics of thiopental in alcoholics after 1 month of abstinence. Again, no differences were found.

(B) *Incorrect.* While there is a greater incidence of wheezing in asthmatic patients receiving thiopental over propofol for induction, there is no evidence that asthma affects the pharmacokinetics of thiopental.

(C) *Incorrect.* Fever can increase heart rate and metabolic rate. There is no evidence that it will increase the duration of narcosis with thiopental.

(D) *Correct.* If thiopental is given as a large dose or is delivered by infusion over a period of time, termination of effect is prolonged because clearance will depend more on uptake into adipose tissue rather than lean tissue that has reached equilibrium with the blood compartment. This is in contrast to the rapid redistribution to brain and lean tissue that explains the termination of effect of an induction dose.

(E) *Incorrect.* Appetite suppressants include drugs with different mechanisms of action, including serotonin-reuptake inhibitors such as fenfluramine or phentermine, serotonin and norepinephrine reuptake inhibitors such as sibutramine, and amphetamines. While these drugs have various side effects such as primary pulmonary hypertension for fenfluramine, they do not include increased narcosis with thiopental.

**REASONING:**

Key concepts for answering this question are an understanding of the pharmacokinetics and pharmacodynamics of thiopental. Choice A can be easily ruled out either based on the common misconception that chronic alcoholics require a greater dose of barbiturates for induction, or knowledge of the fact that there is no difference between alcoholics and nonalcoholics. The pulmonary system is not involved in the metabolism of thiopental, so choice B can be ruled out. Choices C and E both increase metabolic rate that logically might increase metabolism of drugs. There is no evidence that either has any effect on thiopental, so both can be eliminated. Finally, obesity increases the potential adipose reservoir in which thiopental can accumulate when infused over 3 hours. Thus choice D is the correct answer.

**BIBLIOGRAPHY:**

Miller, 7th Edition, pg 722-734.

Morgan GE, Mikhail MS, Murray MJ. *Clinical Anesthesiology.* 4th ed. New York, NY: McGraw-Hill; 2006:185-187.

Stoelting RK, Dierdorf SF. *Anesthesia and Co-existing Disease.* 5th ed. Philadelphia, PA: Churchill Livingstone; 2008:167, 306, 549.

Swerdlow BN, Holley FO, Maitre PO, Stanski DR. Chronic alcohol intake does not change thiopental anesthetic requirement, pharmacokinetics, or pharmacodynamics. *Anesthesiology.* 1990;72:455-461.

---

**BOOK B:**      **QUESTION 66**

---

*Answer D*

Clinical Anesthesia

**QUESTION (Choose single best answer):**

A previously healthy 60-kg, 17-year-old boy is undergoing emergency surgery for a gunshot wound involving the iliac vein. Ventilation is controlled with a tidal volume of 700 mL/breath, rate of 10/min, and peak inspiratory pressure of 30 cmH$_2$O. Body temperature is normal. The most likely cause of an end-tidal carbon dioxide partial pressure of 16 mm Hg is

(A) Endobronchial intubation.
(B) Excessive expiratory time.
(C) Excessive tidal volume.
(D) Low cardiac output.
(E) Pulmonary aspiration.

**CORRECT ANSWER: D**

**SUMMARY:**

*An ET$_{CO_2}$ of 16 mm Hg is abnormally low. Causes of low ET$_{CO_2}$ include an increased A–a CO$_2$ gradient or mechanical/measurement artifacts. Causes of artifacts include a partial or complete circuit disconnection, esophageal intubation, improper aspiration rate of the sidestream capnography line, and water precipitation in the sampling tubing. An increased A–a CO$_2$ gradient can be due to any significant increase in alveolar dead space (ventilation without perfusion) such as low cardiac output or pulmonary embolism.*

**EXPLANATION:**

(A) *Incorrect.* Endobronchial intubation results in increased pulmonary shunting (perfusion without ventilation) that should not significantly increase dead space (ventilation without perfusion) or change end-tidal CO$_2$.

(B) *Incorrect.* A prolonged expiratory time would not be expected to decrease ET$_{CO_2}$. Decreased MV may occur as a result of decreased inspiratory time, but that would increase end-tidal CO$_2$ rather than decrease it.

(C) *Incorrect.* The tidal volume in a patient with normal lung function during mechanical ventilation as part of a routine general anesthetic is kept between 8 and 11 mL/kg to avoid atelectasis. A 700-mL tidal volume is acceptable in this 60-kg patient and does not explain such a low ET$_{CO_2}$.

(D) **Correct.** The A–a $CO_2$ gradient is increased in a low cardiac output state because decreased pulmonary perfusion increases alveolar dead space (ventilated, nonperfused alveoli). A lower end-tidal $CO_2$ is expected.

(E) **Incorrect.** Pulmonary aspiration results in impaired alveolar gas exchange and ventilation. This may lead to increased pulmonary shunting (perfusion without ventilation) and does not increase dead space or significantly affect the A–a $CO_2$ gradient.

## REASONING:

This question tests knowledge of A–a $CO_2$ gradient and associated etiologies for decreased measured $ET_{CO_2}$. It is important to note that increased alveolar dead space is the primary etiology for a widened A–a $CO_2$ gradient, although other artifacts also can lead to incorrect $ET_{CO_2}$ measurement. D is the best answer.

## BIBLIOGRAPHY:


Barash PG, Cullen BF, Stoelting RK. *Clinical Anesthesia*. 4th ed. Philadelphia, PA: Lippincott Williams & Wilkins; 2001:802-803.

Morgan GE, Mikhail MS, Murray MJ. *Clinical Anesthesiology*. 3rd ed. New York, NY: McGraw-Hill; 2002:111-112.


---

**BOOK B:**      **QUESTION 67**

---

*Answer A*

Equipment/Physics

## QUESTION (Choose single best answer):

Which of the following statements concerning anesthetic management for MRIs is true?

(A) ECG wires are associated with patient burns.
(B) Mechanical ventilation of the lungs is not feasible.
(C) Monitors with ferromagnetic components may be used.
(D) Oxygen analysis of inspired gas is inaccurate.
(E) Pulse oximetry is not reliable near the MR scanner.

## CORRECT ANSWER: A

## SUMMARY:

*Anesthesia for patients undergoing magnetic resonance imaging (MRI) examinations poses significant problems and threats to patient safety. First and foremost, all ferromagnetic objects must be removed from the patient because the scanner acts as a powerful magnet to attract these objects. Patients with pacemakers, prosthetic joints, and surgical clips must not undergo MRI. In addition, all external metal objects (credit cards, watches, jewelry, pens, etc) must be removed from the patient. ECG wires with metal leads and pulse oximeters with wire cables can cause patient burns. The wires can attract high radiofrequency energy and transmit that energy to the patient in the form of heat. MRI does not interfere with the monitoring of inspired oxygen or with the ability to measure oxygen saturation adequately by pulse oximetry. Special $O_2$ cylinders and ventilators are available to enable mechanical ventilation of the lungs in the MRI suite.*

## EXPLANATION:

(A) **Correct.** Regular ECG wires have been associated with patient burns because they attract energy in the form of radiofrequency waves and may transmit that energy in the form of heat.

(B) **Incorrect.** Mechanical ventilation of the lungs is possible with a nonmetal endotracheal tube and an aluminum oxygen cylinder. Special MRI-compatible mechanical ventilators are also available.

(C) *Incorrect.* The ferromagnetic components of patient monitors are attracted by the MRI magnet and pose a safety hazard to the patient and MRI staff.

(D) *Incorrect.* MRI scanners do not interfere with the analysis of oxygen in inspired air.

(E) *Incorrect.* Pulse oximetry is reliable in the MRI suite because it uses spectrophotometric measurement of transmitted light to determine oxygen saturation. It is not affected by magnetic energy.


**REASONING:**

This question tests knowledge of anesthesia safety in the MRI scanner. Choices B and E can be eliminated because these options imply that MRI scans are not safe for patients requiring airway and oxygenation monitoring. This is certainly not the case because intubated patients are commonly taken to the MRI suite. Pulse oximetry is mandatory in the MRI suite because adequate oxygenation otherwise cannot be assessed adequately while patients are in the scanner. Choice C cannot be true because MRI uses powerful magnetic fields to create images of different tissues, and these magnetic fields attract metallic objects. Choice D is false because electromagnetic energy does not interfere with the process used to analyze inspired oxygen (electrochemical gas analysis). This leaves A as the best answer.


**BIBLIOGRAPHY:**

Barash PG, Cullen BF, Stoelting RK, Cahalan M, Stock M. *Clinical Anesthesia*. 6th ed. Philadelphia, PA: Lippincott Williams & Wilkins; 2009:868-869.

Morgan GE, Mikhail MS, Murray MJ. *Clinical Anesthesiology*. 4th ed. New York, NY: McGraw-Hill; 2006:152-154.

---

**BOOK B:** | **QUESTION 68**

---

*Answer C*

Physiology

**QUESTION (Choose single best answer):**

Intraocular pressure is

(A) Decreased by glycopyrrolate.
(B) Increased by hyperventilation.
(C) Decreased by halothane.
(D) Increased by nondepolarizing muscle relaxants.
(E) Increased by phenylephrine eye drops.


**CORRECT ANSWER: C**


**SUMMARY:**

*The ocular globe is exquisitely sensitive to volume and intraocular pressure (IOP). An increase in arterial pressure, Paco$_2$, or CVP and topical anticholinesterase agents effectively raise IOP by increasing aqueous volume or decreasing its drainage. IOP also increases with coughing and the Trendelenburg and prone positions, laryngoscopy, and decreased Pao$_2$. In contrast, most inhalational and intravenous anesthetic agents lower IOP, with the exception of succinylcholine, which raises it. The effect of ketamine on IOP remains controversial.*


**EXPLANATION:**

(A) *Incorrect.* Glycopyrrolate and atropine are used often to attenuate the oculocardiac reflex during eye surgeries. They have been shown to have no significant effect on IOP when used as premedications and even reduce IOP during a general anesthesia.

(B) *Incorrect.* Hyperventilation decreases $Paco_2$ and thus decreases IOP.

(C) *Correct.* Inhalational anesthetics, including halothane, reduce IOP in a dose-related fashion.

(D) *Incorrect.* With the exception of succinylcholine, neuromuscular blocking drugs directly decrease IOP by muscle relaxation. This effect may be attenuated if the resulting apnea elevates $Paco_2$ sufficiently to raise IOP.

(E) *Incorrect.* Capillary decongestion caused by the topical application of phenylephrine improves aqueous drainage from the eye, thereby decreasing IOP. Phenylephrine eye drops should be administered with caution because they can exhibit significant systemic absorption and lead to hypertension.

### REASONING:

This question tests knowledge of determinants of IOP and the drugs that may influence changes in IOP. The reader should ensure that the side effects of common drugs used for eye surgery are reviewed carefully. Some examples include phenylephrine (can lead to systemic hypertension), sulfur hexafluoride (can increase IOP in the presence of $N_2O$ for up to 10 days), and echothiophate (can inhibit pseudocholinesterase activity for 3-14 days). The best answer is C.

### BIBLIOGRAPHY:

Barash PG, Cullen BF, Stoelting RK. *Clinical Anesthesia.* 4th ed. Philadelphia, PA: Lippincott Williams & Wilkins; 2001:286, 487, 972-973.

Cozanitis DA, Dundee JW, Buchanan TA, Archer DB. Atropine versus glycopyrrolate: a study of intraocular pressure and pupil size in man. *Anaesthesia.* 1979;34(3):236-238.

Morgan GE, Mikhail MS, Murray MJ. *Clinical Anesthesiology.* 3rd ed. New York, NY: McGraw-Hill; 2002:761-763 (Tables 38-1 and 38-3).

Salem MG, Ahearn RS. The effects of atropine and glycopyrrolate on intra-ocular pressure in anaesthetised elderly patients. *Anaesthesia.* 1984;39(8):809-812.

---

## BOOK B:  QUESTION 69

*Answer B*

Physiology

### QUESTION (Choose single best answer):

Compared with adult hemoglobin, which of the following is a characteristic of fetal hemoglobin?

(A) It has a greater oxygen-carrying capacity.

(B) It has a lower $P_{50}$.

(C) It is more likely to cause an artifactual increase in $Spo_2$.

(D) It is more likely to sickle.

(E) It unloads oxygen more readily at the tissues.

### CORRECT ANSWER: B

### SUMMARY:

*Fetal hemoglobin (HbF) is present at birth and is gradually replaced by adult hemoglobin in the 6 months after birth. HbF has low levels of 2,3-diphosphoglycerate (2,3-DPG) and a $P_{50}$ of 18 mm Hg compared to 27 mm Hg in adults. The lower $P_{50}$ means greater oxygen affinity. This allows the fetus to bind more oxygen at low placental oxygen tension and makes it more difficult to unload at the tissue level, but it makes unloading oxygen in tissues more difficult. Infants compensate for their anemia and lower $P_{50}$ of fetal hemoglobin by increasing cardiac output to deliver adequate oxygenation.*

### EXPLANATION:

(A) *Incorrect.* Although fetal hemoglobin has a greater affinity for oxygen, its oxygen-carrying capacity compared to adult hemoglobin is the same. Each hemoglobin molecule can bind up to four molecules of oxygen.
(B) *Correct.* Fetal hemoglobin has a lower $P_{50}$ of approximately 18 to 19 mm Hg when compared to normal adult hemoglobin $A_1$ that is 26 mm Hg.
(C) *Incorrect.* Fetal hemoglobin can produce an artifactual decrease in $SpO_2$ due to less unloading of oxygen in the periphery.
(D) *Incorrect.* Hemoglobin F has been showed to prevent sickling in sickle cell anemia. Sickle cell infants and patients with higher levels of HbF have milder disease.
(E) *Incorrect.* The hemoglobin-oxygen dissociation curve for fetal hemoglobin is shifted to the left in comparison to adult hemoglobin. As a result, hemoglobin F unloads oxygen less readily at the tissues.

### REASONING:

The correct choice is B. This question is easy to answer with a good understanding of the hemoglobin-oxygen dissociation curve. The left shift of the oxygen dissociation curve for hemoglobin F has an important role in fetal life because a high oxygen affinity facilitates transfer of maternal oxygen across the placenta.

### BIBLIOGRAPHY:

Morgan GE, Mikhail MS, Murray MJ. *Clinical Anesthesiology*. 4th ed. New York, NY: McGraw-Hill; 2006:562-563.

---

**BOOK B:**
**QUESTION 70**

*Answer A*

Clinical Anesthesia

### QUESTION (Choose single best answer):

Which of the following is most effective in decontaminating an anesthesia machine that was splattered with HIV-contaminated blood?

(A) Bleach.
(B) Deionized water.
(C) Ethylene oxide.
(D) Hydrogen peroxide.
(E) Isopropyl alcohol.

### CORRECT ANSWER: A

### SUMMARY:

*Vectors implicated in human immunodeficiency virus (HIV) transmission include blood products, body fluids, and tissues. Although the risk of environmentally mediated HIV transmission is negligible, it is theoretically possible. Fortunately, HIV is easily inactivated or killed from surfaces. Multiple reports recommend first cleaning a surface contaminated with HIV to reduce the organic load prior to attempted disinfection. Bleach, 70% isopropyl alcohol, ultraviolet (UV) light, and aldehyde preparations are among the possible options. The cheapest and most convenient remains a 1:10 or 1:100 dilution of household bleach.*

### EXPLANATION:

(A) *Correct.* Sodium hypochlorite (bleach) has been proven to be effective in inactivating HIV virus when used in appropriate concentration and in the presence of a low amount of serum. Cleaning a surface prior to disinfection with bleach is recommended to reduce the organic load. In cases where prior cleaning is impossible, care must be taken to use a higher bleach concentration (a minimum of 10,000 ppm [parts per million] available chlorine).

(B) *Incorrect.* Water is deionized when all anions and cations are removed. No disinfectant property exists.

(C) *Incorrect.* Ethylene oxide is a colorless flammable gas used in steam sterilization such as an autoclave and is not a practical agent for decontamination of an anesthesia machine.

(D) *Incorrect.* Hydrogen peroxide is a poor antiseptic that reacts with the enzyme catalase to yield water and oxygen.

(E) *Incorrect.* Isopropyl alcohol 70% has been shown to rapidly deactivate high titers of HIV in suspension but only partially inactivated virus dried onto a surface. Alcohol also quickly evaporates when sprayed and is an unreliable chemical disinfectant for surfaces contaminated with HIV virus.

### REASONING:

This question tests knowledge of best practices for chemical disinfection of HIV surface contamination. Choice B is incorrect because it has no disinfectant property, whereas choice D is a poor antiseptic. Choice C can be eliminated because it is an inappropriate method for decontamination of an anesthesia machine. Choices A or E are both plausible answers. However, alcohol evaporates quickly from surfaces and only partially inactivates the virus. A is the best answer.

### BIBLIOGRAPHY:


Crutcher JM, Lamm SH, Hall TA. Procedures to protect health-care workers from HIV infection: category I (health-care) workers. *Am Ind Hyg Assoc J*. 1991;52(2):A100-A103.

Rutala, WA, Weber DJ; Healthcare Infection Control Practices Advisory Committee. Guideline for disinfection and sterilization in healthcare facilities: recommendations of the CDC. *MMWR Morb Mortal Wkly Rep*. 2008:41.

Van Bueren J, Larkin DP, Simpson RA. Inactivation of human immunodeficiency virus type 1 by alcohols. *J Hosp Infect*. 1994;28(2):137-148.

Van Bueren J, Simpson RA, Salman H, et al. Inactivation of HIV-1 by chemical disinfectants: sodium hypochlorite. *Epidemiol Infect*. 1995;115(3):567-579.


---

| BOOK B: | QUESTION 71 |
|---|---|

## *Answer B*

Physiology

### QUESTION (Choose single best answer):

Which of the following is greater in an obese patient than in a nonobese patient of equal height?

(A) Milliliters of local anesthetic required for epidural block.
(B) Milligrams of succinylcholine required for intubation.
(C) Clearance of diazepam.
(D) Clearance of fentanyl.
(E) Oxygen consumption per body surface area.

### CORRECT ANSWER: B

### SUMMARY:

*Pharmacokinetics in obese patients are difficult to predict. High fat stores, larger volumes of distribution, increased cardiac output and GFR, and other derangements of obesity can all have variable effects on drug distribution, binding, metabolism, and elimination. In general, the most prudent approach is to dose drugs based on ideal body weight rather than actual body weight which can lead to gross overdosing. An increased dose of succinylcholine (1.5-2 times) is usually recommended to achieve optimal intubating conditions. For neuraxial anesthesia the obese patient should receive 10% to 20% less local anesthetic. Oxygen consumption increases directly with increasing size.*

**EXPLANATION:**

(A) *Incorrect.* Obese patients require less local anesthetic for epidurals. This is probably due to a smaller epidural space from increased fat and engorged epidural veins.

(B) *Correct.* With an increased blood volume and an increase in pseudocholinesterase activity, a higher bolus dose of succinylcholine may be indicated to achieve adequate levels at the NMJ.

(C) *Incorrect.* Diazepam is lipophilic so it has a large volume of distribution and a longer-elimination half-life. Clearance, however, is similar to the nonobese.

(D) *Incorrect.* Fentanyl has similar pharmacokinetics in the obese and nonobese.

(E) *Incorrect.* Oxygen consumption is higher for the obese, but after correcting for BSA it is roughly equal at rest.

**REASONING:**

This question is difficult given the many and often conflicting effects of obesity on pharmacokinetics and dynamics. A is clearly incorrect. The lipophilic (diazepam, thiopental) drugs do take longer to remove from the body (elimination) because of increased stores in the fat, but removal from the blood (clearance) is the same in obese and nonobese patients. Obese patients have higher basal metabolic rates and increased demand for oxygen, but this is directly related to size.

**BIBLIOGRAPHY:**

Longnecker, 1st Edition, p 384.
Morgan GE, Mikhail MS, Murray MJ. *Clinical Anesthesiology.* 4th ed. New York, NY: McGraw-Hill; 2006:814-815.
Stoelting RK, Dierdorf SF. *Anesthesia and Co-existing Disease.* 5th ed. Philadelphia, PA: Churchill Livingstone; 2008:305.

---

**BOOK B:**  **QUESTION 72**

---

*Answer D*

Pharmacology

**QUESTION (Choose single best answer):**

The best premedication regimen for a known active narcotic addict would include

(A) Secobarbital.
(B) Diazepam.
(C) Nalbuphine.
(D) Morphine.
(E) Droperidol.

**CORRECT ANSWER: D**

**SUMMARY:**

*Opiate withdrawal from acute drug cessation is an important preoperative concern for patients with narcotic addiction or dependency. Opiate withdrawal is characterized by an increased sympathetic and parasympathetic response that results in hypertension, tachycardia, diaphoresis, abdominal cramping, and diarrhea. The incidence of withdrawal symptoms peaks 1 to 3 days after acute cessation of opiates such as morphine, heroin, or meperidine. Anesthesiologists should attempt to maintain opioid medications at their usual level to prevent acute opiate withdrawal. Administration of opioid antagonist agents such as naloxone should be avoided.*

### EXPLANATION:

(A) *Incorrect.* Secobarbital, like other barbiturates, can cause mild stimulation at low doses and can lead to sedation and unconsciousness with higher doses. It acts at the γ-aminobutyric acid (GABA) receptor and would not be useful for withdrawal prophylaxis in an opioid addict.

(B) *Incorrect.* Diazepam is a benzodiazepine that also acts at the GABA receptor. It would not be useful for withdrawal prophylaxis in an opioid addict.

(C) *Incorrect.* Nalbuphine is an opioid agonist-antagonist and can precipitate acute opioid withdrawal in patients dependent on opiates.

(D) *Correct.* Morphine is an opioid agonist agent that is suitable for maintenance of a patient's usual narcotic dose and provides prophylaxis against opioid withdrawal symptoms.

(E) *Incorrect.* Droperidol is a dopamine antagonist that acts centrally to interfere with serotonin, norepinephrine, and GABA transmissions. It would not be useful for withdrawal prophylaxis in an opioid addict.

### REASONING:

This question tests knowledge of preoperative management of patients with opiate addiction. The best premedication regimen to prevent acute opiate withdrawal in these patients is administration of an opiate agonist medication such as morphine or methadone. Barbiturates, benzodiazepines, and butyrophenones like droperidol do not act at the opioid receptor and would not be useful for opioid withdrawal prophylaxis. Mixed opioid agonist-antagonist agents such as nalbuphine or buprenorphine also should be avoided because their antagonist properties have the potential to precipitate acute withdrawal. Morphine is the only option that is a pure opioid agonist. D is the best answer.

### BIBLIOGRAPHY:

Barash PG, Cullen BF, Stoelting RK, Cahalan M, Stock M. *Clinical Anesthesia.* 6th ed. Philadelphia, PA: Lippincott Williams & Wilkins; 2009:489, 587-588, 594, 1498-1499.

Morgan GE, Mikhail MS, Murray MJ. *Clinical Anesthesiology.* 4th ed. New York, NY: McGraw-Hill; 2006:185-187, 202-204, 285, 658-659.

Noble J, Greene HL, et al. *Textbook of Primary Care Medicine.* 3rd ed. St. Louis, MO: Mosby; 2001:447.

---

| **BOOK B:** | **QUESTION 73** |
| --- | --- |

## *Answer D*

Cardiovascular

### QUESTION (Choose single best answer):

During cardiopulmonary bypass (CPB) at a nasopharyngeal temperature of 28°C and a hematocrit of 20%, temperature-corrected $Paco_2$ is 50 mm Hg and uncorrected $Paco_2$ is 60 mm Hg. The most appropriate management is to

(A) Administer additional opioid.

(B) Administer packed red blood cells to increase the hematocrit to 25%.

(C) Further decrease the patient's temperature.

(D) Increase fresh gas flow to the oxygenator.

(E) Institute mechanical ventilation.

**CORRECT ANSWER: D**

## SUMMARY:

*Acid-base management during hypothermic CPB (ie, alpha-stat vs pH-stat) is controversial. pH-stat acid-base management uses temperature-corrected blood gases to guide management, whereas alpha-stat management uses temperature-uncorrected blood gas analysis. In a normal patient, ventilation is controlled by varying the delivered MV. Ventilation and perfusion can be controlled separately during CPB. Perfusion is controlled by varying flow rates and ventilation is controlled by varying total gas flow through the oxygenator. Regardless of which method of acid-base management is used during hypothermic CPB, $Paco_2$ is controlled by varying total gas flows. Hypercarbia should be treated by increasing the total gas flow through the oxygenator.*

## EXPLANATION:

(A) **Incorrect.** Additional opioid will not affect hypercarbia during CPB. If sympathetic stimulation is suspected, opioid may be given, but the ventilation still needs to be increased.

(B) **Incorrect.** A hematocrit of 20% is well tolerated under hypothermic conditions. Low hematocrit decreases blood viscosity and improves the rheology of the microcirculation. Administration of packed red blood cells would not help correct the underlying respiratory acidosis.

(C) **Incorrect.** The magnitude of hypothermia used during CPB is determined by type of surgery and the duration and magnitude of flows during bypass. Hypothermia will not help correct the significant respiratory acidosis.

(D) **Correct.** Increasing the fresh gas flow to the oxygenator will increase ventilation and help correct the respiratory acidosis.

(E) **Incorrect.** The pulmonary circulation is isolated during CPB. There is no benefit to the ventilating lungs that are not perfused. Mechanical ventilation would not correct the respiratory acidosis.

## REASONING:

This question tests knowledge of acid-base management during hypothermic CBP. Discussions of the interpretation of blood gas analysis in hypothermic patients are often difficult to understand because many readers find certain concepts confusing. It is important to understand that the partial pressure of a gas in a liquid is defined as the partial pressure of that gas that would be present in a gas mixture in equilibrium with the liquid. Therefore, $Paco_2$ is a measure of the partial pressure of $CO_2$ in a gas mixture in equilibrium with blood. It is not a direct measure of the $CO_2$ content in the blood itself.

Interpretation of blood gas results during hypothermia is difficult because the solubility of $CO_2$ in solution increases, as does $CO_2$ binding to hemoglobin. As a result, a larger amount of $CO_2$ gas will dissolve into blood as temperature decreases. In a closed system (ie, sealed heparinized blood gas syringe), the total amount of $CO_2$ must remain the same. When temperature decreases, $CO_2$ solubility and hemoglobin binding increase, causing additional $CO_2$ gas to dissolve into blood. Because this is a closed system, the partial pressure of $CO_2$ must decrease as the concentration in solution increases. This explains why the $Paco_2$ decreases as temperature decreases. (Note that although more $CO_2$ is dissolved in blood at lower temperatures, the molecular interaction between water and $CO_2$ is decreased with hypothermia, and therefore formation of H is minimal.)

Because blood samples are heated to 37°C prior to measuring gas tensions, they will overestimate the true arterial $CO_2$ gas tension in a hypothermic patient. Temperature-corrected values can be generated to estimate the true arterial $CO_2$ gas tension and pH at the patient's actual temperature. Management of acid-base status during hypothermic CPB can be achieved through either pH-stat or alpha-stat management. pH-stat management uses temperature-corrected values to guide management, whereas alpha-stat uses temperature-uncorrected measurements. The goal in both is the same: to maintain a normal arterial $Paco_2$ of 40 mm Hg and a pH of 7.40. In this question we are given a temperature-corrected $Paco_2$ value of 50 mm Hg and a temperature-uncorrected value of

60 mm Hg. Regardless of management technique, the hypercarbia should be treated by increasing "ventilation." Accordingly, fresh gas flow to the oxygenator should be increased. D is the best answer.


**BIBLIOGRAPHY:**
Alston T. Blood gases and pH during hypothermia: the "-Stats." *Int Anesthesiol Clin.* 2004 Fall;42(4):73-80.
Hensley WJ, Loblay RH, Tiller DJ. *Fluid, Electrolyte and Acid-Base Disturbances*: A Practical Guide for Interns. New York, NY: Wiley; 1976:488.
Kaplan JA. *Cardiac Anesthesia.* 4th ed. Philadelphia, PA: Saunders; 1999:1069-1070.
Kofstad J. Blood gases and hypothermia: some theoretical and practical considerations. *Scand J Clin Lab Invest.* 1996;56(suppl 224):21-26.
Miller RD, Miller ED, Reves JG, et al. *Anesthesia.* 7th ed. New York, NY: Churchill Livingstone; 2009;1918-1919.
Morgan GE, Mikhail MS, Murray MJ. *Clinical Anesthesiology.* 4th ed. New York, NY: McGraw-Hill; 2005.


---

## BOOK B:    QUESTION 74

*Answer B*

Clinical Anesthesia

**QUESTION (Choose single best answer):**

Two days after coronary artery bypass grafting, a 62-year-old man remains sedated, tracheally intubated, and mechanically ventilated with full neuromuscular block. Over the next 3 hours, $Pao_2$ decreases from 90 to 70 mm Hg at an $Fio_2$ of 0.7, peak inspiratory pressure measured proximally in the ventilatory circuit increases from 40 to 66 $cmH_2O$, and plateau pressure remains unchanged at 30 $cmH_2O$. Which of the following is the most likely cause of these changes?

(A) Adult respiratory distress syndrome
(B) Bronchial mucus plugging
(C) Left ventricular failure
(D) Lobar pneumonia
(E) Tension pneumothorax

**CORRECT ANSWER: B**

**SUMMARY:**

*Peak inspiratory pressure (PIP) measures dynamic lung compliance. Plateau pressure (PP) is measured at end inspiration (zero gas flow) and reflects static lung compliance. Both PIP and PP are increased when tidal volume is increased or lung compliance is decreased. Increased PIP with unchanged PP is seen with increased inspiratory gas flow or increased airway resistance (eg, bronchospasm, mucus plugging, airway compression, etc).*

**EXPLANATION:**
(A) *Incorrect.* ARDS results in increased PIP and PP owing to decreased lung compliance.
(B) *Correct.* Increased PIP with unchanged PP is seen with increased inspiratory gas flow and increased airway resistance (eg, bronchospasm, mucus plugging, kinked endotracheal tube, foreign-body aspiration, airway compression, and endotracheal tube cuff herniation).
(C) *Incorrect.* Left ventricular failure leading to pulmonary edema would result in decreased lung compliance and a corresponding increase in PIP and PP.
(D) *Incorrect.* Lobar pneumonia would lead to decreased lung compliance and a corresponding increase in PIP and PP.
(E) *Incorrect.* Both PIP and PP would be expected to rise with a tension pneumothorax.

## REASONING:

This question tests knowledge of the differences between PIP and PP and corresponding differences in dynamic versus static lung compliance. PIP is the highest pressure generated in the breathing circuit during inspiration and reflects dynamic compliance. PP is measured during inspiratory pause and reflects static lung compliance. Normally, PIP is equal to or slightly more than PP. If PIP and PP are both increased, this suggests a decrease in lung compliance or increased tidal volumes (Trendelenburg position, pleural effusion, ascites, tension pneumothorax, endobronchial intubation, abdominal packing, retractors, insufflation, alveolar diseases such as ARDS, PNA, or pulmonary edema). Alternatively, an increase in airway resistance or inspiratory gas flow likely has occurred if PIP is increased but PP is unchanged. The best answer is B.

## BIBLIOGRAPHY:



Barash PG, Cullen BF, Stoelting RK, Cahalan M, Stock M. *Clinical Anesthesia*. 6th ed. Philadelphia, PA: Lippincott Williams & Wilkins; 2009:794-795.

Miller RD, Miller ED, Reves JG, et al. *Anesthesia*. 7th ed. New York, NY: Churchill Livingstone; 2010:1429-1431.

Morgan GE, Mikhail MS, Murray MJ. *Clinical Anesthesiology*. 4th ed. New York, NY: McGraw-Hill; 2005:47.



---

**BOOK B:**

# QUESTION 75

*Answer A*

OB/Regional

## QUESTION (Choose single best answer):

A combined epidural and general anesthetic is used for aortofemoral bypass surgery. Just prior to extubation, the patient received morphine 5 mg through the epidural catheter. Eleven hours later, he is unresponsive while breathing 40% oxygen from a face mask. Respiratory rate is 6 breaths/min and $Spo_2$ is 92%. Arterial blood gas analysis shows a $Pao_2$ of 80 mm Hg, a $Paco_2$ of 84 mm Hg, and a pH of 7.16. Which of the following statements concerning this patient is true?

(A) Hypercarbia is contributing to the decreased level of consciousness.
(B) Naloxone is ineffective for reversing the respiratory depression.
(C) The oxygen saturation is higher than expected because of the pH.
(D) The risk for respiratory depression would have been lower with subarachnoid administration of 0.5 mg morphine.
(E) Residual local anesthetic is contributing to the respiratory depression.

## CORRECT ANSWER: A

## SUMMARY:

*Epidural opiates are effective agents for postoperative pain relief. Morphine given in epidural doses up to 10 mg has an onset of 1 to 2 hours and duration of 12 to 24 hours. Side effects are dose-dependent and include pruritus, nausea and vomiting, urinary retention, and respiratory depression. All can be ameliorated by administration of naloxone, which also will decrease the analgesic properties. It is important to remember that these side effects can occur at any point in the duration of the action, and delayed respiratory depression can occur. Because of the dose-dependent nature of side effects and limited analgesic efficacy with increased doses, the recommended dose of epidural morphine is approximately 3 to 5 mg.*

## EXPLANATION:

(A) *Correct.* Increased $Paco_2$ is associated with agitation, sedation, and even coma. These mental status changes are thought to be due to intracranial hypertension secondary to increased cerebral blood flow and severe intracellular acidosis.

(B) *Incorrect.* Naloxone *is* effective for reversing respiratory depression from epidural morphine.
(C) *Incorrect.* Based on the oxyhemoglobin dissociation curve, an oxygen saturation of 90% corresponds to a $PaO_2$ of 60 mm Hg. This patient has a $PaO_2$ of 80 mm Hg, and the oxygen saturation is 92%, which is slightly lower than would be expected.
(D) *Incorrect.* The risk of respiratory depression is higher with intrathecal narcotics than with epidural narcotics.
(E) *Incorrect.* Local anesthetics do not cause respiratory depression.

### REASONING:

This patient is experiencing delayed respiratory depression from epidural narcotics resulting in alveolar hypoventilation. He has a pure respiratory acidosis and impaired level of consciousness with relatively normal oxygenation. Choice C is incorrect because the saturation is not higher than expected. Choice B is incorrect because naloxone can reverse respiratory depression secondary to neuraxial narcotic administration, and choice E is incorrect because local anesthetics are not associated with respiratory depression. This makes A the best answer.

### BIBLIOGRAPHY:

Barash PG, Cullen BF, Stoelting RK, Cahalan M, Stock M. *Clinical Anesthesia.* 6th ed. Philadelphia, PA: Lippincott Williams & Wilkins; 2101:470-473.
Miller RD, Eriksson LI, Fleisher LA, Wiener-Kronish JP, William YL. *Miller's Anesthesia.* 7th ed. Philadelphia, PA: Churchill Livingstone; 2010:2765-2766.

---

**BOOK B:**     **QUESTION 76**

*Answer B*

Physiology

### QUESTION (Choose single best answer):

A rapid, shallow ventilatory pattern is most energy efficient for a patient who

(A) Has a low ratio of forced expiratory volume in 1 second to vital capacity ($FEV_1/VC$).
(B) Has a high ratio of tidal volume to vital capacity and diminished vital capacity.
(C) Has increased pulmonary compliance.
(D) Is using the accessory muscles of respiration.
(E) Has increased airway resistance.

### CORRECT ANSWER: B

### SUMMARY:

*Work of breathing in most conditions is largely due to inspiration with expiration being normally passive. Factors to overcome with breathing include the elastic recoil of the chest wall and lung, frictional airway resistance, and tissue resistance. As tidal volume (Vt) increases, the work to overcome the elastic forces increases. In contrast, as respiratory rate (RR) increases, the work to overcome airway resistance increases. Patients can minimize the work of breathing by altering Vt and RR. In patients with decreased compliance (restrictive lung disease), rapid shallow breathing patterns decreases the work of breathing. In patients with increased airflow resistance (obstructive diseases), slow deep breathing patterns are more efficient. All lung volumes are typically reduced on spirometry with vital capacity affected to a greater extent than tidal volume. The $FEV_1/FVC$ ratio remains normal because both are decreased proportionally.*

(A) *Incorrect.* A low ratio of $FEV_1$ to vital capacity is characteristic of obstructive lung disease. Patients with obstructive lung disease do not benefit from a rapid shallow ventilatory pattern.

(B) *Correct.* This describes a patient with restrictive lung disease. All lung volumes are decreased with vital capacity being more affected to a greater extent than tidal volume. These patients benefit most from rapid shallow breathing.

(C) *Incorrect.* Increased pulmonary compliance is seen in chronic obstructive lung disease and acute asthma. A slow and deeper breathing pattern would be more energy efficient.

(D) *Incorrect.* Patients using accessory muscles of respiration may be in respiratory distress. This may be seen in obstructive disease in an attempt to preserve or increase Vt.

(E) *Incorrect.* Patients with increased airway resistance show an obstructive lung disease pattern and would not benefit from rapid shallow breathing.

REASONING:

Only choice B describes a pattern with restrictive lung disease who may benefit from a rapid shallow breathing pattern. This question emphasizes the differences between obstructive and restrictive lung disease. The characteristic features of restrictive lung disease result from reduced lung compliance: smaller lung volumes and a rapid shallow breathing pattern.

BIBLIOGRAPHY:

Barash PG, Cullen BF, Stoelting RK, Cahalan M, Stock M. *Clinical Anesthesia*. 6th ed. Philadelphia, PA: Lippincott Williams & Wilkins; 2010:793-794.
Morgan GE, Mikhail MS, Murray MJ. *Clinical Anesthesiology*. 4th ed. New York, NY: McGraw-Hill; 2006:550-551.

---

**BOOK B:**          **QUESTION 77**

---

*Answer E*

Clinical Anesthesia

QUESTION (Choose single best answer):

A 70-year-old patient has absence of the left radial pulse 1 month after repair of an aortic aneurysm. Arterial pressure was monitored perioperatively with a 20-gauge left radial artery catheter. Which of the following statements concerning this complication is true?

(A) A preoperative Allen test would have predicted this complication.
(B) Stellate ganglion block should be performed.
(C) This complication would have been less likely with an 18-gauge catheter.
(D) This patient has poor collateral circulation in the hand.
(E) The pulse likely will return.

CORRECT ANSWER: E

SUMMARY:

*The radial artery is most often used for continuous blood pressure monitoring because the location is accessible and there is usually good collateral circulation in the hand. This is often assessed with the Allen test, which has been found to be unreliable as there are documented instances of ischemia despite normal Allen tests, as well as uncomplicated catheterizations despite abnormal Allen tests. In addition to thromboses, complications can include median nerve dysfunction, hematoma, infection, blood or air emboli, hand ischemia, skin necrosis, and arteriovenous fistula formation. Avoidance of larger size of catheter, longer duration of catheterization, and use of polypropylene-tapered catheters can help decrease the incidence of complications.*

**EXPLANATION:**

(A) *Incorrect.* The Allen test does not reliably predict adverse outcomes from radial artery catheterization. Moreover, radial artery cannulations have been safely performed despite abnormal Allen test.

(B) *Incorrect.* Stellate ganglion block is used to treat head, neck, arm, and upper chest pain. It can also be used to treat pain after accidental intra-arterial injection of thiopental. However, there is no evidence that such a block is indicated.

(C) *Incorrect.* Complications would be more likely with an 18-gauge catheter. The larger the catheter, the greater the risk of thrombosis.

(D) *Incorrect.* The fact that the radial artery is occluded does not necessarily mean that there is poor collateral circulation of that hand. The ulnar artery may be normal, patent, and supplying adequate blood to the rest of the hand even with the radial artery occluded. The patient described has absence of radial pulse, not ischemia of the entire hand.

(E) *Correct.* In a study by Slogoff, of 1700 patients who had radial artery cannulation, 25% had evidence of radial artery occlusion after decannulation. However, there were no ischemic complications. Blood flow usually normalizes in 3 to 70 days.

**REASONING:**

Key concepts to answering this question include understanding the indications, procedure, complications, and treatment for radial arterial catheters. Knowing that the Allen test is unreliable should allow choice A to be eliminated. Stellate ganglion block may help vasodilate the artery, but there is no evidence that this should be performed, so choice B can be ruled out. Choice C can be ruled out because catheter size is related to incidence of complications. Absence of pulse does not mean that there is poor circulation of that hand, so choice D can be eliminated. Finally, even though it may take time, recanalization of the artery usually occurs, making choice E the correct answer.

**BIBLIOGRAPHY:**

Barash PG, Cullen BF, Stoelting RK. *Clinical Anesthesia.* 6th ed. Philadelphia, PA: Lippincott Williams & Wilkins; 2009:704-705.
Miller, 7th Edition, pg 1272-1284.
Morgan GE, Mikhail MS, Murray MJ. *Clinical Anesthesiology.* 4th ed. New York, NY: McGraw-Hill; 2006:91-93, 332-333.

---

**BOOK B:** | **QUESTION 78**

---

*Answer A*

OB/Regional

**QUESTION (Choose single best answer):**

Five minutes after intrathecal administration of tetracaine 12 mg in hyperbaric solution, a 60-year-old man has a weak hand grasp. Respirations are normal, heart rate has decreased from 80 to 45 bpm, and blood pressure has decreased from 150/80 to 90/50 mm Hg. The most appropriate management at this time is

(A) Administration of atropine.
(B) Administration of ephedrine.
(C) Administration of phenylephrine.
(D) Placement of the patient in the head-down position.
(E) Observation.

**CORRECT ANSWER: A**

**SUMMARY:**

*With neuraxial anesthesia, the most readily anesthetized fibers are the small sympathetic nerves, followed by the unmyelinated and then the myelinated fibers associated with pain and touch, and finally, the myelinated motor neurons. When patients with spinal or epidural anesthesia exhibit decreased hand strength, the block is at least to the high thoracic and low cervical levels because the motor innervation to the hand is derived from C5-T1. This situation will result in significant decreases in blood pressure and heart rate owing to blockade of the sympathetic vasomotor fibers at T5-L1 and cardioaccelerator fibers at T1-4. Hypotension and bradycardia leading to full arrest are possible in this situation, especially in patients with high vagal tone. The anesthesiologist must be prepared to treat the patient with fluids and medications such as atropine, ephedrine, and possibly epinephrine to increase cardiac output and systemic perfusion.*

**EXPLANATION:**

(A) *Correct.* The blockade of the cardioaccelerator fibers is causing severe bradycardia. When combined with the decreased vasomotor tone associated with sympathectomy, cardiac arrest is possible. Atropine is the medication of choice for this patient, as it is a competitive antagonist of muscarinic receptors in the heart, therefore blocking vagal input.

(B) *Incorrect.* Ephedrine is an indirect-acting $\alpha$- and $\beta$-agonist. It may be a second-line agent for treating this patient after atropine.

(C) *Incorrect.* Phenylephrine is a direct $\alpha$-agonist that will provide vasoconstriction, possibly resulting in a reflex bradycardia that would not be optimal in this patient.

(D) *Incorrect.* The solution is hyperbaric, which means that its spread in the intrathecal space depends on gravity. Placing this patient in the head-down position potentially could cause the block to move even higher.

(E) *Incorrect.* This patient requires careful observation for signs that his block is compromising respiratory function, but not in the absence of treating his current problems.

**REASONING:**

This question is testing what you should do *first*. The high level of neuraxial blockade is evidenced by the decreased grip strength in the hands, indicating that the block has reached the cervical-thoracic junction. The cardiovascular effects of the spinal are manifested by decreased heart rate and blood pressure. In the setting of spinal (or epidural) anesthesia, bradycardia combined with the decreased venous return to the heart from the sympathectomy can lead to complete cardiac arrest. The first course of action should be to increase the heart rate. The drug of choice for this is atropine, followed by ephedrine and/or epinephrine if it is not effective. A is the best answer.

**BIBLIOGRAPHY:**

Limongi JA, Lins RS. Cardiopulmonary arrest in spinal anesthesia. *Rev Bras Anestesiol.* 2011 Jan-Feb;61(1):110-120.

Morgan GE, Mikhail MS, Murray MJ. *Clinical Anesthesiology.* 4th ed. New York, NY: McGraw-Hill; 2006:317-318.

## Answer B

### Equipment/Physics

**QUESTION (Choose single best answer):**

A burn is found at the site of the electrocautery pad. Which of the following is most likely?

(A) The electrosurgical unit was in the bipolar mode.
(B) The electrocautery pad became partially detached.
(C) The electrosurgical unit ground wire was severed.
(D) The line-isolation monitor alarmed.
(E) The patient became grounded.

**CORRECT ANSWER: B**

**SUMMARY:**

*The great majority of patient burns in the operating room are caused by incorrect or inadequate placement of the electrocautery pad on the patient. Electrocautery devices send ultrahigh-frequency current from the machine to the tip of the cauterizing electrode. The current has a high density at the electrocautery tip and is able to exert coagulation and cutting at the tissue level. The current enters the patient at the cautery tip and exits through the electrocautery pad. The pad should be placed on skin that is devoid of bony protuberances and should cover a large surface area. It is the large surface area of the electrocautery pad that prevents concentration of electric current in a small area that would cause a burn. Inadequate surface-area coverage or placement over a bony protuberance that attracts current in high density can lead to unintended thermal injury in the operating room.*

**EXPLANATION:**

(A) ***Incorrect.*** The bipolar mode of the electrocautery unit returns current through an adjacent return electrode in close proximity to the cautery tip. This confines the current flow to a few millimeters and eliminates the need for an electrocautery pad.

(B) ***Correct.*** Inadequate surface-area contact between the electrocautery pad and the patient can concentrate electric current on the exit limb of the circuit and lead to a patient burn at the site of the electrocautery pad.

(C) ***Incorrect.*** If an electrosurgical ground unit wire becomes severed, the isolation transformer (installed in most operating rooms in the United States) will protect the patient from electric shock. Because isolation transformers create a second ungrounded circuit loop, patient contact with a single live wire will not cause a shock or burn because no electric circuit is completed.

(D) ***Incorrect.*** The line-isolation monitor (LIM) alarm indicates that a single fault between a power line and ground has occurred. Because most operating rooms have isolation transformers, two faults have to occur in order for electric shock to occur. The most likely cause of thermal injury in this patient is a partially detached electrocautery pad. This event would not cause the LIM to alarm.

(E) ***Incorrect.*** If the patient becomes grounded in a modern operating room setting, an isolation transformer would prevent electric shock or burns by isolating the patient from completing an electric circuit.

**REASONING:**

This question tests knowledge of electrical safety in the operating room and causes of inadvertent thermal injury from electrocautery. Choice A can be eliminated because bipolar mode does not use an electrocautery pad. Choices C, D, and E are associated with electric shock and not burns or diathermy. Therefore, B is the best choice because it relates to burn injuries, and the mechanism involved clearly increases the risk for thermal injury (a smaller surface area of electric current causing a burn).

**BIBLIOGRAPHY:**
Barash PG, Cullen BF, Stoelting RK, Cahalan M, Stock M. *Clinical Anesthesia.* 6th ed. Philadelphia, PA: Lippincott Williams & Wilkins; 2009:181-182.
Morgan GE, Mikhail MS, Murray MJ. *Clinical Anesthesiology.* 4th ed. New York, NY: McGraw-Hill; 2006:23-26 (Figures 2-6, 2-7, 2-8, and 2-10).

---

**BOOK B:** | **QUESTION 80**

*Answer C*

Equipment/Physics

**QUESTION (Choose single best answer):**

Which property of oxygen is detected by the fail-safe device on the anesthesia machine?

(A) Concentration.
(B) Flow.
(C) Pressure.
(D) Partial pressure.
(E) Reserve volume.

**CORRECT ANSWER: C**

**SUMMARY:**

*The fail-safe device on an anesthesia machine helps prevent delivery of a hypoxic mixture of gas to patients. The device measures the pressure of oxygen across a valve near the oxygen flowmeter. Should the pressure of oxygen fall below 25 psig (pounds per square inch gauge) (normal is approximately 50 psig), the fail-safe valve will shut off automatically or proportionally decrease flow of all other gases. When this occurs, an alarm will sound. The fail-safe mechanism does not protect against all causes of hypoxic gas mixtures such as insufficient $O_2$ concentration in the oxygen supply, inadvertent switching of the gas pipeline supplies, or hypoxic proportioning of gases at the flowmeter assembly (in the absence of a flow-proportioning system).*

**EXPLANATION:**

(A) *Incorrect.* The fail-safe mechanism does not measure concentration of $O_2$. It measures the pressure in the oxygen pipeline across the valve.
(B) *Incorrect.* The flow of gases does not determine whether the gas mixture is hypoxic. Low flow can occur at 100% concentration of $O_2$, and there would be no need to shut off the delivery of other gases in this situation.
(C) *Correct.* The device measures the pressure of $O_2$ across the fail-safe valve. When it falls below 25 psig, it will shut off or proportionally decrease flow of all other gases, and an alarm will sound.
(D) *Incorrect.* The fail-safe valve measures the pressure of $O_2$ across a valve near the $O_2$ flowmeter, not the partial pressure of oxygen.
(E) *Incorrect.* The fail-safe device does not measure the reserve volume of oxygen in either the cylinders or the central supply.

**REASONING:**

This question tests knowledge of the fail-safe valve in an anesthesia machine. Choice A can be eliminated because the fail-safe valve does not measure the concentration of oxygen in the pipeline. Choice B potentially could be normal even when a gas mixture is hypoxic (ie, if the flow of other gases is very high), so B is not a good answer. Choice E does not make sense because the fail-safe device is in the machine itself and not at the level of the oxygen tank or central supply of oxygen (where volume would have to be measured). This leaves choices C and D. The concentration of inspired oxygen is measured by an oxygen sensor in the inspiratory limb. The partial pressure of expired oxygen is measured by the gas analyzer. The pressure of oxygen (in psig) is measured by the fail-safe device. The best answer is C.

**BIBLIOGRAPHY:**
Barash PG, Cullen BF, Stoelting RK, Cahalan M, Stock M. *Clinical Anesthesia.* 6th ed. Philadelphia, PA: Lippincott Williams & Wilkins; 2009:654-655.
Morgan GE, Mikhail MS, Murray MJ. *Clinical Anesthesiology.* 4th ed. New York, NY: McGraw-Hill; 2006:50-59.

---

| **BOOK B:** | **QUESTION 81** |
|---|---|

*Answer A*

OB/Regional

**QUESTION (Choose single best answer):**

Which of the following nerves should be blocked for an operation at the medial aspect of the lower leg?

(A) Femoral.
(B) Sciatic.
(C) Obturator.
(D) Common peroneal.
(E) Tibial.

**CORRECT ANSWER: A**

**SUMMARY:**

*Lower extremity nerve blocks are effective at providing both intraoperative and postoperative analgesia to patients undergoing surgery of the thigh, knee, or ankle. Blocking the femoral nerve at a level approximately 2 cm below the inguinal ligament (just lateral to the arterial pulse) will provide analgesia to the medial and anterior aspects of the thigh, as well as to the patellar region. The saphenous nerve comes off the posterior branch of the femoral nerve and supplies the medial portion of the lower leg to the level of the malleolus. Blocking the femoral nerve also will block areas of the lower extremity innervated by the saphenous nerve. Femoral nerve blockade is useful for surgeries of the anterior thigh and anterior/medial aspects of the lower leg. For surgeries below the knee, femoral nerve blocks often are combined with sciatic and/or lateral femoral cutaneous nerve blocks to increase the lateral and posterior distributions of analgesia.*

**EXPLANATION:**

(A) **Correct.** The femoral nerve supplies the anterior and medial aspects of the thigh and leg below the knee. It also supplies the knee joint and the ligaments within the joint. Blocking the femoral nerve is the single best regional technique for surgeries of the medial aspect of the lower leg. Combining femoral and sciatic nerve block is best for surgeries below the knee.

(B) **Incorrect.** The sciatic nerve supplies the posterior aspect of the thigh and gluteal region. Its branches supply the lateral aspect of the lower leg and the dorsolateral aspect of the foot. Sciatic nerve blocks by themselves will not provide analgesia for the medial aspect of the lower leg.

(C) *Incorrect.* The obturator nerve innervates the hip, the deep adductor muscles, and the lower aspect of the inner thigh. Obturator nerve block is indicated as a supplement to femoral, sciatic, and lateral femoral cutaneous nerve blocks. Alone it does not provide adequate surgical analgesia for procedures of the lower limb. The most common use of the obturator nerve block is in diagnosis of painful conditions of the hip or relief of adductor muscle spasms.

(D) *Incorrect.* The common peroneal nerve supplies the lateral (not medial) aspect of the lower leg.

(E) *Incorrect.* The tibial nerve supplies the lateral aspect of the ankle and the plantar surface of the foot.

## REASONING:

This question tests knowledge of the nerve supply to the lower limb and differences in innervation to the medial and lateral aspects of the lower leg. Choices C and E can be eliminated because they do not supply the lower leg at all. Choice D can be eliminated if the reader knows that the peroneal nerve runs on the lateral aspect of the leg (derived from the sciatic nerve branches). This leaves choices A and B (femoral and sciatic). The sciatic nerve runs posteriorly, and branches wrap around to supply the lateral aspect of the leg. Thus the femoral nerve, choice A, is the best answer.

## BIBLIOGRAPHY:

Miller RD, Eriksson LI, Fleisher LA, Wiener-Kronish JP, William YL. *Miller's Anesthesia.* 7th ed. Philadelphia, PA: Churchill Livingstone; 2010:1651-1653.

Morgan GE, Mikhail MS, Murray MJ. *Clinical Anesthesiology.* 4th ed. New York, NY: McGraw-Hill; 2006:344-346.

---

**BOOK B:**      **QUESTION 82**

---

*Answer B*

Equipment/Physics

## QUESTION (Choose single best answer):

Which of the following is most effective in preventing intraoperative hypothermia in adults?

(A) Heating and humidifying inspired gases.
(B) Maintaining a warm operating room.
(C) Using a circulating warm-water mattress.
(D) Using reflective coverings.
(E) Warming intravenous fluids.

## CORRECT ANSWER: B

## SUMMARY:

*Intraoperative hypothermia is a common complication in patients undergoing surgery. Heat loss occurs primarily through radiation, conduction, and convection from the patient's skin and open-body cavities to surrounding ambient air and surfaces in contact with skin. Convection is by far the most important mechanism of heat loss. Methods to prevent intraoperative hypothermia include administration of warm intravenous fluids; use of warmed and humidified inspired gases; maintaining a warm operating room environment; and use of forced-air warming blankets (Bair Huggers), circulating warm-water mattresses, resistive heating pads, and reflective coverings. Of these, maintaining a warm operating room environment and forced-air warming (addressing convective heat loss) are the most efficient methods. Circulating warm-water mattresses and warming intra-venous fluids are somewhat effective, whereas warm inspired gases and reflective coverings have been shown to be relatively ineffective at preventing hypothermia. Newer methods using resistive heating techniques have been shown to be as effective as forced-air warming.*

## EXPLANATION:

(A) ***Incorrect.*** Heating and humidification of inspired gases are a relatively ineffective method of preventing intraoperative hypothermia.

(B) ***Correct.*** Conductive heat loss will not occur if the operating room environment is warmer than the patient's core temperature. However, this is difficult to accomplish while surgeons work under heavily gowned conditions. For this reason, other methods of preventing hypothermia must be used.

(C) ***Incorrect.*** Circulating warm-air mattresses are used commonly in the pediatric operating room suite and are effective at providing conductive heat transfer. However, only the side of the body in contact with the mattress is treated, and therefore this method is not as effective as maintaining high ambient air temperatures.

(D) ***Incorrect.*** Use of reflective coverings is relatively ineffective at preventing hypothermia.

(E) ***Incorrect.*** Warming intravenous fluids is relatively ineffective at preventing hypothermia by itself because the total body surface area addressed by the intravascular system is small compared with skin.

## REASONING:

This question is challenging because it requires comparing several different warming methods and fails to provide the most commonly used method (forced-air warming) as an answer option. Common sense can help eliminate choices that are not used commonly in the operating room suite (choices A and D). The most efficient methods to prevent heat loss involve transfer of heat to the patient over a large surface area. Methods that provide contact between warm fluid and air with skin have the greatest surface-area exposure and therefore would be the best answers. Choice E can be eliminated by realizing that the total surface area of the intravascular system is relatively small compared with skin and that warming is limited by the total amount of intravenous fluid administered. This leaves choices B and C. B is the best answer because it involves contact with the largest surface area.

## BIBLIOGRAPHY:

Bennett J, Ramachandra V, Webster J, Carli F. Prevention of hypothermia during hip surgery: effect of passive compared with active skin surface warming. *Br J Anaesth.* 1994;73(2):180-183.

Buggy DJ, Crossley AWA. Thermoregulation, mild perioperative hypothermia and post-anaesthetic shivering. *Br J Anaesth.* 2000;84(5):615-628.

Morgan GE, Mikhail MS, Murray MJ. *Clinical Anesthesiology.* 4th ed. New York, NY: McGraw-Hill; 2006:160-161.

Ng SF, Oo CS, Loh KH, et al. A comparative study of three warming interventions to determine the most effective in maintaining perioperative normothermia. *Anesth Analg.* 2003;96(1):171-176.

# QUESTION 83

*Answer C*

Equipment/Physics

**QUESTION (Choose single best answer):**

Which of the following shaded areas most accurately represents the dead space of a properly functioning circle system?

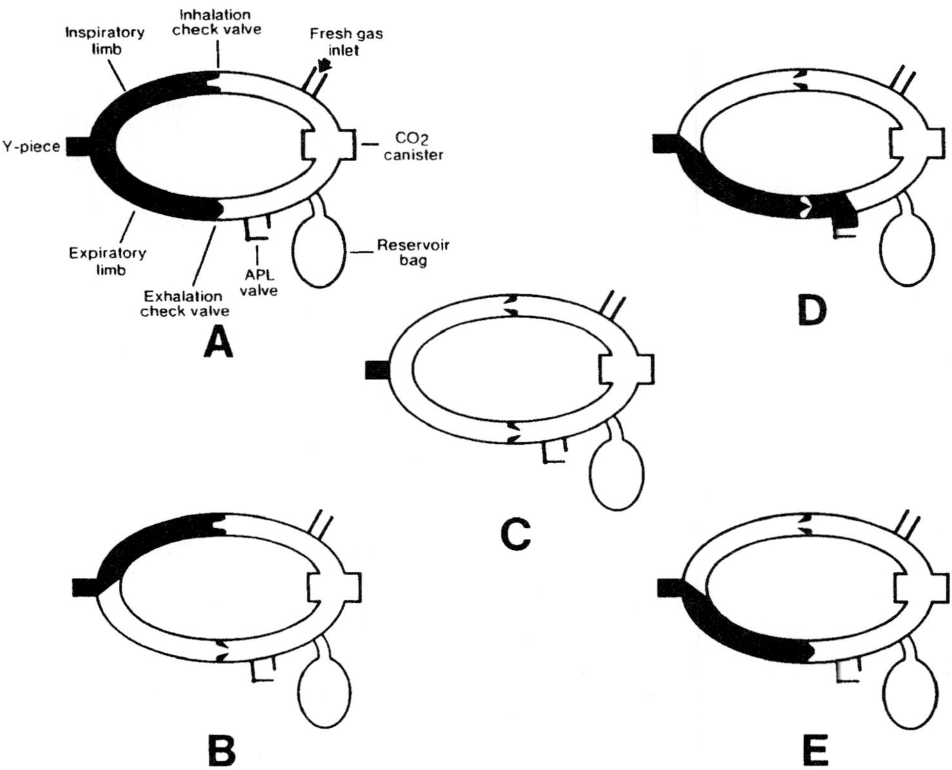



**CORRECT ANSWER: C**

**SUMMARY:**

*The circle system used on most modern anesthesia machines was developed in an attempt to address the inefficiencies of the Mapleson and Bain circuits. Most important the circle system overcomes the problem of rebreathing exhaled gases. In the circle system, the expiratory and inspiratory limbs are separated proximal to the Y-piece, and a unidirectional valve is used in both limbs. This allows fresh gases to enter the system and exhaled gases to exit the system in separate limbs proximal to the Y-piece. The area of the circle system distal to the Y-piece is the only dead space of the circle system because it is the only place where inspired and exhaled gases are mixed. Areas of the circuit proximal to the Y-piece do not represent dead space.*

**EXPLANATION:**

(A) *Incorrect.* The areas in the inspiratory and expiratory limbs that are proximal to the Y-piece do not represent dead space (see items B and E here).

(B) *Incorrect.* Because inspired gas only moves unidirectionally (toward the patient), the area between the inspiratory valve and the Y-piece is not dead space.

(C) *Correct.* Only the area distal to the Y-piece is dead space in the circle system. This is so because there is no mixing of inspired and expired gases proximal to the Y-piece.

(D) ***Incorrect.*** Neither the exhaled gas between the Y-piece and the expiratory valve nor that between the expiratory valve and the APL valve is dead space because no remixing of inspired and expired gas occurs.

(E) ***Incorrect.*** Because exhaled gases do not move backward across the expiratory valve, the area between the Y-piece and the expiratory valve is not dead space.

**REASONING:**

This question tests knowledge of dead space in the circle system. *Dead space* as it relates to breathing systems is defined as the part of tidal volume that does not participate in alveolar ventilation. Careful examination of the diagrams in this question should reveal that the volumes of gas in the inspiratory and expiratory limbs participate in alveolar ventilation during some part of their transit. Only the area in diagram C distal to the Y-piece contains mixed inspiratory and expiratory gases that do not undergo alveolar ventilation. Therefore, C is the best answer.

**BIBLIOGRAPHY:**

Barash PG, Cullen BF, Stoelting RK, Cahalan M, Stock M. *Clinical Anesthesia*. 6th ed. Philadelphia, PA: Lippincott Williams & Wilkins; 2009:671-673.

Morgan GE, Mikhail MS, Murray MJ. *Clinical Anesthesiology*. 4th ed. New York, NY: McGraw-Hill; 2006:40.

---

| **BOOK B:** | **QUESTION 84** |
|---|---|

## *Answer B*

## Pharmacology

**QUESTION (Choose single best answer):**

The effect of succinylcholine is terminated at postsynaptic effector cells by

(A) Binding and uptake by effector cells.
(B) Diffusion into capillaries.
(C) Hydrolysis by junctional cholinesterase.
(D) Hydrolysis by pseudocholinesterase.
(E) Spontaneous degradation to succinylmonocholine.

**CORRECT ANSWER: B**

**SUMMARY:**

*Succinylcholine is a rapidly acting depolarizing muscle relaxant that binds to receptors in the NMJ and mimics the action of acetylcholine. Succinylcholine works by inducing a long period of depolarization at the postsynaptic receptor such that acetylcholine cannot bind and cause muscle contraction. Succinylcholine undergoes rapid hydrolysis in the circulation by plasma cholinesterases. Its primary clinical effect occurs when drug that is not degraded in plasma reaches and binds to receptors at the level of the NMJ. Once bound, there is little available cholinesterase in the NMJ to terminate drug effect. Drug bound to postsynaptic NMJ receptors undergoes diffusion from the NMJ into the extracellular fluid. Degradation of succinylcholine occurs both at the level of the plasma (rapid hydrolysis) and at postsynaptic receptor cells (slow diffusion). This question specifically asks for the mechanism at postsynaptic cells.*

**EXPLANATION:**

(A) ***Incorrect.*** The action of succinylcholine is terminated by hydrolysis at the level of the plasma and NMJ and by diffusion of unbound drug from the NMJ into capillaries.

Binding of succinylcholine at effector cells would result in depolarizing blockade, not drug termination.

(B) **Correct.** Once succinylcholine is bound to receptor cells, termination of action occurs by diffusion into capillaries. This reduces the amount of available succinylcholine in the NMJ but does not terminate drug action once bound.

(C) **Incorrect.** Cholinesterases are not present in sufficiently large quantities in the NMJ to contribute to termination of action at the level of the postsynaptic receptors.

(D) **Incorrect.** Hydrolysis by pseudocholinesterases occurs in plasma with respect to unbound drug, not to drug already bound to NMJ receptors.

(E) **Incorrect.** Although succinylmonocholine is a major metabolite of succinylcholine, this metabolite is produced primarily in the circulation after hydrolysis, not at the level of the postsynaptic effector cells.

## REASONING:

This question tests knowledge of the three sites at which succinylcholine is metabolized. Choice A can be eliminated because uptake and binding at effector cells likely would produce drug action, not termination. Choices D and E describe degradation of unbound drug in plasma, not at effector cells. Choice C is not a good choice because cholinesterases are not present in sufficient quantities in the NMJ. The vast amount of succinylcholine that reaches the NMJ and binds to receptors is removed via diffusion into extracellular fluid and capillaries. B is the best answer.

## BIBLIOGRAPHY:

Morgan GE, Mikhail MS, Murray MJ. *Clinical Anesthesiology.* 4th ed. New York, NY: McGraw-Hill; 2006;212.

Stoelting RK. *Pharmacology and Physiology in Anesthetic Practice.* 4th ed. Philadelphia, PA: Lippincott Williams & Wilkins; 2006:218.

---

**BOOK B:**　　　　**QUESTION 85 (OPTIONAL)**

---

*Answer D*

OB/Regional

**QUESTION (Choose single best answer):**

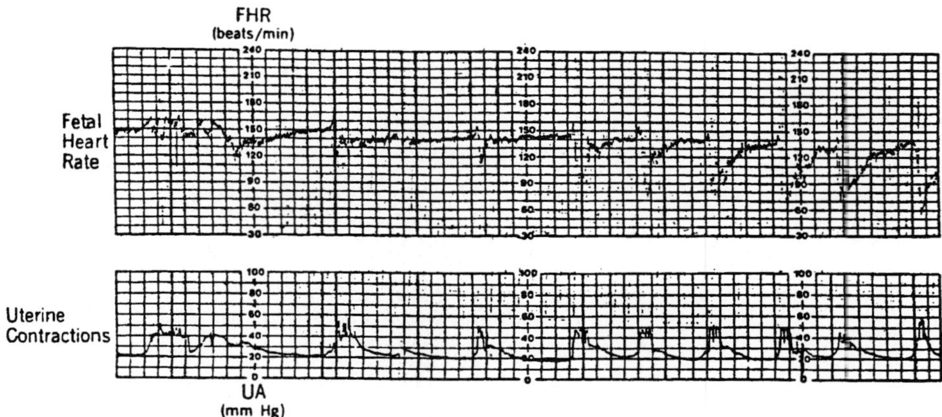


The fetal heart rate and uterine contraction tracings shown here are most consistent with

(A) Fetal acidosis.
(B) Fetal cerebral hemorrhage.
(C) Fetal head compression.
(D) Fetal hypoxia.
(E) Uteroplacental insufficiency.

**CORRECT ANSWER: D**

**SUMMARY:**

*It is essential for the anesthesiologist to possess an understanding of fetal heart rate (FHR) monitoring because it is a useful tool for measuring fetal oxygenation and well-being. The FHR tracing should be measured in conjunction with uterine contractions. U-shaped decelerations that predictably occur with contractions are referred to as "early" or "late" depending on when they occur. Early decelerations have their onset with the contraction, nadir at the peak, and return to baseline by the end of the contraction. These decelerations are a reassuring pattern associated with fetal head compression. Late decelerations begin after the onset of the contraction, nadir after the peak, and return to baseline after the contraction. This pattern is associated with uteroplacental insufficiency and is commonly a nonreassuring pattern depending on the fetal baseline heart rate and variability. Variable decelerations have an abrupt onset and variable association with contractions, and the change from baseline is greater than with other types of decelerations. This pattern tends to be nonreassuring and is associated with acute interruptions in umbilical cord blood flow. Over time, fetal hypoxia can develop with both variable and late patterns owing to a decreased ability of the fetus to compensate for the interruptions in blood flow.*

*The nomenclature for FHR tracings was changed in 2009 to improve communication among obstetrical care providers. The new nomenclature is represented in Table 1. Characteristics are as follows: Category I FHR tracings are normal and no immediate intervention is necessary; category III FHR tracings are abnormal and require immediate intervention, beginning with conservative measures such as optimization of maternal condition. If these are ineffective, delivery is recommended; and category II FHR tracings are indeterminate and require reevaluation.*

**EXPLANATION:**

(A) *Incorrect.* While lactic acidosis can develop over time in a compromised fetus, there is no predictable pattern associated with fetal acidosis.

(B) *Incorrect.* There is currently no reliable method to detect fetal cerebral hemorrhage from the FHR tracing.

(C) *Incorrect.* Fetal head compression is associated with early decelerations. While the onset of this patient's decelerations occurs with contractions and the nadir is close to the peak in a couple of the decelerations, the lowest heart rate is much lower than what is usually associated with early decelerations and the return to baseline is long after the contraction is over. This is the "official" answer to this question. The authors disagree with this answer because the depth of FHR is too low to be consistent with only head compression.

(D) *Correct.* The fetus is exhibiting variable decelerations in the second stage of labor (one can see that the patient is pushing based on the up-and-down pattern with the uterine contractions). This is a common pattern in this stage of labor. However, the slow return to baseline as the labor progresses indicates a decreased ability to tolerate the acute decreases in umbilical cord blood flow, and the decelerations become more profound and the return to baseline becomes slower. This is a pattern associated with fetal hypoxia.

(E) *Incorrect.* Uteroplacental insufficiency is associated with late decelerations, which are not seen in this tracing.

**REASONING:**

This is a difficult question because the FHR tracing is not straightforward. This is an example of a category II FHR tracing. Choice B can be eliminated immediately because there is not a pattern associated with cerebral hemorrhage. The next step is to determine what types of decelerations are displayed. Because they have an abrupt onset and low nadir, they are variables. Why not early or late? It is possible that the first few decelerations are early, but the overwhelming pattern is one with acute decelerations, gradually getting lower, and a return to baseline that is getting slower. This pattern is associated with variable decelerations, and the slow return to baseline over time is associated with hypoxia. Table 2 lists the characteristics of early and variable decelerations. Knowing this, one can eliminate choices C and E. The baby may be compromised, but we would not know it was acidotic without performing a blood gas analysis. Choice A can be eliminated. The best answer is D. The reader should not be discouraged by the difficulty of this question. We were only able to interpret this tracing correctly after extensive research and consultation with senior maternal-fetal medicine specialists at Stanford.

**Table 1  Fetal Heart Rate Categories**

| Category I FHR Tracing (Normal) | Category II FHR Tracing (Indeterminate) | Category III FHR Tracing (Abnormal) |
|---|---|---|
| Baseline FHR 110-160 | Bradycardia not accompanied by absent variability | Absent baseline variability *and* any of the following: |
| Moderate variability | Tachycardia | Recurrent late decelerations |
| Late or variable decelerations absent | Variability: absent without decelerations<br>Minimal or marked baseline variability | Recurrent variable decelerations |
| Early decelerations and accelerations present or absent | Recurrent variable decelerations | Bradycardia |
| | Recurrent late decelerations with moderate baseline variability | Sinusoidal pattern |

Modified from: ACOG Practice Bulletin No. 106. *Obstet Gynecol.* 2009;114(1):192-202.

**Table 2  Early Versus Variable Decelerations**

| Early Deceleration | Variable Deceleration |
|---|---|
| Visually apparent usually symmetrical gradual decrease and return of the FHR associated with a uterine contraction | Visually apparent abrupt decrease in FHR |
| A gradual FHR decrease is defined as from the onset to the FHR nadir of $\geq 30$ s | An abrupt FHR decrease is defined as from the onset of the deceleration to the beginning of the FHR nadir of $< 30$ s. |
| The decrease in FHR is calculated from the onset to the nadir of the deceleration | The decrease in FHR is calculated from the onset to the nadir of the deceleration |
| The nadir of the deceleration occurs at the same time as the peak of the contraction | The decrease in FHR is $\geq 15$ bpm lasting $\geq 15$ s, and $< 2$ min duration |
| In most cases the onset, nadir, and recovery of the deceleration are coincident with the beginning, peak, and ending of the contraction, respectively. | When variable decelerations are associated with uterine contractions, their onset, depth, and duration commonly vary with successive uterine contractions. |

Modified from: ACOG Practice Bulletin No. 106. *Obstet Gynecol* 2009;114(1):192-202.

**BIBLIOGRAPHY:**

ACOG Practice Bulletin No. 117. Intrapartum fetal heart rate monitoring: nomenclature, interpretation, and general management principles. *Obstet Gynecol.* 2009;114(1) 192-202.

Chestnut DH, Polley LS, Tsen LC, Wong CA. *Chestnut's Obstetric Anesthesia Principles and Practice.* 4th ed. Philadelphia, PA: Mosby Elsevier; 2009;144-147.

Gibb D, Arulkumaran S. *Fetal Monitoring in Practice.* 2nd ed. Oxford, UK: Butterworth Heinemann; 1997:45-70, 130-131.


---

**BOOK B:**

**QUESTION 86 (OPTIONAL)**

*Answer None*

Basic Science

**QUESTION (Choose single best answer):**

The cardiovascular effects of an inhalational anesthetic are evaluated in 10 normal volunteers in the awake resting state and after 15 minutes of constant inspired concentration. Results were analyzed by *t* test for paired data and are presented below as mean ± standard deviation.

| | Mean Arterial Pressure (mm Hg) | Heart Rate (bpm) | Cardiac Output (L/min) |
|---|---|---|---|
| Awake | 94 ± 5 | 82 ± 2 | 4.2 ± 0.5 |
| Anesthetized | 83 ± 9 | 90 ± 2[a] | 3.9 ± 0.7 |

[a]$p < .05$.

Based on these data, which of the following conclusions is most valid?

(A) A decrease in cardiac output would have been evident if more subjects were included in the study.
(B) The anesthetic decreases mean arterial pressure.
(C) The anesthetic does not cause cardiac depression.
(D) The anesthetic is unsafe for patients with coronary artery disease.
(E) There is a 95% to 100% chance that the anesthetic increases heart rate.

**CORRECT ANSWER: None of the choices are correct.**

**SUMMARY:**

*Anesthesiologists should have a basic understanding of epidemiology and statistics to interpret the quality of evidence presented in scientific journals. Anesthetic practice should be guided by evidence-based principles that are supported by high-quality research. This question describes a crossover study in which the patient serves as his or her own control. Measurements first were performed awake and then repeated while the patient was anesthetized. The outcome measures (mean arterial pressure, heart rate, and cardiac output) are all continuous variables and can be described by their average value (mean) and standard deviation (a measure of variance from the mean). The correct statistical test for analyzing continuous variables in a crossover study is the paired* t *test because it accounts for the decreased sample variance when a subject is used as his or her own control. A* p *value indicates the probability of committing a type I error, that is, the chance that we reject the null hypothesis, H0, when it is actually true. In this case, the H0 would state: "There is no significant change in heart rate when a patient is anesthetized." The p < .05 for the heart rate variable indicates that this H0 can be rejected with a 5% chance of committing a type I error. Restated, we can be at least 95% certain that anesthesia increases heart rate.*

**EXPLANATION:**

(A) *Incorrect.* This study did not show a statistically significant difference in cardiac output when the patient was anesthetized. Negative findings should prompt the reader to question the power of the study to resolve the difference it observed. Statistical power is the probability of concluding that there was a difference when a difference truly exists. In other words, power reflects our confidence that we could detect a difference in cardiac output if there were truly a difference. The computed post hoc power for this study is approximately 20%. Thus we are only 20% confident that we could detect a difference in cardiac output if a difference truly exists. Therefore, it is possible that we may find a difference if a larger cohort of patients were studied. However, we cannot conclude with certainty that this would be the case.

(B) *Incorrect.* The difference on this measure did not reach statistical significance ($p < .05$), and we cannot reject the H0.

(C) *Incorrect.* We cannot make a conclusion on this measure because this study did not evaluate "cardiac depression." We presume that cardiac depression means negative inotropy, although this is not specified.

(D) *Incorrect.* We cannot make this conclusion based on the current study design. The cohort used in this study did not have coronary artery disease. In addition, the outcome measure "anesthetic is unsafe" would need to be defined more clearly (eg, incidence of perioperative myocardial infarction, drop in MAP > 20 mm Hg with induction, etc).

(E) *Incorrect.* The difference on this measure did reach statistical significance ($p < .05$), and we can reject the H0 with 95% certainty. Therefore, we can say that the anesthetic increases heart rate with at least 95% certainty. Please note, however, that this is not the same as saying, "There is a 95% to 100% chance that the anesthetic increases heart rate." In truth, the anesthetic either increases heart rate or it does not. This is truth, and it is fixed. Therefore, there is not a 95% chance that the anesthetic increases heart rate; it simply does or it does not. Scientific methods and statistical analysis allow us to report that we can be 95% certain that we captured the truth. In addition, it should be noted that nothing can be proven to have a 100% certainty of being correct.

**REASONING:**

This question tests knowledge of basic epidemiology and statistics for interpretation of experimental evidence. Choice D can be eliminated immediately because patients with coronary artery disease were not studied in this experiment. Choice A can be eliminated even though the study did not have adequate power to resolve the observed difference in cardiac output. We cannot know with certainty that a difference would be found if a larger cohort were studied. Choice B can be eliminated because we did not achieve statistical significance ($p < .05$) on this measure. Choice C can be eliminated because "cardiac depression" was not measured in this study. The only outcome measure that was statistically significant was an increase in heart rate. Choice E is not correct because the anesthetic cannot have a "chance" of increasing heart rate—it either does or does not. We can report that we have a 95% certainty that it increases heart rate, but we can never claim that we have 100% certainty in resolving the truth. On an actual examination, we would choose choice E because it best reflects the intent of the question. However, none of the answers are correct.

**BIBLIOGRAPHY:**


Norman GR, Streiner DL. *Biostatistics: The Bare Essentials.* Ontario, BC: Decker; 2000:62-68 (Chapter 7).

Vacanti CA. *Essential Clinical Anesthesia.* Cambridge University Press; 2011:374-876 (Chapter 142).

## *Answer D*

### Clinical Anesthesia

**QUESTION (Choose single best answer):**

A patient with alcoholic cirrhosis, ascites, and gastrointestinal bleeding receives 4 units of red blood cells prior to anesthesia with isoflurane in oxygen for emergency exploratory laparotomy. After the peritoneum is opened and the fluid is drained, blood pressure decreases to 60/40 mm Hg and $SpO_2$ decreases to 90%. The most likely cause of the hypoxemia is

(A) Acute myocardial ischemia.
(B) Decreased 2,3-diphosphoglycerate in transfused blood.
(C) Increased intrapulmonary shunting.
(D) Relative hypovolemia.
(E) Venous air embolism.

**CORRECT ANSWER: D**

**SUMMARY:**

*Liver cirrhosis is characterized by a hyperdynamic circulatory state with systemic and pulmonary arteriovenous shunting. Low blood viscosity due to chronic anemia and hypo-albuminemia further contributes to this hyperdynamic state of high cardiac output and low peripheral vascular resistance. Ascites fluid increases intra-abdominal pressure on the diaphragm, decreases FRC, and creates a restrictive pulmonary physiology. Hypoxemia results from a combination of pulmonary arteriovenous (AV) communications and V/Q mismatch. Although the circulatory and ventilatory systems generally are compensated, infection, blood loss, rapid volume shifts, and cardiac dysfunction can quickly upset this fragile balance and lead to circulatory collapse.*

**EXPLANATION:**

(A) *Incorrect.* Myocardial infarction can cause hypotension and hypoxemia. However, in this patient, the symptoms presented during decompression of the peritoneum on opening the abdomen. The most likely clinical explanation is that abdominal decompression from the rapid drainage of blood caused an intravascular volume shift to the extravascular space, creating a relative hypovolemia. Decreased venous return to the heart lowers pulmonary perfusion and increases alveolar dead space, which results in hypoxemia.

(B) *Incorrect.* Transfused packed red blood cells are depleted of 2,3-diphosphoglycerate (2,3-DPG) and cause a leftward shift of the oxyhemoglobin dissociation curve, impeding unloading of oxygen from hemoglobin. This would not lead to hypoxemia. Also, the transfusion was given prior to anesthesia with no apparent change in the $SpO_2$, with the change coming acutely after abdominal decompression. The timing of the symptoms makes this an unlikely cause of hypoxemia in this patient.

(C) *Incorrect.* Increased intrapulmonary shunting would exacerbate hypoxia. However, the abdominal decompression is expected to relieve the pressure on the diaphragm and improve pulmonary gas exchange instead of making it worse.

(D) *Correct.* Intra-abdominal bleeding can be extensive in a patient with liver failure and presumed coagulopathy. More than 1 L of blood can accumulate before any change in abdominal girth occurs, and more when accounting for displacement of the diaphragm. Although bleeding may have been slowed temporarily by a tamponade effect, hypovolemia can be unmasked rapidly once the peritoneum is opened and bleeding resumes.

(E) *Incorrect.* Venous air embolism is a rare complication that is unlikely in this patient.

This question tests knowledge of the pathophysiology of alcoholic cirrhosis and liver failure. The clinical scenario of hypotension and hypoxemia can happen in the setting of myocardial infarction, VAE, and hypovolemia. The most likely cause in this patient is relative hypovolemia, choice D.


**BIBLIOGRAPHY:**

Barash PG, Cullen BF, Stoelting RK, Cahalan M, Stock M. *Clinical Anesthesia*. 6th ed. Philadelphia, PA: Lippincott Williams & Wilkins; 2009:907, 1260-1262.

Morgan GE, Mikhail MS, Murray MJ. *Clinical Anesthesiology*. 4th ed. New York, NY: McGraw-Hill; 2006:562-563, 699, 792-796, 869.

---

**BOOK B:**      **QUESTION 88**

---

*Answer D*

Neuroanesthesia

**QUESTION (Choose single best answer):**

Which of the following statements concerning barbiturate protection from cerebral ischemia is true?

(A) It may be achieved with dosages low enough to avoid cardiovascular effects.
(B) It is linearly dose-related.
(C) It improves neurologic outcome following cardiac arrest.
(D) It is most useful in patients with focal ischemia.
(E) It is unrelated to EEG activity.


**CORRECT ANSWER: D**


**SUMMARY:**

*Cerebral protection by barbiturates is limited to focal ischemic events with no significant benefit following global ischemia due to cardiac arrest. Barbiturates may provide cerebral protection by decreasing cerebral metabolism. Additionally, barbiturates can cause inverse steal by vasoconstricting blood vessels in areas of healthy brain and shunting blood to ischemic brain tissue, reduce calcium influx, block sodium channels, and inhibit free radical formation. Barbiturates at these doses are high enough to induce an isoelectric EEG and decrease cardiac contractility and produce hypotension.*


**EXPLANATION:**

(A) *Incorrect.* Decreased cardiac contractility and hypotension are seen.
(B) *Incorrect.* The cerebral protective effect of barbiturates plateaus with the onset of burst suppression with increased side effects and no additional benefits at higher doses.
(C) *Incorrect.* Barbiturates have not been shown to be effective in protecting the brain from global ischemic events such as cardiac arrest.
(D) *Correct.* The protective efficacy of barbiturates in focal cerebral ischemia but not in global ischemia has been demonstrated and is attributed to suppression of CMR.
(E) *Incorrect.* The cerebral protective effect of barbiturates is directly related to the onset of burst suppression. Maximal reduction in $CMRO_2$ is achieved when the EEG is isoelectric.


**REASONING:**

Choice D is the best answer. Remember, the benefit of barbiturates is limited to focal ischemic events with no significant benefit following global ischemia. Choice C is incorrect. Choices A, B, and E incorrectly assert that cardiac events are not seen with barbiturate use, have linear dose-related effects, or are not closely related to EEG suppression in focal cerebral protection.

**BIBLIOGRAPHY:**
Morgan GE, Mikhail MS, Murray MJ. *Clinical Anesthesiology*. 4th ed. New York, NY: McGraw-Hill; 2006:625.

| BOOK B: | QUESTION 89 |
|---|---|

## *Answer D*

### Clinical Anesthesia

**QUESTION (Choose single best answer):**

A 77-year-old woman is still intubated and breathing spontaneously following a total hip replacement. The muscle relaxant has been reversed. Tidal volume is 400 mL, end-tidal carbon dioxide tension is 45 mm Hg, and $Spo_2$ is 98% at an $Fio_2$ of 1.0. On transfer from the operating table to the gurney, her heart rate increases from 65 to 100 bpm, and her blood pressure decreases from 130/80 to 80/50 mm Hg. End-tidal carbon dioxide tension ($ETco_2$) is 30 mm Hg, and $Spo_2$ is 94%. The most likely diagnosis is

(A)  Anaphylactic reaction.
(B)  Bronchospasm.
(C)  Myocardial infarction.
(D)  Pulmonary embolism.
(E)  Unreplaced blood loss.

**CORRECT ANSWER: D**

**SUMMARY:**

*Three potentially life-threatening complications associated with total hip replacement (THR) are bone cement implantation syndrome (BCIS), thromboembolism, and intraoperative hemorrhage. BCIS occurs with the use of methyl methacrylate, an acrylic cement compound used to fuse the joint prosthesis to bone in arthroplastic procedures. It is characterized by hypoxia, hypotension, or both, and/or unexpected loss of consciousness occurring around the time of cementation, prosthesis insertion, reduction of the joint, or, occasionally, limb tourniquet deflation in a patient undergoing cemented bone surgery. The etiology is now thought to be related to embolization of fat, marrow, cement particles, air, bone particles, and aggregates of platelets and fibrin. Deep venous thrombosis (DVT) is the most frequent postoperative complication associated with hip replacement surgery, with a prevalence of 42% to 57%, and a 0.9% to 28% prevalence of pulmonary embolism. The incidence of fatal pulmonary embolism after hip arthroplasty is 0.14% to 2%.*

**EXPLANATION:**
(A)  *Incorrect.* Anaphylactic reaction to the cement or anesthetic can occur, but it is a rare complication. Anaphylactic reactions often are correlated temporally with a specific exposure. This patient's sudden hypotension in the absence of an inciting exposure makes this choice less likely.
(B)  *Incorrect.* Bronchospasm is characterized by increased expiratory effort and polyphonic expiratory wheezes that usually are accompanied by coughing, shortness of breath, or complaints of chest tightness. We are not given any other information to suspect this finding.
(C)  *Incorrect.* A sudden acute myocardial infarction leading to hemodynamic compromise and collapse could explain the observed findings, but it is not the most likely diagnosis in this patient.

(D) **Correct.** Patients undergoing hip replacement surgery have a high incidence of developing DVT. They also have an increased risk of developing clinically significant and/or fatal pulmonary embolism. Pulmonary embolism acutely increases PVR, causing a localized or generalized reflex bronchoconstriction to areas affected by the embolic event. The result is an increase in pulmonary shunting and hypoxemia. Tachycardia, elevated CVP, and hypotension also may occur owing to progressive right ventricular failure.

(E) **Incorrect.** Only hypovolemia owing to rapid blood loss could explain these acute cardiovascular changes. We have no reason to suspect it in this patient.

### REASONING:

This question tests knowledge of common complications following hip replacement surgery. It is important to understand that these patients are at increased perioperative risk for developing clinically significant and/or fatal pulmonary embolism from DVT. Cement implantation syndrome also places these patients at increased risk of hypotension, hypoxia, and pulmonary embolism during cementation, prosthesis insertion, reduction of the joint, or, occasionally, limb tourniquet deflation in a patient undergoing cemented bone surgery. The temporal association of the patient's hypotension with transfer from the operating table makes dislodgment of a DVT and subsequent pulmonary embolism the most likely diagnosis. D is the best answer.

### BIBLIOGRAPHY:


Barash PG, Cullen BF, Stoelting RK, Cahalan M, Stock M. *Clinical Anesthesia*. 6th ed. Philadelphia, PA: Lippincott Williams & Wilkins; 2009:907, 1388-1389.

Donaldson AJ, Thomson HE, Harper NJ, et al. Bone cement implantation syndrome. *Br J Anaesth*. 2009;102(1):12-22.

Feeley BT, Lieberman JR. Venous thromboembolism following total hip arthroplasty. In: Callaghan JJ, Rosenberg AG, Rubash HE, eds. *The Adult Hip*. Philadelphia, PA: Lippincott-Raven Publishers; 2006:654-671.

Morgan GE, Mikhail MS, Murray MJ. *Clinical Anesthesiology*. 4th ed. New York, NY: McGraw-Hill; 2006:849-856


---

## BOOK B:     QUESTION 90

*Answer D*

Pain

### QUESTION (Choose single best answer):

A 40-year-old woman has continuous nondermatomal burning pain of the distal foot 4 weeks after sustaining a metatarsal fracture. On examination, the foot is mildly swollen, tender, and cool. Which of the following statements concerning this condition is true?

(A) A radiograph of the distal bones of the painful foot will show severe osteoporosis.
(B) A technetium scan of the distal joints of the painful foot will show decreased uptake.
(C) Early use of the opioid analgesia will prevent progression of the symptoms.
(D) Intravenous phentolamine will relieve the pain.
(E) The chance of spontaneous recovery within 8 weeks is greater than 80%.

### CORRECT ANSWER: D

### SUMMARY:

*The question describes the syndrome of reflex sympathetic dystrophy now known as complex regional pain syndrome (CRPS) type I. During the acute phase a technetium bone scan will show increased uptake and x-ray will be normal. Opioids have no effect on the course of the disease, but the pain is sympathetically maintained and blockade with the α-blocker phentolamine will relieve the pain. The chance of recovery has been reported to be high only if treatment is initiated within a month of symptom onset.*

## EXPLANATION:

(A) **Incorrect.** The condition has only been ongoing for 4 weeks, during which only minimal changes would be expected if any.

(B) **Incorrect.** As stated above the classic finding would be increased uptake on technetium scan.

(C) **Incorrect.** Opioids do not prevent progression of the disease and are controversial in the treatment of this disease as they are often not effective.

(D) **Correct.** Intravenous phentolamine will relieve the pain. This effect is dose dependent and correlates highly with relief provided by local anesthetic sympathetic block.

(E) **Incorrect.** To achieve a high rate of recovery requires aggressive treatment with physical therapy and sympathetic blockade.

## REASONING:

The diagnosis of CRPS requires the presence of regional pain and sensory changes following a noxious event either a serious or trivial injury. Further, the pain is associated with findings such as abnormal skin color, temperature change, abnormal sudomotor activity, or edema. The combination of these findings exceeds their expected magnitude in response to known physical damage during and following the inciting event. These changes occur in the setting of no other concomitant conditions to account for the findings. Two types of CRPS have been recognized: Type I corresponds to RSD (reflex sympathetic dystrophy) and occurs without a definable nerve lesion, and type II, formerly called *causalgia*, refers to cases where a definable nerve lesion is present. More recently, a third type has been added, namely CRPS not otherwise specified (NOS), involving a syndrome that only partially complies with the diagnostic criteria, but where no other diagnosis can be made. A hallmark of these conditions is the presence of sympathetically maintained pain, which can be relieved by regional sympathetic block, intravenous regional block, or infusion of the α-blocker phentolamine. The estimated incidence varies from 5.46 to 26.2 per 100,000 person years. Although the phentolamine technique will relieve the pain, this technique has not gained widespread use. The more common and time-tested approach is to perform a local anesthetic sympathetic trunk block. No specific test is available for CRPS. Plain radiographs can show patchy osteoporosis as early as 2 weeks after the onset of CRPS. As the disease progresses, the bones may have a ground-glass appearance and cortical erosions may be present. A technetium scan of the affected joints has been studied for CRPS. It has been reported to be highly sensitive but relatively nonspecific. Classic findings include increased periarticular uptake, though in some patients the reverse can be seen. Aggressive early intervention is needed to produce a high rate of recovery. The likelihood of a cure is high (over 90%) if treatment is initiated within 1 month of symptoms and appears to decease with time.


## BIBLIOGRAPHY:

McMahon SB, Koltzenburg M. *Wall and Melzack's Textbook of Pain*. 5th ed. Philadelphia, PA: Churchill Livingstone; 2006:29.

Morgan GE, Mikhail MS, Murray MJ. *Clinical Anesthesiology*. 4th ed. New York, NY: McGraw-Hill; 2006:406-407.

Raja SN, Treede RD, Davis KD, Campbell JN. Systemic alpha-adrenergic blockade with phentolamine: a diagnostic test for sympathetically maintained pain. *Anesthesiology*. 1991;74:691-698.

Rho RH, Brewer RP, Lamer TJ, Wilson PR. Complex regional pain syndrome. *Mayo Clin Proc*. 2002 Feb;77(2):174-180.

Rowbotham MC. Pharmacologic management of complex regional pain syndrome. *Clin J Pain*. 2006;22:425-429.

van Eijs F, Stanton-Hicks M, Van Zundert J, et al. Evidence-based interventional pain medicine according to clinical diagnoses. 16. Complex regional pain syndrome. *Pain Pract*. 2011;11:70-87.

*Answer D*

Clinical Anesthesia

**QUESTION (Choose single best answer):**

Evaluation of a postoperative neurologic deficit discloses an inability to oppose the thumb and little finger, weakness of abduction of the thumb, and loss of flexion of the distal phalanx of the index finger. This problem is most likely related to

(A)  Paresthesia occurring during an interscalene brachial plexus block.
(B)  Attempted radial artery cannulation at the wrist.
(C)  Inadequate padding under the elbow.
(D)  Attempted venipuncture in the antecubital fossa.
(E)  Abduction of the upper humerus against an "ether screen."

**CORRECT ANSWER: D**

**SUMMARY:**

*The median nerve lies next to the medial cubital and basilic veins in the antecubital fossa and may be traumatized by attempts at cannulation or by the extravasation of intravenous medications such as thiopental. This nerve is rarely injured by improper positioning, that is, extreme dorsiflexion at the wrist). A median nerve injury will result in the inability to oppose the thumb and little finger, weakness of thumb abduction, loss of flexion of the distal phalanx of the index finger, and decreased sensation over the palmar surface of the thumb, index, and lateral half of the middle finger.*

**EXPLANATION:**

(A)  *Incorrect.* An interscalene brachial plexus block affects the C5-T1 dermatomes and is useful for surgery on the shoulder, arm, and forearm. Paresthesias elicited during the performance of this block will result in isolated median nerve palsy.
(B)  *Incorrect.* Radial artery cannulation attempts have been associated with hematomas, thrombosis, air embolization, or infection, and would be more likely to harm the radial nerve.
(C)  *Incorrect.* Inadequate padding under the elbow may result in an ulnar neuropathy, the most common perioperative peripheral nerve injury. This nerve is most frequently injured when the forearm is flexed or pronated. There is usually elbow pain and impairment of flexion at the proximal finger joints and abduction/adduction of the fingers. Risk factors for ulnar neuropathies include male gender, prolonged bed rest, a hospital stay greater than 2 weeks, and a very large or very thin body habitus. Ulnar nerve injury is minimized in the supine position with the arm abducted on an arm board and the forearm supinated with the palm facing up.
(D)  *Correct.* Attempts at venipuncture in the cubital fossa may result in median nerve palsy as described above.
(E)  *Incorrect.* Compression of the upper lateral humerus predisposes to a radial nerve injury leading to wrist drop, inability to extend at the metacarpophalangeal joints, and weak abduction of the thumb.

**REASONING:**

Choice D is clearly correct because the question describes a neurologic deficit consistent with a median nerve injury, given the distribution of the injury. It is also important to realize that trauma from venipuncture attempts is the most likely mechanism of injury.

**BIBLIOGRAPHY:**

Lobato E, Gravenstein N, Kirby RR. *Complications in Anesthesiology*. Philadelphia, PA: Lippincott-Raven Publishers; 2008;726, 822-828, 858.

Morgan GE, Mikhail MS, Murray MJ. *Clinical Anesthesiology*. 4th ed. New York, NY: McGraw-Hill; 2006:963-964, 966t.

---

**BOOK B:**

*Answer B*

OB/Regional

**QUESTION 92**

---

**QUESTION (Choose single best answer):**

Arterial oxyhemoglobin desaturation develops more rapidly following apnea in a pregnant patient at term than in a nonpregnant patient with a large intra-abdominal tumor. Which of the following findings in pregnancy is the most likely cause?

(A) Higher cardiac output.
(B) Higher oxygen consumption.
(C) Larger anatomic dead space.
(D) Smaller blood volume.
(E) Smaller functional residual capacity.

**CORRECT ANSWER: B**

**SUMMARY:**

*Many physiologic changes occur during pregnancy. Changes affecting the cardiorespiratory system include increased blood volume by 35%, increased plasma volume by 45%, increased cardiac output by 40%, increased oxygen consumption by up to 50%, increased tidal volume by 40%, increased MV by 50%, and decreased functional residual capacity (FRC) by 20%. Under normal circumstances, increased MV and tidal volume compensate for the increased oxygen consumption. However, when parturients become apneic, the increased oxygen consumption combined with the smaller FRC causes rapid arterial oxyhemoglobin desaturation, even when compared with a patient with a large intra-abdominal tumor of comparable size to the gravid uterus.*

**EXPLANATION:**

(A) *Incorrect.* Parturients have an increase in cardiac output by up to 40% at term. This serves to increase oxygen delivery to the tissues and does not contribute to arterial desaturation.

(B) *Correct.*

$$\text{Apneic time} = (\text{FRC} \times \text{FIO}_2)/\dot{V}\text{O}_2$$

where apneic time is the period of time from the beginning of apnea until arterial oxyhemoglobin desaturation occurs, FRC is the functional residual capacity, $\text{FIO}_2$ is the alveolar oxygen concentration, and $\dot{V}\text{O}_2$ is the rate of oxygen consumption. $\dot{V}\text{O}_2$ increases by 20% to 50% in pregnancy mainly owing to fetal consumption. Patients who have a large intra-abdominal tumor do have decreased FRC secondary to increased intra-abdominal pressure but do not have an increased $\dot{V}\text{O}_2$ and therefore do not desaturate as quickly as a parturient.

(C) *Incorrect.* Anatomic dead space is not changed in parturients.

(D) *Incorrect.* Parturients have a 35% increase in blood volume at term.

(E) *Incorrect.* FRC is decreased by 20% in parturients, and any patient with a large intra-abdominal tumor will also likely have decreased FRC.

This question requires knowledge of the major cardiopulmonary physiologic changes in pregnancy. These include decreased FRC, increased oxygen consumption, increased cardiac output, and increased blood volume. These facts eliminate choice D. Anatomic dead space is a parameter that does not change in pregnancy, which eliminates answer C. While a patient with a large intra-abdominal tumor will have a decreased FRC and possibly an increased cardiac output depending on the vascularity of the tumor, these patients do not have a significant source of oxygen consumption such as a growing fetus, which eliminates answers A and E. B is the best answer.

**BIBLIOGRAPHY:**

Bucklin B, Gambling DR, Wlody DJ. *A Practical Approach to Obstetric Anesthesia.* Philadelphia, PA: Lippincott Williams & Wilkins; 2009:3-14.

Chestnut DH, Polley LS, Lawrence CT, Wong CA. *Chestnut's Obstetrical Anesthesia Principles and Practice.* 4th ed. Philadelphia, PA: Mosby Elsevier; 2009:15-26.

---

## BOOK B:      QUESTION 93

---

*Answer D*

Neuroanesthesia

**QUESTION (Choose single best answer):**

Which of the following best describes the relationship between cerebral perfusion pressure and CBF in a patient with untreated chronic hypertension?

(A)  It is constant at mean blood pressures between 50 and 150 mm Hg.
(B)  It is linear for all blood pressures.
(C)  The flow-versus-pressure curve is hyperbolic.
(D)  The flow-versus-pressure curve is shifted to the right.
(E)  The flow-versus-pressure curve is shifted to the left.

**CORRECT ANSWER: D**

**SUMMARY:**

*The relationship between cerebral perfusion pressure (CPP) and cerebral blood flow (CBF) is determined by cerebral autoregulation. As CPP changes, cerebrovascular resistance adjusts to maintain stable flow. The CPP over which autoregulation is maintained, or autoregulatory plateau, is generally quoted as MAP range of 60 to 150 mm Hg although there is some variability between individuals. Flow becomes pressure-dependent above or below these limits. In patients with chronic hypertension, the entire curve shifts rightward. Thus higher CPPs are required to maintain CBF in patients with untreated chronic hypertension. The clinical implication is that hypertensive patients are more likely to experience cerebral hypoperfusion at "normal" blood pressure ranges. Intraoperative blood pressure management in these patients should account for this rightward shift in the cerebral autoregulation curve to ensure adequate cerebral perfusion.*

**EXPLANATION:**

(A)  ***Incorrect.*** This relationship is true for normotensive patients. Patients with untreated chronic hypertension may require higher mean blood pressures to ensure constant CBF.

(B)  ***Incorrect.*** Flow increases and decreases linearly with pressure only at the extremes of pressure.

(C)  ***Incorrect.*** The basic shape of the curve is similar for normotensive and hypertensive patients.

(D) *Correct.* Patients with untreated chronic hypertension may need higher CPPs to ensure constant CBF. This causes the flow-versus-pressure curve to shift to the right.

(E) *Incorrect.* The flow-versus-pressure curve is shifted to the right, not the left.

### REASONING:

This question tests knowledge of cerebral autoregulation of blood flow and the flow-versus-pressure curve that describes that relationship. The cerebral vasculature modulates vascular resistance to maintain a constant flow within a certain range of CPPs. CBF becomes pressure-dependent outside this range. Untreated chronic hypertension modifies this relationship, shifting the flow-versus-pressure curve to the right. The best answer is D.

### BIBLIOGRAPHY:


Barash PG, Cullen BF, Stoelting RK, Cahalan M, Stock M. *Clinical Anesthesia.* 6th ed. Philadelphia, PA: Lippincott Williams & Wilkins; 2009:1007-1008, 1008f.

Morgan GE, Mikhail MS, Murray MJ. *Clinical Anesthesiology.* 4th ed. New York, NY: McGraw-Hill; 2006:616, 616f.


---

**BOOK B:**      **QUESTION 94**

*Answer B*

Equipment/Physics

### QUESTION (Choose single best answer):

The accuracy of oxyhemoglobin saturation determined by digital pulse oximetry is affected significantly by each of the following *except*

(A) Movement of the patient.
(B) Isovolemic hemodilution to a hematocrit of 23%.
(C) Position of the operating room light.
(D) Intravenous administration of methylene blue.
(E) Infusion of phenylephrine.

### CORRECT ANSWER: B

### SUMMARY:

*Pulse oximeters are noninvasive monitors that use a combination of plethysmography and oximetry to estimate Spo$_2$, the oxyhemoglobin saturation of arterial blood. These monitors transmit light in the red (660 nm) and infrared (960 nm) wavelengths, absorbed by deoxyhemoglobin and oxyhemoglobin, respectively. An algorithm corrects for light absorbed by nonpulsatile tissue. Low perfusion caused by peripheral vasoconstriction, increased vascular resistance, low cardiac output, hypovolemia, or hypothermia can cause a loss of signal. Excessive ambient light, patient motion, carboxyhemoglobin, methemoglobin, dyes such as methylene blue, venous pulsations, low oxyhemoglobin states, or poor sensor positioning can also result in an inaccurate Spo$_2$ reading.*

### EXPLANATION:

(A) *Incorrect.* Patient motion may interfere with plethysmography, making it difficult for the pulse oximeter to isolate arterial pulsations and to correct for light absorption by nonpulsatile venous tissue.

(B) *Correct.* Isovolemic hemodilution to a Hct of 23%, as that found in patients with chronic anemia, will not reduce perfusion and should not affect the accuracy of pulse oximetry.

(C) *Incorrect.* An operating room light may provide excessive ambient light interfering with red and infrared light absorption.

(D) *Incorrect.* Methylene blue will produce a transient false drop in $Spo_2$.
(E) *Incorrect.* Impaired perfusion resulting from noninvasive oscillometric blood pressure (NIBP) cuff inflation, hypothermia, low cardiac output, Raynaud disease, hypovolemia, or an infusion of vasoactive drugs such as phenylephrine (an $\alpha_1$-adrenergic agonist that causes peripheral vasoconstriction) may result in falsely low or absent $Spo_2$ signals.

### REASONING:

Choices A,C, and D are clearly incorrect. The key to answering this question is knowing that a phenylephrine infusion may cause prolonged vasoconstriction that may decrease tissue perfusion leading to inaccurate $Spo_2$ readings. Choice B describes an isovolemic state with normal tissue perfusion, which will not affect the accuracy of $Spo_2$ readings.

### BIBLIOGRAPHY:

Dorsch J, Dorsch S. *Understanding Anesthesia Equipment.* 5th ed. Baltimore, MD: Lippincott Williams & Wilkins; 2007:775-795.
Morgan GE, Mikhail MS, Murray MJ. *Clinical Anesthesiology.* 4th ed. New York, NY: McGraw-Hill; 2006:140-141.

---

## BOOK B:      QUESTION 95

*Answer B*

Pharmacology

### QUESTION (Choose single best answer):

The use of droperidol as a preanesthetic medication has been associated with each of the following *except*

(A) Acute anxiety.
(B) Anterograde amnesia.
(C) Hypotension.
(D) Extrapyramidal signs.
(E) Catalepsy.

### CORRECT ANSWER: B

### SUMMARY:

*Droperidol is a derivative of haloperidol, which is the first butyrophenone, a class of drug designed to produce an "artificial hibernation" without circulatory or respiratory depression. It submaximally inhibits GABAA $\alpha_1$, $\beta_1$, and $\gamma_2$ acetylcholine receptors and fully inhibits $\alpha_2$ acetylcholine receptors in the CNS, therefore interfering with the dopamine, serotonin, norepinephrine system. This results in the sedative and antiemetic effects, in addition to side effects of hypotension, extrapyramidal symptoms, and catalepsy. Droperidol has also been reported to cause neuroleptic malignant syndrome. Recently, use of droperidol has decreased due to an FDA black-box warning linking the drug to prolonged QT intervals and resultant torsade de pointes ventricular dysrhythmias.*

### EXPLANATION:
(A) *Incorrect.* Used as a preanesthetic medication, droperidol may cause patients to appear sedate, but on further examination, they will admit to feeling dysphoric, restless, and may even refuse surgery.
(B) *Correct.* At usual doses droperidol does not cause unconsciousness, analgesia, or amnesia.

(C) *Incorrect.* Droperidol has α-adrenergic blocking effects that can cause hypotension. Droperidol is also contraindicated in patients with pheochromocytoma because it can cause release of catecholamines from the adrenal medulla, resulting in severe hypertension.

(D) *Incorrect.* Use of droperidol can cause extrapyramidal reactions such as oculogyric crisis, torticollis, and agitation due to antidopaminergic effects. These symptoms may be treated with diphenhydramine. Droperidol can also antagonize the effects of levodopa, and it should be avoided in patients with Parkinson disease.

(E) *Incorrect.* Droperidol can cause a cataleptic immobility manifested by a trance-like state with mobile but stiff extremities.

### REASONING:

This is a straightforward questions if the reader understands the pharmacology of droperidol. Knowing that droperidol is a butyrophenone, which is fluorinated derivatives of phenothiazines, the reader should be able to rule out choices A, D, and E that are known side effects of phenothiazines. Next, choice C, hypotension, is a known cardiovascular effect of droperidol, so it can also be eliminated. This leaves choice B, anterograde amnesia, which is not associated with droperidol.

### BIBLIOGRAPHY:

Miller, 7th Edition, pg 757-758.

Morgan GE, Mikhail MS, Murray MJ. *Clinical Anesthesiology.* 4th ed. New York, NY: McGraw-Hill; 2006:202-203.

---

| **BOOK B:** | **QUESTION 96** |
|---|---|

*Answer E*

Physiology

### QUESTION (Choose single best answer):

Each of the following changes is expected with deliberate hypothermia *except*

(A) Decreased unloading of oxygen from hemoglobin.
(B) A 5% decrease in MAC for each 1°C decrease in temperature.
(C) Increased arterial oxygen and carbon dioxide contents.
(D) A 50% decrease in cerebral metabolic rate at 28°C.
(E) Spike and dome EEG activity at temperatures below 30°C.

### CORRECT ANSWER: E

### SUMMARY:

*Hypothermia will shift the hemoglobin-oxygen dissociation curve to the left, increasing the affinity of hemoglobin for oxygen and making it less available to the tissues. Reduction of 1°C in temperature will result in about a 5% decrease in MAC and a 6% to 7% drop in CMRO$_2$. Hypothermia will increase the solubility of gases in blood so arterial oxygen and carbon dioxide will increase. Spike and dome EEG activity is related to specific epileptic states and not to hypothermia, which would tend to slow and then suppress brain waves.*

### EXPLANATION:

(A) *Incorrect.* With hypothermia, there is decreased unloading of oxygen to the tissues.

(B) *Incorrect.* There is a 5% decrease in MAC for each Celsius degree drop in temperature.

(C) *Incorrect.* The solubility of gases increases with hypothermia. However, while the content of dissolved $O_2$ ($Cao_2$) and $CO_2$ ($Cao_2$) in arterial blood will increase, their partial pressures, the $Po_2$ and $Pco_2$, will decrease. Arterial blood with a $Pco_2$ of 40 mm Hg and a pH of 7.4, when cooled to 25°C, will have a $Pco_2$ of 23 mm Hg and a pH of 7.60, but an unchanged $Caco_2$. Correction of the respiratory alkalosis in a hypothermic patient will result in severe acidosis upon rewarming.

(D) **Incorrect.** A temperature of 28°C (a 9°C reduction in normal body temperature) will result in an approximately 50% reduction in $CMRO_2$.

(E) **Correct.** Hypothermia is associated with EEG slowing, burst suppression and then an isoelectric pattern with the progressive suppression of neuronal activity.

## REASONING:

The key to answering this type of question is recognizing the single wrong answer; that is, that hypothermia is associated with EEG slowing, burst suppression, and isoelectric activity, not "spike and dome," an EEG pattern that is rarely, if ever, associated with the practice of anesthesiology.

## BIBLIOGRAPHY:

Miller. 7th edition, 2010, p 1507.

Morgan GE, Mikhail MS, Murray MJ. *Clinical Anesthesiology*. 4th ed. New York, NY: McGraw-Hill; 2006:148-150, 616-617, 623-624.

Schubert A. Symposium article: side effects of mild hypothermia. *J Neurosurg Anesthesiol.* 1995;7(2):141.

Sessler DI. Hypothermia, mild (core temperature 34-36°C). In: Roizen MF, Fleischer LA, eds. *Essence of Anesthesia Practice*. 2nd ed. Philadelphia, PA; WB Saunders; 2002:189.

---

| **BOOK B:** | **QUESTION 97** |
|---|---|

*Answer E*

Pharmacology

## QUESTION (Choose single best answer):

Each of the following drugs is a cause of central anticholinergic syndrome *except*

(A) Amitriptyline.
(B) Atropine.
(C) Diphenhydramine.
(D) Promethazine.
(E) Ranitidine.

## CORRECT ANSWER: E

## SUMMARY:

*Central anticholinergic syndrome (CAS) is referred to as CNS effects ranging from stupor and coma to anxiety, delirium, and seizures that occur with the administration of medications having antimuscarinic properties. These include antihistamines, tricyclic antidepressants, topical cycloplegic eyedrops, GI antispasmodics, synthetic opioids, and antipsychotics. The CNS effects are related to the degree to which these drugs cross the blood-brain barrier and antagonize brain muscarinic Ach receptors. While all of the medications listed in the question fall into the above classes, ranitidine only has weak penetration into the CNS and would be unlikely to cause CAS. The treatment is physostigmine, a lipid-soluble tertiary amine cholinesterase inhibitor.*

## EXPLANATION:

(A) **Incorrect.** Amitryptyline, a tricyclic antidepressant, works by blocking the reuptake of norepinephrine and serotonin. Among the tricyclics, amitriptyline has high antimuscarinic activity and tends to be the most sedating. It can also potentiate other centrally acting anticholinergic agents and contribute to postoperative delirium.

(B) *Incorrect.* CAS is also known as atropine toxicity. Atropine, a tertiary amine and belladonna alkaloid, readily crosses the blood brain barrier to cause mild postoperative memory loss at the usual dose, and delirium and CNS excitation at toxic doses.

(C) *Incorrect.* Diphenhydramine, an ethanolamine and $H_1$-receptor antagonist, readily crosses the blood-brain barrier. Its antimuscarinic and antiserotoninergic activity confers hypnotic and antiemetic properties.

(D) *Incorrect.* Promethazine, like diphenhydramine, diphendyrinate, and chlorpheniramine, is an $H_1$ blocker with sedative and antiemetic properties that has been implicated in CAS.

(E) *Correct.* While $H_2$ blockers such as cimetidine have been associated with lethargy, hallucinations, and seizures especially in elderly patients, ranitidine, famotidine, and nizatidine penetrate the blood-brain barrier poorly and have minimal CNS effects.

**REASONING:**

All of the medications listed in this question fall into classes of drugs that have antimuscarinic effects. However, choice E lists the only medication that does not have CNS effects because it does not cross the blood-brain barrier.

**BIBLIOGRAPHY:**

Barash PG, Cullen BF, Stoetling RK, Cahalan M, Stock M. *Clinical Anesthesia.* 6th ed. Philadelphia, PA: Lippincott-Raven Publishers; 2009:347-348, 348t.

Morgan GE, Mikhail MS, Murray MJ. *Clinical Anesthesiology.* 4th ed. New York, NY: McGraw-Hill; 2006:239-240, 276-279, 390, 655-657.

---

| **BOOK B:** | **QUESTION 98** |
| --- | --- |

## *Answer E*

### Pharmacology

**QUESTION (Choose single best answer):**

A 24-year-old woman requires anesthesia for emergency repair of open fractures of the tibia and fibula. She used cocaine 2 hours ago. Blood pressure is 170/110 mm Hg. Each of the following is useful in managing the hypertension *except*

(A) Hydralazine.
(B) Labetalol.
(C) Nitroprusside.
(D) Phentolamine.
(E) Propranolol.

**CORRECT ANSWER: E**

**SUMMARY:**

*Cocaine is an ester local anesthetic. It is unique among local anesthetics in that it inhibits the reuptake of norepinephrine in adrenergic nerve terminals and potentiates the effects of adrenergic stimulation. Norepinephrine is a potent agonist to $\alpha_1$ and $\alpha_2$ receptors and somewhat less of an agonist to $\beta_1$ receptors. The patient in this question is hypertensive. Both $\alpha$-blockade and $\beta$-blockade are necessary when treating cocaine-induced hypertension. Sole $\beta$-blockade therapy could result in lethal hypertension owing to unopposed $\alpha$-adrenergic tone. Cocaine-induced hypertension can be potentiated by other sympathomimetic agents such as epinephrine and phenylephrine, as well as by tricyclic antidepressants and monoamine oxidase inhibitors.*

**EXPLANATION:**

(A) **Incorrect.** Hydralazine is a direct-acting vasodilator that would decrease SVR. It would be useful in treating the hypertension.

(B) **Incorrect.** Labetalol blocks $\alpha_1$, $\beta_1$, and $\beta_2$ receptors at a ratio of 1:7 $\alpha$-to-$\beta$-blockade. Unlike hydralazine, labetalol lowers overall peripheral vascular resistance without reflex tachycardia because of its combined effect.

(C) **Incorrect.** Nitroprusside relaxes both arterial and venous smooth muscle. It primarily reduces preload. It could be used to treat the hypertension.

(D) **Incorrect.** Phentolamine lowers blood pressure by competitively blocking $\alpha$ receptors nonselectively. Reflex tachycardia and postural hypotension limit its utility in this patient.

(E) **Correct.** Propranolol is a nonselective $\beta$-blocker that lowers blood pressure by decreasing myocardial contractility and decreasing heart rate. This would lead to unopposed alpha effects and exacerbate this patient's hypertension. This drug should not be administered in the setting of cocaine-induced hypertension.

**REASONING:**

This question tests knowledge of the pathophysiology and treatment of acute cocaine intoxication. All the choices can be used to treat hypertension, but certain drugs should not be administered in the setting of acute cocaine intoxication. The high levels of circulating norepinephrine possess $\alpha$- and $\beta$-adrenergic agonist properties. Therapy should be directed at blocking both receptor sites. Choice D may lead to reflex tachycardia and postural hypotension. However, choice E is clearly the most incorrect choice because it will worsen the patient's malignant hypertension. The complications of pure $\beta$-blockade during acute cocaine intoxication are well known. E is the best answer.

**BIBLIOGRAPHY:**

Barash PG, Cullen BF, Stoelting RK, Cahalan M, Stock M. Clinical Anesthesia. 4th ed. Philadelphia, PA: Lippincott Williams & Wilkins; 2001:277 (Table 12-13), 975.

Morgan GE, Mikhail MS, Murray MJ. *Clinical Anesthesiology*. 3rd ed. New York, NY: McGraw-Hill; 2002:239, 591.

---

**BOOK B:**          **QUESTION 99**

---

*Answer B*

Clinical Anesthesia

**QUESTION (Choose single best answer):**

Carbon monoxide poisoning with a carboxyhemoglobin concentration of 20% is characterized by each of the following *except*

(A) Decreased oxygen-carrying capacity of hemoglobin.
(B) Decreased $PaO_2$.
(C) Shift of the oxyhemoglobin dissociation curve to the left.
(D) Normal minute volume of ventilation.
(E) Headache and nausea.

**CORRECT ANSWER: B**

**SUMMARY:**

*Carbon monoxide combines with hemoglobin to form carboxyhemoglobin, interfering with oxygen binding and resulting in a leftward shift in the oxyhemoglobin dissociation curve. Carbon monoxide poisoning occurs when carboxyhemoglobin concentrations exceed 15% in the blood. Levels approaching 20% or more cause altered mental status, headaches, nausea, vomiting, and eventually progress to coma and shock. Carboxyhemoglobin levels greater than 40% to 60% can be fatal. Carbon monoxide poisoning does not affect the arterial oxygen tension. Normal carboxyhemoglobin levels are 1.5% in nonsmokers and up to 15% in chronic smokers.*

**EXPLANATION:**

(A) *Incorrect.* Carbon monoxide has a 200-fold greater affinity for hemoglobin than oxygen. When carboxyhemoglobin is formed, it shifts the oxyhemoglobin dissociation curve leftward, reducing the oxyhemoglobin concentration and impairing the delivery and release of oxygen to tissues.

(B) *Correct.* The $Pao_2$ remains normal. It is important to note that the $Pao_2$ plays a relatively small contribution to the overall oxygen content of the blood given the oxygen content equation: $Cao_2 = (1.34 \times Hg \times O_2sat) + (0.003 \times Pao_2)$. Although the $Pao_2$ remains normal, carbon monoxide poisoning decreases the oxygen-hemoglobin saturation which markedly reduces the oxygen content of the blood.

(C) *Incorrect.* Carbon monoxide toxicity interferes with the unloading of oxygen at the tissues, shifting the oxyhemoglobin curve to the left.

(D) *Incorrect.* Carbon monoxide toxicity can occur without lung injury. The $Pao_2$ should be normal if lung injury has not occurred. The carotid bodies are sensitive to $Pao_2$, not to the $O_2$ content of the blood. $CO_2$ elimination and the ventilatory response to $Paco_2$ and $Pao_2$ remain unchanged. Minute ventilation should be normal in the absence of lung injury.

(E) *Incorrect.* Severity of carbon monoxide poisoning depends on the amount of carboxyhemoglobin present, the patient's tissue oxygen demands, and hemoglobin concentration. Mild carbon monoxide poisoning (15%-20%) results in headache, dizziness, and occasional confusion. Levels between 20% and 40% result in nausea, vomiting, and disorientation, whereas levels between 40% and 60% result in agitation, combativeness, and hallucinations that eventually progress to coma, shock, and death as levels reach 60% or greater.

**REASONING:**

This question tests knowledge of the pathophysiology of carbon monoxide poisoning. Choice D is somewhat correct. Carbon monoxide poisoning accompanied by lung injury will reduce the arterial oxygen tension and will result in tachypnea. However, we cannot assume that this patient has concurrent lung injury. B is the single best answer.

**BIBLIOGRAPHY:**

Barash PG, Cullen BF, Stoelting RK. *Clinical Anesthesia*. 5th ed. Philadelphia, PA: Lippincott Williams & Wilkins; 2006:1275 (Table 36-8).
Morgan GE, Mikhail MS, Murray MJ. *Clinical Anesthesiology*. 3rd ed. New York, NY: McGraw-Hill; 2002:801-802.

---

**BOOK B:**

*Answer E*

Pharmacology

**QUESTION 100**

**QUESTION (Choose single best answer):**

A 40-year-old woman receives alfentanil 75 µg/kg followed by an infusion of 1.5 µg/kg/min for a 1-hour cholecystectomy and cholangiogram. This regimen could be associated with each of the following *except*

(A) Muscle rigidity.
(B) Increased biliary tract pressure.
(C) Inadequate anesthesia.
(D) Postoperative respiratory depression.
(E) 2 to 4 hours of postoperative analgesia.

**SUMMARY:**

*Alfentanil is a synthetic opioid that is characterized by a very rapid onset and brief duration of action. Approximately 90% of the drug is in a lipid-soluble nonionized form at physiologic pH owing to a low $pK_a$ of 6.8. The typical loading dose of alfentanil is 8 to 100 $\mu g/kg$, with maintenance infusion rates of 0.5 to 3 $\mu g/kg/min$. Side effects of alfentanil are similar to those of other opioids and include nausea and vomiting, chest wall rigidity, respiratory depression, increased biliary pressure, and decreased peristalsis.*

**EXPLANATION:**

(A) *Incorrect.* All opioids potentially can cause muscle rigidity following rapid bolus administration. Chest wall rigidity occurs more commonly with alfentanil  sufentanil, and fentanyl.

(B) *Incorrect.* Opioids such as alfentanil can cause spasm of the sphincter of Oddi. This can produce a rise in biliary tract pressure and result in symptoms of biliary colic.

(C) *Incorrect.* Although opioids can produce intense analgesia and sedation, they do not reliably provide amnesia and can result in inadequate anesthesia when used alone. One also must assume that alfentanil is the sole anesthetic agent being administered to this patient.

(D) *Incorrect.* Opioids shift the $CO_2$ response curve to the right, resulting in higher resting $Paco_2$, decreased ventilatory response to $CO_2$, and higher apneic threshold. These effects can persist for up to 2 hours into the postoperative period. Opioid-induced respiratory depression is increased in the elderly and in combination with other sedatives.

(E) *Correct.* The context-sensitive half-time for alfentanil is approximately 60 minutes for infusions of up to 10 hours. The terminal half-life of alfentanil is 84 to 90 minutes.

**REASONING:**

This question tests knowledge of the unique pharmacology of alfentanil. Its rapid onset and minimal accumulation make it an ideal opioid for continuous intravenous infusion. Choices A through D are true for all opioids including alfentanil. However, it is not associated with significant postoperative analgesia after discontinuation, making choice E incorrect. E is the best answer.

**BIBLIOGRAPHY:**

Barash PG, Cullen BF, Stoelting RK, Cahalan M, Stock M. *Clinical Anesthesia*. 6th ed. Philadelphia, PA: Lippincott Williams & Wilkins; 2009:482-484, 491-492.

Morgan GE, Mikhail MS, Murray MJ. *Clinical Anesthesiology*. 4th ed. New York, NY: McGraw-Hill; 2006:192-197, 193 (Figure 8-6 Uses and doses of common opioids), 196 (Table 8-6).

Stoelting RK, Miller RD. *Basics of Anesthesia*. 5th ed. New York, NY: Churchill Livingstone; 2007;116, 119.

---

**BOOK B:**  **QUESTION 101**

---

*Answer B*

Neuroanesthesia

**QUESTION (Choose single best answer)**

Monitoring sensory evoked potentials may be useful in detecting functional derangement of each of the following *except*

(A) Cranial nerve pathways during posterior fossa operations.
(B) Motor pathways during anterior cervical diskectomy.
(C) Dorsal column pathways during operations for spinal tumors.
(D) Visual pathways during operations on the sphenoid wing.
(E) Cortical pathways during carotid artery operations.

## SUMMARY:

*Sensory evoked potential (SEP) monitoring is a noninvasive method to assess neurologic function. For example, an electric current is delivered to the tibial nerve. If the neural pathway is intact, an evoked potential will be transmitted to the contralateral sensory cortex. There are three types of SEPs in clinical use: somatosensory evoked potentials (SSEPs), visual evoked potentials (VEPs), and brain stem auditory evoked potentials (BAEPs). It is important to note that intact sensory evoked potentials do not ensure normal motor function.*

## EXPLANATION:

(A) *Incorrect.* Cranial nerves (eg, optic nerve) carry sensory information. These pathways are monitored by SEPs.

(B) *Correct.* SEPs evaluate dorsal spinal column pathways, whereas motor evoked potentials (MEPs) evaluate ventral spinal cord function. Because of this differing anatomy, normal SEPs do not ensure normal motor function.

(C) *Incorrect.* Dorsal column pathways carry sensory information. These pathways are monitored by SEPs.

(D) *Incorrect.* Visual pathways carry sensory information. These pathways are monitored by SEPs.

(E) *Incorrect.* Cortical pathways carry sensory information. These pathways are monitored by SEPs.

## REASONING:

SEPs are influenced by anesthetics and drugs in a dose-dependent fashion. SEPs are altered by hypothermia, volatile anesthetics, and multiple intravenous anesthetic agents, including benzodiazepines and barbiturates. The reader should review these pharmacologic effects on SEPs carefully. Of the SEPs listed above, BAEPs are the most resistant to anesthetics. Functional derangement is suggested by an increase in latency and a decrease in amplitude in the evoked potential. SEPs evaluate ascending sensory pathways, whereas MEPs are useful in assessing descending motor pathways. Choice B should stand out because it states "motor pathways." The others refer to sensory pathways. B is the single best answer.

## BIBLIOGRAPHY:

Barash PG, Cullen BF, Stoelting RK. *Clinical Anesthesia*. 5th ed. Philadelphia, PA: Lippincott Williams & Wilkins; 2006:760-763 (Table 27-8).

Morgan GE, Mikhail MS, Murray MJ. *Clinical Anesthesiology*. 3rd ed. New York, NY: McGraw-Hill; 2002:115-116.

---

**BOOK B:**      **QUESTION 102**

---

*Answer E*

OB/Regional

## QUESTION (Choose single best answer):

Which of the following drug is *least* likely to cross the placenta?

(A) Lidocaine.
(B) Meperidine.
(C) Midazolam.
(D) Thiopental.
(E) Vecuronium.

**CORRECT ANSWER: E**

**SUMMARY:**

*Assuming constant uterine artery blood flow, transfer of free drug (non–protein-bound) from the maternal to fetal circulation can be described by the Fick equation*

$$\frac{\Delta q}{\Delta t} = \frac{KA(C_m - C_f)}{X}$$

*where $\Delta q/\Delta t$ represents rate of transfer of the drug, A is the surface area of the membrane, $C_m$ is the maternal drug concentration, $C_f$ is the fetal drug concentration, X is the thickness of the membrane, and K is a diffusion constant determined by drug properties such as molecular weight, lipid solubility, degree of ionization, and spatial configuration. Because the surface area and membrane thickness of the placenta will remain constant, nonionized, lipid-soluble, non–protein-bound drugs will cross the placenta more readily. Examples of lipid-soluble agents that readily cross the placenta and enter the fetal circulation include thiopental, benzodiazepines, and opiates. Highly water-soluble agents such as muscle relaxants do not cross the placenta in significant amounts. This is why babies delivered by cesarean section from mothers who have been given muscle relaxants do not exhibit neuromuscular blockade.*

**EXPLANATION:**
(A) *Incorrect.* Lidocaine has little maternal protein binding and therefore crosses the placenta easily.
(B) *Incorrect.* Meperidine is a lipid-soluble opiate and has been shown to cross the placenta.
(C) *Incorrect.* Midazolam is a benzodiazepine, and all benzodiazepines are lipid-soluble and cross the placenta. Midazolam is water soluble at a pH of less than 6.0 but lipid soluble at a pH greater than 6.0. This allows it to readily cross the placenta at physiologic pH.
(D) *Incorrect.* Thiopental is not frequently used (propofol and etomidate are more common these days), but is highly lipid soluble and readily crosses the placenta, reaching fetal circulation within 30 seconds of an intravenous dose. Interestingly, the incidence of neonatal depression is minimal in babies whose mothers are given less than 4 mg/kg.
(E) *Correct.* Vecuronium is an NDMR. This class of drugs is highly water soluble, and therefore such drugs do not cross the placenta in significant amounts.

**REASONING:**

This question tests knowledge of the pharmacology of anesthetic drugs across the placenta. The first thing to note about this question is the format. It asks which drug is the *least* likely to cross the placenta. This means that there must be something very different about one of the drugs in the list. Keeping in mind that ionized, water-soluble, protein-bound drugs will not cross the placenta, one can eliminate midazolam, meperidine, and thiopental owing to their lipid solubility. Lidocaine can be eliminated because it has little protein binding. Alternatively, one can answer the question by knowing that the drug on the list that is the most water soluble, vecuronium, will cross the placenta the least. E is the best answer.

**BIBLIOGRAPHY:**
Bucklin B, Gambling DR, Wlody DJ. *A Practical Approach to Obstetric Anesthesia.* Philadelphia, PA: Lippincott Williams & Wilkins; 2009:17-24.
Chestnut DH, Polley LS, Lawrence CT, Wong CA. *Chestnut's Obstetric Anesthesia Principles and Practice.* 4th ed. St. Louis, MO: Mosby; 2009:63-68.

*Answer D*

Physiology

**QUESTION (K-type):**

Characteristics of a depolarizing neuromuscular block include

(1)  Tetanic fade at 50 Hz for 5 seconds.
(2)  Decreased train-of-four ratio.
(3)  Posttetanic facilitation.
(4)  Decreased twitch height.

**CORRECT ANSWER: D (4 only is correct.)**

**SUMMARY:**

*Depolarizing neuromuscular blockers such as succinylcholine bind to acetylcholine receptors and generate continuous muscle endplate depolarization. This prevents the reopening of perijunctional sodium channels, resulting in muscle relaxation. Phase 1 depolarizing neuromuscular blockade such as that elicited by the usual intubating doses of succinylcholine exhibits constant but decreased twitch height responses (ie, no fade) to train-of-four, tetanic, and double-burst peripheral nerve stimulation. Furthermore, post-tetanic potentiation is also absent in depolarizing blockade.*

**EXPLANATION:**
(1)  *Incorrect.* There would be a constant but reduced height evoked response to a 5-second 50-Hz tetanic stimulus in a depolarizing block.
(2)  *Incorrect.* The height of all four twitches in a train-of-four stimulus (0.2-millisecond 2-Hz twitches over 2 seconds) would be diminished but equal.
(3)  *Incorrect.* Post-tetanic potentiation or the ability of a tetanic stimulus to increase the height of a subsequent twitch response is characteristic of a nondepolarizing or phase 2 blockade only.
(4)  *Correct.* A typical depolarizing blockade would result in a decreased twitch height without fade.

**REASONING:**

This question is K-type. Answer C is clearly incorrect because post-tetanic facilitation is seen only in nondepolarizing or a phase 2 depolarizing block. (We should assume that this question refers to a phase 1 depolarizing block that is achieved with the usual doses of succinylcholine.) This rules out answers A, B, and E. Choice 2 is incorrect because the train-of-four ratio in a phase 1 depolarizing block would have a short twitch height but the same ratio from the first to the fourth twitch, leaving D as the only valid answer.

**BIBLIOGRAPHY:**
Barash PG, Cullen BF, Stoelting RK, Cahalan M, Stock M. *Clinical Anesthesia*. 6th ed. Philadelphia, PA: Lippincott Williams & Wilkins; 2009:504-505.
Morgan GE, Mikhail MS, Murray MJ. *Clinical Anesthesiology*. 4th ed. New York, NY: McGraw-Hill; 2006:208-215, 210t.

*Answer A*

OB/Regional

**QUESTION (K-type):**

Before awake nasal intubation in a patient who has been NPO, areas to be anesthetized are supplied by which of the following nerves?

(1)  Glossopharyngeal.
(2)  Superior laryngeal.
(3)  Recurrent laryngeal.
(4)  Hypoglossal.

**CORRECT ANSWER: A (1, 2, and 3 are correct.)**

**SUMMARY:**

*Anesthetizing the naso-, oro-, and hypopharynx and larynx will facilitate an awake nasal intubation. Branches of the trigeminal nerve provide sensation to the mucous membranes of the nose and anterior tongue. The glossopharyngeal nerve provides sensation to the back of the tongue, pharynx, tonsils, and soft palate. The vagus nerve, which branches into the superior laryngeal nerve and the recurrent laryngeal nerve, provides sensory innervation to the hypopharynx and larynx.*

**EXPLANATION:**

(1)  ***Correct.*** The glossopharyngeal nerve, cranial nerve (CN) IX, provides sensory innervation to the posterior third of the tongue with branches to the soft palate and oropharynx. This nerve may be blocked by the application of aerosolized lidocaine or by bilateral injection of local anesthetic at the base of the anterior tonsillar pillars.

(2)  ***Correct.*** The superior laryngeal nerve, which is a branch of the vagus nerve (CN X), provides sensory innervation to the lower pharynx and the larynx above the vocal cords. This nerve can be blocked in between the greater cornu of the hyoid bone and the superior cornu of the thyroid cartilage or by instillation of topical lidocaine by transtracheal injection through the cricothyroid ligament.

(3)  ***Correct.*** The recurrent laryngeal nerve, another branch of the vagus nerve, provides sensation to the vocal cords and the larynx.

(4)  ***Incorrect.*** The hypoglossal nerve (CN XII) is the motor nerve of the tongue and does not need to be anesthetized prior to an awake nasal intubation.

**REASONING:**

This question tests knowledge of the innervation of the larynx and nasopharynx. Recognizing that the hypoglossal nerve is purely a motor nerve rules out choice 4 and answers C, D, and E. Therefore, choices 1 and 3 must be correct. The superior laryngeal nerve typically is blocked in an awake nasal or oral fiberoptic intubation (FOI), so choice 2 also must also be correct. The best answer is A.

**BIBLIOGRAPHY:**

Barash PG, Cullen BF, Stoelting RK, Cahalan M, Stock M. *Clinical Anesthesia*. 6th ed. Philadelphia, PA: Lippincott Williams & Wilkins; 2010:775, 1317-1319.
Morgan GE, Mikhail MS, Murray MJ. *Clinical Anesthesiology*. 4th ed. New York, NY: McGraw-Hill; 2006:92-93 (Figure 5-3 Sensory nerve supply of the airway).

*Answer A*

Pain

**QUESTION (K-type):**

A 40-year-old patient is referred to a pain clinic for evaluation of right upper quadrant pain 6 months after cholecystectomy performed through a subcostal incision. Which of the following procedures would provide diagnostic information?

(1)  Intercostal nerve blocks.
(2)  Celiac plexus block.
(3)  Differential spinal block.
(4)  Lumbar sympathetic block.

**CORRECT ANSWER: A (1, 2, and 3 are correct.)**

**SUMMARY:**

*Intercostal nerve block inhibits nociceptive signals of somatic origin on the body wall but not visceral nociceptive signals. Celiac plexus blocks inhibit transmission of visceral nociceptive signals from all of the abdominal viscera but will not block somatic nociception. Differential spinal blockade helps distinguish between psychogenic, somatic, sympathetic, and central pain states. Thus, these three tests can be used to help determine the anatomic location and mechanism of the patient's pain. Lumbar sympathetic block is used for diagnosis and treatment of pain, and vascular insufficiency in the lower extremity.*

**EXPLANATION:**

Intercostal nerve blocks block the ventral rami of spinal nerves, resulting in a block of sensation from the abdominal wall. Therefore, if this block produced pain relief for the patient, a visceral origin of the pain would be excluded. Celiac plexus block will block sensation transmitted by the visceral afferents that run along with sympathetic efferent nerves through the celiac plexus. The celiac plexus block will block nociception from virtually all of the abdominal viscera except the left side of the colon and the pelvic viscera. Pain relief following a celiac plexus block would thus exclude a musculoskeletal cause of the pain. Differential spinal blockade (Winnies conventional technique) is predicated upon the differential sensitivity of nerve fibers to local anesthetic. Classically, four different intrathecal sequential injections were given.

1.  *Saline:* Pain relief suggests a placebo responder or psychogenic pain.
2.  *Procaine 0.25%:* Pain relief suggests a sympathetic mechanism to the pain (only preganglionic $\beta$ fibers blocked).
3.  *Procaine 0.5%:* Pain relief suggests a somatic origin or organic pain.
4.  *Procaine 5%:* Lack of pain relief suggests a CNS mechanism for the pain.

Thus, this could be used to provide further diagnostic information regarding this patient's pain. Lumbar sympathetic block inhibits the transmission of sympathetic efferent signals to the lower extremity and blocks visceral afferent information from the lower extremity. It would, therefore, have very little utility in the assessment of right upper quadrant pain.

**REASONING:**

Choices 1 and 2 (intercostal and celiac plexus block) more clearly provide diagnostic information than differential spinal blockade. However, once choices 1 and 2 are known to be correct, choice 3 must be correct and the only question remaining is whether choice 4 is correct. As outlined above choice 4 (lumbar sympathetic block) is used for lower extremity sympathetic block and is not likely to be useful. Therefore, the answer must be A—1, 2, 3 only.

BIBLIOGRAPHY:
Cousins MJ, Carr DB, Horlocker TT, Bridenbaugh PO. *Cousins & Bridenbaugh's Neural Blockade in Clinical Anesthesia and Pain Medicine.* 4th ed. Philadelphia, PA: Lippincott Williams & Wilkins; 2009:386-390, 617-620, 839-840, 1124-1131.
McMahon SB, Koltzenburg M. *Wall and Melzack's Textbook of Pain.* 5th ed. Philadelphia, PA: Churchill Livingstone; 2006:508.
Morgan GE, Mikhail MS, Murray MJ. *Clinical Anesthesiology.* 4th ed. New York, NY: McGraw-Hill; 2006:266 (Table 14-1), 387-388 (Table 18-8).

---

## BOOK B:

*Answer D*

Pain

## QUESTION 106

### QUESTION (K-type):

Compared with intermittent injections of intramuscular opioids for postoperative pain relief, patient-controlled analgesia is associated with

(1) A lower incidence of nausea and vomiting.
(2) An increased risk for ventilatory depression.
(3) A greater variability in opioid pharmacokinetics.
(4) A lower total opioid requirement.

### CORRECT ANSWER: D (4 only is correct.)

### SUMMARY:

*Patient-controlled analgesia (PCA) is associated with many advantages when compared with the IM route of opioid administration. PCA use is associated with a lower total opioid requirement, superior analgesia, less sleep disturbance, and less sedation and concomitant ventilatory depression. Intramuscular opioids are associated with marked variability in opioid pharmacokinetics.*

### EXPLANATION:

PCA has been associated with a lower total opioid requirement, and less variability in pharmacokinetics than intramuscular opioid administration. IM administration of opioids is characterized by significant variability in opioid pharmacokinetics. PCA by requiring patient activation of drug delivery is less likely to produce the sedation that results from unpredictable absorption of IM boluses. PCA does not reliably lower the incidence of nausea and vomiting.

### REASONING:

If you are going to remember one thing about PCA, it should be that their use results in less overall opioid consumption. Therefore, choice 4 is correct and you can eliminate answers A and B. The principal criticism of IM use of opioids has been the erratic absorption that often results. Therefore, choice 3 is incorrect and answer E is thereby eliminated. Now one needs only to decide if choice 2 is correct. PCA decreases the risk of ventilatory depression compared to IM administration of opioids. Therefore, answer C may be eliminated, leaving D as the correct answer.

### BIBLIOGRAPHY:

Miller RD, Eriksson LI, Fleisher LA, Wiener-Kronish JP, William YL. *Miller's Anesthesia.* 7th ed. Philadelphia, PA: Churchill Livingstone; 2010:2761-2762.
Morgan GE, Mikhail MS, Murray MJ. *Clinical Anesthesiology.* 4th ed. New York, NY: McGraw-Hill; 2006:396 (Table 18-14).
Palmer PP, Miller RD. Current and developing methods of patient-controlled analgesia. *Anesthesiol Clin.* 2010 Dec;28(4):587-599.

## Answer E

### Pharmacology

**QUESTION (K-type):**

Adverse reactions to protamine include

(1) Markedly increased pulmonary vascular resistance.
(2) Anaphylaxis.
(3) Decreased systemic vascular resistance.
(4) Noncardiogenic pulmonary edema.

**CORRECT ANSWER: E (All are correct.)**

**SUMMARY:**

*Protamine is a polycationic protein isolated from salmon sperm that is used to bind and neutralize heparin, a highly negatively charged polysaccharide. These heparin-protamine complexes are then cleared by the reticuloendothelial system. Adverse reactions to protamine include anaphylactic as well as anaphylactoid reactions, characterized by a decrease in systemic vascular resistance (SVR). Rapid administration of protamine has also been associated with the sudden onset of profound pulmonary hypertension and systemic hypotension. Noncardiogenic pulmonary edema is not characteristic of protamine administration.*

**EXPLANATION:**

(1) **Correct.** Markedly increased pulmonary vascular resistance (PVR), which occurs in approximately 1% of patients, is a sudden, devastating yet short-lived complication of protamine administration. The deposition of protamine-heparin complexes mediates pulmonary vasoconstriction through the release of thromboxane and C5a anaphylatoxin. This reaction is accompanied by an elevation in CVP and systemic hypotension. Protamine administered slowly, that is, up to 50 mg over 10 minutes, usually has minimal effects.

(2) **Correct.** Anaphylaxis may occur with protamine administration, especially in patients sensitized to protamine in previous cardiac catheterizations, cardiac surgeries, dialysis, NPH (neutral protamine Hagedorn) or protamine zinc insulin therapy. This reaction is characterized by increased airway pressures, cutaneous flushing, systemic hypotension, and decreased SVR.

(3) **Correct.** Decreased SVR may accompany an anaphylactic or pulmonary hypertensive response to protamine.

(4) **Correct.** Noncardiogenic pulmonary edema does not typically result from protamine administration.

**REASONING:**

Choices 1 and 2 are well-known complications of intravenously administered protamine. Choice 3 is associated with both of these complications. Choice 4 is a red herring. The answer is A.

**BIBLIOGRAPHY:**

Barash PG, Cullen BF, Stoetling RK, Cahalan M, Stock M. *Clinical Anesthesia*. 6th ed. Philadelphia, PA: Lippincott-Raven Publishers; 2009;1100.

Morgan GE, Mikhail MS, Murray MJ. *Clinical Anesthesiology*. 4th ed. New York, NY: McGraw-Hill; 2006:519.

*Answer B*

Physiology

**QUESTION (K-type):**

Causes of the hypoxemia that occurs in patients with advanced cirrhosis include

(1)  Decreased total lung capacity.
(2)  Decreased cardiac output.
(3)  Right-to-left pulmonary shunting.
(4)  Decreased 2,3-diphosphoglycerate concentration in erythrocytes.

**CORRECT ANSWER: B (1 and 3 are correct.)**

**SUMMARY:**

*Patients with hepatic cirrhosis are prone to hypoxemia for several reasons. Some of these reasons include (1) hypoventilation due to decreased lung volumes and increased intra-abdominal pressures from ascites, (2) right-to-left pulmonary shunts, (3) abnormalities from impaired hypoxic vasoconstriction, and (4) decreased pulmonary diffusing capacity from increased extracellular fluid. A rightward shift of the oxyhemoglobin dissociation curve due to increased 2,3-diphosphoglycerate (2,3-DPG) can also occur.*

**EXPLANATION:**

(1)  ***Correct.*** The presence of ascites in the abdomen causes mechanically induced restriction of the diaphragm, which reduces all lung volumes and all lung capacities. Furthermore, hepatic hydrothorax occurs in 4% to 10% of cirrhotic patients and can further worsen lung volumes. This can lead to hypoventilation, atelectasis, and hypoxemia.

(2)  ***Incorrect.*** End-stage liver disease is characterized by a hyperdynamic state that includes an increased cardiac output and low peripheral vascular resistance in the setting of normal heart rates and filling pressures.

(3)  ***Correct.*** Right-to-left shunting across the lungs is seen in advanced cirrhotics owing to portopulmonary-pulmonary communications, spider angiomas in the lungs, and the secretion of vasodilatory substances such as glucagons, vasoactive intestinal protein (VIP), and ferritin. These vasodilatory substances are thought to impair hypoxic vasoconstriction and contribute to ventilation-perfusion abnormalities.

(4)  ***Incorrect.*** Because of the propensity toward hypoxemia, advanced cirrhotics must compensate by unloading oxygen more readily than normal individuals. This is accomplished by a rightward shift in the oxyhemoglobin dissociation curve. Factors that cause a rightward shift in the oxyhemoglobin curve include acidosis, hyperthermia, and an increase in 2,3-DPG concentration.

**REASONING:**

This question tests knowledge of pulmonary physiology contributing to hypoxemia in the setting of hepatic failure. The reader should carefully review factors that contribute to hypoxemia in patients with hepatic cirrhosis. It is helpful to remember the physiologic mechanisms that help compensate for hypoxemia. A rightward shift of the oxyhemoglobin dissociation curve decreases the affinity of hemoglobin for oxygen. This facilitates unloading of oxygen from hemoglobin and the delivery of oxygen to end organs. A decrease in 2,3-DPG would cause a leftward shift of the oxyhemoglobin curve, so choice 4 is wrong. The best answer is B.

**BIBLIOGRAPHY:**
Barash PG, Cullen BF, Stoelting RK. *Clinical Anesthesia*. 4th ed. Philadelphia, PA: Lippincott Williams & Wilkins; 2001:1085-1087 (Table 39-5).
Barash PG, Cullen BF, Stoelting RK. *Clinical Anesthesia*. 5th ed. Philadelphia, PA: Lippincott Williams & Wilkins; 2006:1093.
Morgan GE, Mikhail MS, Murray MJ. *Clinical Anesthesiology*. 3rd ed. New York, NY: McGraw-Hill; 2002:502, 726-728, 945.

---

## BOOK B:  QUESTION 109

*Answer A*

Clinical Anesthesia

**QUESTION (K-type):**

In a patient who is breathing room air spontaneously at the conclusion of a nitrous oxide(70%)–opioid anesthetic, causes of hypoxemia include

(1)  Decreased functional residual capacity.
(2)  Dilution of alveolar oxygen by outpouring of nitrous oxide.
(3)  Opioid-induced respiratory depression.
(4)  Increased physiologic dead space.

**CORRECT ANSWER: A (1, 2, and 3 are correct.)**

**SUMMARY:**

*All patients undergoing general anesthesia are at risk for hypoxemia during emergence. The combined effects of residual potent inhalational anesthetic agent and opioid medications attenuate the ventilatory response to hypoxemia and hypercarbia. Restrictive changes in pulmonary function after surgery result in a decreased functional residual capacity (FRC). A decreased FRC can contribute to atelectasis and shunting that can lead to hypoxemia. Rapid elimination of nitrous oxide from the lungs at the end of surgery can dilute alveolar $O_2$ and $CO_2$, leading to diffusion hypoxia.*

**EXPLANATION:**

(1)  **Correct.** The most important predictor of the degree of restrictive lung physiology and postoperative pulmonary complications is the site of the surgical wound. All healthy patients when placed supine have a 10% to 15% reduction in FRC. Inducing general anesthesia consistently decreases this further by 5% to 10% for most operative sites other than thoracic or abdominal. Lower abdominal and thoracic operations decrease FRC by 30%, whereas nonlaparoscopic abdominal surgeries have the most profound effect, leading to a 40% to 50% decrease in FRC from preoperative levels.

(2)  **Correct.** At the end of a general anesthetic, significant hypoxemia can result from the rapid elimination of nitrous oxide, which can dilute oxygen and $CO_2$ in the alveoli. Administering 100% oxygen at the conclusion of a general anesthetic can easily prevent this diffusion hypoxia.

(3)  **Correct.** Opioid medications attenuate the ventilatory response to hypoxia and hypercarbia. The carbon dioxide–ventilatory response curve is shifted to the right. The typical opioid-induced ventilatory pattern is a decreased respiratory rate with increased tidal volumes.

(4)  **Incorrect.** Physiologic dead space is composed of anatomic and alveolar dead space. Anatomic dead space involves the parts of the respiratory tree that do not exchange gas; it includes the oropharynx and extends to the terminal and respiratory bronchioles. Factors that alter anatomic dead space are tracheal intubation, tracheostomy, the ventilator Y-piece, and excessive ventilator tubing. Alveolar dead space arises from areas of the lung that are ventilated but not perfused. Alveolar dead space would increase in any disease state that decreases the overall perfusion to the lungs. At the conclusion

of a general anesthetic, there is collapse of alveoli (atelectasis), resulting in increased shunting (perfused and unventilated alveoli). Dead space ventilation, however, is not increased.

## REASONING:

This question tests knowledge of the changes in respiratory physiology associated with surgery and anesthesia. The key phrase in this question is "spontaneously breathing room air at the conclusion of nitrous oxide (70%)–opioid anesthetic." We assume that the patient is supine. Decreased FRC is a well-known complication of surgery and anesthesia. Diffusion hypoxia also can occur during emergence and in the immediate postoperative period owing to rapid dilution of alveolar oxygen with nitrous oxide (diffusion hypoxia). Furthermore, at the conclusion of a general anesthesia, the reader should expect increased shunting (areas that are perfused but not ventilated), not increased dead space. The best answer is A.

## BIBLIOGRAPHY:

Barash PG, Cullen BF, Stoelting RK. *Clinical Anesthesia*. 5th ed. Philadelphia, PA: Lippincott Williams & Wilkins; 2006:799 (Table 28-4), 809-810.
Fink BR. Diffusion anoxia. *Anesthesiology*. 1955;6(4):511-519.
Morgan GE, Mikhail MS, Murray MJ. *Clinical Anesthesiology*. 3rd ed. New York, NY: McGraw-Hill; 2002:945, 133.

---

| BOOK B: | QUESTION 110 (OPTIONAL) |
|---|---|

## *Answer A*

### Clinical Anesthesia

### QUESTION (K-type):

Compared with an induction dose of midazolam, an induction dose of thiopental causes a greater decrease in

(1) Blood pressure.
(2) Cerebral blood flow (CBF).
(3) Cerebral metabolic rate.
(4) Cortical EEG activity.

### CORRECT ANSWER: A (1, 2, and 3 are correct.)

### SUMMARY:

*Midazolam and thiopental are both intravenous anesthetics useful for induction of anesthesia that exert their clinical CNS effects by interacting with GABA receptors. When used for induction, benzodiazepines produce minimal cardiovascular depression. Barbiturates reduce $CMRO_2$, cerebral blood flow (CBF), and intracranial pressure (ICP) to a greater extent than benzodiazepines. Thiopental can produce electrical silence on the EEG. Unlike midazolam, this effect is not apparent at typical induction doses.*

### EXPLANATION:

(1) **Correct.** Induction doses of thiopental can produce hypotension from peripheral vasodilation and tachycardia owing to vagolysis. Hypovolemic patients are more prone to the cardiovascular effects of this drug. In contrast, midazolam and other benzodiazepines have minimal effects on blood pressure.
(2) **Correct.** Benzodiazepines decrease CBF to a lesser extent than barbiturates. Barbiturates are potent cerebral vasoconstrictors and reduce CBF in a dose-dependent fashion.

(3) **Correct.** Midazolam has a ceiling on its effect on $CMRO_2$ corresponding to its EEG effect. Thiopental reduces $CMRO_2$ uniformly throughout the brain to a greater extent than midazolam.

(4) **Incorrect.** Thiopental can produce burst suppression on EEG, whereas midazolam is not able to produce similar EEG effects. However, this difference is not apparent at typical induction doses.

### REASONING:

This answer to this question is controversial because commonly used textbooks disagree. Barbiturates exert a greater effect on blood pressure, CBF, and $CMRO_2$ than benzodiazepines at typical induction doses. Choice 4 is also somewhat vague. At 3 mg/kg of thiopental, one probably would only see activation of the EEG, which also would be seen with midazolam. However, at 5 mg/kg, the biphasic EEG pattern of thiopental would be evident with EEG slowing, whereas midazolam still would show only EEG activation. If choice 4 were worded "dose-dependent cortical EEG inhibition," it would be correct. However, because of the vague wording, A is the best answer.

### BIBLIOGRAPHY:

Barash PG, Cullen BF, Stoelting RK, Cahalan M, Stock M. *Clinical Anesthesia.* 6th ed. Philadelphia, PA: Lippincott Williams & Wilkins; 2009:1515.

Morgan GE, Mikhail MS, Murray MJ. *Clinical Anesthesiology.* 4th ed. New York, NY: McGraw-Hill; 2006:187-189, 200 (Table 8-8 Summary of Nonvolatile Anesthetic Effects on Organ Systems), 620 (Table 25-1 Comparative Effects of Anesthetic Agents on Cerebral Physiology), 619-621.

Stoelting RK, Miller RD. *Basics of Anesthesia.* 5th ed. New York, NY: Churchill Livingstone; 2007:106.

---

## BOOK B:                QUESTION 111

*Answer E*

Equipment/Physics

### QUESTION (K-type):

The $F_{IO_2}$ achieved by nasal prongs with oxygen flowing at 8 L/min depends on

(1) Tidal volume.
(2) Respiratory frequency.
(3) Inspiratory flow rate.
(4) Volume of the nasopharynx.

### CORRECT ANSWER: E (All are correct.)

### SUMMARY:

*Two types of equipment can provide supplemental oxygen: low-flow (variable-performance) or high-flow (fixed-performance) equipment. Low-flow or variable-performance equipment includes nasal cannulas, nasal masks, nonreservoir oxygen masks, and reservoir masks. Fixed-performance equipment includes anesthesia bag/bag-mask valve systems, air entrainment venturi masks, and air entrainment nebulizers. Additionally, newer high-flow nasal cannula devices are available that have been shown to deliver equal or higher $F_{IO_2}$ than traditional mask devices. High-flow nasal cannula delivers $O_2$ at similar rates (10-40 L/min) through the nasopharynx and can produce a CPAP effect from the higher gas flow, further enhancing oxygen delivery. Fixed-performance delivery systems provide a consistent and predictable delivered $F_{IO_2}$ but require flow rates three to four times the patient's minute ventilation. Variable-performance equipment supplies oxygen at a lower flow, and these devices are appropriate for patients with stable breathing patterns.*

**EXPLANATION:**

(1) *Correct.* Inspired oxygen will be diluted by various amounts of entrained room air as ventilatory demand changes. Oxygen fills the nasopharynx during exhalation. However, during inspiration, both oxygen and air are drawn into the respiratory system. The fractional concentration of inspired oxygen therefore is lowered.

(2) *Correct.* With rapid respiration rates, inspired gas flows will exceed oxygen supply because nasal prongs deliver oxygen at fixed flows. The respiratory frequency affects the fractional concentration of inspired oxygen when nasal prongs are used.

(3) *Correct.* The $F_{IO_2}$ decreases with decreased oxygen flow rates.

(4) *Correct.* The nasopharynx acts as an oxygen reservoir when nasal prongs are used.

**REASONING:**

This question tests knowledge of anesthetic equipment and respiratory physiology. Low-flow oxygen delivery devices such as nasal prongs are used commonly in the perioperative care of surgical patients. The approximate values of delivered $F_{IO_2}$ for these devices should be reviewed by the reader. In patients with normal, stable breathing patterns, each L/min increase in oxygen delivered by nasal prongs increases the $F_{IO_2}$ by approximately 0.04. Therefore, nasal prongs can achieve an $F_{IO_2}$ of 0.24 to 0.44 (1-6 L/min), oxygen mask 0.40 to 0.60 (5-8 L/min), and a mask with reservoir bag 0.6 to 0.80 or more (6-10 L/min). All the options are correct, and E is the best answer.

**BIBLIOGRAPHY:**

Miller RD, Erikkson LI, Fleisher LA, et al. *Anesthesia*. 7th ed. New York, NY: Churchill Livingstone; 2010:2715.

Morgan GE, Mikhail MS, Murray MJ. *Clinical Anesthesiology*. 4th ed. New York, NY: McGraw-Hill; 2006:1024.

---

**BOOK B:** | **QUESTION 112**

---

*Answer C*

Pharmacology

**QUESTION (K-type):**

The administration of mannitol 1 g/kg over 15 minutes produces an acute increase in

(1) Serum potassium concentration.
(2) Central venous pressure.
(3) Systemic vascular resistance.
(4) Serum osmolality.

**CORRECT ANSWER: C (Traditionally 2 and 4 are correct; evidence suggests 1, 2, and 4 correct.)**

**SUMMARY:**

*Mannitol is an osmotic diuretic that typically is used in anesthesia for decreasing brain volume and ICP during neurosurgical procedures. It also increases renal blood flow and scavenges free radicals and has been used to provide putative renal protection during aortic cross-clamping. Acutely, mannitol increases the plasma osmolality, causing an extracellular shift of water resulting in intravascular volume expansion. Mannitol is believed to cause an increase in serum potassium at high dose levels (2 g/kg) although there have been several recent case reports indicating that clinically significant hyperkalemia may also occur at standard 1 g/kg levels.*

**EXPLANATION:**

(1) *Correct.* Traditionally, increased serum potassium levels were believed to occur only when higher doses such as 2 g/kg of mannitol are used. However, several recent published case reports suggest that even at standard doses of mannitol, clinically significant hyperkalemia can be observed.

(2) *Correct.* Mannitol administration is associated with an increase in intravascular volume. This will increase the central venous pressure (CVP). Increased intravascular volume can precipitate acute CHF in patients with limited cardiac reserve.

(3) *Incorrect.* A transient decrease in mean arterial pressure (MAP) after administration of mannitol owing to decreased systemic vascular resistance is not uncommon. The phenomenon has been studied in animal models, but the exact mechanism is unclear.

(4) *Correct.* Mannitol is a hypertonic solution. It will increase the serum osmolality.

**REASONING:**

This is a somewhat challenging question that tests knowledge of the acute effects of mannitol administration. Mannitol is an osmotic diuretic that should be administered slowly ($\geq$ 10 minutes) to prevent a transient increase in ICP in patients with intracranial hypertension. Caution also should be used in patients with impaired cardiac function because the increased preload associated with rapid mannitol administration can precipitate left ventricular failure and acute CHF. Mannitol can cause hyperkalemia at even standard 1 g/kg doses, though traditionally it was believed to only occur at higher doses. A decrease in potassium can be seen with repeated administration. The best answer is C.

**BIBLIOGRAPHY:**


Barash PG, Cullen BF, Stoelting RK. *Clinical Anesthesia*. 4th ed. Philadelphia, PA: Lippincott Williams & Wilkins; 2001:762.

Cote CJ, Greenhow DE, Marshall BE. The hypotensive response to rapid intravenous administration of hypertonic solutions in man and in the rabbit. *Anesthesiology*. 1979;50(1):30-35.

Flynn BC. Hyperkalemic cardiac arrest with hypertonic mannitol infusion: the strong ion difference revisited. *Anesth Analg*. 2007 Jan;104:225-226.

Hirota K, Hara T, Hosoi S, et al. Two cases of hyperkalemia after administration of hypertonic mannitol during craniotomy. *J Anesth*. 2005;19:75-77.

Manninen PH, Lam AM, Gelb AW, Brown SC. The effect of high dose mannitol on serum and urine electrolytes and osmolality in neurosurgical patients. *Can J Anaesth*. 1987;34(5):442-446.

Miller RD, Miller ED, Reves JG, et al. *Anesthesia*. 5th ed. New York, NY: Churchill Livingstone; 2000:686.

Morgan GE, Mikhail MS, Murray MJ. *Clinical Anesthesiology*. 3rd ed. New York, NY: McGraw-Hill; 2002:674.

Seto A, Murakami M, Fukuyama H, et al. Ventricular tachycardia caused by hyperkalemia after administration of hypertonic mannitol. *Anesthesiology*. 2000;93:1359-1361.

Stiff JL, Munch DF, Bromberger-Barnea B. Hypotension and respiratory distress caused by rapid infusion of mannitol or hypertonic saline. *Anesth Analg*. 1979;58(1):42-48.


---

**BOOK B:**         **QUESTION 113**

*Answer C*

Pediatrics

**QUESTION (K-type):**

Compared with a term infant, an infant born at 32 weeks' gestation who receives anesthesia at 2 months of age is at increased risk for

(1) Pulmonary oxygen toxicity.
(2) Postoperative apnea.
(3) Renal failure.
(4) Retrolental fibroplasia.

**SUMMARY:**

*Premature infants are at increased risk for retrolental fibroplasia and postoperative apnea. Anesthesiologists caring for infants younger than 44 weeks postconceptional age should attempt to maintain normal neonatal Pao$_2$ between 60 and 80 mm Hg intraoperatively to prevent retinopathy. Infants younger than 50 weeks postconceptional age are not good candidates for elective or outpatient surgery and should be admitted at least 12 hours postoperatively for apnea monitoring.*

**EXPLANATION:**

(1) *Incorrect.* High alveolar oxygen tensions for prolonged periods of time may generate oxygen-free radicals. Bronchopulmonary dysplasia is a chronic disorder that presents with pulmonary dysfunction in the first year of life.

(2) *Correct.* Premature infants are at increased risk for postoperative apnea up to 60 weeks of postconceptional age. Other risk factors for postoperative apnea include anemia (hematocrit < 30%), hypothermia, infection, and CNS disease.

(3) *Incorrect.* Prematurity alone is not a risk factor for renal failure.

(4) *Correct.* Retrolental fibroplasia, also known as *retinopathy of prematurity*, is a disease associated with hyperoxia in infants younger than 44 weeks postconceptional age. Normal Pao$_2$ in the neonate is between 60 and 80 mm Hg. Maintaining the Pao$_2$ at less than 140 mm Hg generally is considered safe.

**REASONING:**

This question highlights the special diseases particular to premature neonates: retrolental fibroplasia and apnea of prematurity. Choices 1 and 3 can be eliminated because oxygen toxicity and renal failure are not problems that are specific to premature neonates. The best answer is C.

**BIBLIOGRAPHY:**

Morgan GE, Mikhail MS, Murray MJ. *Clinical Anesthesiology.* 4th ed. New York, NY: McGraw-Hill; 2006:924, 939-940.

Stoelting RK, Miller RD. *Basics of Anesthesia.* 5th ed. New York, NY: Churchill Livingstone; 2007:507-508.

---

**BOOK B:**      **QUESTION 114**

---

*Answer A*

OB/Regional

**QUESTION (K-type):**

Advantages of performing spinal anesthesia via the lateral approach include

(1) Larger opening for needle insertion than for the midline approach.

(2) Avoidance of the calcified interspinous ligament in the elderly.

(3) Less flexion of the spine required than for the midline approach.

(4) Less likelihood of peridural vein puncture than for the midline approach.

**CORRECT ANSWER: A (1, 2, and 3 are correct.)**

**SUMMARY:**

*Spinal anesthesia may be performed by the midline or lateral paramedian approach. The midline technique is done in the sitting or lateral position and is facilitated by the patient flexing his or her back. The spinous processes are palpated, and the needle is placed in the middle of the interspinous space. As the needle is advanced, the layers encountered are skin, subcutaneous tissue, supraspinous ligament, interspinous ligament, ligamentum flavum, epidural space, dura, and finally the subarachnoid space. The paramedian approach is helpful in patients who have calcified ligaments or may be uncooperative with flexion of the spine. Owing to the sharp angle of the thoracic spinous processes, the paramedian technique may be useful when performing a thoracic epidural. The needle is inserted 1 cm lateral to the lower border of the desired interspace and angled 45 degrees cephalad and approximately 15 degrees medial. In contrast to the midline approach, the first significant resistance encountered is ligamentum flavum. It is also important to note that the incidence of venous puncture is higher with the paramedian approach because veins travel anterior and lateral in the epidural space.*

**EXPLANATION:**
(1) *Correct.* The opening into the spinal canal is larger laterally rather than via the midline approach.
(2) *Correct.* Elderly patients often have calcified interspinous ligaments that can make the midline approach difficult.
(3) *Correct.* Flexion of the spine facilitates the midline approach by making the intervertebral spaces larger and has limited effect when one uses the paramedian approach.
(4) *Incorrect.* The epidural and spinal veins traverse laterally in the spinal canal and therefore are more likely to be punctured with the lateral paramedian approach.

**REASONING:**

This question tests knowledge of vertebral anatomy. The paramedian technique is used by many practitioners when the interspinous ligaments are calcified or the patient is uncooperative or unable to flex the spine to facilitate the midline technique. Choices 1, 2, and 3 are all advantages of the technique. Choice 4 can be eliminated because the veins are located laterally in the spinal column. A is the correct answer.

**BIBLIOGRAPHY:**
Barash PG, Cullen BF, Stoelting RK, Cahalan M, Stock M. *Clinical Anesthesia.* 6th ed. Philadelphia, PA: Lippincott Williams & Wilkins; 2010:932-935.
Morgan GE, Mikhail MS, Murray MJ. *Clinical Anesthesiology.* 4th ed. New York, NY: McGraw-Hill; 2006:301-305.

---

**BOOK B:**  **QUESTION 115**

---

*Answer B*

Pain

**QUESTION (K-type):**

In meralgia paresthetica

(1) There is pain in the anterolateral aspect of the thigh.
(2) The obturator nerve is involved.
(3) Obesity is an associated factor.
(4) Neurolytic alcohol block is the treatment of choice.

**CORRECT ANSWER: B (1 and 3 are correct.)**

**SUMMARY:**

*Meralgia paresthetica is an entrapment neuropathy involving the lateral femoral cutaneous nerve. The site of entrapment is the anterior iliac spine under the inguinal ligament. There is usually pain, paresthesias, or numbness in the anterolateral thigh distal to this site. Meralgia paresthetica can be diagnosed with nerve conduction studies, electromyography, or by blockade of this nerve with local anesthetics, which also provides temporary pain relief. The treatment of choice is symptomatic with NSAIDs or corticosteroid injections. Intractable symptoms may require surgery.*

**EXPLANATION:**

(1) **Correct.** The lateral femoral cutaneous nerve provides sensation to the anterolateral thigh and meralgia paresthetica typically involves pain in this area.

(2) **Incorrect.** Entrapment of the obturator nerve usually occurs in the obturator canal, which results in pain in the upper medial thigh.

(3) **Correct.** Obesity increases the likelihood of nerve entrapment and is an associated factor.

(4) **Incorrect.** Neurolytic alcohol blocks cause temporary nonselective destruction of nerve fibers and ganglia. They are used as treatments of last resort for severe intractable cancer pain. NSAIDs and rest are the treatments of choice in meralgia paresthetica.

**REASONING:**

This question is K-type. Choice 2 is obviously incorrect because this syndrome involves the lateral femoral cutaneous nerve. This rules out answers A, C, and E. Because choice 1 is correct, D is incorrect and B is the only possible answer.

**BIBLIOGRAPHY:**

Morgan GE, Mikhail MS, Murray MJ. *Clinical Anesthesiology.* 4th ed. New York, NY: McGraw-Hill; 2006:346-348, 388-389, 400-401.

---

| **BOOK B:** | **QUESTION 116** |
|---|---|

*Answer E*

Neuroanesthesia

**QUESTION (K-type):**

In patients undergoing transsphenoidal hypophysectomy for acromegaly, anesthesia is complicated by

(1) Decreased subglottic diameter.
(2) Temporomandibular joint dysfunction.
(3) Glucose intolerance.
(4) Diabetes insipidus.

**CORRECT ANSWER: E (All are correct.)**

**SUMMARY:**

*Acromegaly is an endocrine disorder that involves oversecretion of growth hormone. Though it has an overall population prevalence of 50 to 70 cases per million with an annual incidence rate of only three to four cases per million people, the incidence may in fact be double in areas of better surveillance . It is a multisystem disease that affects the viscera, skeletal muscles, and soft and connective tissues. Diabetes, hypertension, heart disease, and sleep apnea are physical manifestations of acromegaly that are particularly concerning to the anesthesiologist. A difficult airway should be anticipated in patients with acromegaly. Enlargement of the tongue and epiglottis, as well as the increased length of the mandible, predisposes to difficult upper airway management and endotracheal intubation. Moreover, the recurrent laryngeal nerve may be paralyzed because of excessive stretching caused by overgrowth of cartilaginous structures. A decrease in subglottic diameter also should be anticipated if the patient complains of dyspnea on exertion. Excessive growth hormone affects carbohydrate metabolism and may lead to glucose intolerance. Because of connective tissue overgrowth, these patients also may have temporomandibular joint dysfunction. An important complication of transsphenoidal hypophysectomy is increased risk of pituitary hypofunction. Immediate postoperative diabetes insipidus (DI) occurs in about 20% of patients and is strongly associated with intra-operative CSF leak, but it is usually transient; only 10% of patients with postoperative DI require persistent desmopressin treatment.*

## EXPLANATION:

(1) **Correct.** Stridor on examination is suggestive of tissue overgrowth in the subglottic region.

(2) **Correct.** Acromegaly causes an overgrowth of connective tissue that would affect all joints, including the temporomandibular joint.

(3) **Correct.** Alteration in carbohydrate metabolism caused by excessive growth hormone may predispose these patients to develop diabetes mellitus. Insulin therapy may be required in severe cases.

(4) **Correct.** While not a complication of acromegaly, DI may develop as a complication of the surgical procedure. DI typically is seen during the first 12 hours postoperatively and lasts for 2 to 4 days. It is characterized by polyuria (2-15 L/d), hyponatremia, and decreased urine osmolality and specific gravity.

## REASONING:

This question tests knowledge of the anesthetic complications associated with acromegaly. It is a multisystemic disease that can manifest all the findings presented in choices 1, 2, and 3. DI is a complication associated with the surgical procedure, transsphenoidal hypophysectomy. All the choices are correct, and the best answer is E.

## BIBLIOGRAPHY:


Barash PG, Cullen BF, Stoelting RK. *Clinical Anesthesia.* 4th ed. Philadelphia, PA: Lippincott Williams & Wilkins; 2001;769.

Nemergut EC, Zuo Z, Jane JA Jr, Laws ER Jr. Predictors of diabetes insipidus after transsphenoidal surgery: a review of 881 patients. *J Neurosurg.* 2005 Sep;103(3): 448-454.

Daly AF, Rixhon M, Adam C, Dempegioti A, Tichomirowa MA, Beckers A. High prevalence of pituitary adenomas: a cross-sectional study in the province of Liege, Belgium. *J Clin Endocrinol Metab.* 2006;91:4769-4775.

Fernandez A, Karavitaki N, Wass JA. Prevalence of pituitary adenomas: a community-based, cross-sectional study in Banbury (Oxfordshire, UK). *Clin Endocrinol.* 2010;72: 377-382.

Melmed S. Acromegaly. *N Engl J Med.* 1990;322(14):966-977.

Morgan GE, Mikhail MS, Murray MJ. *Clinical Anesthesiology.* 3rd ed. New York, NY: McGraw-Hill; 2002:581.

Seidman PA, Kofke WA, Policare R, Young M. Anaesthetic complications of acromegaly. *Br J Anaesth.* 2000;84(2):179-182.

Stoelting R, Dierdorf S. *Anesthesia and Co-existing Disease.* 4th ed. New York, NY: Churchill Livingstone; 2002:437-438.

*Answer B*

Pediatrics

**QUESTION (K-type):**

In which of the following ways does the infant airway differ from that of the adult?

(1)  The larynx is more cephalad.
(2)  The vocal cords are perpendicular to the plane of the trachea.
(3)  The cricoid cartilage is the narrowest part of the airway.
(4)  The larynx is more anterior.

**CORRECT ANSWER: B (1 and 3 correct.)**

**SUMMARY:**

*Several features differentiate the infant airway from the adult airway and may contribute to difficult tracheal intubation: a more cephalad larynx, a long and stiff epiglottis, a short trachea and neck, and a proportionately larger head and tongue. The larynx in infants actually is not anterior compared with adults, contrary to common perception.*

**EXPLANATION:**

(1)  *Correct.* The larynx is found at the level of C4 in infants and C6 in adults.
(2)  *Incorrect.* In the adult larynx, the vocal cords are more perpendicular to the tracheal plane. The vocal cords in infants are angled in relation to the tracheal plane.
(3)  *Correct.* The narrowest portion of the infant airway is the cricoid ring.
(4)  *Incorrect.* The larynx is more cephalad but not more anterior in infants compared with adults. Sometimes overextension of the infant head can displace the larynx anteriorly during endotracheal intubation.

**REASONING:**

This commonly tested question asks for comparisons between pediatric and adult airways. This may be a controversial question owing to choice 4 because textbooks disagree on this point. However, choice 2 is definitely not correct, making B the best answer.

**BIBLIOGRAPHY:**

Barash PG, Cullen BF, Stoelting RK. *Clinical Anesthesia*. 6th ed. Philadelphia, PA: Lippincott Williams & Wilkins; 2009:1177-1178 (Figures 44-7 and 44-8).
Cote CJ. *A Practice of Anesthesia for Infants and Children*. 4th ed. Philadelphia, PA: Saunders; 2009:237.
Gregory GA. *Pediatric Anesthesia*. 4th ed. New York, NY: Churchill Livingstone; 2002:224.
Morgan GE, Mikhail MS, Murray MJ. *Clinical Anesthesiology*. 4th ed. New York, NY: McGraw-Hill; 2006:923-924, 925 (Table 44-1 Sagittal Section of Adult and Infant Airway).



*Answer D*

OB/Regional

**QUESTION (K-type):**

The duration of an epidural block can be increased clinically by

(1)  Use of a local anesthetic with low protein binding.
(2)  Use of a local anesthetic with a low $pK_a$.
(3)  Addition of sodium bicarbonate to the local anesthetic.
(4)  Increasing the total dose of the local anesthetic.

**CORRECT ANSWER: D (4 only is correct.)**

### SUMMARY:

*The duration of epidural or spinal anesthesia depends on the properties of the local anesthetic used and the total drug concentration administered. Drugs that have high protein binding such as etidocaine and bupivacaine have a longer duration than those with less protein binding such as lidocaine. The addition of sodium bicarbonate to lidocaine can hasten onset by increasing the pH of the solution (depending on the $pK_a$ of the local anesthetic), whereas adding epinephrine to a local anesthetic increases the duration by causing local vasoconstriction and decreased tissue uptake; however, epinephrine effect on concentrated forms of bupivacaine or ropivacaine is limited, probably because the local anesthetic duration is longer than the duration of the epinephrine.*

### EXPLANATION:

(A) *Incorrect.* Local anesthetics with high protein binding will have longer duration.

(B) *Incorrect.* All local anesthetics are weak bases and have $pK_a$ values greater than physiologic pH. Those with comparably lower pH have a faster onset owing to a higher concentration of drug in the nonionized form, but this property does not correlate with duration, solely onset.

(C) *Incorrect.* The addition of sodium bicarbonate to local anesthetic increases the pH of the solution. This increases the nonionized free-base form of local anesthetics, which hastens the onset of the drug but does not prolong the duration.

(D) *Correct.* Higher total doses of local anesthetic correlate with prolonged duration. However, one must take into consideration other properties of the agent used and determine the toxic dose prior to attempting to increase the duration of an epidural based on total dose alone.

### REASONING:

This question tests knowledge of the pharmacokinetics of local anesthetics. It is common practice to add sodium bicarbonate to a local anesthetic solution to hasten onset of analgesia. However, this does not increase the duration of action. Other additives such as epinephrine are added for this purpose. This eliminates choice 3, and thus choice 1 can be eliminated as well, even if the reader is unsure of the relationship between protein binding and duration. Choice 2 is incorrect because the $pK_a$ relates to *onset* rather than duration. Thus D the best answer.

### BIBLIOGRAPHY:


Barash PG, Cullen BF, Stoelting RK, Cahalan M, Stock M. *Clinical Anesthesia*. 6th ed. Philadelphia, PA: Lippincott Williams & Wilkins; 2010:943-944 (Table 37.5 Local Anesthetics Used for Surgical Blocks).

Morgan GE, Mikhail MS, Murray MJ. *Clinical Anesthesiology*. 4th ed. New York, NY: McGraw-Hill; 2006:313-314.


---

## BOOK B:                    QUESTION 119

*Answer D*

OB/Regional

### QUESTION (K-type):

Prior to vaginal delivery at term, a primiparous woman receives epidural anesthesia administered through a catheter inserted at L2-3. The following day she has left footdrop and sensory loss over the left outer calf. Causes of these complications include

(1)  Compression of the obturator nerve by excessive thigh flexion.
(2)  Compression of the lumbosacral trunk by the fetal head.
(3)  Nerve root injury by the epidural needle.
(4)  Compression of the common peroneal nerve by the stirrup.

**CORRECT ANSWER: C (2 and 4 are correct.)**

### SUMMARY:

*Peripartum nerve injuries can occur after vaginal delivery with or without neuraxial analgesia. It is important to distinguish peripheral from central nerve injuries by recognizing the distribution of lower extremity peripheral nerves and dermatomes of the lumbar and sacral nerve roots. Examples of nerve distributions are obturator—medial upper thigh, lateral femoral cutaneous—lateral upper thigh; saphenous—medial lower leg; and common peroneal— lateral lower leg and medial foot. The inguinal region corresponds to the L1 dermatome, whereas L4 is the knee and L5 is the lateral lower leg and medial foot. Epidural anesthesia can contribute to peripheral nerve injuries by allowing a patient to tolerate a position that compromises the nerve and otherwise would be painful. Examples include femoral neuropathy from prolonged extreme lithotomy position during the second stage of labor or common peroneal neuropathy from excessive pressure on the lateral lower leg owing to stirrups.*

### EXPLANATION:

(1)  **Incorrect.** Obturator nerve injury would cause sensory loss over the medial upper leg.

(2)  **Correct.** Compression of the lumbosacral trunk by the fetal head should result in sensory loss over the inguinal region, upper thigh, knee, and medial foot. However, in theory, selective compression of lumbosacral branches could result in foot drop and sensory loss selective to the lateral calf as the only presenting symptoms.

(3)  **Incorrect.** The epidural was placed at L2-3. If a nerve root is injured at this level, the sensory loss would occur over the upper thigh.

(4)  **Correct.** The foot drop and distribution of the sensory loss correspond with the common peroneal nerve, which can be compressed by stirrups. It is important to note that this also can happen to patients placed in the lithotomy position in the operating room, and the reader must monitor carefully for compression over this nerve.

### REASONING:

The key to correctly answering this question is knowledge of the dermatomal distribution of the nerve roots and the sensory distribution of the peripheral nerves in the leg. These should be reviewed carefully by the reader. The only possible answers that correspond to the correct anatomic position are choices 2 and 4, making the correct answer C.

### BIBLIOGRAPHY:

Miller RD, Eriksson LI, Fleisher LA, Wiener-Kronish JP, Young WL. *Miller's Anesthesia.* 7th ed. Philadelphia, PA: Churchill Livingstone; 2010:1649-1658.

Morgan GE, Mikhail MS, Murray MJ. *Clinical Anesthesiology.* 4th ed. New York, NY: McGraw-Hill; 2006:344.

---

**BOOK B:**      **QUESTION 120**

---

*Answer D*

Pediatrics

### QUESTION (K-type):

A 2-year-old boy with tetralogy of Fallot is scheduled for repair of bilateral inguinal hernias. True statements concerning this child include the following:

(1)  Oxygen saturation will improve with crying.
(2)  Cyanosis will increase with use of halothane.
(3)  Resistance to pulmonary outflow will be fixed.
(4)  An increased red cell mass will compensate for right-to-left shunt.

**CORRECT ANSWER: D (4 only is correct.)**

**SUMMARY:**
Tetralogy of Fallot is composed of a ventricular septal defect, overriding aorta, right ventricular outflow tract (RVOT) obstruction, and right ventricular hypertrophy. It is the most common congenital cardiac anomaly that results in right-to-left shunting and cyanosis. RVOT obstruction is dynamic and increases with sympathetic stimulation. The management of patients with uncorrected tetralogy of Fallot should include maintenance of intravascular volume and hematocrit and avoidance of low SVR and high PVR.

**EXPLANATION:**
(1) *Incorrect.* Crying actually can trigger hypercyanotic episodes or "tet spells." Infundibular spasm increases the magnitude of right-to-left shunting and worsens cyanosis.
(2) *Incorrect.* Volatile anesthetics are indicated in anesthetizing children with tetralogy of Fallot because they relax RVOT dynamic obstruction by decreasing myocardial contractility. It is true that decreased SVR can lead to an increase in right-to-left shunting. However, halothane has very little impact on SVR and can be administered safely to these children.
(3) *Incorrect.* In most patients, RVOT obstruction is due to hypertrophy of infundibular muscle. The resistance to pulmonary outflow is dynamic and can be increased by sympathetic tone.
(4) *Correct.* Patients with tetralogy of Fallot tend to have higher hematocrits to compensate for their chronic right-to-left shunt.

**REASONING:**
This question tests knowledge of the pathophysiology and anesthetic management of tetralogy of Fallot. A similar question is virtually guaranteed to be asked on the reader's board examination. Fortunately, this question is fairly straightforward. It is important to understand that the management of patients with right-to-left shunts always depends on balancing PVR and SVR. The best answer is D.

**BIBLIOGRAPHY:**
Morgan GE, Mikhail MS, Murray MJ. *Clinical Anesthesiology.* 4th ed. New York, NY: McGraw-Hill; 2006:482
Stoelting RK, Miller RD. *Basics of Anesthesia.* 5th ed. New York, NY: Churchill Livingstone; 2007:399-400 (Table 26-5).

---

**BOOK B:**  **QUESTION 121**

*Answer D*

Neuroanesthesia
Clipping: Anesthetic
Management

**QUESTION (K-type):**

A previously healthy 28-year-old woman who had a subarachnoid hemorrhage 2 days ago is scheduled for a craniotomy and clipping of an anterior communicating artery aneurysm. She is awake, oriented, and neurologically intact. True statements concerning anesthetic management include the following:

(1) The arterial pressure should be maintained above the preoperative values during induction.
(2) Hyperventilation to a $Paco_2$ of 25 to 30 mm Hg should be initiated prior to endotracheal intubation.
(3) Mannitol should be given immediately following induction.
(4) The mean arterial pressure (MAP) should be decreased to 50 mm Hg if necessary for surgical exposure.

**CORRECT ANSWER: D (4 only is correct.)**

**SUMMARY:**

*Appropriate anesthetic management of a patient undergoing cerebral aneurysm clipping includes avoiding increases in transmural pressure that can lead to aneurysm rupture, maintaining cerebral perfusion pressure and facilitating surgical exposure. Transmural pressure is defined as MAP − ICP. Increases in MAP during induction or decreases in ICP prior to opening of the dura can lead to aneurysm rupture. Hyperventilation may dramatically decrease ICP and compromise CBF and should be avoided especially in patients with vasospasm. Any technique that permits proper control of MAP is acceptable. In the face of increased ICP or a tight surgical field, an inhaled agent technique may be less suitable. The prevention of paroxysmal hypertension is the only absolute requirement in patients undergoing aneurysm clipping.*

**EXPLANATION:**

(1) *Incorrect.* MAP should be maintained at or below preoperative values during induction. Hypertension during induction will increase transmural pressure and potentially cause aneurysm rupture.

(2) *Incorrect.* Hyperventilation prior to intubation may increase the risk of aneurysm rupture by reducing ICP and increasing transmural pressure.

(3) *Incorrect.* Mannitol is often given intraoperatively to facilitate exposure and reduce tissue trauma after the dura is opened and not immediately after induction. An osmotic diuretic given immediately following induction offers no advantage and may worsen dehydration in patients following a subarachnoid hemorrhage (SAH).

(4) *Correct.* This otherwise healthy patient should tolerate MAPs as low as 50 mm Hg without complications making rupture less likely and facilitating clipping.

**REASONING:**

Goals during induction include avoiding sudden increases in MAP and decreases in ICP. Hyperventilation, osmotic diuresis, and deliberate hypotension are all techniques used to facilitate surgical exposure once the dura is open. Controlled hypotension may be used to facilitate exposure during surgical dissection as long as the benefit outweighs the risk. Patients with cardiovascular disease, renal insufficiency, or other end-organ disease may not be good candidates for controlled hypotension.

**BIBLIOGRAPHY:**

Barash PG, Cullen BF, Stoelting RK, Cahalan M, Stock M. *Clinical Anesthesia*. 6th ed. Philadelphia, PA: Lippincott Williams & Wilkins; 2010:728.

Morgan GE, Mikhail MS, Murray MJ. *Clinical Anesthesiology*. 4th ed. New York, NY: McGraw-Hill; 2006:578-579.

*Answer E*

Clinical Anesthesia

**QUESTION (K-type):**

A 45-year-old man is scheduled for elective antrectomy and vagotomy. He has drunk six packs of beer daily for 20 years. Laboratory evaluation shows the following findings:

|  | **Patient** | **Normal** |
|---|---|---|
| AST (SGOT) (U/L) | 75 | 0-45 |
| ALT (SGPT) (U/L) | 56 | 0-45 |
| LDH (U/L) | 300 | 50-250 |
| Alkaline phosphatase (U/L) | 120 | 25-115 |
| Bilirubin (mg/dL) | 1.2 | 0.1-1.2 |

Based on these laboratory findings, anticipated problems in anesthetic management include

(1)  Increased risk for halothane hepatotoxicity.
(2)  Coagulation disorders.
(3)  Large peripheral arteriovenous shunts.
(4)  Increased anesthetic requirements.

**CORRECT ANSWER: E (All are correct.)**

**SUMMARY:**

*In alcoholic hepatitis, the aspartate aminotransferase (AST) is usually higher than the alanine aminotransferase (ALT), usually by a factor of 2, partly because of depletion of pyridoxine (vitamin $B_6$). An AST lower than the ALT may suggest viral hepatitis. The patient has had long-standing alcohol abuse resulting in transaminitis, and the assumption of decreased synthetic function of the liver should be made. Patients with cirrhosis and portal hypertension develop arteriovenous collaterals in the splanchnic organs, skin, and lungs. A possible coagulopathy secondary to decreased liver synthetic function should be considered in this patient. Chronic alcohol consumption generally increases a patient's inhalational/intravenous anesthetic requirement whereas acute alcoholic intoxication will decrease the anesthetic requirements.*

**EXPLANATION:**

(1)  ***Correct.*** Halothane-induced hepatotoxicity is a well-known clinically entity, resulting in part form general cardiorespiratory depression as well as from decreased hepatic arterial flow caused by halothane. The resulting hepatic hypoxia is especially harmful to a cirrhotic liver with venous congestion. In addition, a hypermetabolic effect on the liver causes a marked increase in hepatic oxygen consumption, thus predisposing the liver to relative hypoxia at the microvascular level.
(2)  ***Correct.*** Prothrombin time (PT) is the best indicator of hepatic synthetic dysfunction. An INR (international normalized ratio) of 1.5 or greater after administration of vitamin K suggests severe hepatic synthetic dysfunction.
(3)  ***Correct.*** In patients with cirrhosis and portal hypertension, arteriovenous collaterals can develop in various tissues, including the lungs, skin, splanchnic organs, and muscles.
(4)  ***Correct.*** Chronic alcohol abuse increases anesthetic requirements, whereas acute alcoholic intoxication decreases anesthetic requirements.

**REASONING:**

When answering this question, the assumption of alcoholic cirrhosis was made based on the chronicity of alcohol use and the elevated AST and ALT. Although there is no empirical evidence showing that choice 1 is true, based on the theoretical basis for an increased risk of halothane induced hepatotoxicity and because choices 2, 3, and 4 are clearly true, E is the best answer.

**BIBLIOGRAPHY:**

Barash PG, Cullen BF, Stoelting RK, Cahalan M, Stock M. *Clinical Anesthesia*. 6th ed. Philadelphia, PA: Lippincott Williams & Wilkins; 2010:1248-1276 (Chapter 48).

Morgan GE, Mikhail MS, Murray MJ. *Clinical Anesthesiology*. 4th ed. New York, NY: McGraw-Hill; 2006:658-659.

---

**BOOK B:**

## QUESTION 123

*Answer C*

Cardiovascular

### QUESTION (K-type)

Causes of the pulmonary artery pressure and pulmonary artery occlusion pressure waveforms shown here include

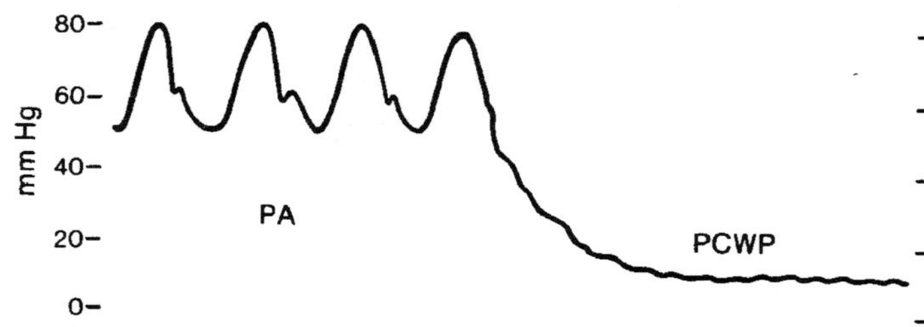


(1) Catheter overwedging.
(2) Protamine reaction.
(3) Acute mitral regurgitation.
(4) Primary pulmonary hypertension.

### CORRECT ANSWER: C (2 and 4 are correct.)

### SUMMARY:

*Flow-directed pulmonary artery catheters (PACs) can be used to provide estimates of left ventricular end-diastolic pressures. Flotation of the catheter into the pulmonary artery allows the pulmonary arterial (PA) pressure waveform to be transduced. When the balloon at the tip of the catheter is inflated and "wedged" into the distal PA circulation, a pulmonary catheter wedge pressure (PCWP) waveform can be recorded. The PCWP (also sometimes referred to as the* pulmonary artery occlusion pressure *[PAOP]) provides an estimate of left ventricular end-diastolic pressure (LVEDP), assuming that the path from the catheter tip to the left ventricle is unobstructed and ventricular compliance is normal. Ideally, the pulmonary artery diastolic pressure will approximate the PCWP. This PAC tracing is abnormal. It indicates very high PA pressures (normal PA pressures 10-25 mm Hg/ 5-15 mm Hg) with a normal PCWP. This relationship is seen in any disease state that increases PVR, such as primary pulmonary hypertension or protamine reaction. A protamine reaction can cause acute pulmonary vasoconstriction. (See also question 107, Book B.)*

### EXPLANATION:

(1) ***Incorrect.*** An overwedged catheter would produce a ramp-like trace with loss of pulsatile flow. The PA pressures would be normal.
(2) ***Correct.*** See below.

(3) *Incorrect.* Acute mitral regurgitation (MR) would produce prominent $v$ waves on the PA tracing. The predictive value of prominent V waves for acute MR has been confirmed.

(4) *Correct.* Elevated PA systolic and diastolic pressure (80/45 mm Hg) with normal wedge pressure (15 mm Hg) is seen in any condition that can produce elevated PVR, such as cor pulmonale, pulmonary embolism, and collagen-vascular disease. This results in right ventricular hypertrophy (RVH) and elevated right ventricular and pulmonary artery pressures over time. A similar presentation can be seen with protamine reaction secondary to thromboxane release producing pulmonary vasoconstriction.


**REASONING:**

This question tests knowledge of the interpretation of a PAC tracing and the effects of pulmonary hypertension on PAP and PCWP. The reader should review the criteria for placement and interpretation of PAC monitoring and its limitations carefully. Choices 1 and 3 can be ruled out based on this knowledge. C is the best answer.


**BIBLIOGRAPHY:**

Barash PG, Cullen BF, Stoelting RK. *Clinical Anesthesia.* 6th ed. Philadelphia, PA: Lippincott Williams & Wilkins; 2009:705-708.

Miller RD, Miller ED, Reves JG, et al. *Anesthesia.* 7th ed. New York, NY: Churchill Livingstone; 2010:1301-1303.

Snyder RW 2nd, Glamann DB, Lange RA, et al. Predictive value of prominent pulmonary arterial wedge v waves in assessing the presence and severity of mitral regurgitation. *Am J Cardiol.* 1994;73(8):568-570.

Stoelting RK, Dierdorf SF. *Anesthesia and Co-existing Diseases.* 3rd ed. New York, NY: Churchill Livingstone; 1993:103-106.

---

## BOOK B:     QUESTION 124

*Answer C*

Pediatrics

**QUESTION (K-type):**

Electrolyte profiles consistent with pyloric stenosis in a 6-week-old infant include the following:

| | $Na^+$ (mEq/L) | $K^+$ (mEq/L) | $Cl^-$ (mEq/L) | $HCO_3^-$ (mEq/L) |
|---|---|---|---|---|
| (1) | 145 | 3.5 | 108 | 24 |
| (2) | 145 | 2.5 | 85 | 15 |
| (3) | 160 | 5.5 | 120 | 36 |
| (4) | 128 | 2.5 | 85 | 32 |

**CORRECT ANSWER: C (2 and 4 are correct.)**


**SUMMARY:**

*Pyloric stenosis is usually seen in the first 3 to 6 weeks of life. It is a medical emergency and not a surgical emergency. Persistent vomiting in pyloric stenosis depletes sodium, potassium, chloride, hydrogen ions, and water. The electrolyte pattern commonly seen in untreated infants is a hyponatremic, hypokalemic, and hypochloremic metabolic alkalosis with a compensatory respiratory acidosis. Initial-stage electrolyte changes may reflect renal excretion of bicarbonate to compensate for alkalosis. Hyponatremia and dehydration continues to worsen progressively; sodium is conserved even at the expense of hydrogen ion excretion.*

(1)  *Incorrect.* No significant electrolyte disturbance is seen.
(2)  *Correct.* This pattern may represent an initial pattern of electrolyte changes in pyloric stenosis.
(3)  *Incorrect.* This pattern shows hypernatremia, hyperkalemia, and hyperchloremia.
(4)  *Correct.* This set of electrolytes is most consistent with pyloric stenosis: low sodium, potassium, and chloride with high bicarbonate.

## REASONING:

Only choices 2 and 4 are correct. The electrolyte abnormalities in pyloric stenosis are due to chronic vomiting. Because gastric fluid contains water and hydrochloric acid, severe vomiting results in a hypokalemic hypochloremic metabolic alkalosis.

## BIBLIOGRAPHY:

Barash PG, Cullen BF, Stoelting RK, Cahalan M, Stock M. *Clinical Anesthesia*. 6th ed. Philadelphia, PA: Lippincott Williams & Wilkins; 2010:1201.
Morgan GE, Mikhail MS, Murray MJ. *Clinical Anesthesiology*. 4th ed. New York, NY: McGraw-Hill; 2006:942.

---

**BOOK B:**　　　　　　　**QUESTION 125**

---

*Answer B*

## Regional Anesthesia

## QUESTION (K-type):

True statements concerning regional anesthesia with peripheral nerve blocks for an operation on a knee using a tourniquet include the following:

(1)  The inguinal perivascular block includes the obturator nerve.
(2)  Paresthesias are required during sciatic block.
(3)  The lateral femoral cutaneous nerve must be blocked.
(4)  Block of the lumbar plexus in the psoas compartment provides adequate anesthesia.

## CORRECT ANSWER: B (1 and 3 are correct.)

## SUMMARY:

*Operations on the knee using a tourniquet require anesthesia of the anterior, medial, lateral, and posterior aspects of the thigh. These areas are innervated by the femoral, obturator, lateral femoral cutaneous, and posterior cutaneous nerves of the thigh, respectively. These are the nerves that must be blocked. Inguinal perivascular block and block of the lumbar plexus in the psoas compartment both aim to block the femoral, obturator, and lateral femoral cutaneous nerves, but not the posterior cutaneous nerve of the thigh.*

## EXPLANATION:

(1)  *Correct.* An inguinal perivascular block aims to have local anesthetic spread proximally along the facial compartment containing the femoral nerve to include the obturator and lateral femoral cutaneous nerves, also called the *3-in-1 block.*
(2)  *Incorrect.* A sciatic block may be accomplished without paresthesias.
(3)  *Correct.* The lateral thigh must be anesthetized with blockade of the lateral femoral cutaneous nerve, particularly if a tourniquet is to be used.
(4)  *Incorrect.* Blockade of the lumbar plexus will not block the posterior cutaneous nerve of the thigh and thus will be inadequate for knee surgery using a tourniquet.

**REASONING:**

This question tests knowledge of the innervation of the lower leg and thigh. The reader hopefully will note by now the frequency with which innervation to the lower extremity is tested. The importance of this topic for careful review by the reader cannot be overstated. Choices 1 and 3 are correct and therefore B is the correct answer. The most obvious incorrect choice is 2. If choice 2 is wrong, only answers B and C are possibilities. Answer B should be more attractive to the unsure test taker. It is important to note the use of the tourniquet to identify the entire area of anesthesia required for surgery. B is the best answer.

**BIBLIOGRAPHY:**

Barash PG, Cullen BF, Stoelting RK, Cahalan M, Stock M. *Clinical Anesthesia.* 6th ed. Philadelphia, PA: Lippincott Williams & Wilkins; 2010:987-992.

Cousins MJ, Carr DB, Horlocker TT, Bridenbaugh PO. *Cousins & Bridenbaugh's Neural Blockade in Clinical Anesthesia and Pain Medicine.* 4th ed. Philadelphia, PA: Lippincott Williams & Wilkins; 2009:577-578.

Miller RD, Eriksson LI, Fleisher LA, Wiener-Kronish JP, William YL. *Miller's Anesthesia.* 7th ed. Philadelphia, PA: Churchill Livingstone; 2010:2251-2252.

Morgan GE, Mikhail MS, Murray MJ. *Clinical Anesthesiology.* 4th ed. New York, NY: McGraw-Hill; 2006:342-348, 856-857.

Raj PP. *Textbook of Regional Anesthesia.* Philadelphia, PA: Churchill Livingstone; 2002:453-454.

www.neuraxiom.com.

www.nysora.com.

---

**BOOK B:**

*Answer E*

OB/Regional

**QUESTION 126**

**QUESTION (K-type):**

Proximal spread of a local anesthetic solution placed in the axillary perivascular space is promoted by

(1) Increased volume of the local anesthetic agent.
(2) Digital pressure distal to the injection site.
(3) Cephalad direction of the needle.
(4) Adduction of the shoulder after the injection.

**CORRECT ANSWER: E (All are correct.)**

**SUMMARY:**

*Factors affecting spread of local anesthetic during placement of axillary blocks are important because proximal spread of local anesthetic leads to more complete and reliable blockade. Interventions that promote proximal spread of local anesthetic include the following: increased volume of local anesthetic, digital pressure distal to the injection site, cephalad direction of the needle, and adduction of the shoulder after the injection.*

**EXPLANATION:**

(1) *Correct.* Large-volume injection promotes spread in all directions.
(2) *Correct.* Factors leading to inadequate axillary block include the septation of the axillary perivascular space and the proximal departure of the musculocutaneous nerve from the axillary sheath. Proximal spread of the local anesthetic helps overcome both these problems and achieves a more effective block. Digital pressure

distal to the site of injection has been advocated to encourage spread proximally rather than distally.

   (3)  *Correct.* Cephalad direction of the needle has been advocated for promoting proximal spread but may incur a small risk of pneumothorax.

   (4)  *Correct.* Multiple authors note that overabduction of the arm during placement of the block may cause forward displacement of the humeral head leading to an attenuated axillary pulse. Similarly, adduction of the shoulder after injection can reduce the pressure caused by forward displacement of the humeral head that may reduce proximal spread of local anesthetic.

### REASONING:

This question tests knowledge of the placement of an axillary block. Factors that affect proximal spread of local anesthetic in the sheath include the volume of anesthetic used, digital pressure distal to the injection, cephalad direction of the needle, and adduction of the shoulder after the injection. All choices are correct, and therefore the best answer is E.

### BIBLIOGRAPHY:

Barash PG, Cullen BF, Stoelting RK, Cahalan M, Stock M. *Clinical Anesthesia.* 6th ed. Philadelphia, PA: Lippincott Williams & Wilkins; 2010:968-971, 976-977, 1491.

Cousins MJ, Carr DB, Horlocker TT, Bridenbaugh PO. *Cousins & Bridenbaugh's Neural Blockade in Clinical Anesthesia and Pain Medicine.* 4th ed. Philadelphia, PA: Lippincott Williams & Wilkins; 2009:613-614.

Morgan GE, Mikhail MS, Murray MJ. *Clinical Anesthesiology.* 4th ed. New York, NY: McGraw-Hill; 2006:334.

Raj PP. *Textbook of Regional Anesthesia.* Philadelphia, PA: Churchill Livingstone; 2002:350-351, 514-515.

www.neuraxiom.com.

www.nysora.com.

---

**BOOK B:**  **QUESTION 127**

---

*Answer D*

Pain

### QUESTION (K-type):

Indications for neurolytic celiac plexus ablation include pain due to carcinoma of the

   (1)  Sigmoid colon.
   (2)  Kidney.
   (3)  Ovary.
   (4)  Pancreas.

### CORRECT ANSWER: D (4 only is correct.)

### SUMMARY:

*Celiac plexus neurolysis is indicated for pain control in upper abdominal and retroperitoneal malignancy. It is generally thought to be helpful for pain originating in the distal esophagus, stomach, duodenum, small intestines, and ascending and proximal transverse colon. In addition, the organs supplied by the celiac artery receive contributions from the celiac plexus, including the liver, biliary system, spleen, and pancreas. Textbooks differ on whether the visceral afferents from the kidney course through the celiac plexus. However, a PubMed search up to mid-2011 resulted in no reports of celiac plexus blockade for renal cell carcinoma. Carcinoma of the sigmoid colon, ovaries, and other pelvic viscera may be treated with hypogastric plexus blocks.*

**EXPLANATION:**

(1) *Incorrect.* Celiac plexus block will relieve intestinal pain related to the mid transverse colon and higher but does not cover the sigmoid colon, which may be covered with other blocks such as a superior hypogastric plexus block.

(2) *Incorrect.* While texts differ on whether visceral afferent fibers from the kidneys travel through the celiac plexus, cancer of the kidney is clearly not an indication for a neurolytic celiac plexus block and no cases of such treatment could be found in an extensive PubMed search.

(3) *Incorrect.* Ovaries are thought to be innervated by fibers originating lower than the celiac plexus.

(4) *Correct.* There is extensive literature supporting use of neurolytic celiac plexus block for pancreatic cancer with reported success rates of pain relief in 74% of patients with pancreatic carcinoma.

**REASONING:**

A hallmark of celiac plexus block is that it does not cover the sigmoid colon. Therefore, choice 1 is incorrect and answers A, B, and E are thus eliminated. Choosing between answers C and D requires only a determination of whether pain due to carcinoma of the kidney is an indication for neurolytic celiac plexus block. There is no literature in PubMed to support this indication.

**BIBLIOGRAPHY:**

Barash PG, Cullen BF, Stoelting RK, Cahalan MK, Stock MC. Clinical Anesthesia. 6th ed. Philadelphia, PA: Lippincott Williams & Wilkins; 2009:1518-1519.

Cousins MJ, Carr DB, Horlocker TT, Bridenbaugh PO. *Cousins & Bridenbaugh's Neural Blockade in Clinical Anesthesia and Pain Medicine*. 4th ed. Philadelphia, PA: Lippincott Williams & Wilkins; 2009:1124-1131.

Miller RD, Eriksson LI, Fleisher LA, Wiener-Kronish JP, William YL. *Miller's Anesthesia*. 7th ed. Philadelphia, PA: Churchill Livingstone; 2010:1669, 1808-1809.

Morgan GE, Mikhail MS, Murray MJ. *Clinical Anesthesiology*. 4th ed. New York, NY: McGraw-Hill; 2006:385, 400 (Figure 18-16).

Polati E, Luzzani A, Schweiger V, Finco G, Ischia S. The role of neurolytic celiac plexus block in the treatment of pancreatic cancer pain. *Transplant Proc*. 2008 May;40(4):1200-1204.

Raj PP. *Textbook of Regional Anesthesia*. Philadelphia, PA: Churchill Livingstone; 2002:995-997.

Rykowski JJ, Hilgier M. Efficacy of neurolytic celiac plexus block in varying locations of pancreatic cancer: influence on pain relief. *Anesthesiology*. 2000;92:347-354.

---

**BOOK B:**                    **QUESTION 128**

---

*Answer A*

Pharmacology

**QUESTION (K-type):**

Compared with a 20-year-old patient, an 80-year-old patient will

(1) Have similar EEG sensitivity to the same blood concentrations of thiopental.
(2) Require lower induction doses (mg/kg) of thiopental.
(3) Have increased sensitivity to volatile anesthetics.
(4) Require lower doses (mg/kg) of succinylcholine.

**CORRECT ANSWER: A (1, 2, and 3 are correct.)**

**SUMMARY:**

*Pharmacokinetic and pharmacodynamic changes occur with aging. These changes exert clinical effects that alter induction doses and duration of anesthetics. In general, the geriatric patient has a decrease in total body water because of a decrease in muscle mass and an increase in body fat. This is because fat contains less water than muscle. This results in a decreased volume of distribution for water-soluble drugs, while an increase in volume of distribution is seen for more lipid-soluble drugs. Plasma concentrations of the drug parallel the changes in volume of distribution. Moreover, because hepatic and renal function is generally decreased in the elderly, elimination and clearance are reduced, which results in a prolongation of drug effect.*

*Barbiturates are highly soluble drugs. Even though they are highly protein bound, their clinical effect is achieved in 30 seconds because of their lipid solubility and highly non-ionized fraction. Redistribution to peripheral components such as muscle reduces the plasma and brain concentration, while hypovolemia, hypoalbuminemia, and acidosis will result in higher plasma and, ultimately, higher brain concentrations. Lower induction doses should be used in the elderly because of the slower redistribution of the drug to peripheral components.*

## EXPLANATION:

(1) ***Correct.*** Thiopental causes dose-dependent changes in the EEG regardless of age, assuming the same blood concentration in both demographics.

(2) ***Correct.*** If given the same induction dose of a young healthy adult, an octogenarian will achieve higher plasma levels because of the slower redistribution of the drug to peripheral compartments. "A typical octogenarian requires less than half the induction dose of thiopental than that required by a 20-year-old."

(3) ***Correct.*** The MAC for inhalational agents is reduced for the geriatric patient. In general, a 4% reduction per decade is seen in MAC for those over age 40. Also, in those patients with depressed cardiac function, the rate of induction will be increased with an inhalational agent.

(4) ***Incorrect.*** The response to both nondepolarizing and depolarizing muscle relaxants is unaltered in the elderly. However, the onset of action may be prolonged due to slower circulation times.

## REASONING:

This is a straight forward question. Choices 1, 2, and 3 are correct. Choice 4 is can be somewhat correct in that elderly men may have decreased synthesis of pseudocholinesterase and could exhibit a slightly prolonged effect from succinylcholine. Clinically, succinylcholine is rarely used to maintain paralysis during a surgical procedure, and dosing for the onset of paralysis should be the same for the young and elderly.

## BIBLIOGRAPHY:

Morgan GE, Mikhail MS, Murray MJ. *Clinical Anesthesiology.* 4th ed. New York, NY: McGraw-Hill; 2006:157-158, 875-881.

---

| **BOOK B:** | **QUESTION 129 (OPTIONAL)** |
| --- | --- |

*Answer D*

Clinical Anesthesia

## QUESTION (K-type):

Induction of anesthesia with usual drug dosages and concentrations may lead to cardiovascular signs of overdose in patients with hypothyroidism because of expected decreases in

(1) Respiratory quotient.
(2) Minute volume of breathing.
(3) Circulating blood volume.
(4) Cardiac output.

CORRECT ANSWER: D (3 and 4 are correct.)

**SUMMARY:**

*Hypothyroidism occurs in up to 0.8% of the adult population, and may result from inadequate levels of free thyroxine ($T_4$) and/or triiodothyronine ($T_3$). A deficiency of thyroid hormones results in a general reduction in metabolic activity, resulting in decreased oxygen consumption and carbon dioxide production. This decrease in carbon dioxide production indirectly decreases minute ventilation. The cardiovascular and respiratory systems are generally depressed. Cardiac output, stroke volume, myocardial contractility, and heart rate are decreased, while ventilatory responses to hypoxia and hypercarbia are depressed. Hypothyroid patients may also have decreased intravascular volume.*

**EXPLANATION:**

(1) *Incorrect.* The respiratory quotient is the ratio of carbon dioxide production to oxygen consumption and generally reflects the type of fuel being used. The hypometabolic state of hypothyroidism results in a decrease of both carbon dioxide production and oxygen consumption; there are no studies quantifying the change in respiratory quotient with hypothyroidism, but an anesthetic overdose would not be expected.

(2) *Incorrect.* The decreased metabolic rate results in decreased carbon dioxide production, which indirectly results in decreased minute ventilation, but this should not cause cardiovascular signs of anesthetic overdose.

(3) *Questionable.* Some sources report that hypothyroid patients may have decreased intravascular volume and hypotension; this may cause an exaggerated hypotensive response to induction agents. Other sources offer hypertension as a possibility from increased peripheral vascular resistance.

(4) *Correct.* Hypothyroid patients have decreased cardiac output, which results in a faster onset of action and possible overdose of an agent used for inhalational induction.

**REASONING:**

Choice 4 is clearly correct as explained above, making C or D the only options. Choice 2 is not correct as explained above, so choice 4 is the best option. Regarding choice 3, although intravascular depletion is commonly cited as a possibility in severe hypothyroidism leading to myxedema coma, no primary literature demonstrates that hypothyroid patients are in general hypovolemic.

**BIBLIOGRAPHY:**

Barash PG, Cullen BF, Stoelting RK, Cahalan M, Stock M. *Clinical Anesthesia.* 6th ed. Philadelphia, PA: Lippincott Williams & Wilkins; 2010:1130-1134.

Morgan GE, Mikhail MS, Murray MJ. *Clinical Anesthesiology.* 4th ed. New York, NY: McGraw-Hill; 2006:806-809.

Surks M. Clinical manifestations of hypothyroidism: up to date (7th ed). *Big Miller.* 2010 Jun 16:1023.

---

**BOOK B:**

**QUESTION 130**

---

*Answer D*

Pharmacology

**QUESTION (K-type):**

The duration of the anticoagulant effect of heparin is

(1) Independent of body temperature.
(2) Determined primarily by renal excretion.
(3) Prolonged two to three times with hypoalbuminemia.
(4) Dose dependent.

**CORRECT ANSWER: D (4 only is correct.)**

**SUMMARY:**

*Heparin is a polyanionic glycosaminoglycan that acts as an anticoagulant by binding to and increasing 1000-fold the activity of serine protease antithrombin III. ATIII irreversibly binds and inhibits activated clotting factors thrombin, Xa, XIa, XIIa, and XIIIa. Most of the anticoagulant effect is derived from the inhibition of thrombin and Xa. The in vivo half-life of heparin varies among individuals and is dose and temperature dependent. Heparin does not bind albumin and its activity is unaffected by hypoalbuminemia. Heparin is eliminated primarily by the reticuloendothelial system. A small percentage is excreted unchanged by the kidneys.*

**EXPLANATION:**
(1) *Incorrect.* The rate of clearance of heparin from the plasma decreases in proportion to the degree of hypothermia.
(2) *Incorrect.* Heparin is primarily degraded and cleared by the reticuloendothelial system. A small amount of undegraded heparin appears in the urine. The half-life of heparin may be mildly increased in patients with significant renal or hepatic disease.
(3) *Incorrect.* Heparin does not bind albumin and is unaffected by low albumin states. Plasma proteins vitronectin and platelet factor 4 bind heparin and competitively inhibit heparin binding to ATIII. These heparin-binding proteins account for the variation in heparin dosing among individuals to reach a therapeutic aPTT.
(4) *Correct.* The anticoagulant effect of heparin is directly dose dependent. The approximate half-lives for 100, 400, and 800 U/kg of intravenous heparin administered at normal body temperature are 60, 180, and 300 minutes, respectively.

**REASONING:**
This question is K-type. Choice 4 is obviously correct, ruling out answers A and B. Because choice 2 is incorrect, D is the only valid answer.

**BIBLIOGRAPHY:**
Barash PG, Cullen BF, Stoetling RK, Cahalan M, Stock M. *Clinical Anesthesia.* 6th ed. Philadelphia, PA: Lippincott-Raven Publishers; 2009:400, 1088.
Evers A, Maze M, Kharasch E. Anesthetic Pharmacology. 2nd ed. Cambridge University Press, 915-919.
Hardman JG, Gilman AG, Limbird LE. *Goodman & Gilman's The Pharmacological Basis of Therapeutics.* 9th ed. New York, NY: McGraw-Hill; 1996:1343-1346.
Morgan GE, Mikhail MS, Murray MJ. *Clinical Anesthesiology.* 4th ed. New York, NY: McGraw-Hill; 2006:510-511, 513f.

---

**BOOK B:**  **QUESTION 131**

*Answer B*

Clinical Anesthesia

**QUESTION (K-type):**

During general endotracheal anesthesia, early signs of an acute asthma attack include

(1) Alteration of the expiratory plateau on capnography.
(2) Increased $Pa_{CO_2}$.
(3) Increased peak airway pressure.
(4) Hypoxemia.

**CORRECT ANSWER: B (1 and 3 are correct.)**

**SUMMARY:**

*Early signs of an acute bronchospasm intraoperatively will usually manifest as increased PIPs, decreased exhaled tidal volumes and end-tidal $CO_2$, an upsloping capnograph, and wheezing. Of note, the severity of the obstruction is inversely correlated to the rate of rise of the carbon dioxide capnograph. During an acute attack, the TLC, residual volume, and FRC are all increased. In light of this, hypoxemia occurs later as the alveolar units with low ventilation/perfusion ratios increase. Other signs of a severe asthma attack include pulsus paradoxus and right heart strain (RBBB, RAD, ST-changes). One should avoid the use of PEEP in patients with moderate-severe asthma.*

**EXPLANATION:**

(1) ***Correct.*** A slow rising waveform or a sloping waveform on the capnograph results during an acute asthma attack.
(2) ***Incorrect.*** Carbon dioxide is readily diffusible across the alveolus (about 20 times more so than oxygen). As such, a rise in the partial pressure of arterial carbon dioxide will not be an early sign.
(3) ***Correct.*** Bronchoconstriction will result in increased peak airway pressure, but unchanged plateau pressure.
(4) ***Incorrect.*** In a patient who is mechanically ventilated, hypoxemia will not be an early sign of an acute asthma attack.

**REASONING:**

All of the signs listed in choices will occur in a spontaneously breathing patient, but this question involves a mechanically ventilated patient. Furthermore, this question is asking about *early* signs of an acute asthma attack.

**BIBLIOGRAPHY:**

Morgan GE, Mikhail MS, Murray MJ. *Clinical Anesthesiology.* 4th ed. New York, NY: McGraw-Hill; 2006:513-516.

---

| **BOOK B:** | **QUESTION 132** |
|---|---|

*Answer B*

OB/Regional

**QUESTION (K-type):**

At the placental interface, the efficiency of oxygen transport to the fetus is enhanced by

(1) Movement of the maternal oxyhemoglobin dissociation curve to the right.
(2) Diffusion of carbon dioxide from fetal blood.
(3) Movement of the fetal oxyhemoglobin dissociation curve to the left.
(4) Maternal hyperventilation.

**CORRECT ANSWER: B (1, 2, and 3 are correct.)**

**SUMMARY:**

*Because the fetus is unable to store oxygen, placental transfer of respiratory gases is critically important. Oxygen transfer depends on maternal and fetal placental blood flow and maternal and fetal oxygen tension. The oxyhemoglobin dissociation curve in the mother is shifted to the right, thereby decreasing affinity and increasing unloading of oxygen to the fetus. Conversely, the fetal oxyhemoglobin dissociation curve is shifted to the left, resulting in increased oxygen affinity. This physiologic state facilitates oxygen transfer to the fetus. Any maternal condition that decreases oxygen tension or shifts the maternal oxyhemoglobin dissociation curve to the left (maternal hyperventilation and alkalosis) will decrease oxygen delivery to the fetus, potentially resulting in fetal asphyxia.*

## EXPLANATION:

(1) ***Correct.*** As stated above, the maternal oxyhemoglobin curve is shifted to the right.
(2) ***Correct.*** Carbon dioxide readily diffuses from the fetus into the maternal circulation. This increases the pH, which shifts the fetal oxyhemoglobin curve to the left. The left shift facilitates oxygen uptake into the fetal circulation.
(3) ***Correct.*** The fetal oxyhemoglobin curve is shifted to the left.
(4) ***Incorrect.*** While the maternal $Paco_2$ decreases slightly during pregnancy, there is little acid-base disturbance owing to renal compensation. However, maternal hyperventilation resulting in hypocarbia and alkalosis causes decreased uterine blood flow and a shift of the oxyhemoglobin curve to the left, both of which impair oxygen delivery to the fetus.

## REASONING:

The reader should review the conditions that result in changes in the oxyhemoglobin dissociation curve carefully. One of these conditions is pregnancy. The goal of the fetus is to take the nutrients and oxygen it needs for survival, and the maternal physiology changes to accomplish this goal. The maternal curve shifts to the right, and the fetal curve shifts to the left. Knowing that alkalosis will shift the curve to the left eliminates choice 4 and answers D and E. Carbon dioxide and oxygen diffuse across the placenta independently, which eliminates choice 2 and answer A. B is the best answer.

## BIBLIOGRAPHY:

Chestnut DH, Polley LS, Tsen LC, Wong CA. *Chestnut's Obstetric Anesthesia Principles and Practice.* 4th ed. Philadelphia, PA: Mosby Elsevier; 2009:61-62.
Miller RD, Eriksson LI, Fleisher LA, Wiener-Kronish JP, Young WL. *Miller's Anesthesia.* 7th ed. Philadelphia, PA: Churchill Livingstone; 2010:1746-1747.

---

| **BOOK B:** | **QUESTION 133** |
|---|---|

*Answer C*

Physiology

### QUESTION (K-type):

During a carbon dioxide challenge test in a healthy patient, the $Paco_2$ increases to 60 mm Hg. Expected effects include

(1) Decreased pulmonary vascular resistance.
(2) Increased cardiac output.
(3) Renovascular dilatation.
(4) Sympathetic stimulation.

### CORRECT ANSWER: C (2 and 4 are correct.)

### SUMMARY:

*Hypercapnia has multiple systemic effects. Hypercapnia activates the sympathetic system, which typically results in increased cardiac output, increased arterial blood pressure, and increased propensity towards dysrhythmias. As the arterial partial pressure of carbon dioxide increases, cerebral blood flow increases proportionally. In general, for every 1 mm Hg increase in $Paco_2$, CBF increases 1 mL/100 g/min. Partial pressures of carbon* *dioxide greater than 80 mm Hg will lead to unconsciousness as the cerebral pH becomes more acidotic. Furthermore, hypercapnia is a strong respiratory stimulant. For each 1 mm Hg increase in $Paco_2$, minute ventilation increases up to 3 L/min in awake subjects.*

### EXPLANATION:

(1) *Incorrect.* In the pulmonary vasculature, hypoxia, hypercapnia, and metabolic acidosis are stimulants for vasoconstriction, while hypocapnia causes pulmonary vasodilation.

(2) *Correct.* Although carbon dioxide by itself is a myocardial depressant, the sympathetic response to hypercapnia masks these effects.

(3) *Incorrect.* Sympathetic stimulation releases adrenergic substances such as norepinephrine that cause renal vasoconstriction.

(4) *Correct.* See above.

### REASONING:

The words *carbon dioxide challenge test* are a red herring. Without knowing what it is used for, this question asks for the systemic effects of hypercapnia, which are straight forward.

### BIBLIOGRAPHY:

Morgan GE, Mikhail MS, Murray MJ. *Clinical Anesthesiology*. 4th ed. New York, NY: McGraw-Hill; 2006:38-39, 493, 671.

---

## BOOK B:                    QUESTION 134

*Answer B*

OB/Regional

### QUESTION (K-type):

Which of the following peripheral nerves must be blocked for removal of a glass splinter from the plantar surface of the heel?

(1) Tibial.
(2) Saphenous.
(3) Sural.
(4) Superficial peroneal.

### CORRECT ANSWER: B (1 and 3 are correct.)

### SUMMARY:

*The posterior tibial nerve provides sensory innervation to the medial and anterolateral sole of the foot and most of the heel. It is a continuation of the tibial nerve, entering the foot posterior to the medial malleolus, where it branches into the lateral and medial plantar nerves. The rest of the heel is innervated by the sural nerve, which provides sensation to the lateral foot. None of the other three nerves that supply cutaneous sensation to the foot—the superficial peroneal nerve, the deep peroneal nerve, and the saphenous nerve—innervates the heel.*

### EXPLANATION:

(1) *Correct.* The tibial nerve is the major nerve to the plantar surface of the foot and provides sensation to all but the lateral heel. The posterior tibial nerve may be blocked posterior to the medial malleolus behind the posterior tibial artery.

(2) **Incorrect.** The saphenous nerve, which is a continuation of the femoral nerve and the only nerve to the foot and does not branch from the sciatic nerve system, is responsible for sensation to the anteromedial foot. It is found most consistently anterior to the medial malleolus.

(3) **Correct.** The sural nerve, which branches off from the tibial nerve, supplies sensation to the lateral heel. It may be blocked by deep subcutaneous fan infiltration of local anesthetic between the Achilles tendon and the lateral malleolus.

(4) **Incorrect.** The superficial peroneal nerve, which branches from the common peroneal nerve, enters the foot lateral to extensor digitorum longus at the medial malleolus and provides cutaneous sensation to the dorsum of foot and to the five toes.

## REASONING:

The key to answering this question is understanding the anatomy of the nerves that supply sensation to the ankle and the foot. The sensation to the plantar surface of the foot is mostly supplied by the posterior tibial nerve with a small area of the lateral heel innervated by the sural nerve and a small area of the anteromedial foot by the saphenous nerve. The superficial and deep peroneal nerves innervate only the dorsal foot.

## BIBLIOGRAPHY:


Barash PG, Cullen BF, Stoelting RK, Cahalan M, Stock M. *Clinical Anesthesia*. 6th ed. Philadelphia, PA: Lippincott Williams & Wilkins; 2010:987-999.

Hadzic A, Vloka JD. *Peripheral Nerve Blocks Principles and Practice*. New York, NY: McGraw-Hill; 2004:316-329 (Chapter 24 Ankle Block).

Morgan GE, Mikhail MS, Murray MJ. *Clinical Anesthesiology*. 4th ed. New York, NY: McGraw-Hill; 2006:352-353, 352f.


---

**BOOK B:**      **QUESTION 135**

---

*Answer E*

Clinical Anesthesia

## QUESTION (K-type):

A 26-year-old woman is to undergo emergency laparotomy for a ruptured appendix. She has been taking propylthiouracil and an oral β-adrenergic blocker for 2 days for acute hyperthyroidism. Appropriate perioperative therapy includes administration of

(1) Potassium iodide.
(2) Hydrocortisone.
(3) Propranolol.
(4) Propylthiouracil.

**CORRECT ANSWER: E (All are correct.)**

## SUMMARY:

*Any patient who is acutely hyperthyroid should be made euthyroid prior to any elective surgery. The goal of medical treatment in hyperthyroidism is threefold and includes (1) inhibition of hormone synthesis with drugs such as propylthiouracil or methimazole, (2) prevention of hormone release with iodide salts or steroids (such as hydrocortisone), and (3) prevention of the hemodynamic consequences of adrenergic activation with β-blockade (such as propranolol). Preoperative preparation ideally requires 7 to 14 days. When surgery cannot be postponed, the main goal of an anesthetic is to maintain hemodynamic stability and control the blood pressure with an esmolol infusion. All perioperative medications treating hyperthyroidism should be continued.*

**EXPLANATION:**

(1) ***Correct.*** Potassium or sodium iodide can be administered perioperatively to prevent hormone release. Iodide ions are actively transported into the thyroid gland and immediately oxidized to iodine, which combines with tyrosine to form the two thyroid hormones, triiodothyronine ($T_3$) and thyroxine ($T_4$). The ingestion of large amounts of inorganic iodide inhibits iodide organification and thus thyroid hormone release, in an autoregulatory process called the *Wolff-Chaikoff effect.* Antithyroid drugs should be started prior to iodide treatment to decrease the chance of an exacerbation of thyrotoxicosis.

(2) ***Correct.*** Patients who are hyperthyroid often have increased production and utilization of cortisol. If persistent hypotension is present intraoperatively, one should consider the administration of IV cortisol. Also, glucocorticoids may also reduce thyroid hormone secretion and peripheral conversion of $T_4$ to $T_3$.

(3) ***Correct.*** In acute hyperthyroidism, patients have a hyperdynamic circulation that results in tachycardia, dysrhythmias, and increased cardiac output. This increased activity of the sympathetic system can be attenuated with β-blockers.

(4) ***Correct.*** Propylthiouracil is a thiourea derivative that inhibits iodide organification, and thus synthesis of thyroid hormone.

**REASONING:**

All medications listed are appropriate medications in the treatment of acute hyperthyroidism and thus are appropriate perioperative therapies.

**BIBLIOGRAPHY:**


Barash PG, Cullen BF, Stoelting RK, Cahalan M, Stock M. *Clinical Anesthesia.* 6th ed. Philadelphia, PA: Lippincott Williams & Wilkins; 2010:1130-1133.

Morgan GE, Mikhail MS, Murray MJ. *Clinical Anesthesiology.* 4th ed. New York, NY: McGraw-Hill; 2006:807-808.


---

| **BOOK B:** | **QUESTION 136** |
|---|---|

## *Answer B*

Pharmacology

**QUESTION (K-type):**

A previously healthy 55-year-old patient is spontaneously breathing oxygen, nitrous oxide, and halothane during a minor surgical procedure. The end-tidal halothane concentration measured by mass spectrometry is 0.7%, end-tidal nitrous oxide concentration is 50%, and end-tidal carbon dioxide concentration is 9%. Findings consistent with these concentrations include

(1) Tachycardia.
(2) Decreased requirement for halothane.
(3) Premature ventricular contractions.
(4) Serum bicarbonate concentration of 35 mEq/L.

**CORRECT ANSWER: B (1 and 3 correct.)**

**SUMMARY:**

*Because of medullary depression and peripheral mechanisms, halothane typically causes rapid shallow breathing, a rise in the apneic threshold, and a diminished ventilatory response to hypercarbia. This patient is hypercarbic, as the $ET_{CO_2}$ of 9% exceeds the typical value of 5%. Physiologic signs of hypercarbia include tachycardia, hypertension, arrhythmias, and pulmonary hypertension. The conversion of 9% $CO_2$ to the more common expressed value of millimeters of mercury, assuming a sea-level pressure of 760 mm, yields*

*0.09 × 760 mm Hg = 68 mm Hg. $HCO_3^-$ acutely increases only about 1 mEq/L for each 10 mm Hg increase in $Paco_2$ above 40 mm Hg. Here, the expected $HCO_3^-$ would be 24 + (68 – 40) × 0.1 = 26.8 mEq/L.*

## EXPLANATION:

(1) ***Correct.*** Tachycardia is a well-known complication associated with hypercarbia.

(2) ***Incorrect.*** Hypercarbia at this level does not affect MAC and would not decrease the halothane requirements.

(3) ***Correct.*** Arrhythmias are associated with hypercarbia.

(4) ***Incorrect.*** Renal compensation for an acute respiratory acidosis is limited and would not explain a serum bicarbonate concentration of 35 mEq/L.

## REASONING:

The key to the question is to first recognize that the patient has an elevated $ETco_2$ by converting from percent composition of expired gas to partial pressure in millimeters of mercury. Hypercarbia causes tachycardia (1) and arrhythmias (3). Acute hypercarbia to 68 mm Hg would not cause a bicarbonate level of 35 as explained above. Regarding choice 2, Barash reports that hypercarbia does not influence MAC. Although some older texts list hypercarbia of greater than 90 mm Hg as a factor that can decrease MAC, hypercarbia to 68 mm Hg would still be insufficient to decrease MAC. The best answer is thus B.

## BIBLIOGRAPHY:

Barash PG, Cullen BF, Stoelting RK. *Clinical Anesthesia*. 6th ed. Philadelphia, PA: Lippincott Williams & Wilkins; 2009:425.

Morgan GE, Mikhail MS, Murray MJ. *Clinical Anesthesiology*. 4th ed. New York, NY: McGraw-Hill; 2006:166-168.

---

**BOOK B:**        **QUESTION 137**

---

*Answer C*

Clinical Anesthesia

## QUESTION (K-type):

A 48-year-old man who is undergoing a right upper lobectomy for cancer has a $Pao_2$ of 67 mm Hg while his left lung is being ventilated at 10 mL/kg at a rate of 10 breaths/min. Measures to increase $Pao_2$ include

(1) Hyperventilation to a $Paco_2$ of 30 mm Hg.

(2) Insufflation of the right lung with continuous positive airway pressure.

(3) Application of positive end-expiratory pressure of 15 $cmH_2O$ to the left lung.

(4) Partial occlusion of right pulmonary blood flow.

**CORRECT ANSWER: C (2 and 4 correct.)**

## SUMMARY:

*Hypoxemia is a known risk during one-lung ventilation. Effective measures to increase the $Pao_2$ include applying continuous positive airway pressure (CPAP) (5-10 $cmH_2O$) to the collapsed lung, periodic inflation of the collapsed lung, and early ligation or clamping of the ipsilateral pulmonary artery to decrease the ventilation-perfusion mismatch. Other measures that are only marginally effective in improving hypoxemia include applying PEEP to the ventilated lung, continuous insufflation of oxygen into the collapsed lung, and changing the tidal volume or ventilatory rate. Persistent or clinically significant hypoxemia may require reexpansion of the collapsed lung.*

## EXPLANATION:

(1) *Incorrect.* Changing the minute ventilation would not greatly improve oxygenation.
(2) *Correct.* CPAP to the collapsed lung will consistently improve oxygenation.
(3) *Incorrect.* PEEP to the ventilated lung will not greatly improve the ventilation-perfusion mismatch of the collapsed lung
(4) *Correct.* Ligation or clamping of the ipsilateral pulmonary artery will decrease shunting.

## REASONING:

Choices 2 and 4 are measures that are consistently effective in improving oxygenation during one-lung ventilation. Choices 1 and 3, though occasionally employed clinically, do not consistently improve oxygenation.

## BIBLIOGRAPHY:

Morgan GE, Mikhail MS, Murray MJ. *Clinical Anesthesiology*. 4th ed. New York, NY: McGraw-Hill; 2006:588-599.

---

**BOOK B:**      **QUESTION 138**

*Answer C*

OB/Regional

## QUESTION (K-type):

Uterine contractility is decreased by

(1) Epidural lidocaine.
(2) Terbutaline.
(3) Ketamine anesthesia.
(4) Halothane.

**CORRECT ANSWER: C (2 and 4 are correct.)**

## SUMMARY:

*Agents that decrease uterine tone are used to treat preterm labor and uterine hypertonus or to facilitate removal of a retained placenta. The uterus contracts due to a rise in myometrial cell calcium concentration that occurs in response to an enzyme cascade set in motion by circulating hormones or other mediators. Uterine $\beta_2$-receptor activation results in an increase in cAMP, decreasing intracellular calcium and inhibiting the myosin light-chain kinase. $\beta$-Agonists such as terbutaline and ritodrine act via this mechanism. Magnesium sulfate and calcium channel blockers such as nifedipine relax the uterus by decreasing intracellular calcium. Nitroglycerin causes nitric oxide–mediated uterine relaxation. Halogenated anesthetic agents also provide uterine relaxation, although their mechanism is less well understood.*

## EXPLANATION:

(1) *Incorrect.* Epidural lidocaine has not been shown to inhibit uterine contractility. In fact, at clinically relevant intravenous concentrations, lidocaine and bupivacaine did not show any effect on uterine tone in pregnant ewes.
(2) *Correct.* Terbutaline is a $\beta$-agonist with $\beta_1$ and $\beta_2$ activity. It results in uterine relaxation via its $\beta_2$ effects.
(3) *Incorrect.* Ketamine has been shown to increase uterine contractions, especially in the second trimester. When given closer to delivery (ie, at cesarean section), ketamine has little effect on uterine tone.

(4) *Correct.* Halothane and all other volatile agents cause a dose-dependent decrease in uterine tone and are useful for situations requiring uterine relaxation as with retained placenta.

**REASONING:**
This question tests knowledge of the pharmacologic effects of various anesthetics on uterine tone. Choices 2 and 4 are agents used commonly to provide uterine relaxation in obstetric practice and therefore are correct. The reader must determine whether the remaining two choices are correct in order to differentiate between answers E and C. Epidural lidocaine does not decrease uterine contractility, which eliminates both choices 1 and 3 (alternatively, if the reader knows that ketamine does not provide uterine relaxation, choice 1 could be eliminated). The best answer is C.

**BIBLIOGRAPHY:**
Chestnut DH, Polley LS, Lawrence CT, Wong CA. *Chestnut's Obstetric Anesthesia Principles and Practice.* 4th ed. St. Louis, MO: Mosby; 2009:256, 758-759.
Morgan GE, Mikhail MS, Murray MJ. *Clinical Anesthesiology.* 4th ed. New York, MY: McGraw-Hill; 2006:883-884.

---

**BOOK B:**

*Answer B*

Neuroanesthesia

**QUESTION 139**

**QUESTION (K-type):**
During induction of anesthesia for removal of a large intracranial tumor, effects of adding 1 MAC of isoflurane at normocarbia include

(1) Decreased cerebral metabolic rate.
(2) Attenuated cerebrovascular response to $Paco_2$.
(3) Increased intracranial pressure.
(4) Abolished cerebral autoregulation.

**CORRECT ANSWER: B (1 and 3 are correct.)**

**SUMMARY:**
*The effect of inhalational agents on cerebral metabolic activity and blood flow is important to consider during neuroanesthesia. Isoflurane increases CBF and thus ICP at higher concentrations (most prominently above 1 MAC, but the changes occur in a dose-dependent manner). Isoflurane also reduces cerebral metabolic oxygen requirements in a dose-dependent manner and produces a silent EEG at 2 MAC. It also impairs autoregulation in a dose-dependent manner, but at 1 MAC autoregulation will not be abolished. The cerebral vasculature will maintain responsiveness to arterial carbon dioxide tension, so hyperventilation will help offset the increased CBF with high MAC levels.*

**EXPLANATION:**
(1) *Correct.* Isoflurane administration results in a decrease in CMR.
(2) *Incorrect.* The cerebral vasculature maintains its response to carbon dioxide in the presence of volatile anesthetics.
(3) *Correct.* Unless simultaneous hyperventilation is present, cerebral vessels will dilate and increase ICP.
(4) *Incorrect.* 1 MAC of isoflurane will not abolish autoregulation.

**REASONING:**

Choices 1 and 3 are correct, as explained above.


**BIBLIOGRAPHY:**

Morgan GE, Mikhail MS, Murray MJ. *Clinical Anesthesiology*. 4th ed. New York, NY: McGraw-Hill; 2006:168-172.


| **BOOK B:** | **QUESTION 140** |
| --- | --- |

## *Answer A*

### Physiology

**QUESTION (K-type):**

Intraoperative events that may cause an increased arterial to end-tidal carbon dioxide tension difference include

(1)  Pulmonary embolus.
(2)  Induced hypotension.
(3)  Application of positive end-expiratory pressure.
(4)  Atelectasis.


**CORRECT ANSWER: A (1, 2, and 3 are correct.)**


**SUMMARY:**

*End-tidal carbon dioxide tension ($ETco_2$) is clinically used as an estimate of $Paco_2$. The normal gradient between alveolar carbon dioxide tension and end-tidal carbon dioxide is 5 mm Hg. This gradient is due to the dilution of alveolar gas with carbon dioxide from alveolar and anatomic dead space. Increases in the $Paco_2$–$PETco_2$ are seen with decreases in lung perfusion or increases in alveolar dead space. Dead space refers to lung units that are ventilated but not perfused. Significant decreases in lung perfusion will increase this gradient as seen with air embolism, decreased cardiac output, decreased blood pressure, or upright position. Furthermore, increases in alveolar dead space will also increase this gradient. PEEP can actually increase alveolar dead space by overdistending alveoli, mimicking a West zone 1 scenario. Other factors that increase dead space include neck extension, increasing age, positive-pressure ventilation, anticholinergic drugs, and emphysema.*


**EXPLANATION:**

(1)  ***Correct.*** See above.
(2)  ***Correct.*** See above.
(3)  ***Correct.*** See above.
(4)  ***Incorrect.*** Atelectasis or collapse of alveoli decreases dead space and therefore would decrease arterial to $ETco_2$ differences.


**REASONING:**

To answer this question correctly, one must remember that increases arterial to end-tidal carbon dioxide differences can be achieved with either decreases in lung perfusion or increases in alveolar ventilation.


**BIBLIOGRAPHY:**

Morgan GE, Mikhail MS, Murray MJ. *Clinical Anesthesiology*. 4th ed. New York, NY: McGraw-Hill; 2006:111-112, 501.

*Answer C*

OB/Regional

**QUESTION (K-type):**

Factors that decrease beat-to-beat variability of the fetal heart rate include

(1)  Epidural administration of lidocaine.
(2)  Maternal hypotension.
(3)  Intravenous administration of ephedrine.
(4)  Intravenous administration of glycopyrrolate.

**CORRECT ANSWER: (Only 2 is correct and there is no corresponding letter.)**

**SUMMARY:**

*Fetal heart rate (FHR) monitoring is the most widely available method for assessing fetal status during pregnancy and labor. One of the most important parameters is beat-to-beat variability. Variability is measured clinically by visual recognition of a "wavy baseline" that normally has an amplitude range of 5 to 25 bpm. It represents an intact pathway between the fetal CNS, vagus nerve, and cardiac conduction system. Minimal variability alone usually is unrelated to fetal academia. However, loss of variability in association with tachycardia or decelerations is the most sensitive indicator of metabolic acidosis. Conditions associated with decreased variability include fetal sleep state, congenital neurologic or cardiac abnormalities, severe asphyxia, extreme prematurity, and idiopathic causes. Drugs known to decrease variability include opiates, general anesthesia, barbiturates, diazepam, and phenothiazines.*

**EXPLANATION:**

(1)  *Incorrect.* Epidural lidocaine has not been shown to change beat-to-beat variability; however, bupivacaine has been shown to cause transient abnormalities in FHR and beat-to-beat variability.

(2)  *Correct.* Persistent maternal hypotension can lead to decreased oxygen delivery to the fetus. This can result in asphyxia and lead to decreased beat-to-beat variability.

(3)  *Incorrect.* Ephedrine is an indirect- and direct-acting sympathomimetic drug and increases FHR and beat-to-beat variability.

(4)  *Incorrect.* Parasympatholytic drugs such as atropine and glycopyrrolate have been shown to increase maternal heart rate, but they have no effect on fetal beat-to-beat variability.

**REASONING:**

A compromised fetus has decreased beat-to-beat variability. Maternal hypotension leads to decreased oxygen delivery, so choice 2 is correct. In the absence of hypotension, epidural lidocaine does not cause fetal depression or decreased oxygen delivery. Choice 1, therefore, is incorrect. For many years, including the time frame when these questions were published, ephedrine was the drug of choice for treatment of maternal hypotension. Because of concerns associated with decreased fetal umbilical pH representing fetal metabolic acidosis, presumably due to increased fetal metabolism, ephedrine is no longer the favored drug for treatment of maternal hypotension. Ephedrine causes increased fetal beat-to-beat variability, which is likely due to increased fetal metabolism. Therefore, this section of this question is dated and no longer valid, making choice 3 incorrect. Parasympatholytics have been shown to increase maternal heart rate, but no change in FHR or variability; therefore choice D is incorrect as well.

**BIBLIOGRAPHY:**

Abboud TK, Khoo SS, Miller F, Doan T, Henriksen EH. Maternal, fetal, and neonatal responses after epidural anesthesia with bupivacaine, 2-chloroprocaine, or lidocaine. *Anesth Analg.* 1982 Aug;61(8):638-644.

Abboud T, Raya J, Sadri S, Grobler N, Stine L, Miller F. Fetal and maternal cardiovascular effects of atropine and glycopyrrolate. A*nesth Analg.* 1983 Apr;62(4):426-430.

Chestnut DH, Polley LS, Tsen LC, Wong CA. *Chestnut's Obstetric Anesthesia Principles and Practice.* 4th ed. Philadelphia, PA: Mosby Elsevier; 2009:143-144.

Ngan Kee WD. Placental transfer and fetal metabolic effects of phenylephrine and ephedrine during spinal anesthesia for cesarean delivery. *Anesthesiology.* 2009;111(3):506-512.

Ngan Kee WD. Prevention of maternal hypotension after regional anaesthesia for caesarean section, *Curr Opin Anaesthesiol.* 2010;23(3):304-309.

Wright RG, Shnider SM, Levinson G, Rolbin SH, Parer JT. The effect of maternal administration of ephedrine on fetal heart rate and variability. *Obstet Gynecol.* 1981 Jun;57(6):734-738.

---

## BOOK B: QUESTION 142

*Answer C*

Pain

**QUESTION (K-type):**

Neural fibers that transmit pain include

(1) B fibers.
(2) C fibers.
(3) Aα fibers.
(4) Aδ fibers.

**CORRECT ANSWER: C (2 and 4 are correct.)**

**SUMMARY:**

*In mammals, nerve fibers are divided in A, B, and C groups. The A group has four subdivisions, namely α (alpha), ß (beta), γ (gamma), and δ (delta). Pain information is transmitted within the nervous system by either small unmyelinated C fibers (nociception) or myelinated Aδ fibers (high-threshold mechanoreceptors). The stimulation of C fibers generates a dull, aching, and poorly localized pain. Aδ fibers transmit a sharp, well-localized pain. Aα fibers are large myelinated motor neurons, and B fibers are preganglionic myelinated sympathetic fibers.*

**EXPLANATION:**

(1) *Incorrect.* B fibers are preganglionic sympathetic fibers and do not carry pain signals.
(2) *Correct.* C fibers are unmyelinated (therefore slow) small nerves that carry pain, temperature, and some mechanoreception.
(3) *Incorrect.* Aα fibers are myelinated large (therefore fast) axons carrying somatic motor, and proprioception.
(4) *Correct.* Aδ fibers transmit pain, cold temperature, and touch signals.

**REASONING:**

This question is a straight-forward anatomy, checking facts without any extra challenge. It shows the importance of mastering the basic knowledge for the examination.

**BIBLIOGRAPHY:**

Miller RD, Eriksson LI, Fleisher LA, Wiener-Kronish JP, William YL. *Miller's Anesthesia.* 7th ed. Philadelphia, PA: Churchill Livingstone; 2009:2519-2521.

Morgan GE, Mikhail MS, Murray MJ. *Clinical Anesthesiology.* 4th ed. New York, NY: McGraw-Hill; 2006:218, 276-283.

Vadivelu N, Urman RD, Hines RL. *Essentials of Pain Management.* New York, NY: Springer; 2011:31-35.

---

| **BOOK B:** | **QUESTION 143 (OPTIONAL)** |
|---|---|

## *Answer A*

### Basic Science

**QUESTION (K-type):**

Gas flow through an endotracheal tube is

(1)  Directly related to the change in pressure along the length of the tube.
(2)  Inversely related to the viscosity of the gas.
(3)  Inversely related to the length of the tube.
(4)  Directly related to the square of the radius of the tube.

**CORRECT ANSWER: A (1, 2, and 3 are correct.)**

**SUMMARY:**

*Laminar flow, where the gas flow has a predictable flow velocity profile (with velocity highest in the center and decreasing parabolically toward the periphery), is represented by the equation:*

$$Flow = \frac{pressure\ gradient}{airway\ resistance}$$

*where airway resistance is given by the equation:*

$$Airway\ resistance = \frac{8 \times length \times gas\ viscosity}{Pi \times (radius)\,4}$$

*Factors favoring laminar flow include a low flow velocity, low viscosity, and large diameter of the receptacle. High flow through irregular, branched, or small tubes results in turbulent flow. In turbulent flow, the relationship between flow versus the pressure gradient and radius are nonlinear.*

$$Flow\,2 = \frac{pressure\ gradient \times radius\,5}{gas\ density}$$

**EXPLANATION:**

(1)  *Correct.* Flow is proportional to the pressure gradient in laminar flow.
(2)  *Correct.* Airway resistance is proportional to viscosity. Flow is inversely related to airway resistance and thus inversely related to viscosity.
(3)  *Correct.* Airway resistance is proportional to length. Flow is inversely related to airway resistance and thus inversely related to viscosity.
(4)  *Incorrect.* Flow is proportional to the fourth power of the radius.

**REASONING:**

This problem requires us to assume laminar flow, as if turbulent flow were assumed, none of the answer choices would be correct. Knowing the relationship flow = pressure/resistance and knowing the factors affecting resistance in laminar flow, we can see that choices 1, 2, and 3 are correct.

**BIBLIOGRAPHY:**
Barash PG, Cullen BF, Stoelting RK, Cahalan M, Stock M. *Clinical Anesthesia*. 6th ed. Philadelphia, PA: Lippincott Williams & Wilkins; 2010:795.
Morgan GE, Mikhail MS, Murray MJ. *Clinical Anesthesiology*. 4th ed. New York, NY: McGraw-Hill; 2006:546.

---

**BOOK B:**

*Answer C*

Pharmacology

**QUESTION 144**

**QUESTION (K-type):**

Hetastarch

(1)  Produces a hypercoagulable state.
(2)  Complicates blood cross-matching.
(3)  Is contraindicated in patients with diabetes mellitus.
(4)  Is metabolized by amylase.

**CORRECT ANSWER: C (2 and 4 are correct.)**

**SUMMARY:**

*Hetastarch, or hydroxyethyl starch is a synthetic colloid. A hemodilution of more than 30% with hetastarch has been shown to affect platelet function and fibrin formation, thus leading to a state of hypocoagulation. Furthermore, hetastarch complicates blood cross-matching. Larger molecules require amylase to be broken down. Hetastarch does not significantly affect blood glucose levels and is not contraindicated in diabetics.*

**EXPLANATION:**

(1)  *Incorrect.* Hetastarch causes hypocoagulation via a dilution of coagulation factors, interfering with factor VIII, platelet dysfunction, and ultimately decreased fibrin meshwork formation. Hetastarch coats the surface of platelets, "reducing the availability of the functional receptor for fibrinogen on the platelet surface."
(2)  *Correct.* Increased rouleaux formation of hetastarch-containing blood samples has been shown to cause difficulties in the interpretation of typing and screening of blood samples in the blood bank.
(3)  *Incorrect.* Studies done on diabetic and nondiabetic rats have shown that hetastarch does not cause or aggravate hyperglycemia. One could assume that this data is transferable to humans.
(4)  *Correct.* Smaller molecules of hetastarch can be eliminated directly by the kidneys, while larger ones must be degraded by amylase first.

**REASONING:**

This is a relatively straightforward question if one knows about the clinical effects and metabolism of synthetic colloids. Clinically, the main point about hetastarch is that it does interfere with factor VIII-platelet interaction and prolong bleeding times. Thus, in a patient who is actively bleeding, some anesthesiologists would prefer to use albumin for volume expansion rather than hetastarch.

**BIBLIOGRAPHY:**
Barash PG, Cullen BF, Stoelting RK. *Clinical Anesthesia*. 3rd ed. Philadelphia, PA: Lippincott-Raven Publishers; 1997:168.
Daniels MJ, Strauss RG, Smith-Floss AM. Effects of hydroxyethyl starch on erythrocyte typing and blood crossmatching. *Transfusion*. 1982 May-Jun;22(3):226-228.

Franz A, Bräunlich P, Gamsjäger T, Felfernig M, Gustorff B, Kozek-Langenecker SA. The effects of hydroxyethyl starches of varying molecular weight on platelet function. *Anesth Analg.* 2001 Jun;92(6):1402-1407.

Hofer RE, Lanier WL. Effect of hydroxyethyl starch solutions on blood glucose concentrations in diabetic and nondiabetic rats. *Crit Care Med.* 1992 Feb;20(2):211-215.

Mishler JM. Pharmacological effects produced by the acute and chronic administration of hydroxyethyl starch. *J Clin Apheresis.* 1984;2(1):52-62. http://www.drugs.com/pro/hetastarch.html.

Morgan GE, Mikhail MS, Murray MJ. *Clinical Anesthesiology.* 4th ed. New York, NY: McGraw-Hill; 2006:630.

---

**BOOK B:**      **QUESTION 145 (OPTIONAL)**

---

*Answer A*

Physiology

**QUESTION (K-type):**

During pelvic laparoscopy under epidural anesthesia, the patient is placed in the Trendelenburg position, and the abdomen is distended by insufflation of carbon dioxide. Anticipated responses include

(1) Hyperpnea to maintain normal minute ventilation.
(2) Pain despite sensory block to T4.
(3) Decreased venous return and cardiac output.
(4) Metabolic acidosis from absorption of carbon dioxide.

**CORRECT ANSWER: A (1, 2, and 3 are correct.)**

**SUMMARY:**

*Laparoscopic surgery is made possible by the creation of a pneumoperitoneum using insufflation of carbon dioxide gas. This pneumoperitoneum has many important physiologic and metabolic consequences. First, carbon dioxide is absorbed by the abdominal vasculature because it is highly soluble. This can lead to higher arterial carbon dioxide levels and a resulting respiratory acidosis. The increase in intra-abdominal pressure (IAP) from the pneumoperitoneum results in cephalad displacement of the diaphragm, leading to decreased lung compliance and increased PIPs. The Trendelenburg position also contributes to the resulting atelectasis, decreased compliance, decreased FRC, and increased ventilation-perfusion mismatch that leads to impaired arterial oxygenation. Expected cardiovascular consequences of pneumoperitoneum with high insufflation pressures include decreased preload (compression of the abdominal IVC) and cardiac output. While laparoscopic surgery is performed most commonly under general anesthesia, other anesthetics have been used, such as local anesthesia with monitored anesthesia care or neuraxial blockade. A patient undergoing laparoscopic surgery using an epidural or spinal technique requires a high level of blockade to facilitate complete muscle relaxation and the prevention of diaphragmatic irritation.*

**EXPLANATION:**

(1) ***Possibly correct.*** Increased IAP from pneumoperitoneum and Trendelenburg position contributes to decreased tidal volumes. Hyperpnea can help maintain normal minute ventilation (MV). However, increased $Paco_2$ from insufflation with $CO_2$ gas will increase the ventilatory drive. An *increased* MV is expected.

(2) ***Correct.*** A T2 level is needed to optimize muscle relaxation and prevent diaphragmatic irritation. Diaphragmatic irritation sometimes can present as referred shoulder pain.

(3) ***Correct.*** Insufflation is associated with a transient increase in venous return followed by an impedance of flow. Cardiac output decreases proportionately with IAP. One study found a 30% reduction in cardiac index (CI) after insufflation to 15 mm Hg.

(4) **Incorrect.** Carbon dioxide is highly absorbable via the peritoneal vasculature and can result in a respiratory acidosis, not metabolic acidosis.


### REASONING:

This question tests knowledge of the physiologic changes associated with laparoscopy and pneumoperitoneum. It is somewhat challenging because choice 1 is not entirely correct. Decreased tidal volumes requiring hyperpnea to maintain normal MV might be anticipated as a consequence of increased IAP and Trendelenburg positioning. However, it is not entirely clear that normal MV should be anticipated because increased $Paco_2$ from the pneumoperitoneum should increase the ventilatory drive and MV. Most readers would find choices 2 and 3 correct, providing additional confidence that choice 1 is also correct. Therefore, A is the best answer.


### BIBLIOGRAPHY:

Barash PG, Cullen BF, Stoelting RK. *Clinical Anesthesia.* 4th ed. Philadelphia, PA: Lippincott Williams & Wilkins; 2001;1058-1061.

Morgan GE, Mikhail MS, Murray MJ. *Clinical Anesthesiology.* 3rd ed. New York, NY: McGraw-Hill; 2002:522-524.

Westerband A, Van De Water J, Amzallag M, et al. Cardiovascular changes during laparoscopic cholecystectomy. *Surg Gynecol Obstet.* 1992;175(6):535-538.


## BOOK B:  QUESTION 146

## *Answer A*

## Cardiovascular

### QUESTION (K-type):

When triggered by the R wave, the intra-aortic balloon pump is likely to be ineffective with

(1) Prolonged use of electrocautery.
(2) Development of rapid atrial fibrillation.
(3) Sudden onset of aortic regurgitation.
(4) Sudden onset of mitral regurgitation.


**CORRECT ANSWER: A (1, 2, and 3 are correct.)**


### SUMMARY:

*To provide optimal counterpulsation, an intra-aortic balloon pump (IABP) should be inflated right after the dichrotic notch, to augment diastolic blood pressure and thus coronary blood flow. IABP is contraindicated in patients with acute or severe aortic regurgitation as the increased diastolic pressure may worsen the magnitude of regurgitation. The deflation just prior to systole decreases myocardial oxygen consumption and improves forward flow by afterload reduction. Errors in the timing of an IABP can be as seen with conditions that alter the ECG or rhythm, such as electrocautery artifacts on ECG, rapid heart rates, and dysrhythmias.*


### EXPLANATION:

(1) **Correct.** Prolonged use of electrocautery would distort the ECG and result in improper timing of the IABP.
(2) **Correct.** Rapid atrial fibrillation also would distort the ECG and result in improper timing of the IABP.
(3) **Correct.** The use of an IABP may exacerbate acute aortic regurgitation as inflation of the balloon during diastole would worsen the regurgitant fraction into the left ventricle.

(4) *Incorrect.* The management of mitral regurgitation includes improving forward flow, which is what occurs when the IABP deflates during systole.


**REASONING:**

Choices 1, 2, and 3 are correct, and 4 is clearly incorrect as explained above. The answer is thus A.


**BIBLIOGRAPHY:**

Morgan GE, Mikhail MS, Murray MJ. *Clinical Anesthesiology*. 4th ed. New York, NY: McGraw-Hill; 2006:516-517.

---

**BOOK B:** | **QUESTION 147**

---

*Answer D*

Cardiovascular

**QUESTION (K-type):**

An asymptomatic 40-year-old woman with a systolic click and a late systolic murmur is scheduled for total abdominal hysterectomy. Anesthetic considerations include the following:

(1) Prophylactic antibiotics are recommended.
(2) Intraoperative fluid restriction is indicated.
(3) Myocardial depressant inhalational agents are contraindicated.
(4) The patient is predisposed to tachyarrhythmias.


**CORRECT ANSWER: D (4 only is correct.)**


**SUMMARY:**

*Mitral valve prolapse (MVP) is the most common valvular disorder of the heart and occurs in 5% to 17% of otherwise healthy individuals. Most patients are asymptomatic but can present with palpitations, syncope, shortness of breath, and atypical chest pain. There is a higher incidence in females. The only clinical finding may be a midsystolic click, with or without the late systolic murmur of mitral regurgitation. Anesthetic considerations include maintaining adequate preload and prevention of sympathetic stimulation, which can accentuate left ventricular emptying and worsen the severity of MVP. These patients are also at risk for dysrhythmias. Supraventricular arrhythmias occur in more than 50% of patients, and ventricular arrhythmias occur in 45% of these patients. Prophylaxis for infective endocarditis is no longer recommended.*

(1) *Incorrect.* Prophylaxis for infective endocarditis is no longer recommended. Patients with MVP benefit from antibiotics as prophylaxis against endocarditis.
(2) *Incorrect.* These patients need to have adequate preload and benefit from fluid loading.
(3) *Incorrect.* There is no contraindication to inhalational agents. Good depth of anesthesia can help prevent a sympathetic response to surgical stimulus and the tachyarrhythmias associated with increased sympathetic stimulation in these patients. Myocardial depression by inhalational agents is not a specific concern for these patients. Increased myocardial contractility actually can exacerbate the severity of MVP by facilitating left ventricular emptying.
(4) *Correct.* Patients with MVP are at increased risk of supraventricular, ventricular, and bradyarrhythmias, and this may explain the observed sudden cardiac death in some of these patients.

**REASONING:**

This question tests knowledge of the mechanism of mitral regurgitation (MR) in MVP and the anesthetic implications and pathophysiology associated with MVP. The important anesthetic implications for patients with MVP are to ensure maintenance of normovolemia and avoid factors that increase left ventricular emptying (ie, sympathetic stimulation, increased myocardial contractility, tachycardia, prolonged afterload reduction). The best answer is D.

**BIBLIOGRAPHY:**

Miller RD, Miller ED, Reves JG, et al. *Anesthesia.* 7th ed. Philadelphia, PA: Churchill Livingstone; 2010:1016.

Morgan GE, Mikhail MS, Murray MJ. *Clinical Anesthesiology.* 3rd ed. New York, NY: McGraw-Hill; 2002:414-416.

---

## BOOK B:        QUESTION 148

*Answer B*

OB/Regional

**QUESTION (K-type):**

A 24-year-old woman who is receiving magnesium sulfate for severe preeclampsia requires emergency cesarean delivery. True statements concerning succinylcholine-induced muscle relaxation in this patient include the following:

(1) It will be potentiated by the magnesium sulfate.
(2) Fasciculations will be absent following succinylcholine administration.
(3) It will be prolonged.
(4) It can be antagonized by calcium chloride.

**CORRECT ANSWER: B (1 and 3 are correct.)**

**SUMMARY:**

*Magnesium sulfate is used in obstetrics for seizure prophylaxis in patients with preeclampsia and for tocolysis in those with preterm labor. It acts at the cellular level, decreasing nerve transmission and uterine activity and antagonizing the effects of calcium on smooth muscle cells. Profound muscular weakness results from decreased release of acetylcholine and sensitivity of the motor end plate to acetylcholine. Patients receiving magnesium treatment who require neuromuscular blockade for cesarean section or other surgical procedures have increased sensitivity to depolarizing and nondepolarizing neuromuscular blockade. Other side effects of magnesium include pulmonary edema, altered sensorium, respiratory paralysis, impaired cardiac conduction, and even death.*

**EXPLANATION:**

(1) ***Correct.*** Patients receiving magnesium have increased sensitivity to nondepolarizing and depolarizing neuromuscular blocking drugs owing to decreased neuromuscular transmission at the motor end plate and excitability of the muscle membrane. However, studies in preeclamptic and normal patients receiving magnesium demonstrate that the initial intubating dose required should not be changed in the presence of magnesium.

(2) ***Incorrect.*** The incidence of succinylcholine-induced fasciculations is decreased in parturients. However, fasciculations are not eliminated completely, even in the presence of magnesium. In a recent study comparing vecuronium, magnesium, and saline, magnesium was associated with the lowest fasciculation scores. It did not eliminate fasciculations completely.

(3) ***Correct.*** Prolongation of succinylcholine in patients receiving magnesium is due to development of a phase II block and is most common with repeated doses of succinylcholine or continuous infusion of magnesium.

(4) ***Incorrect.*** Calcium antagonizes the effects of magnesium, but it has not been shown to antagonize the effects of succinylcholine.

### REASONING:

This question is difficult because it addresses controversial topics in clinical obstetric anesthesia, many of which have been studied in animals but not humans. The important point to remember is that magnesium alters neuromuscular transmission, prolonging the effects of depolarizing and nondepolarizing muscle relaxants. This makes choices 1 and 3 correct. As a general rule, it is best to avoid statements such as those in choice 2 ("will be absent"), and indeed, this statement is incorrect. Choice 4 is incorrect because calcium only antagonizes magnesium. The best answer is B.

### BIBLIOGRAPHY:


Bucklin B, Gambling DR, Wlody DJ. *A Practical Approach to Obstetric Anesthesia.* Philadelphia, PA: Lippincott Williams & Wilkins; 2009:356-357.

Morgan GE, Mikhail MS, Murray MJ. *Clinical Anesthesiology.* 4th ed. New York, NY: McGraw-Hill; 2006:884.

Sakuraba S. Pretreatment with magnesium sulfate is associated with less succinylcholine-induced fasciculation and subsequent tracheal intubation-induced hemodynamic changes than precurarization with vecuronium during rapid sequence induction. *Acta Anaesthesiol Belg.* 2006;57(3):253-257.


---

**BOOK B:**      **QUESTION 149 (OPTIONAL)**

---

*Answer D*

Neuroanesthesia

QUESTION (K-type)

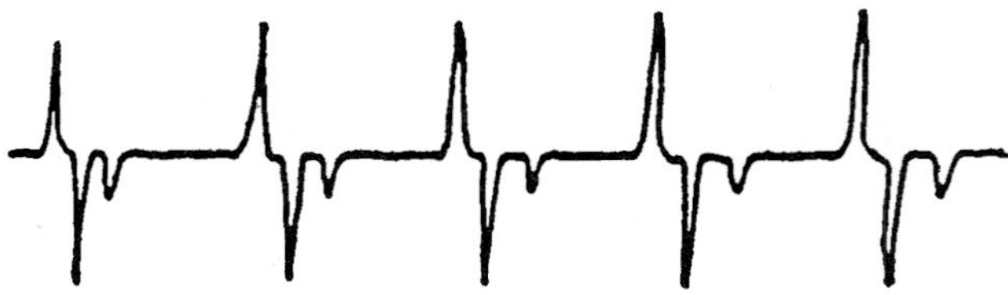

**Figure 1** Transition from normal P wave (arrows) to intra-atrial P waves (P-atriale). (*Source: Corsten et al [1994].*)

During posterior fossa surgery in the sitting position

(1) A single-lumen central venous catheter should display the ECG shown above.

(2) Pulmonary artery occlusion pressures greater than 10 mm Hg prevent paradoxical air embolism.

(3) If venous air embolism occurs, pulmonary artery pressure increases before precordial Doppler sounds change.

(4) If venous air embolism occurs, aspiration of air from the distal lumen of a pulmonary artery catheter is less effective than aspiration from a multiorificed central venous catheter.

**CORRECT ANSWER: D (4 only is correct.)**

**SUMMARY:**

*Venous air embolism (VAE) is a concern whenever the operative site is above the level of the heart such as the sitting position during a craniotomy, as the venous pressure is less than atmospheric pressure favoring intravascular entry of gas. A VAE of sufficient size may present with hemodynamic collapse due to impaired filling and the creation of an air lock that impairs the transmission of fluid pressure, and can be sensitively detected by TEE or precordial Doppler. If a VAE is suspected, treatment includes irrigating and packing the operative site, administering 100% oxygen, as well as aspiration of the entrained air through a right atrial catheter. Central lines are placed during craniotomies for infusion of vasoactive substances. The optimal position of the CVP is at the junction of the superior vena cava and the right atrium. A multiorifice catheter central venous catheter may be superior to single-orifice pulmonary artery catheter for aspiration.*

*The ECG technique is an old and infrequently used technique introduced in 1949 to determine the position of the tip of a central venous catheter. This technique involves the attachment of the ECG lead to the tip of the catheter. The P wave becomes peaked (P-atriale) as the catheter enters the right atrium, because of the adjacent atrial wall tissue that increases the voltage of the P wave (Figure 1). Once the P-atriale is seen, the catheter can be withdrawn 3 cm, or until a normal P wave is observed, which would leave the tip at the junction of the SVC and right atrium*


**EXPLANATION:**

(1) ***Incorrect.*** As explained above, the tip of the catheter in the ECG technique should be withdrawn slightly after a peaked P wave (P atriale) is shown, indicating that the tip is in the right atrium. The ECG in the question shows what appears to be a P atriale (perhaps in $V_1$) and the catheter is not in the ideal position.

(2) ***Incorrect.*** Paradoxical air embolism can occur in patients with patent foramen ovales when the right atrial pressure is greater than the left atrial pressure. An intra-arterial pressure of 10 $cmH_2O$ or greater may lead to paradoxical air embolism.

(3) ***Incorrect.*** The most sensitive indicators of intracardiac air is the precordial Doppler, which will first demonstrate an erratic high-pitched swishing roar and can detect 0.05 mL/kg of air, and TEE, which can detect as little as 0.02 mL/kg of air. Elevated pulmonary artery pressure may develop later, and a pulmonary artery catheter is thus much less sensitive (requiring 0.25 mL/kg of air for detection). Other findings characteristic of VAE occur later. Changes in end-tidal nitrogen concentrations occur before the decrease in end-tidal $P_{CO_2}$ and increased pulmonary artery pressures. The classic "mill wheel" or "drumlike" murmur is a late sign of VAE indicating cardiovascular decompensation.

(4) ***Correct.*** Right atrial multiorifice catheters allow for larger volumes of intracardiac air to be aspirated as opposed to pulmonary artery catheters that have a very small lumen.

**REASONING:**

Although the efficacy of aspiration attempts through a central multiorifice catheter versus a pulmonary artery catheter has not been clinically proven in the primary literature (and would depend on the location of the intracardiac air bubble), choices 1, 2, and 3 are clearly incorrect. Choice 4, and thus D, is the best answer.

**BIBLIOGRAPHY:**

Corsten SA, van Dijk B, Bakker NC, de Lange JJ, Scheffer GJ. Central venous catheter placement using the ECG-guided Cavafix-Certodyn SD catheter. *J Clin Anesth.* 1994;6:469-472.

Hoffman MA, Langer JC, Pearl RH, Filler RM. Electrocardiographic guided placement of central venous catheters. *Br J Surg.* 1989 Oct;76:1032-1033.

Mirski MA, Lele AV, Fitzsimmons L, Toung TJ. Diagnosis and treatment of vascular air embolism. *Anesthesiology.* 2007;106:164-177.

Morgan GE, Mikhail MS, Murray MJ. *Clinical Anesthesiology.* 4th ed. New York, NY: McGraw-Hill; 2006:638-639.

## Answer C

### Clinical Anesthesia

**QUESTION (K-type):**

A patient undergoing strabismus repair develops acute bradycardia during traction on an eye muscle. This response is

(1)  Mediated by a facial nerve afferent.
(2)  Also manifested by ventricular ectopy.
(3)  Prevented by preanesthetic intramuscular administration of atropine.
(4)  Treated by stopping the surgical stimulus.

**CORRECT ANSWER: C (2 and 4 correct.)**

**SUMMARY:**

*The oculocardiac reflex occurs with traction on extraocular muscles or pressure applied to the ocular globe, through a trigeminal afferent ($V_1$) and a vagal efferent pathway. This reflex is commonly seen in pediatric patients undergoing strabismus surgery, but it can occur in all patient populations undergoing a variety of ophthalmologic procedures such as enucleation, cataract extraction, retinal detachment repair, and even placement of a retrobulbar block. Bradycardia is a common presentation, but other forms of cardiac dysrhythmias such as ventricular ectopy, sinus arrest, or ventricular fibrillation are possible. Awake patients may present with somnolence or nausea. One of the first steps in managing cardiac dysrhythmias associated with this reflex is to temporarily cease surgical stimulus immediately.*

**EXPLANATION:**

(1)  *Incorrect.* The afferent pathway is via the trigeminal nerve, and the efferent pathway is via the vagus.
(2)  *Correct.* The oculocardiac reflex can elicit a wide variety of cardiac dysrhythmias such as ventricular ectopy.
(3)  *Incorrect.* Intramuscular premedication with anticholinergics is not as effective as intravenous administration in the prevention of the oculocardiac reflex; the need for routine prophylaxis is controversial, and it cannot ensure the lack of an arrhythmias or bradycardia.
(4)  *Correct.* Intraoperative management of the oculocardiac reflex includes supportive care, cessation of surgical stimulus, administration of anticholinergics, and infiltration of the rectus muscles with local anesthetics.

**REASONING:**

As explained above, the oculocardiac reflex can cause ventricular ectopy (choice 2) and can be immediately treated by cessation of surgical stimulus (choice 4).

**BIBLIOGRAPHY:**
Morgan GE, Mikhail MS, Murray MJ. *Clinical Anesthesiology*. 4th ed. New York, NY: McGraw-Hill; 2006:828.

## *Answer A*

### Clinical Anesthesia

**QUESTION (K-type):**

In a patient treated with propranolol and phenoxybenzamine prior to resection of a solitary pheochromocytoma, factors contributing to postoperative hypotension include

(1) Residual $\alpha$-adrenergic block.
(2) Heart failure.
(3) Residual $\beta$-adrenergic block.
(4) Adrenal insufficiency.

**CORRECT ANSWER: A (1, 2, and 3 are correct.)**

**SUMMARY:**

*Pheochromocytomas are norepinephrine- and epinephrine-secreting tumors of chromaffin tissues; 90% originate in the adrenal medulla. The clinical symptoms are related to the effects of catecholamines. $\alpha_1$ Stimulation results in increased peripheral vascular resistance and hypertension (usually sustained, with occasional paroxysmal spikes in blood pressure). There is often corresponding hypovolemia. $\beta_1$ Stimulation results in tachycardia and can cause dysrhythmias and ventricular ectopy. Cardiomyopathy may develop resulting from prolonged $\alpha_1$ and $\beta_1$ stimulation. Prior to resection, these patients are placed on long-acting $\alpha_1$ antagonists (such as phenoxybenzamine) and $\beta$-blockers (given after $\alpha$-blockade to prevent unopposed $\alpha$ stimulation).*

*Hypotension, not hypertension, is the primary problem postresection, and it can occur quite rapidly after resection or venous clamping. Aside from the lack of the extra catecholamine supply, causes of hypotension after pheochromocytoma resection include hypovolemia, prior tolerance to endogenous catecholamines, and persistent adrenergic blockade. Fluid resuscitation and possible adrenergic support with norepinephrine or phenylephrine may be necessary.*

**EXPLANATION:**
(1) *Correct.* Residual $\alpha$-adrenergic blockade can result in post-operative hypotension.
(2) *Correct.* Prolonged exposure to catecholamines can result in catecholamine-induced cardiomyopathy. Furthermore, the increased peripheral vascular resistance predisposes individuals to ventricular hypertrophy and CHF because of increased myocardial work.
(3) *Correct.* Residual $\beta$-blockade can also result in postoperative hypotension.
(4) *Incorrect.* Pheochromocytomas involve the adrenal medulla, which secretes catecholamines. The adrenal cortex, which secretes androgens, mineralocorticoids, and glucocorticoids, remains unaffected. Adrenal insufficiency, in which there would be decreased steroid hormone production, does not thus occur with pheochromocytoma resections.

**REASONING:**

Residual $\alpha$-blockade (choice 1), heart failure (choice 2), and residual $\beta$-blockade (choice 3) can all cause postoperative hypotension. Adrenal insufficiency does not occur with pheochromocytoma or its resection.

**BIBLIOGRAPHY:**

Barash PG, Cullen BF, Stoelting RK, Cahalan M, Stock M. *Clinical Anesthesia*. 6th ed. Philadelphia, PA: Lippincott Williams & Wilkins; 2010:1142-1144.

Morgan GE, Mikhail MS, Murray MJ. *Clinical Anesthesiology*. 4th ed. New York, NY: McGraw-Hill; 2006:254, 812-813.

## Answer B

Physiology

**QUESTION (K-type):**

Anesthesia is induced with isoflurane and nitrous oxide in a patient with low cardiac output. Compared with a patient with normal cardiac function, which of the following will occur?

(1)  Alveolar isoflurane concentration will approach the inspired concentration more rapidly.
(2)  Total uptake of isoflurane will be higher during the first 11 minutes.
(3)  The rate of rise in the alveolar concentration of isoflurane will be affected more than that of nitrous oxide.
(4)  Induction will be slower.

**CORRECT ANSWER: B (1 and 3 are correct.)**

**SUMMARY:**

*Brain tissue concentration determines the clinical effect of inhalational agents. The brain tissue concentration is directly proportional to the partial pressure of the anesthetic in the brain. Brain partial pressure is approximated by alveolar partial pressure of the inhalational agent. Therefore, the clinical effect of an inhalational agent is proportional to the alveolar partial pressure. The greater the uptake of inhalational agent, the greater the difference between inspired and alveolar concentration and the slower the rate of induction. The factors that affect anesthetic uptake are the following: solubility in the blood, alveolar blood flow (cardiac output), and the partial pressure difference between gas in the alveolus and venous blood. The effect of changing cardiac output on rate of induction is more pronounced with soluble inhalational agents. As cardiac output decreases, there will be less uptake of the inhalational agent by the blood, and therefore a quicker rise in the alveolar partial pressure. Because alveolar partial pressure approximates brain tissue concentration of the inhalational agents, this results in a quicker induction in those with low cardiac outputs as compared with those with normal cardiac outputs.*

**EXPLANATION:**

(1)  *Correct.* Alveolar isoflurane concentration approaches inspired concentration more rapidly in low cardiac output states compared with normal cardiac output states. This is because less volatile anesthetic is taken up by the blood in low cardiac output states.
(2)  *Incorrect.* Uptake of isoflurane will be less during low cardiac output states as compared to normal cardiac output states.
(3)  *Correct.* The rate of rise of the alveolar concentration of isoflurane is increased during low cardiac output states for reasons stated above. Nitrous oxide uptake is not significantly affected by changing cardiac output because it is highly insoluble compared to isoflurane.
(4)  *Incorrect.* Induction will be faster. See above.

**REASONING:**

The uptake of a volatile anesthetic is directly proportional to the cardiac output, blood-gas solubility coefficient of the anesthetic in question, and the difference between the alveolar partial pressure of the anesthetic compared to that in the pulmonary capillaries. However, the speed of induction is inversely proportional to the uptake of a volatile anesthetic. Thus, one can mathematically understand the relationship between the factors that contribute to uptake and the speed of induction.

BIBLIOGRAPHY:
Morgan GE, Mikhail MS, Murray MJ. *Clinical Anesthesiology*. 4th ed. New York, NY: McGraw-Hill; 2006:129-130.

---

**BOOK B:**

*Answer C*

Pediatrics

## QUESTION 153 (OPTIONAL)

**QUESTION (K-type):**

Factors associated with postintubation croup in children include

(1) Age less than 3 months.
(2) History of recent upper respiratory infection.
(3) Use of a nasotracheal tube.
(4) Surgery of the head and neck.

**CORRECT ANSWER: C (2 and 4 are correct.)**

**SUMMARY:**

*Pediatric patients are at increased risk for laryngospasm and postintubation. Croup results from glottic or tracheal edema, and in pediatric patients it usually occurs at the level of the cricoid. Postintubation croup is a complication that most commonly affects children ages 1 to 4 years. Factors associated with increased risk include traumatic or repeated intubations, large endotracheal tubes (no leak over 25 cmH$_2$O), prolonged surgery, head and neck procedures, and excessive movement with the tube in place. Unlike laryngospasm, postintubation croup is seen some time after extubation, usually within 3 hours.*

**EXPLANATION:**

(1) *Incorrect.* Postintubation croup occurs most commonly in children 1 to 4 years of age.
(2) *Correct.* A child with an upper respiratory infection (URI) has an irritable airway and is at increased risk for laryngospasm, bronchospasm, postintubation croup, atelectasis, pneumonia, and episodes of desaturation.
(3) *Incorrect.* Use of a nasotracheal tube is not associated with increased risk compared to an orotracheal tube.
(4) *Correct.* Procedures involving the head and neck are known risk factors for postintubation croup.

**REASONING:**

Only choices 2 and 4 are correct, and the correct answer is C. Children younger than 1 year are not independently at increased risk until the ages of 1 to 4 years old—nor is the use of a nasotracheal tube. Most risk factors of postintubation croup include age of 1 to 4 years, traumatic or repeated intubations, large endotracheal tubes, prolonged surgery, head and neck procedures, and excessive movement with the tube in place.

**BIBLIOGRAPHY:**
Cote CJ. *A Practice of Anesthesia for Infants and Children*. 4th ed. Philadelphia, PA: Saunders; 2009:93.
Miller RD, Eriksson LI, Fleisher LA, Wiener-Kronish JP, Young WL. *Miller's Anesthesia*. 7th ed. Philadelphia, PA: Churchill Livingstone; 2010.
Morgan GE, Mikhail MS, Murray MJ. *Clinical Anesthesiology*. 4th ed. New York, NY: McGraw-Hill; 2006:939.
Morgan GE, Mikhail MS, Murray MJ. *Clinical Anesthesiology*. New York, NY: Lange Medical Books/McGraw-Hill Medical Publishing Division; 2006.

*Answer A*

Pharmacology

**QUESTION (K-type):**

True statements concerning the effects of amrinone include the following:

(1)  Systemic vascular resistance is decreased.
(2)  Intracellular levels of cyclic adenosine monophosphate (cAMP) are increased.
(3)  It acts independently of $\beta_1$-adrenergic receptors.
(4)  Simultaneous administration of norepinephrine enhances ventricular dysrhythmias.

**CORRECT ANSWER: A (1, 2, and 3 are correct.)**

**SUMMARY:**

*Amrinone and its newer derivative milrinone are phosphodiesterase type III inhibitors. The clinical effect is positive inotropy with peripheral vasodilation. The mechanism is cAMP mediated. Amrinone acts at the cell membrane and impedes the breakdown of cAMP. As cAMP increases, protein kinase is activated. This promotes the phosphorylation of the sarcoplasmic reticulum. Phosphorylation increases the slow inward movement of calcium current, increasing intracellular calcium stores, thus increasing inotropism in cardiac muscle. In peripheral smooth muscle cells of the vascular system, increased cAMP levels lead to vasodilation.*

**EXPLANATION:**

(1)  ***Correct.*** Amrinone causes peripheral vasodilation, and thus a decrease in systemic vascular resistance should be expected.
(2)  ***Correct.*** See above.
(3)  ***Correct.*** Amrinone acts independently of catecholamine ($\beta/\alpha$) receptors. It is a phosphodiesterase type III inhibitor.
(4)  ***Incorrect.*** Norepinephrine is a direct $\alpha$- and $\beta$-agonist. While administration of norepinephrine with amrinone may prevent vasodilation, there is no evidence to suggest that the combination enhances ventricular dysrhythmias.

**REASONING:**

This is straight forward pharmacology. Important side effects of amrinone include dose-related thrombocytopenia and centrilobular hepatic necrosis. The latter was seen in canine subjects who received high doses over several weeks. Milrinone is a derivative of amrinone with nearly 20 times the potency. It is more widely used in clinical practice today compared to amrinone.

**BIBLIOGRAPHY:**

Barash PG, Cullen BF, Stoelting RK, Cahalan M, Stock M. *Clinical Anesthesia*. 6th ed. Philadelphia, PA: Lippincott Williams & Wilkins; 2010:288.
Morgan GE, Mikhail MS, Murray MJ. *Clinical Anesthesiology*. 4th ed. New York, NY: McGraw-Hill; 2006:317.

*Answer A*

Clinical Anesthesia

**QUESTION (K-type):**

Deflation of a leg tourniquet after 2 hours of inflation decreases

(1) Mixed venous oxygen saturation.
(2) Core temperature.
(3) Systemic vascular resistance.
(4) End-tidal carbon dioxide tension.

**CORRECT ANSWER: A (1, 2, and 3 are correct.)**

**SUMMARY:**

*Tourniquets are often used to minimize the blood loss in peripheral orthopedic procedures. Typically, the tourniquet is inflated to 100 mm Hg above systolic blood pressure. Deleterious effects of tourniquets are time and pressure dependent. Damage to nerves, skeletal muscles, and vessels have all been reported with prolonged usage. According to Barash, "clinical examination, electromyography, and effluent blood analysis all show completely reversible changes for inflations of 1 to 2 hours...." The physiologic changes seen are due to washout of lactic acid and potassium from the isolated limb. Physiologic derangements expected with tourniquet release include (1) transient metabolic acidosis (due to accumulation of lactic acid), (2) increased arterial carbon dioxide tensions (1-8 mm Hg), (3) increase in heart rate (10%-15%), (4) increased serum potassium (5%-10%), and (5) decreased SVR.*

**EXPLANATION:**

(1) ***Correct.*** Mixed venous oxygen tension represents the overall balance between oxygen consumption and oxygen delivery. A decreased mixed oxygen venous tension is seen during periods of increased oxygen consumption or decreased oxygen delivery. After 2 hours of tourniquet time, a patient's ischemic limb is full of cells that are oxygen starved. Once the tourniquet is released, these starving cells will maximally extract oxygen from the arterial blood, resulting in a decreased mixed venous oxygen tension.

(2) ***Correct.*** Reestablishment of circulation to the exsanguinated limb would mix warm blood with that of a cold extremity, thus possibly lowering core body temperature.

(3) ***Correct.*** The transient metabolic acidosis seen with deflation of a leg tourniquet would result in a transient decrease in systemic vascular resistance. Expected cardiovascular changes also include a decrease in CVP and MAP, with an increase in heart rate and propensity for dysrhythmias, the latter exacerbated by electrolyte abnormalities.

(4) ***Incorrect.*** An increase in the $ETCO_2$ would be expected due to the "washout" of acid from the ischemic limb. One would see an increase in MV if the patient is not paralyzed.

**REASONING:**

I could not find any references stating explicitly what happens to core body temperature upon release of the tourniquet. The clinical significance does not seem relevant. The key to this question is to remember what occurs with reperfusion of ischemic tissue, namely acid and potassium washout, and the associated physiologic changes.

**BIBLIOGRAPHY:**

Barash PG, Cullen BF, Stoelting RK, Cahalan M, Stock M. *Clinical Anesthesia*. 6th ed. Philadelphia, PA: Lippincott Williams & Wilkins; 2010:1035.

Morgan GE, Mikhail MS, Murray MJ. *Clinical Anesthesiology*. 4th ed. New York, NY: McGraw-Hill; 2006:498, 500.

## *Answer B*

## Pharmacology

**QUESTION (K-type):**

Compared with those of isoflurane, the respiratory effects of enflurane include

(1) Similar decrease in airway resistance.
(2) Greater attenuation of hypoxic pulmonary vasoconstriction.
(3) Greater increase in Paco$_2$ during spontaneous ventilation at 1 MAC.
(4) Less inhibition of hypoxic ventilatory drive at "MAC awake" concentrations.

**CORRECT ANSWER: B (1 and 3 are correct.)**

**SUMMARY:**

*All volatile anesthetics share similar effects on respiratory physiology. Isoflurane and enflurane cause respiratory depression, inhibit hypoxic pulmonary vasoconstriction, cause bronchodilation, and depress the ventilatory response to hypoxia and hypercarbia and inhibit mucociliary function.*

**EXPLANATION:**

(1) **Correct.** Enflurane and isoflurane have similar effects on bronchomotor tone.
(2) **Incorrect.** All volatile anesthetics in animal models cause inhibition of the hypoxic pulmonary constriction reflex. There does not appear to be a difference between the various agents.
(3) **Correct.** Enflurane causes a more profound respiratory depression at 1 MAC compared with isoflurane.
(4) **Incorrect.** All volatile anesthetics cause equal depression of the hypoxic ventilatory drive even at the "MAC awake" concentration.

**REASONING:**

This is a difficult question because enflurane is not used in modern anesthesia. The important point to remember is that all volatile anesthetics suppress the ventilatory response to hypoxia and hypercarbia. Studies show that the ventilatory response to hypoxia is depressed 15% to 75% with as little as 0.1 MAC of volatile anesthetic. This has important clinical implications for patients recovering from anesthesia.

**BIBLIOGRAPHY:**

Barash PG, Cullen BF, Stoelting RK. *Clinical Anesthesia.* 4th ed. Philadelphia, PA: Lippincott Williams & Wilkins; 2001:387, 399-400.

Hirshman CA, McCullough RE, Cohen PJ, Weil JV. Depression of hypoxic ventilatory response by halothane, enflurane and isoflurane in dogs. *Br J Anaesth.* 1977;49(10): 957-963.

Lindahl SG, Johannesson GP. Ventilatory CO$_2$ response, respiratory drive and timing in children anaesthetized with halothane, enflurane or isoflurane. *Eur J Anaesthesiol.* 1987;4(5):313-326.

Morgan GE, Mikhail MS, Murray MJ. *Clinical Anesthesiology.* 3rd ed. New York, NY: McGraw-Hill; 2002:142-143.

*Answer A*

Pharmacology

**QUESTION (K-type):**

Intravenous drugs that produce central nervous system effects by modulating γ-aminobutyric acid (GABA) receptor activity include

(1)  Midazolam.
(2)  Thiopental.
(3)  Flumazenil.
(4)  Ketamine.

**CORRECT ANSWER: A (1, 2, and 3 are correct.)**

**SUMMARY:**

*γ-Aminobutyric acid (GABA) is an important inhibitory neurotransmitter. Many anesthetics are GABA agonists and enhance the inhibitory effects of GABA, while GABA antagonists reverse some anesthetic affects. Many different types of drugs have an effect on GABA receptor activity. Benzodiazepines bind to a specific receptor in the CNS that facilitates GABA receptor binding. Flumazenil is a specific benzodiazepine receptor antagonist that reverses the CNS effects of benzodiazepines. Barbiturates suppress transmission of excitatory neurotransmitters and enhance transmission of inhibitory neurotransmitters (ie, GABA). In addition, both propofol and etomidate's mechanism of action involves modulating GABA receptor activity. Ketamine is an unique intravenous anesthetic. It causes a dissociative anesthesia by dissociating the thalamus through an N-methyl-D-aspartate (NMDA) receptor antagonism. It does not affect GABA activity.*

**EXPLANATION:**
(1)  ***Correct.*** Midazolam is the most commonly used benzodiazepine in anesthesia. It binds to the benzodiazepine receptor that facilitates GABA binding to its receptor.
(2)  ***Correct.*** Thiopental is the most commonly used barbiturate in anesthesia. Thiopental suppresses transmission of excitatory neurotransmitters and enhances transmission of inhibitory neurotransmitters (ie, GABA).
(3)  ***Correct.*** Flumazenil is a benzodiazepine antagonist with an indirect effect on the GABA receptor by reversing the effect of the benzodiazepines.
(4)  ***Incorrect.*** Ketamine is an NMDA antagonist and has no direct or indirect effects on GABA activity.

**REASONING:**

This questions test your knowledge of the mechanism of action of commonly used intravenous anesthetics. Many anesthetics produce their effects via GABA receptors and it is important to recognize that ketamine is a unique anesthetic with a different mechanism of action. It is also important to remember that benzodiazepines such as midazolam can be reversed by a specific antagonist, flumazenil. This is a pretty straight forward K-type question. Because Midazolam is the most likely correct answer, you can eliminate answers C and D. Because Ketamine does not have GABA activity, you are now down to answers A and B. Because choice 3 is linked to both A and B, it is a freebie. The challenge here is remembering that barbiturates have GABA activity, thus making 1, 2, and 3 correct and making answer A the correct response.

**BIBLIOGRAPHY:**
Barash PG, Cullen BF, Stoelting RK, Cahalan M, Stock M. *Clinical Anesthesia.* 6th ed. Philadelphia, PA: Lippincott Williams & Wilkins; 2009;445, 450-456.

Mihic S, Harris R. Hypnotics and sedatives. In: Brunton LL, Chabner BA, Knollmann BC, eds. *Goodman & Gilman's The Pharmacological Basis of Therapeutics*. 12th ed. New York, NY: McGraw-Hill; 2011:chap 17. Retrieved January 25, 2012 from http://www.accessmedicine.com/content.aspx?aID=16663643.

Miller RD, Eriksson LI, Fleisher LA, et al. *Miller: Miller's Anesthesia*. 7th ed. New York, Churchill Livingstone; 2009. Retrieved on January 25, 2012 from http://www.mdconsult.com/books/linkTo?type=bookPage&isbn=978-0-443-06959-8&eid=4-u1.0-B978-0-443-06959-8..00026-1--s0150.

Morgan GE, Mikhail MS, Murray MJ. *Clinical Anesthesiology*. 4th ed. New York, NY: McGraw-Hill; 2006:156, 160, 169, 184, 187, 197.

---

## BOOK B:

**QUESTION 158**

*Answer A*

Clinical Anesthesia

**QUESTION (K-type):**

Findings consistent with heparin-induced thrombocytopenia include

(1)  Platelet count of 25,000/mm$^3$.
(2)  Subcutaneous route of heparin administration.
(3)  Thrombosis.
(4)  Onset within 4 hours of initiating heparin therapy.

**CORRECT ANSWER: A (1, 2, and 3 are correct.)**

**SUMMARY:**

*Heparin-induced thrombocytopenia (HIT) is an absolute or relative (> 50% reduction) thrombocytopenia in the setting of heparin therapy when other causes of thrombocytopenia have been ruled out. There are two forms. HIT type I is a clinically inconsequential form that usually occurs within 4 days of starting heparin, is non–immune-mediated, results in a milder thrombocytopenia, and usually resolves spontaneously despite continuing on heparin. It is thought to be direct effect of heparin on platelets. HIT type II usually occurs between days 5 and 14 of heparin therapy and is caused by an antibody against platelet factor 4. It can result in thrombosis, both venous and arterial, and is thus sometimes referred to as* heparin induced thrombocytopenia/thrombosis (HIT/T). *It is associated with all forms of heparin, including intravenous, subcutaneous, heparin flushes, and even heparin-coated catheters. Once HIT/T is suspected, all forms of heparin should be stopped. The platelet count should rise following discontinuation, but the patient continues to be at risk of thrombotic events. Anticoagulation with an alternative agent such as argatroban, lepirudin, bivalirudin, or fondaparinux should be started with the consultation of a hematologist.*

**EXPLANATION:**

(1)  *Correct.* A platelet count of 25,000/mm$^3$ is likely to represent a 50% decline from baseline.
(2)  *Correct.* All forms of heparin administration have been associated with HIT/T.
(3)  *Correct.* Thrombosis is clinical feature of HIT/T.
(4)  *Incorrect.* It takes several days for HIT/T to occur.

**REASONING:**

This question tests knowledge of the pathophysiology of HIT/T. Because thrombosis is the most correct answer, choices C and D can be eliminated. Because it takes several days of heparin therapy to cause HIT/T, answer E can be eliminated. Because all forms of heparin cause HIT/T, the only correct answer is A.

**BIBLIOGRAPHY:**

Baglin TP. Heparin-induced thrombocytopenia thrombosis (HIT/T) syndrome. *J Clin Pathol.* 2001;54(4):272-274.

Miller RD, Eriksson LI, Fleisher LA, Wiener-Kronish JP, Young WL. *Miller's Anesthesia.* 7th ed. Philadelphia, PA: Churchill Livingstone; 2010:1899-1902.

Morgan GE, Mikhail MS, Murray MJ. *Clinical Anesthesiology.* 4th ed. New York, NY: McGraw-Hill; 2006:450.

---

## BOOK B:  QUESTION 159

*Answer B*

Clinical Anesthesia

**QUESTION (K-type):**

An anephric 12-year-old patient with a large pericardial effusion is to have pericardiocentesis under general anesthesia. Appropriate anesthetic management includes

(1)  Maintenance of a high venous pressure.
(2)  Prevention of tachycardia.
(3)  Avoidance of positive end-expiratory pressure.
(4)  Reduction of systemic vascular resistance.

**CORRECT ANSWER: B (1 and 3 are correct.)**

**SUMMARY:**

*Without evidence to the contrary, one should treat this patient as if they have tamponade physiology. Goals of management include maintenance of high sympathetic tone, which maintains a high venous pressure, relatively high heart rate, and a relatively high afterload. Peep will diminish preload that must remain high and should thus be avoided.*

**EXPLANATION:**

Maintenance of high venous pressure is desirable to maintain filling of the heart in a patient with a large pericardial effusion. The effusion exerts pressure on the right atria, which will prevent diastolic filling unless venous pressures are maintained. Because the effusion impedes diastolic filling, stroke volume is relatively fixed and reductions in heart rate will result in decreased cardiac output and may precipitate cardiac arrest. Increases in airway pressure (like PEEP) will add to the intrathoracic pressure retarding diastolic filling and should be avoided. As diastolic filling limits cardiac output in tamponade, a reduction in systemic vascular resistance will not be met with increased cardiac output and blood pressure may fall precipitously.

**REASONING:**

Choices 1 and 3 are correct while 2 and 4 are wrong. Therefore, answer B is correct. Local anesthesia only, ketamine induction, and maintenance of spontaneous ventilation should be considered.

**BIBLIOGRAPHY:**

Barash PG, Cullen BF, Stoelting RK, Cahalan MK, Stock MC. *Clinical Anesthesia.* 6th ed. Philadelphia, PA: Lippincott Williams & Wilkins; 2009:1102.

Miller RD, Eriksson LI, Fleisher LA, Wiener-Kronish JP, Young WL. *Miller's Anesthesia.* 7th ed. Philadelphia, PA: Churchill Livingstone; 2010:1948-1951.

Morgan GE, Mikhail MS, Murray MJ. *Clinical Anesthesiology.* 4th ed. New York, NY: McGraw-Hill; 2006:526-527, 868.

*Answer D*

Physiology

## QUESTION (K-type):

Reliable indicators of left ventricular function in a patient with severe chronic obstructive pulmonary disease include

(1)  Left ventricular end-diastolic volume.
(2)  Pulmonary artery diastolic pressure (PADP).
(3)  Left atrial pressure (LAP).
(4)  Cardiac index.

## CORRECT ANSWER: D (4 only is correct.)

## SUMMARY:

*Chronic obstructive pulmonary disease (COPD) is characterized by pulmonary maldistribution of ventilation and perfusion giving rise to areas of intrapulmonary shunt and dead space. The evolution of this disease is chronic hypoxemia, erythrocytosis, pulmonary hypertension, and eventual right ventricular failure or cor pulmonale. Left ventricular function may be impaired secondarily, and hemodynamic parameters normally measured by Swan Ganz catheter no longer may be reliable in patients with severe COPD.*

## EXPLANATION:

(1)  *Incorrect.* The left ventricular end-diastolic volume (LVEDV) can be approximated from the left ventricular end-diastolic pressure (LVEDP), assuming normal ventricular compliance. This relationship is no longer reliable in severe COPD owing to the interventricular interdependence between the right and left ventricles. A distended right ventricle pushes on the interventricular septum, altering the left ventricular compliance and function.

(2)  *Incorrect.* PADP is usually within a few millimeters of mercury of pulmonary catheter wedge pressure (PCWP) except in the setting of pulmonary hypertension. (*See also question 123, Book B.*)

(3)  *Incorrect.* LAP is equivalent to LVEDP when there is no obstruction between the ventricle and atrium. Because PCWP is measured when there is no flow from the catheter tip to the left atrium, PCWP = LAP = LVEDP. The possible presence of pulmonary hypertension in severe COPD makes wedging the catheter difficult, and PCWP can be artificially high, making LAP an unreliable indicator of LV function.

(4)  *Correct.* Cardiac index is derived from the cardiac output measured via thermodilution technique. It reflects the rate of blood flow through the pulmonary artery and, by extension, cardiac output by the left ventricle.

## REASONING:

This question tests knowledge of the pathophysiology of COPD and its effects on cardiovascular function. Complications of severe COPD include pulmonary hypertension and right ventricular failure that change the relationship between PCWP, LAP, LVEDP, and LVEDV. Because these parameters are no longer measured reliably, they are poor indicators of left ventricular function. Cardiac index that is calculated by thermodilution technique is least affected. Thus only choice 4 or D is correct.

## BIBLIOGRAPHY:

Marino PL. *The ICU Book.* 2nd ed. Philadelphia, PA: Lippincott Williams & Wilkins; 1998:247.

Mason RJ, Broaddus VC, Martin T, et al. *Mason: Murray and Nadel's Textbook of Respiratory Medicine.* 5th ed. Philadelphia, PA: Saunders, 2010:1333-1334.

## *Answer B*

### Cardiovascular

**QUESTION (K-type):**

A 38-year-old woman who takes verapamil for idiopathic hypertrophic subaortic stenosis is anesthetized with enflurane, nitrous oxide, oxygen, and fentanyl for laparoscopic cholecystectomy. After inflation of the abdomen with carbon dioxide, her heart rate increases to 140 bpm, blood pressure decreases to 85/60 mm Hg, and ST-segment depression occurs. End-tidal carbon dioxide concentration is unchanged. Appropriate pharmacologic management includes intravenous administration of

(1)  Phenylephrine.
(2)  Nitroglycerin.
(3)  Esmolol.
(4)  Calcium chloride.

**CORRECT ANSWER: B (1 and 3 are correct.)**

**SUMMARY:**

*Idiopathic hypertrophic subaortic stenosis (IHSS) is a dynamic obstruction of the left ventricular outflow tract (LVOT) with the systolic anterior motion (SAM) of the anterior mitral leaflet abutting against the hpertrophic septum. Factors that worsen the LVOT obstruction include increased myocardial contractility, decreased left ventricular preload, and decreased left ventricular afterload. Decreasing the contractility with β-blockers and increasing the afterload with α-agonists and preload augmentation with fluid and release of abdominal insufflation are all appropriate maneuvers.*

**EXPLANATION:**

(1)  *Correct.* Phenylephrine causes peripheral vasoconstriction, increasing central filling volumes, and helps prevent and treat LVOT obstruction in patients with IHSS.
(2)  *Incorrect.* Nitroglycerine causes vasodilatation and decreases preload, worsening LVOT obstruction.
(3)  *Correct.* Esmolol decreases the heart rate, allowing more time for diastolic filling, and decreases myocardial contractility. This helps prevent and treat LVOT obstruction.
(4)  *Incorrect.* Calcium chloride increases myocardial contractility and exacerbates the outlet obstruction.

**REASONING:**

This question tests knowledge of the pathophysiology and anesthetic implications of IHSS. It is important to understand the dynamic nature of the LVOT obstruction in patients with IHSS and factors that modulate the severity of obstruction. A full ventricle decreases obstruction. Factors that impair filling or increase emptying, such as increased myocardial contractility, peripheral vasodilation, and decreased preload, all worsen LVOT obstruction in these patients. B is the best answer.

**BIBLIOGRAPHY:**

Barash PG, Cullen BF, Stoelting RK. *Clinical Anesthesia.* 6th ed. Philadelphia, PA: Lippincott Williams & Wilkins; 2009:1080-1082.
Braunwald D, Zipes P. Heart Disease. *A Textbook of Cardiovascular Medicine.* 6th ed. Philadelphia, PA: Saunders; 2001:207.
Miller RD, Miller ED, Reves JG, et al. *Anesthesia.* 7th ed. Philadelphia, PA: Churchill Livingstone; 2010:1931-1932.
Morgan GE, Mikhail MS, Murray MJ. *Clinical Anesthesiology.* 3rd ed. New York, NY: McGraw-Hill; 2002:418.

## Answer D

### Pharmacology

**QUESTION (K-type):**

Compared with intermittent bolus administration, effects of continuous infusion of a short-acting anesthetic include

(1)  Increased therapeutic index.
(2)  Decreased serum concentration required.
(3)  Prolonged recovery time.
(4)  Decreased total amount of anesthetic required.

**CORRECT ANSWER: D (4 only is correct.)**

**SUMMARY:**

*Continuous infusion of medication during anesthetic administration has several advantages over intermittent bolus administration. Continuous infusions allow more predictable plasma drug concentrations and avoid peak and trough drug levels (peaks produce unwanted side effects, and troughs produce decreased clinical efficacy). Infusions provide the ability to titrate clinical effect more closely and thus give the clinician more precise hemodynamic and therapeutic control. There is some evidence to suggest that infusions decrease the total amount of drug required and may be associated with fewer postoperative side effects. Continuous parenteral infusions do not have an impact on therapeutic index (this property of a drug is relatively constant regardless of route of administration). If anything, continuous infusions decrease recovery time because they allow slow titration of medication. The serum concentration associated with continuous infusions may be higher or lower than with bolus administration, depending on whether the comparison is to peak or trough bolus concentrations.*

**EXPLANATION:**

(1)  *Incorrect.* Continuous parenteral infusions do not affect therapeutic index.
(2)  *Incorrect.* This statement is not correct because it depends on whether you are comparing infusion concentrations with peak bolus drug concentrations or trough bolus drug concentrations.
(3)  *Incorrect.* Continuous infusions are not associated with prolonged recovery times when titrated properly in healthy patients.
(4)  *Correct.* Of all the choices listed, only decreased total amount of drug required is supported by clinical studies.

**REASONING:**

This question tests knowledge of the pharmacokinetics of anesthetic infusions. Answers A, B, and E can be eliminated immediately simply by knowing that choice 1 is incorrect (the therapeutic index of a drug does not change based on the route of administration). This leaves answers C and D. Although it is tempting to say that the serum concentration would be lower with an infusion (choice 2), this is only true when the infusion concentration is compared with the peak bolus concentrations. During the trough phase of bolus injections, the infusion concentration may well be higher. Thus D is the best answer.

**BIBLIOGRAPHY:**

Morgan GE, Mikhail MS, Murray MJ. *Clinical Anesthesiology.* 3rd ed. New York, NY: McGraw-Hill; 2002:887-888.

Newson C, Joshi GP, Victory R, et al. Comparison of propofol administration techniques for sedation during monitored anesthesia care. *Anesth Analg.* 1995;81:486-491.

Reves JG, et al. Continuous infusion of fentanyl and midazolam for cardiac surgery. *Anesth Analg.* 1990;70:S1-S450.

White PF. *Textbook of Intravenous Anesthesia.* Baltimore, Williams & Wilkins, 1997, p. 603.

White PF. Use of continuous infusion versus intermittent bolus administration of fentanyl or ketamine during outpatient anesthesia. *Anesthesiology.* 1983;59:294-300.

---

## BOOK B:

*Answer D*

Pediatrics

## QUESTION 163

### QUESTION (K-type):

During abdominal closure for gastroschisis in a 1-day-old infant, airway pressure increases and oxygen saturation decreases. Breath sounds are bilateral, and endotracheal suctioning does not improve ventilation. After increasing $F_{IO_2}$, appropriate management includes

(1)  Deepening volatile anesthesia.
(2)  Administering additional muscle relaxant.
(3)  Adding positive end-expiratory pressure.
(4)  Foregoing primary abdominal closure.

### CORRECT ANSWER: D (4 only is correct.)

### SUMMARY:

*Gastroschisis is a congenital anomaly characterized by an abdominal wall defect lateral to the umbilicus. It results from occlusion of the omphalomesenteric artery in utero and is not typically associated with other congenital anomalies. The lack of a hernia sac predisposes neonates with this disorder to dehydration, infection, and hypothermia. Primary closure of the defect is not always possible because it can result in a dramatic decrease in pulmonary compliance and hypotension from abdominal compartment syndrome. A staged closure may be indicated if there is increased peak inspiratory (> 20 cmH₂O), intragastric or vesicular pressures.*

### EXPLANATION:

(1)  *Incorrect.* Deepening anesthesia will not necessary help improve ventilation. In fact, higher concentrations of volatile anesthetic may worsen hypotension.
(2)  *Incorrect.* Adequate muscle relaxation is usually necessary to facilitate decreasing abdominal wall tension when attempting primary closure, but it will not improve ventilation.
(3)  *Incorrect.* Adding positive end-expiratory pressure (PEEP) in this setting may worsen oxygen desaturation secondary to a decrease in decrease in venous return and pulmonary blood flow.
(4)  *Correct.* For many neonates, primary closure is not advisable because they will not tolerate drastic decreases in pulmonary compliance and venous return.

### REASONING:

Appropriate management of gastroschisis includes ensuring adequate ventilation and resuscitation. At first glance, choices 1 and 3 sound reasonable. However, the major problem with performing primary closure of a gastroschisis is abdominal compartment syndrome. Increased intra-abdominal pressure results in poor pulmonary compliance, decreased venous return, decreased cardiac output, decreased pulmonary blood flow, and decreased lower extremity perfusion. Administering more volatile anesthetic and PEEP will not improve any of these conditions.

**BIBLIOGRAPHY:**
Cote CJ. *A Practice of Anesthesia for Infants and Children.* 4th ed. Philadelphia, PA: Saunders; 2009:309-310.
Morgan GE, Mikhail MS, Murray MJ. *Clinical Anesthesiology.* 4th ed. New York, NY: McGraw-Hill; 2006:942.

---

| **BOOK B:** | **QUESTION 164 (OPTIONAL)** |

*Answer C*

Clinical Anesthesia

**QUESTION (K-type):**

True statements concerning airway management in a patient with suspected injury to the cervical spine following head and chest trauma include the following:

(1)  Cricothyroidotomy is the preferred method of securing the airway.
(2)  Injuries at C1 or C2 place the patient at greatest risk for neurologic injury during laryngoscopy.
(3)  Cricoid pressure is contraindicated.
(4)  Normal lateral, anteroposterior (AP), and open-mouth views of the cervical spine rule out spinal cord injury.

**CORRECT ANSWER: C (2 only is correct.)**

**SUMMARY:**

*Spinal cord injuries are common, with cervical injury constituting 50% of all spine injuries. Cervical spinal injury is present in 2% of blunt trauma victims. One should assume that all trauma patients have potentially unstable spinal injuries. Extreme care must be taken at all steps when treating these patients to prevent neurologic injury. All trauma patients are at high risk for aspiration and should be treated accordingly. The preferred method of securing the airway is an awake FOI or a rapid sequence induction with cricoid pressure and inline cervical stabilization.*

**EXPLANATION:**

(1)  *Incorrect.* In the early 1990s, Advanced Trauma Life Support (ATLS) recommendations for securing the airway in trauma patients with potential cervical spine injury advocated for nasal intubation or cricothyroidotomy to minimize the risk of neurologic injury. However, convincing data now demonstrate that oral intubation can be performed safely and successfully. Oral intubation with manual inline stabilization is the preferred airway management strategy in most cases.
(2)  *Correct.* Studies of cervical motion measured fluoroscopically during oral intubation with inline stabilization demonstrate the greatest degree of movement at the occiput-C1 and C1-C2 spinal segments, placing patients with high cervical spine injuries at the greatest risk of injury during intubation.
(3)  *Incorrect.* All trauma patients are at significant risk of aspiration, and cricoid pressure should be used for all inductions. In addition, cadaveric studies have demonstrated that application of cricoid pressure does not result in movement of the cervical spine when injury is present.
(4)  *Partially correct.* A series of three plain cervical radiographs detects approximately 90% of cervical spine injuries. Approximately 1% of missed injuries will be clinically significant. However, many medical centers still rely on a series of three radiographs to rule out cervical spine injury. The addition of CT improves the NPV of cervical spine imaging to 99% to 100%.

This question is difficult because only statement 2 is entirely correct. When faced with a question like this, it is best to go with the most correct statement(s) and eliminate the most incorrect. Statement 3 is most incorrect. Your answer choices are now limited to C (statements 2 and 4) or D (statement 4 only). In this case, answer C is the best available choice.

**BIBLIOGRAPHY:**

Crosby ET. Airway management in adults after cervical spine trauma. *Anesthesiology.* 2006;104:1293-1318.

Morgan GE, Mikhail MS, Murray MJ. *Clinical Anesthesiology.* 4th ed. New York, NY: McGraw-Hill; 2006:793, 794.

Turkstra TP, Williams SR, Tremblay MH, Guilbert F, Thériault M, Drolet P. Cervical spine motion during tracheal intubation with manual in-line stabilization: direct laryngoscopy versus GlideScope video laryngoscopy. *Anesth Analg.* 2008;106:935-941.

---

## BOOK B:     QUESTION 165

*Answer B*

Clinical Anesthesia

**QUESTION (K-type):**

A 30-year-old man with gunshot wounds receives an emergency transfusion of 4 units of uncrossmatched O, Rh-negative blood. His blood type is AB, Rh-positive. For further intraoperative transfusions, he should receive

(1)  O, Rh-negative red cells.
(2)  AB, Rh-positive red cells.
(3)  AB, Rh-positive plasma.
(4)  O, Rh-negative plasma.

**CORRECT ANSWER: B (1 and 3 are correct.)**

**SUMMARY:**

*Human red cell membranes are estimated to contain at least 300 different antigenic determinants and there are at least 20 separate blood group antigen systems. A and B antigens are most important clinically, and their presence or absence results in the four major blood types, known as* ABO *classification:*

1.  *Type A blood expresses the A antigen on the RBC surface and these individuals develop natural antibodies to the B antigen.*
2.  *Type B blood expresses the B antigen on the RBC surface and these individuals develop natural antibodies to the A antigen.*
3.  *Type AB blood expresses both the A and B antigens on the RBC surface; these individuals lack natural antibodies to either the A or B antigen and may receive RBCs from any blood type. Type AB blood is the universal recipient.*
4.  *Type O blood expresses neither the A nor the B antigen on the RBC surface; these individuals develop natural antibodies to both the A and B antigen. Because they express neither A nor B antigens, group O blood may be donated to any individual. Type O blood is the universal donor. Unfortunately, all RBC transfusions are contaminated with a small amount of plasma from the donor. The plasma contains antibodies that my result in transfusion reactions when uncrossmatched blood is transfused.*

**EXPLANATION:**

(1)  ***Correct.*** RBC transfusions contain a small amount of plasma from the donor blood group. When more than 2 units of uncrossmatched blood are transfused, the risk of antibodies in donor plasma reacting with type-specific blood increases. In this case,

the donor has received a small volume of serum containing anti-A and anti-B antibodies with the type O RBCs. Subsequent transfusion with AB blood puts him at risk of hemolytic transfusion reaction.

(2) *Incorrect.* See explanation above.

(3) *Correct.* Transfusion of plasma should be ABO compatible. As with RBCs, transfused plasma may contain a very small amount of antibodies to blood antigens. However, because the ABO blood type lacks antibodies to both A and B blood antigens, type AB plasma is preferred for emergency plasma transfusion if the recipient's blood type is not available.

(4) *Incorrect.* Type O plasma may contain small amounts of anti-A and anti-B antibodies and should not be given to an individual with AB blood type.


### REASONING:

Anesthesiologists frequently transfuse blood products and should have a thorough understanding of blood transfusion compatibility, including transfusion of untyped blood products in emergency situations. This question reviews both ABO and Rh compatibility of RBC and plasma transfusion. Note that because this patient is Rh-positive (D antigen-positive), he lacks anti-D antibodies and may receive either Rh-positive or Rh-negative blood. Rh-negative individuals do not produce anti-D antibodies constitutively, but 60% to 70% will develop anti-D antibodies when exposed to Rh-positive blood. Rh compatibility is not necessary for plasma transfusion.


### BIBLIOGRAPHY:


Barash PG, Cullen BF, Stoelting RK, Cahalan M, Stock M. *Clinical Anesthesia*. 6th ed. Philadelphia, PA: Lippincott-Raven Publishers; 2009:384-385.

Morgan GE, Mikhail MS, Murray MJ. *Clinical Anesthesiology*. 4th ed. New York, NY: McGraw-Hill; 2006:633.


---

**BOOK B:**　　　　　**QUESTION 166**

---

*Answer E*

Pharmacology

### QUESTION (K-type):

A 46-year-old man who takes clonidine for essential hypertension undergoes a 12-hour limb reimplantation under general anesthesia. Which of the following should be anticipated during the perioperative course?

(1) Decreased anesthetic requirements.
(2) Postoperative hypertension.
(3) Blunting of tachycardia with tracheal intubation.
(4) Excessive postoperative drowsiness.


### CORRECT ANSWER: E (1, 2, and 3 are correct.)


### SUMMARY:

*Clonidine is a presynaptic $\alpha_2$-adrenergic agonist that acts in the CNS to decrease sympathetic activity. It is used for the treatment of refractory hypertension. In addition to its antihypertensive effects, it also decreases anesthetic and analgesic requirements and produces sedation and anxiolysis. In regional and neuraxial anesthesia, it can be used to produce prolongation of blockade. Patients receiving clonidine for hypertension should continue the medication postoperatively because severe rebound hypertension can result from abrupt discontinuation.*

**EXPLANATION:**
(1) *Correct.* Clonidine has been shown to decrease anesthetic requirements.
(2) *Correct.* Patients receiving clonidine for hypertension are at risk of developing post-operative hypertension from withdrawal of the medication. Signs of withdrawal include hypertension, tachycardia, insomnia, flushing, headache, apprehension, sweating, and tremulousness, and usually occur 18 hours after discontinuing the drug.
(3) *Correct.* Patients receiving clonidine may have a blunting of tachycardia from intubation from the decreased activation of the sympathetic nervous system and increased vagal tone.
(4) *Incorrect.* Orally administered clonidine is typically given as twice daily dosing and has a duration of action of 6 to 10 hours. While a key characteristic of clonidine is its sedative effects, you must take into account the context of the question. It is unlikely that a dose of oral clonidine would continue to have sedative effects 12 hours after administration to the extent that it would lead to excessive postoperative drowsiness.

**REASONING:**
This question tests knowledge of the pharmacology of clonidine. It is important for the reader to have a thorough understanding of the multiple pharmacologic effects of clonidine at its various sites of administration, its duration of action, and to be aware of the hazards of acute clonidine withdrawal. Choices 1, 2, and 3 are correct, and thus A is the best answer.

**BIBLIOGRAPHY:**
Barash PG, Cullen BF, Stoelting RK, Calahan M, Stock MC. *Clinical Anesthesia.* 6th ed. Philadelphia, PA: Lippincott Williams & Wilkins; 2009:446-447.
Morgan GE, Mikhail MS, Murray MJ. *Clinical Anesthesiology.* 4th ed. New York, NY: McGraw-Hill; 2006:247-248, 283-284.
Westfall TC, Westfall DP. Chapter 12. Adrenergic agonists and antagonists. In: Brunton LL, Chabner BA, Knollmann BC, eds. *Goodman & Gilman's The Pharmacological Basis of Therapeutics.* 12th ed. New York, NY: McGraw-Hill; 2011:chap 12. http://www.accessmedicine.com.laneproxy.stanford.edu/content.aspx?aID=16661344.

---

**BOOK B:**      **QUESTION 167**

---

*Answer A*

Equipment/Physics

**QUESTION (K-type):**

Defective expiratory unidirectional valves in a circle system result in

(1) Increased dead space.
(2) Decreased $F_{IO_2}$.
(3) Prolonged anesthetic induction.
(4) Transformation to a non-rebreathing system.

**CORRECT ANSWER: A (1, 2, and 3 are correct.)**

**SUMMARY:**
*The circle system is a rebreathing circuit with inspiratory and expiratory unidirectional valves and a $CO_2$ absorber canister to prevent rebreathing of expired $CO_2$ gas. The inspiratory valve opens on inspiration and closes on expiration, and the expiratory valve has the opposite action. Unidirectional valves prevent rebreathing of expired $CO_2$ and limit*

*the circuit's dead space. Advantages of the circle system over non-rebreathing systems include ability to use lower gas flows while maintaining stable gas concentrations, conservation of heat and moisture, and minimizing operating room contamination. The main disadvantage is its complexity, including big and heavy machines with multiple components that make it prone for disconnections, obstructions, and leaks.*

## EXPLANATION:

(1) ***Correct.*** Unidirectional valves are important in decreasing the dead space of the anesthetic circuit. The only dead space in a circle system is distal to the Y piece. If the expiratory valve is defective, this will add the entire volume of the expiratory limb to the dead space.

(2) ***Correct.*** Because the expiratory valve prevents rebreathing, failure of this valve will allow the exhaled gas to mix with the inspiratory gas and lower the $F_{IO_2}$.

(3) ***Correct.*** Rebreathing exhaled gas causes the inspired gas concentration to be lower. The lower the inspired concentration of anesthetic, the slower is the induction.

(4) ***Incorrect.*** The circle system still has a functioning inspiratory valve and cannot be converted into a non-rebreathing system (ie, Mapleson circuit) because fresh gas flow will not occur during expiration, a requirement for a non-rebreathing system.

## REASONING:

This question tests knowledge of the circle system. Questions regarding the circle system, its advantages and disadvantages, associated dead space, and problems with its components are tested frequently. The reader should review these topics carefully. The best answer is A.

## BIBLIOGRAPHY:

Barash PG, Cullen BF, Stoelting RK. *Clinical Anesthesia.* 6th ed. Philadelphia, PA; Lippincott Williams & Wilkins; 2009:672-673.

Ehrenwerth J, Eisenkraft JB. *Anesthesia Equipment: Principles and Applications.* St Louis, MO: Mosby-Year Book; 1993:93.

Morgan GE, Mikhail MS, Murray MJ. *Clinical Anesthesiology.* 4th ed. New York, NY: McGraw-Hill; 2006:37-41.

---

**BOOK B:**  **QUESTION 168**

---

*Answer E*

Equipment/Physics

### QUESTION (K-type):

In the absence of a change in the ventilator settings, the measured exhaled tidal volume on the machine spirometer decreases when

(1) The endotracheal tube migrates into the right main stem bronchus.
(2) Fresh gas flow is decreased.
(3) A heated humidifier is added.
(4) The endotracheal tube cuff begins to leak.

### CORRECT ANSWER: E (All are correct.)

### SUMMARY:

*The tidal volume that is delivered by the anesthesia machine ventilator is measured by a device known as a spirometer. There are various types of spirometers and they measure the tidal volumes in different ways. They are usually placed in the expiratory limb of the circuit to measure exhaled tidal volume. Changes in measured exhaled tidal volume that are not due to changes in the ventilator settings can be caused by various factors. These factors include circuit leaks, loss of volume through breathing tube expansion, water condensation in the spirometer, and measurement inaccuracies with high or low fresh gas flow.*

## EXPLANATION:

(1) ***Correct.*** As the endotracheal tube migrates into a mainstem bronchus, the PIPs will increase. A mainstem intubation creates a less compliant system, thus less volume per pressure measurement and the resultant decrease tidal volume.

(2) ***Correct.*** Some spirometers use a system not unlike a weather vane to measure the volume of exhaled gas. As the volume of gas passes through the vane, it spins and is translated into a volume of gas that represents the tidal volume. However, the measurement can be inaccurate at either low or high fresh gas flows secondary to friction or inertia of the mechanical apparatus.

(3) ***Correct.*** The spirometers are calibrated at the factory for a specific density of gas. If the temperature of the gas changes, it will result in a change in density of the gas. Adding a heated humidifier will change the density of the gas creating a measurement error.

(4) ***Correct.*** As the endotracheal tube cuff begins to leak, it will result in loss of part of the exhaled tidal volume from around the tube. Because the measurement of exhaled tidal volume occurs within the expiratory limb of the circuit, the lost volume that leaks around the cuff will be lost to measurement.

## REASONING:

There are some factors that would affect the *actual* tidal volume, such as changes in ventilator settings, endobronchial intubation, pneumothorax, pneumoperitoneum, Trendelenburg position, and circuit leaks, disconnections, and/or malfunction. In addition, there are also factors that would affect the spirometer-*measured* tidal volume, including compliance of the circuit, compression, humidity and temperature of the gas, fresh gas flow rate, again circuit leaks, and location of the spirometer, either close to the exhalation valve or at the Y piece. Spirometers, as any other monitoring tool, should be complemented with sound clinical judgment.

## BIBLIOGRAPHY:

Feldman JM, Muller J. Tidal volume measurement errors—the impact of lung compliance and a circuit humidifier. *Anesthesiology.* 1990;A468.

Morgan GE, Mikhail MS, Murray MJ. *Clinical Anesthesiology.* 4th ed. New York, NY: McGraw-Hill; 2006;71-84.

**QUESTION 169**

*Answer D*

**QUESTION (K-type)**

Equipment/Physics

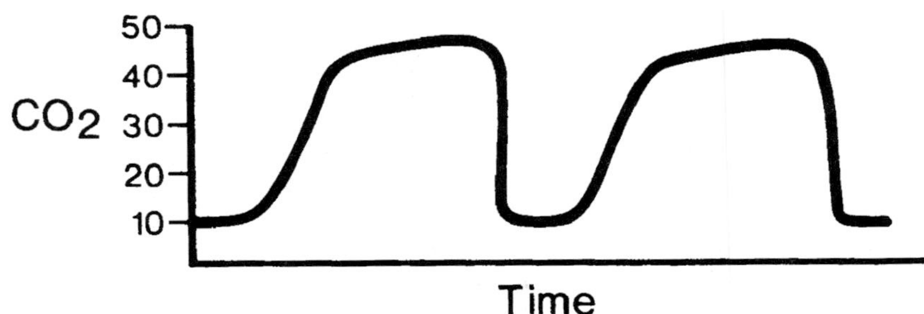



The capnographic waveform shown above was obtained during anesthesia using a semiclosed-circle system and mechanical ventilation. This waveform is consistent with

(1) Increased body temperature to 40°C.
(2) Kinking of the endotracheal tube.
(3) Inadequate minute ventilation.
(4) An incompetent expiratory value.

**CORRECT ANSWER: D (4 only is correct.)**

**SUMMARY:**
*Continuous monitoring of the capnogram has become standard of care in anesthesia. Correct interpretation of the capnogram provides with invaluable information regarding equipment performance, endotracheal tube placement, and patient pulmonary, and cardiac and metabolic function. The normal capnogram starts at zero during the inhalation (phase I), followed by a rapid upstroke representing the beginning of the expiration (phase II); the next phase, the majority of exhalation, is almost flat with a slightly positive slope due to V/Q mismatch (phase III); this is followed by a rapid descent at the start of inhalation (phase 0). The end-tidal $CO_2$ is measured at the peak of the plateau.*

**EXPLANATION:**
(1) *Incorrect.* An elevated body temperature, usually associated with increased metabolic rate, would increase the overall production of $CO_2$ with a resultant increase in the plateau. However, the capnogram should still return to baseline despite the increase $CO_2$ production.
(2) *Incorrect.* Kinking of the ET could cause an increase in airway pressure. It should not affect phase I of the capnogram.
(3) *Incorrect.* Inadequate minute ventilation (MV) will cause the end-tidal $CO_2$ to be elevated, but it would still return to zero in phase I of the capnogram.
(4) *Correct.* Because an elevated phase I is associated with malfunctioning, expiratory or inspiratory valves or exhaustion of the $CO_2$ absorber causing rebreathing, this answer is correct.

**REASONING:**
The differential for rebreathing of $CO_2$, as represented by an increase from zero on the capnograph, is short: malfunctioning valves or exhaustion of $CO_2$ absorber; therefore the only correct answer is choice 4.

**BIBLIOGRAPHY:**

Barash PG, Cullen BF, Stoelting RK. *Clinical Anesthesia*. 6th ed. Philadelphia, PA: Lippincott Williams & Wilkins; 2009:698-700.

Miller RD, Eriksson LI, Fleisher LA, et al. *Miller: Miller's Anesthesia*. 7th ed. New York, NY: Churchill Livingstone; 2009. Retrieved January 24, 2012 from http://www.mdconsult.com/books/linkTo?type=bookPage&isbn=978-0-443-06959-8&eid=4-u1.0-B978-0-443-06959-8.00044-3--s0380.

Morgan GE, Mikhail MS, Murray MJ. *Clinical Anesthesiology*. 4th ed. New York, NY: McGraw-Hill; 2006:141-143.

---

| | |
|---|---|
| **BOOK B:** | **QUESTION 170** |

*Answer A*

Clinical Anesthesia

**QUESTION (K-type):**

A 45-year-old woman is scheduled for a cholecystectomy following an episode of acute cholecystitis. Thirty minutes after premedication with morphine and midazolam, she has nausea and acute right upper quadrant pain. Drugs that alleviate these symptoms include

(1) Glucagon.
(2) Nitroglycerin.
(3) Naloxone.
(4) Flumazenil.

**CORRECT ANSWER: A (1, 2, and 3 are correct.)**

**SUMMARY:**

*Choledochoduodenal sphincter (sphincter of Oddi) spasm can be induced by the administration of opioids. Smooth muscle constriction of the sphincter can cause right upper quadrant pain. The treatment options for the treatment of the spasm include naloxone, glucagon, nifedipine, and nitroglycerin.*

**EXPLANATION:**

(1) *Correct.* Glucagon has been shown to help relax sphincter of Oddi spasm. The dose is usually 1 to 3 mg IV.
(2) *Correct.* Nitroglycerin causes smooth muscle relaxation in vascular tissue and in the gastrointestinal tract and has also shown to alleviate sphincter of Oddi spasm.
(3) *Correct.* Opioids are a common cause of sphincter of Oddi spasm, and pure opioid antagonists such as naloxone can reverse sphincter spasm.
(4) *Incorrect.* Sphincter of Oddi spasm is not caused by the administration of benzodiazepines; therefore flumazenil will have no effect on the spasm.

**REASONING:**

Sphincter of Oddi dysfunction is a commonly described opiate side effect. Glucagon and naloxone are well-known treatments, but nitrates that cause smooth muscle relaxation are less well known but equally effective treatments.

**BIBLIOGRAPHY:**

Morgan GE, Mikhail MS, Murray MJ. *Clinical Anesthesiology*. 4th ed. New York, NY: McGraw-Hill; 2006:716.

Toyoyama H, Kariya N, Hase I, Toyoda Y. The use of intravenous nitroglycerin in a case of spasm of the sphincter of Oddi during laparoscopic cholecystectomy. *Anesthesiology*. 2001;94:708-709.

Velosy B, Madacsy L, Lonovics J, Csernay L. Effect of glyceryl trinitrate on the sphincter of Oddi spasm evoked by prostigmine-morphine administration. *Eur J Gastroenterol Hepatol.* 1997;9:1109-1112.

---

**BOOK B:**                    **QUESTION 171**

---

*Answer E*

Physiology

**QUESTION (K-type):**

During a blood transfusion, a patient develops sudden hypotension and oozing from the puncture sites. Laboratory studies useful in establishing the diagnosis include

(1)  Serum-free hemoglobin concentration.
(2)  Direct antiglobulin (Coombs') test.
(3)  Urine hemoglobin concentration.
(4)  Serum haptoglobin concentration.

**CORRECT ANSWER: E (All are correct.)**

**SUMMARY:**

*The most severe transfusion reaction is the acute hemolytic reaction in which preformed antibodies in the patient's plasma react against donor RBCs. These antibodies are usual anti-A or anti-B but can also be anti-Rh or anti-Jka. The result is a potentially fatal acute intravascular hemolysis. The signs of an acute reaction in an anesthetized patient include increased temperature, tachycardia, hypotension, hemoglobinuria, disseminated intravascular coagulation (DIC), shock, and acute renal failure. If a transfusion reaction is suspected, the transfusion should immediately be stopped, a repeat type and cross performed, and a direct Coombs test sent. Additional useful laboratory tests include serum haptoglobin, urine and serum hemoglobin, complete blood cell count (CBC), and a DIC panel.*

**EXPLANATION:**

(1)  ***Correct.*** Because the principal pathologic event in an acute hemolytic reaction is intravascular hemolysis, any test that shows increased red cell destruction would be helpful in making the diagnosis. Lysed RBCs will release free hemoglobin into the serum.
(2)  ***Correct.*** The direct Coombs test (also known as the *direct antiglobulin test*) is the definitive test to confirm an acute hemolytic reaction.
(3)  ***Correct.*** As the free hemoglobin is cleared from the circulation, it will be excreted in the urine. This will give the urine a characteristic pink color. The patient is at risk for developing acute renal failure.
(4)  ***Correct.*** Initially as the hemoglobin is freed, it is bound to haptoglobin and albumin. Ultimately, these sites are all bound resulting in free hemoglobin in the blood.

**REASONING:**

The key to this question is understanding the pathophysiology of an acute hemolytic transfusion reaction. It is an antibody-mediated lysis of RBCs, which results in the release of free hemoglobin, thus making all of the choices correct.

**BIBLIOGRAPHY:**

Barash PG, Cullen BF, Stoelting RK, Calahan M, Stock MC. *Clinical Anesthesia*, 6th ed. Philadelphia, Lippincott Williams & Wilkins, 2009, pp. 373.
Morgan GE, Mikhail MS, Murray MJ. *Clinical Anesthesiology.* 4th ed. New York, NY: McGraw-Hill; 2006:700.

*Answer B*

Pharmacology

**QUESTION (K-type):**

A continuous infusion of atracurium for 60 hours has been associated with

(1) Seizure activity.
(2) Histamine release.
(3) Increased anesthetic requirements.
(4) Adrenal suppression.

**CORRECT ANSWER: B (1 and 3 are correct.)**

**SUMMARY:**

*Atracurium is an intermediate-acting nondepolarizing neuromuscular blocker agent that has been used more commonly in the United Kingdom for continuous infusion. It is metabolized by two different mechanisms: Hoffman elimination (a spontaneous chemical breakdown depending on pH and temperature) and nonspecific ester hydrolysis. The principal end product is laudanosine; it has been associated with CNS stimulation leading to increased MAC (in humans) and even seizure activity (in animals). When a bolus is administered at doses higher than 0.5 mg/kg, atracurium triggers histamine release. This effect can be avoided by slow injection over 1 to 3 minutes.*

**EXPLANATION:**

(1) *Correct.* The principal metabolite of atracurium is laudanosine, which has been associated with seizure activity in animals at high doses. Such association has not been proven in humans.
(2) *Incorrect.* Although atracurium has been associated with histamine release, it is usually with large and rapid bolus dose of the drug. It is unlikely that a 60-hour continuous infusion of atracurium would be associated with histamine release.
(3) *Correct.* Elimination of laudanosine depends on liver and kidney function. The presence of laudanosine after long-term infusions of atracurium has been associated with CNS stimulation and elevation of MAC.
(4) *Incorrect.* There is no reported link between long-term infusion of atracurium and adrenal suppression.

**REASONING:**

This is quite a controversial question. Even though the most commonly known effect of atracurium is histamine release, this occurs only with rapid administration of a high-dose bolus. The key for answering this question is to focus on the effects caused by long-term administration, which relate to accumulation of laudanosine more than direct effects of Atracurium.

**BIBLIOGRAPHY:**

Barash PG, Cullen BF, Stoelting RK. *Clinical Anesthesia.* 6th ed. Philadelphia, PA: Lippincott Williams & Wilkins; 2009:509-510.

Johnson PN, Miller J, Gormley AK. Continuous-infusion neuromuscular blocking agents in critically ill neonates and children. *Pharmacotherapy.* 2011;31(6):609-620.

Miller RD, Eriksson LI, Fleisher LA, et al. *Miller: Miller's Anesthesia.* 7th ed. New York, NY: Churchill Livingstone; 2009. Retrieved January 24, 2012 from http://www.mdconsult.com/books/linkTo?type=bookPage&isbn=978-0-443-06959-8&eid=4-u1.0-B978-0-443-06959-8.00029-7--s0250.

Morgan GE, Mikhail MS, Murray MJ. *Clinical Anesthesiology.* 4th ed. New York, NY: McGraw-Hill; 2006:220-221.

## QUESTION 173

# *Answer A*

### Pharmacology

**QUESTION (K-type):**

The anesthetic recovery of a newborn infant is complicated by the slow return of neuro-muscular function. Factors that would cause this complication include

(1) An inadequate dose of anticholinesterase.
(2) Active maternal myasthenia gravis.
(3) A core temperature of 35°C.
(4) Intraoperative administration of cefamandole.

**CORRECT ANSWER: A (1, 2, and 3 are correct.)**

**SUMMARY:**

*Anesthetic issues resulting in slow recovery of neuromuscular function include presence of volatile anesthetics, acidosis, hypothermia, inadequate reversal, electrolyte abnormalities, drug interactions, and coexisting diseases. In neonates the response to NDMRs is variable owing to their immature NMJs, large extracellular fluid volume and resulting large volume of distribution, and immature metabolic pathways. Transient neonatal myasthenia gravis occurs in 10% to 20% of infants born to mothers with myasthenia gravis causing these neonates to be more sensitive to the effects of nondepolarizers.*

**EXPLANATION:**

(1) **Correct.** An inadequate dose of anticholinesterase can result in slow return of neuromuscular function. The dose of reversal agent should be determined by response to peripheral nerve stimulation.
(2) **Correct.** Mothers with active myasthenia gravis transfer anti-Ach receptor antibodies across the placenta, causing transient neonatal myasthenia 1 to 3 weeks after birth.
(3) **Correct.** Hypothermia can prolong neuromuscular blockade by decreasing drug metabolism.
(4) **Incorrect.** Many antibiotics, particularly those of the aminoglycoside (neomycin and streptomycin), tetracycline, clindamycin, or polypeptide classes (polymyxin B), are known to increase the effects of neuromuscular blocking agents. However, cephalosporins such as cefamandole have not been shown to have this effect.

**REASONING:**

This question tests knowledge of prolonged neuromuscular blockade. This problem is not specific to pediatric patients, so it is important to consider all potential causes when approaching this question. Choices 1 and 3 should be easy to identify as correct. Choice 4 can be eliminated if the reader recalls which drugs interact with muscle relaxants. Penicillins, macrolides, and cephalosporins are not known to impair functioning at the NMJ. A is the best answer.

**BIBLIOGRAPHY:**

Barash PG, Cullen BF, Stoelting RK. *Clinical Anesthesia*. 5th ed. Philadelphia, PA: Lippincott Williams & Wilkins; 2001;437-439.
Morgan GE, Mikhail MS, Murray MJ. *Clinical Anesthesiology*. 4th ed. New York NY: McGraw-Hill; 2006:215-219, 213 (Table 9-4 Potentiation and Resistance of Neuromuscular Blocking Agents by Other Drugs).

*Answer E*

Pain

**QUESTION (K-type):**

Complications of stellate ganglion block include

(1)  Elevation of the ipsilateral hemidiaphragm.
(2)  Total spinal anesthesia.
(3)  Seizures.
(4)  Hoarseness.

**CORRECT ANSWER: E (All are correct.)**

**SUMMARY:**

*Aberrant needle positioning in the vertebral artery when attempting stellate ganglion block can lead to an intravascular injection resulting in seizures. Similarly injection into the dural sleeve of a nerve root can lead to subarachnoid injection and total spinal anesthesia. Correct placement of the needle may still result in hoarseness or elevated ipsilateral hemidiaphragm with blockade of the recurrent laryngeal and phrenic nerve respectively.*

**EXPLANATION:**

Described complications of Stellate ganglion block include hematoma, hoarseness, phrenic nerve block, spinal block, epidural block, subdural block, pneumothorax, seizures, contamination and infection of bone (vertebral body), and mediastinum due to esophageal puncture.

**REASONING:**

As noted above, choice 1 is correct as elevation of the hemidiaphragm is correct and occurs through incidental block of the phrenic nerve. Choice 2 is correct as total spinal can occur with subarachnoid injection in the dural sleeve. Direct injection of local anesthetic into the vertebral artery delivers a high concentration of local anesthetic to the brain resulting in seizures, and thus choice 3 is correct. Choice 4 is also correct as hoarseness is commonly seen following stellate block with blockade of the recurrent laryngeal nerve. In view of the potential complications, a bilateral block should never be performed.

**BIBLIOGRAPHY:**

Cousins MJ, Carr DB, Horlocker TT, Bridenbaugh PO. *Cousins & Bridenbaugh's Neural Blockade in Clinical Anesthesia and Pain Medicine*. 4th ed. Philadelphia, PA: Lippincott Williams & Wilkins; 2009:1123-1124.

Huntoon MA. The vertebral artery is unlikely to be the sole source of vascular complications occurring during stellate ganglion block. *Pain Pract*. 2010;10(1):25-30.

Miller RD, Eriksson LI, Fleisher LA, Wiener-Kronish JP, Young WL. *Miller's Anesthesia*. 7th ed. Philadelphia, PA: Churchill Livingstone; 2010:1667.

Morgan GE, Mikhail MS, Murray MJ. *Clinical Anesthesiology*. 4th ed. New York, NY: McGraw-Hill; 2006:383-384 (Figure 18-15).

Raj PP. *Textbook of Regional Anesthesia*. Philadelphia, PA: Churchill Livingstone; 2002: 628-629.

# Index

BNTI. *See* blind nasotracheal intubation

bone cement implantation syndrome (BCIS), 103–104, 393–394

brachial plexus

  axillary block of, 256–257

  interscalene block of, 250–251

bradycardia

  **during eye surgery**, 95

  halothane and, 177

  with neuraxial anesthesia, 377–378

  oculocardiac reflex causing, 458

  sinus, 332–333

  with umbilical cord compression, 182

**brain herniation, treatment of**, 345

brain swelling

  hyperventilation for, 130

  **hypocarbia and**, 344–345

breathing, work of, 375–376

breathing-system canisters, carbon dioxide in, 134

bretylium, 208–209

bronchial markings, with emphysema, 152–153

bronchitis, severity of, 313–314

bronchomotor tone, ketamine and, 111

bronchospasm

  β-agonists for, 191–192

  with epidural anesthesia, 149

bullae, 152

bupivacaine, 170

  caudal anesthesia with, 314–315

  complications with, 255–256

  duration of action of, 425

  fetal/maternal plasma ratio of, 346–347

  FHR effects of, 448

  protein binding by, 342–343

  toxicity of, 208–209

buprenorphine, 371

  acute withdrawal response with, 137

burn injuries

  ECG wires causing, 365–366

  electrocautery pad causing, 379–380

  nondepolarizing muscle relaxants in, 289–290

burn patients, pancuronium and, 167

burst suppression, on EEG, 247, 307–308

butyrophenones

  opioid withdrawal and, 371

  side effects of, 400–401

C fibers, pain transmission by, 449

calcium

  in left main coronary artery disease, 361–362

  neomycin and, 184–185

  succinylcholine interactions with, 455–456

calcium channel blockers, 270

  HPV and, 194

  uterine contractility effects of, 445–446

calcium channels, presynaptic voltage-gated, 91

calcium chloride, 469

  CPR indication for, 144

calcium concentration, reduction of, 113

cAMP. *See* cyclic adenosine monophosphate

cancer, lung, 91

**capnography, differential diagnosis of abnormal waveforms**, 478

carbon dioxide ($CO_2$)

  in breathing-system canisters, 134

  in closed-circuit systems, 97

  insufflation of, 452–453

  retention of, 175–176, 248–250

  shivering and, 92

  with TPN and hyperalimentation, 99

carbon dioxide challenge test, 440–441

**carbon dioxide response curve, anesthetic implications**, 221

**carbon monoxide poisoning**, 318, 404–405

carboxyhemoglobin levels, 404–405

  smoking and, 164

cardiac index, 278, 468

cardiac ischemia, with hypothermia, 108–109

cardiac output

  child *vs.* adult, 226–227

  hypothyroidism effects on, 436–437

  isoflurane and nitrous oxide response to, 460

  mixed venous oxygen saturation and, 196

  PEEP and, 90

  in pregnancy, 397–398

  S$\bar{v}o_2$ and, 200–201

cardiac surgery, arrhythmias after, 324–325

cardiac tamponade, 235–236

  **anesthetic management, hemodynamic manipulation**, 467

cardiomyopathy, phosphorus and, 173

cardiopulmonary bypass (CPB)

  acid-base management during, 371–373

  FFP after, 105–106

  ventricular defibrillation during, 104–105

cardiopulmonary resuscitation (CPR)

  calcium chloride indication during, 144

  for PEA, 351

  sodium bicarbonate during, 292

cardiovascular depression, with propofol, 238–239

cardioversion, for VT, 311–312

carotid bodies, injury to, 284–285

carotid endarterectomy (CEA), 284–285

  **carotid body denervation**, 284

  **chemoreceptors after**, 284

  **ventilatory drive following**, 284

carotid sinus, parasympathetic activity and, 155–156

CAS. *See* central anticholinergic syndrome

catheter, for transtracheal jet ventilation, 100

catheterization, arterial, 376–377

caudal anesthesia, in pediatric patients, 314–315

caudal block

  **complications of**, 255–256

  landmarks for, 119–120

causalgia, 161–162

  **diagnosis of**, 394–395

CBF. *See* cerebral blood flow

CEA. *See* carotid endarterectomy

celiac plexus block

  **indications for**, 411, 434–435

  **pancreatic cancer treatment with**, 434–435

  right upper quadrant pain evaluation with, 411

**central anticholinergic syndrome (CAS)**, 147, 222–223

  **toxicity**, 402–403

  **treatment of**, 94

central nervous system (CNS)

  anesthetic effects on, 101

  atropine and, 94–95

central pain state, 203

cerebral aneurysm clipping, 427–428

cerebral blood flow (CBF), 321–322

  **autoregulation, physiologic inferences**, 321–322

  in chronic hypertension, 398–399

  hyperventilation and, 130

  isoflurane effects on, 446–447

  **perioperative regulation of**, 392–393

cerebral ischemia, with hypothermia, 108–109

cerebral metabolic rate

  hyperventilation and, 130

  isoflurane effects on, 446–447

cerebral perfusion pressure (CPP)

  in chronic hypertension, 398–399

  **determinants of**, 360–361

  maintenance of, 360–361

cerebral protection, barbiturates for, 360–361, 392–393

cerebral salt-wasting syndrome, 246–247

cerebral vasospasm, after SAH, 320–321

**cervical spine injury**, airway management in, 472–473